Tumors
of the
Bone Marrow

Atlas
of
Tumor Pathology

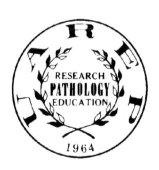

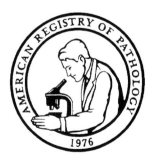

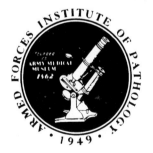

ATLAS OF TUMOR PATHOLOGY

Third Series
Fascicle 9

TUMORS OF THE
BONE MARROW

by

RICHARD D. BRUNNING, M.D.
Head of Hematopathology
Department of Laboratory Medicine and Pathology
University of Minnesota
420 Delaware Street S.E.
Minneapolis, Minnesota 55455-0395

and

ROBERT W. MCKENNA, M.D.
John Childers Professor and Vice Chair of Pathology
University of Texas Southwestern Medical Center
5323 Harry Hines Boulevard
Dallas, Texas 75235-9072

Published by the
ARMED FORCES INSTITUTE OF PATHOLOGY
Washington, D.C.

Under the Auspices of
UNIVERSITIES ASSOCIATED FOR RESEARCH AND EDUCATION IN PATHOLOGY, INC.
Bethesda, Maryland
1994

Accepted for Publication
1993

Available from the American Registry of Pathology
Armed Forces Institute of Pathology
Washington, D.C. 20306-6000
ISSN 0160-6344
ISBN 1-881041-09-3

ATLAS OF TUMOR PATHOLOGY

EDITOR
JUAN ROSAI, M.D.
Department of Pathology
Memorial Sloan-Kettering Cancer Center
New York, New York 10021-6007

ASSOCIATE EDITOR
LESLIE H. SOBIN, M.D.
Armed Forces Institute of Pathology
Washington, D.C. 20306-6000

EDITORS' NOTE

The Atlas of Tumor Pathology has a long and distinguished history. It was first conceived at a Cancer Research Meeting held in St. Louis in September 1947 as an attempt to standardize the nomenclature of neoplastic diseases. The first series was sponsored by the National Academy of Sciences-National Research Council. The organization of this Sisyphean effort was entrusted to the Subcommittee on Oncology of the Committee on Pathology, and Dr. Arthur Purdy Stout was the first editor-in-chief. Many of the illustrations were provided by the Medical Illustration Service of the Armed Forces Institute of Pathology, the type was set by the Government Printing Office, and the final printing was done at the Armed Forces Institute of Pathology (hence the colloquial appellation "AFIP Fascicles"). The American Registry of Pathology purchased the Fascicles from the Government Printing Office and sold them virtually at cost. Over a period of 20 years, approximately 15,000 copies each of nearly 40 Fascicles were produced. The worldwide impact that these publications have had over the years has largely surpassed the original goal. They quickly became among the most influential publications on tumor pathology ever written, primarily because of their overall high quality but also because their low cost made them easily accessible to pathologists and other students of oncology the world over.

Upon completion of the first series, the National Academy of Sciences-National Research Council handed further pursuit of the project over to the newly created Universities Associated for Research and Education in Pathology (UAREP). A second series was started, generously supported by grants from the AFIP, the National Cancer Institute, and the American Cancer Society. Dr. Harlan I. Firminger became the editor-in-chief and was succeeded by Dr. William H. Hartmann. The second series Fascicles were produced as bound volumes instead of loose leaflets. They featured a more comprehensive coverage of the subjects, to the extent that the Fascicles could no longer be regarded as "atlases" but rather as monographs describing and illustrating in detail the tumors and tumor-like conditions of the various organs and systems.

Once the second series was completed, with a success that matched that of the first, UAREP and AFIP decided to embark on a third series. A new editor-in-chief and an associate editor were selected, and a distinguished editorial board was appointed. The mandate for the third series remains the same as for the previous ones, i.e., to oversee the production of an eminently practical publication with surgical pathologists as its primary audience, but also aimed at other workers in oncology. The main purposes of this series are to promote a consistent, unified, and biologically sound nomenclature; to guide the surgical pathologist in the diagnosis of the various tumors and tumor-like lesions; and to provide relevant histogenetic, pathogenetic, and clinicopathologic information on these entities. Just as the second series included data obtained from ultrastructural (and, in the more recent Fascicles, immunohistochemical) examination, the third series will, in addition, incorporate pertinent information obtained with the newer molecular biology techniques. As in the past, a continuous attempt will be made to correlate, whenever possible, the nomenclature used in the Fascicles with that proposed by the World Health Organization's International Histological Classification of Tumors. The format of the third series has been changed in order to incorporate additional items and to ensure a consistency of style throughout. This includes the dropping of the 's possessive in eponymic terms, in accordance with the WHO and the International Nomenclature of Diseases. Close cooperation between the various authors and their respective liaisons from the editorial board will be emphasized to minimize unnecessary repetition and discrepancies in the text and illustrations.

To its everlasting credit, the participation and commitment of the AFIP to this venture is even more substantial and encompassing than in previous series. It now extends to virtually all scientific, technical, and financial aspects of the production.

The task confronting the organizations and individuals involved in the third series is even more daunting than in the preceding efforts because of the ever-increasing complexity of the matter at hand. It is hoped that this combined effort—of which, needless to say, that represented by the authors is first and foremost—will result in a series worthy of its two illustrious predecessors and will be a suitable introduction to the tumor pathology of the twenty-first century.

Juan Rosai, M.D.
Leslie H. Sobin, M.D.

ACKNOWLEDGMENTS

The cases illustrated in this Fascicle represent contributions from several sources. The majority are from patients studied at the University of Minnesota Hospital in Minneapolis and Parkland Hospital in Dallas. We express our appreciation to the clinicians, past and present, at these institutions who have supported our hematopathology endeavors. We are also indebted to the many pathologists from other institutions who have enriched our diagnostic experience by sending us cases for review. Many of these are illustrated in this Fascicle.

We express our gratitude to Dr. Leo T. Furcht, Chairman of the Department of Laboratory Medicine and Pathology at the University of Minnesota and Dr. Errol C. Friedberg, Chairman of the Department of Pathology at the University of Texas, Southwestern Medical School, for their continued support and encouragement during the preparation of this Fascicle.

Many individuals including colleagues, technologists, fellows, and residents have contributed to our education in hematology and hematopathology. We are grateful to them for sharing their experience and knowledge with us. We would particularly like to acknowledge Dr. R. Dorothy Sundberg, former professor of Laboratory Medicine and Pathology at the University of Minnesota, who introduced us to the study of blood cells and nurtured our interest in hematopathology.

We are indebted to Ms. Janet Parkin for the excellent electron micrographs and the printing of the black and white illustrations.

We thank Mss. Carol Ghandour, Patricia Pipes, and Tracy Svea for transcribing the manuscript.

We express our appreciation to the editorial staff of the Fascicle, Ms. Dian Thomas, Mr. Paul Clifford, and Ms. Audrey Kahn, for their extraordinary contributions to the preparation of this Fascicle.

Richard D. Brunning, M.D.
Robert W. McKenna, M.D.

TUMORS OF THE BONE MARROW

Contents

TUMORS OF THE BONE MARROW

INTRODUCTION

The tumors involving the bone marrow can be categorized into two groups: those originating in the marrow hematopoietic cells, the leukemias and multiple myeloma, and those involving the marrow secondarily, the malignant lymphomas and metastatic tumors. The leukemias, which constitute the major group, are categorized morphologically as myeloid or lymphocytic based on the cell of origin and as acute or chronic based on the degree of maturation of the proliferating cells. The terms acute and chronic antedated effective therapy and were in general predictive of biologic course in that patients with the morphologic findings of acute leukemia had a short survival period, usually a few months, and patients with chronic leukemia had a more prolonged survival. This relationship has been substantially altered by contemporary chemotherapy regimens and bone marrow transplantation.

For several decades one of the major problems in leukemia and lymphoma diagnosis was the lack of uniformity in nomenclature. The choice of diagnostic terminology usually reflected the various "schools" of hematology. The first international approach to disciplined classification of the acute leukemias occurred in 1976 with the proposals advanced by the French-American-British (FAB) Cooperative Group (2). These proposals and three subsequent modifications proposed by the FAB Group, and the modifications suggested by a National Cancer Institute working group now serve as the primary basis for the classification of acute leukemias by the international hematology community (1,2,5,7).

The concurrent introduction of the concept of the dysmyelopoietic syndromes, now referred to as myelodysplastic syndromes, was also important for establishing criteria for recognizing a group of bone marrow disorders which share some features with the acute myeloid leukemias but in which the percent of myeloblasts in the bone marrow or blood is less than the 30 percent proposed for a diagnosis of acute leukemia (2,4). The important unifying feature of this group of disorders is the presence of dysplastic maturation in myeloid cells. These changes are usually accompanied by some degree of marrow failure similar to acute myeloid leukemia.

The classification of the various myeloproliferative disorders has been substantially advanced by the recognition of the Philadelphia chromosome or its molecular counterpart, the BCR/abl hybrid gene in chronic myeloid leukemia, and by the contributions of the Polycythemia Vera Study Group, which proposed specific criteria for the diagnosis of polycythemia vera and essential thrombocythemia (6,9).

The FAB proposals for the classification of the chronic lymphoproliferative disorders recognize the contribution of both morphology and immunology to the diagnosis and classification of this group of diseases (3). The combined use of immunology and morphology has resulted in greater precision in the classification of this group of leukemias.

In general, the nomenclature and classification of the leukemias and myeloproliferative disorders included in this Fascicle follow the proposals of the FAB Cooperative Group and the Polycythemia Vera Study Group. The modifications for acute myeloid leukemia proposed by the National Cancer Institute working group are also recognized (7). Additional modifications based on the authors' experience are identified in the appropriate sections.

Standard terminology and criteria for diagnosis are used for the plasma cell dyscrasias and related disorders (8). The terminology for the lymphomas follows the Working Formulation (10). The remainder of the lesions discussed in this Fascicle primarily involve the bone marrow as a secondary process and the terminology is that used in standard pathology literature.

There is an appendix in this Fascicle which details methods of preparation of bone marrow specimens. Optimally, the diagnosis of bone marrow tumors is based on examination of blood and bone marrow smears and bone marrow biopsies. The quality of the preparations is of critical importance in establishing a correct diagnosis. The blast percentages should be based on differential cell counts of both blood and bone marrow. This is particularly relevant to the diagnosis and classification of the acute leukemias, which are predicated on specific numbers of blasts in the blood and marrow smears. A minimum of 100 cells should be enumerated on the blood smear and a minimum of 500 cells on the marrow smears or particle crush preparations.

The bone marrow sections are important for estimation of the degree of cellularity prior to and following therapy and for determining the presence of fibrosis. The sections also serve to confirm the cell percentages derived from the smears. Occasionally, because of fibrosis or inadequate aspirate specimens, the trephine biopsy gives a more accurate assessment of the number of immature cells in the marrow. In several disorders, the features of the lesions in section specimens are sufficiently distinctive to suggest or establish a diagnosis.

Although the major emphasis in this Fascicle is the description of the morphologic features of tumors in the bone marrow and blood, recognition is accorded to recent advances in immunology, cytogenetics, and molecular technology which have had substantial impact in diagnostic hematopathology and which serve as additional resources in the classification of processes that cannot be confidently classified with routine morphology and cytochemistry. In addition, the predictive value of cytogenetic findings for biologic course is becoming increasingly important to therapeutic decisions.

NORMAL BONE MARROW

The hematopoietic system is compromised of two major cell lineages, myeloid and lymphocytic, both of which have their origin in a pluripotential hematopoietic stem cell which is assumed to be bone marrow derived (fig. 1). The origin, differentiation, and maturation of the myeloid cells, which include granulocytes, monocytes, erythroid cells, and megakaryocytes, occur in the bone marrow in normal postnatal life. Lymphocytogenesis is more widespread and takes place in several organs including bone marrow, thymus, lymph nodes, spleen, and lymphatic tissue in various sites.

The myeloid hematopoietic system is unique among organ systems in that its anatomic location shifts during embryogenesis (11). The earliest evidence of myelopoiesis, the mesoblastic phase, occurs in the yolk sac of the embryo. In this phase the hematopoietic tissue consists primarily of mesenchymal-derived primitive erythroblasts. The hepatic stage of myeloid hematopoiesis begins in the second month of fetal life when granulocytes and megakaryocytes appear in the sinusoids of the liver. At 10 to 12 weeks of gestation the liver is the principal site of blood forming tissue and continues as the primary hematopoietic organ until approximately 24 weeks (11,20). Bone marrow hematopoiesis begins at 4 to 5 months of gestation and is the major site of hematopoiesis at birth; the liver and spleen have little or no role in myelopoiesis by the end of fetal life. Myeloid hematopoiesis in normal individuals in the first year of postnatal life occurs in both the axial and radial skeleton. Thereafter, there is a gradual regression of hematopoiesis in the long bones until about age 15 when the flat bones of the central skeleton are the exclusive sites of production of myeloid cells.

The bone marrow in postnatal life comprises 3.5 to 6 percent of total body weight and in aggregate mass approximates the size of the liver (11). The structure of the marrow consists of hematopoietic cells, adipose tissue, and stroma (19). The stroma consists of a delicate framework of connective tissue and vessels. The vascular supply is derived from the nutrient artery which ramifies through the marrow space. The arterioles of the nutrient artery branch into capillaries which are continuous within a system of thin walled sinusoids. The sinusoidal wall consists of a layer of endothelial cells lining the lumen and an outer coat of adventitial reticular cells. The adventitial reticular cells have phagocytic potential and in the process of lipogenesis become adipocytes (13). The adventitial reticular cells synthesize the extravascular collagen and adhesive proteins such

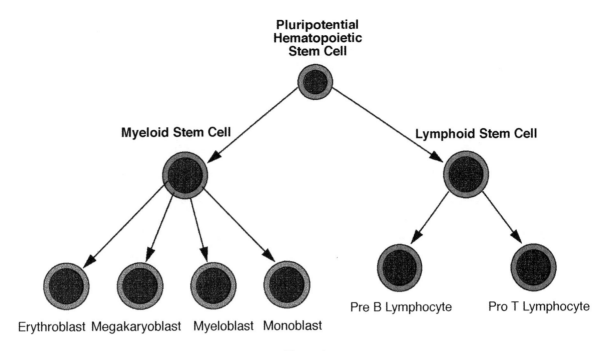

Figure 1
SCHEMATIC DIAGRAM OF EARLY HEMATOPOIETIC CELL DIFFERENTIATION

as laminin, fibronectin, and proteoglycans. The synthesis of type I and III collagen fibers provides a structural framework and compartments for the hematopoietic cells (13).

Bone marrow cellularity, i.e., hematopoietic cells, varies inversely with age (14). In the first decade of life the marrow is markedly hypercellular; about 80 percent of the bone marrow consists of hematopoietic cells (figs. 2, 3). During the first three decades of life there is a gradual decrease in hematopoietic tissue to approximately 50 percent; from the fourth to seventh decade the proportion of hematopoietic cells to fat tissue is relatively stable (figs. 4, 5). Thereafter there is a gradual decrease; the mean cellularity in the eighth decade is approximately 30 percent.

The four major myeloid cell lines, the granulocytes, monocytes, erythroid cells, and megakaryocytes, appear to have their origin in a common myeloid stem cell which has the capacity to replicate and differentiate under the influence of specific cytokines (fig. 6). The earliest cells for each major myeloid cell line are referred to as myeloblasts, monoblasts, proerythroblasts, and megakaryoblasts. The morphologic characteristics of myeloblasts and proerythroblasts in normal marrow are relatively well defined. The morphologic features of the monoblasts and megakaryoblasts in normal marrow are less clearly understood and the descriptions of these cells have been derived primarily from study of leukemias with a predominance of these cell types.

Neutrophil maturation proceeds from the myeloblast to the promyelocyte and ultimately to the segmented neutrophil; the maturation is marked by a decreasing nuclear-cytoplasmic ratio, nuclear segmentation, and granule production. Most schema of myeloid hematopoiesis show the earliest eosinophils and basophils as originating from the myeloblast; alternatively, these cells could originate in a somewhat more immature cell such as the myeloid stem cell. The morphologic evolution of these two cell types during maturation closely parallels neutrophil maturation. Table 1 lists the relative proportions of the various myeloid cells in normal adult bone marrow (18).

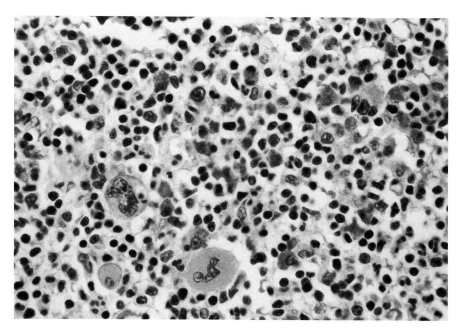

Figure 2
BONE MARROW: 6-MONTH-OLD CHILD

Bone marrow biopsy from a 6-month-old boy being evaluated for metabolic storage disease. The marrow is markedly hypercellular as expected for this age. There is normal myelopoiesis with numerous lymphocytes. There were no abnormal cells noted. (Hematoxylin and eosin stain)

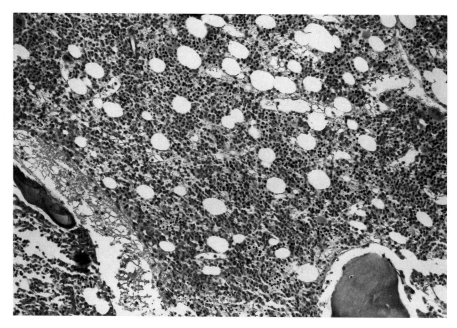

Figure 3
BONE MARROW: 7-YEAR-OLD BOY

Bone marrow from a 7-year-old boy being evaluated for neurologic deterioration. The marrow is hypercellular, within the range of cellularity for the age. There were no abnormalities detected. A dilated sinus is present at the lower left. (Hematoxylin and eosin stain)

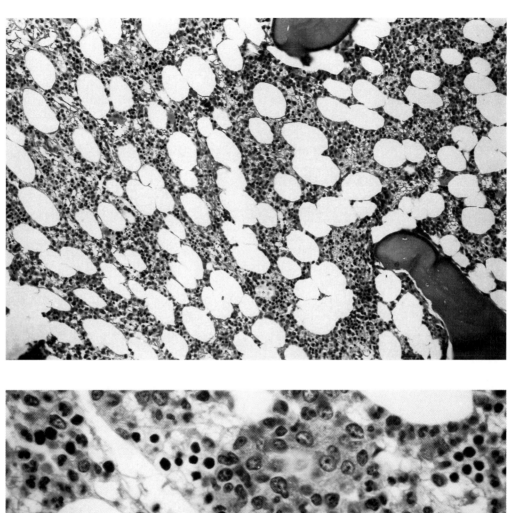

Figure 4
NORMOCELLULAR BONE MARROW FROM A MIDDLE-AGED ADULT
Top: Bone marrow biopsy from a 42-year-old woman being evaluated for extent of lymphoma. The cellularity is within the normal range for the age. (Hematoxylin and eosin stain)
Bottom: High magnification of the specimen on top showing a normal myeloid-erythroid ratio. A small sinus is present at the upper left. There was no evidence of lymphoma. (Hematoxylin and eosin stain)

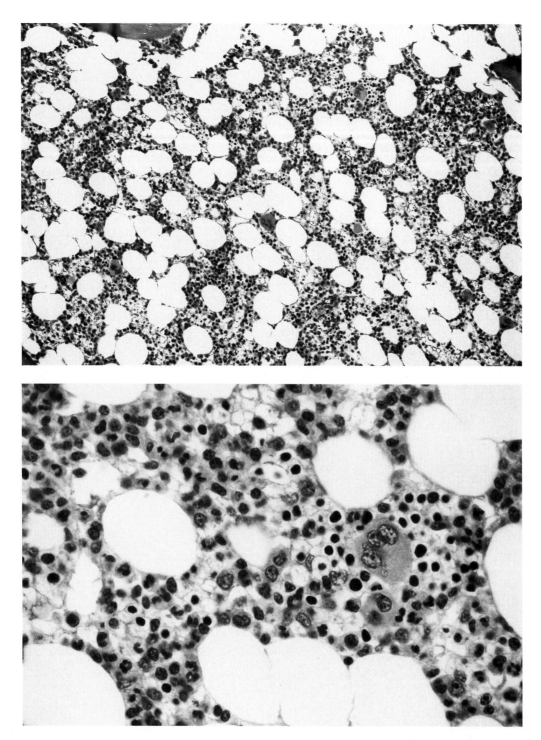

Figure 5
NORMOCELLULAR BONE MARROW IN AN OLDER ADULT

Top: Bone marrow biopsy from a 67-year-old woman with newly diagnosed non-Hodgkin lymphoma. The cellularity is in the range of normal for this age, with the amount of adipose tissue slightly in excess of cellularity. There was no evidence of lymphoma. (Hematoxylin and eosin stain)

Bottom: High magnification of the specimen on top showing essentially normal numbers of granulocytes and erythroid precursors. Normal-appearing megakaryocytes are present. The interstitium is loosely structured, a frequent finding in systemic illness. (Hematoxylin and eosin stain)

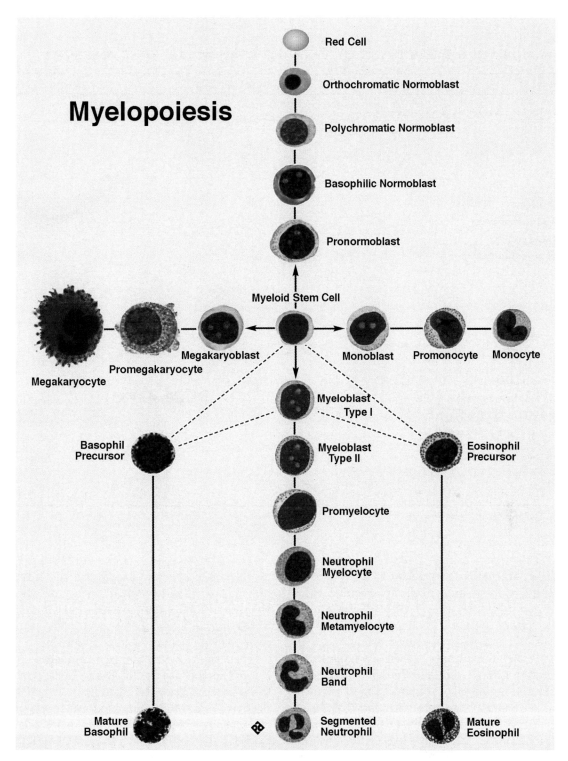

Figure 6
SCHEMATIC DIAGRAM OF MYELOPOIESIS

The four major myeloid cell lineages originate in a common myeloid stem cell. Maturation is marked in all lineages by a decreasing nuclear-cytoplasmic ratio and decreasing cytoplasmic basophilia. Granulocyte, monocyte, and megakaryocyte maturation is accompanied by nuclear lobulation or indentation. The interrupted lines to the basophil and eosinophil precursors indicate the possible origin of these cells from a cell at an earlier stage than the myeloblast.

Table 1

RELATIVE PROPORTION OF CELL TYPES IN ADULT BONE MARROW*

	Percent Cell Type	**Total Percent**
Myeloblasts		3%
Type I	1%	
Type II	2%	
Neutrophils		63%
Promyelocytes	4%	
Myelocytes	13%	
Metamyelocytes	15%	
Band forms	16%	
Segmented neutrophils	15%	
Eosinophils		3%
Basophils		0.5%
Monocytes		1%
Normoblasts		18.5%
Promonoblasts	0.5%	
Basophilic normoblasts	2%	
Polychromatophilic normoblasts	12%	
Orthochromic normoblasts	4%	
Lymphocytes		10%
Megakaryocytes		<1%

*Data obtained from reference 18.

Early neutrophil development in the marrow is anatomically related to paratrabecular and perivascular locations (figs. 7, 8). Myelocytes and promyelocytes are more frequent in these areas. Studies of bone marrow regeneration in mice following irradiation have shown a predilection of undifferentiated cells for the endosteal and periarterial regions. These areas support granulocyte and macrophage differentiation (15). This relationship is often accentuated with the neutrophilic hyperplasia that occurs in chronic myeloid leukemia and may be barely discernable in some normal bone marrows. The pattern may also be less obvious in bone marrow biopsies following bone marrow transplantation and in marrows from patients on granulocyte growth factor in which there may be foci of promyelocytes and myelocytes scattered throughout the interstitium unrelated to endosteal surface or vascular structures (fig. 9). Similar variations in patterns of regeneration may be observed in bone marrows following ablative chemotherapy.

The origin of the monocyte appears closely related to the neutrophil if the concurrence of these two cell lines in leukemic processes is reflective of normal development. Monocyte maturation somewhat parallels neutrophil maturation but distinguishing features for delimiting the monoblast, promonocyte, and monocyte stages are less well defined and are derived primarily from the study of leukemic proliferations (fig. 10). The monoblast and promonocyte, as they occur in acute monocytic leukemia, are not readily recognized in normal bone marrow.

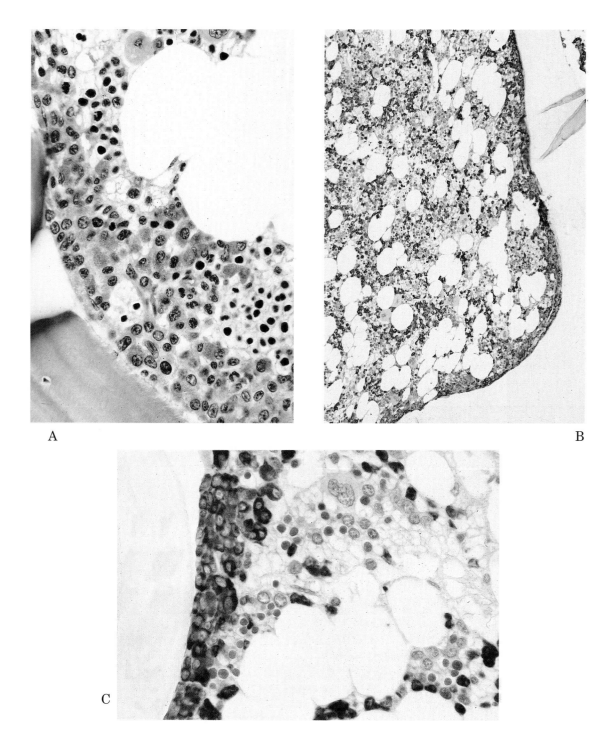

Figure 7
HISTOLOGY OF NEUTROPHIL DEVELOPMENT

A. Bone marrow biopsy showing a margin of neutrophil myelocytes along the endosteum of a bone trabecula. (Hematoxylin and eosin stain)

B. Specimen from A reacted with antibody to myeloperoxidase showing peroxidase-positive neutrophil myelocytes along the endosteal surface and numerous positive neutrophils scattered throughout the interstitium. (Peroxidase-antiperoxidase stain)

C. High magnification of the specimen in B showing primarily neutrophil myelocytes along the endosteal surface. (Peroxidase-antiperoxidase stain)

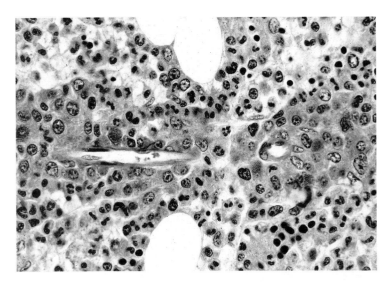

Figure 8
PERIVASCULAR FOCUS OF
NEUTROPHIL PRECURSORS

This photomicrograph illustrates a small perivascular focus of neutrophil myelocytes. (Hematoxylin and eosin stain)

Figure 9
FOCUS OF HEMATOPOIESIS
IN BONE MARROW
ENGRAFTMENT

A focus of hematopoiesis in a bone marrow biopsy 21 days following allogeneic bone marrow transplant in a patient with acute myeloid leukemia. There are numerous promyelocytes and neutrophil myelocytes in the upper portion of the field, unrelated to bone trabeculae or vascular structures. There is minimal evidence of maturation to metamyelocytes and segmented neutrophils. There are numerous red blood cell precursors showing nuclear karyorrhexis secondary to drug therapy. (Hematoxylin and eosin stain)

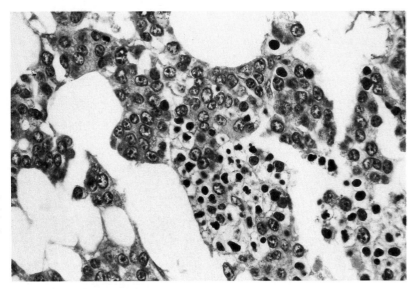

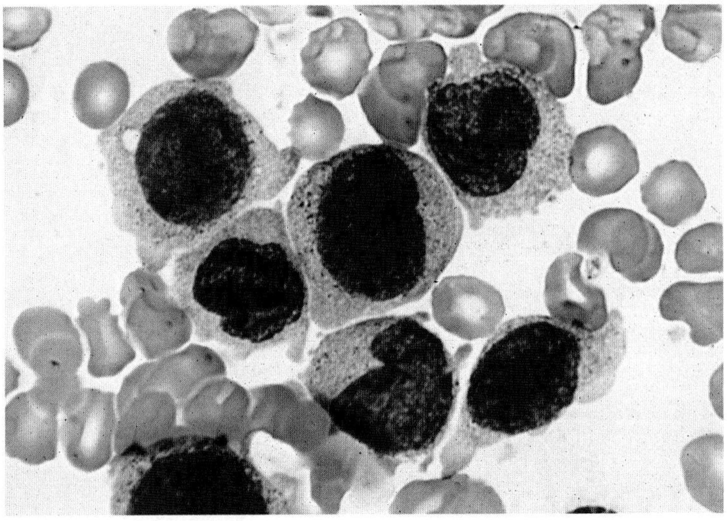

Figure 10
MONOBLASTS AND PROMONOCYTES

Bone marrow smear from a patient with acute monocytic leukemia with monocytes at different stages of maturation. The larger cells with abundant cytoplasm and round nuclei are monoblasts. The cell immediately below the monoblast in the center is also a monoblast. The two cells with folded and creased nuclei juxtaposed to the monoblast in the center are promonocytes. (Wright-Giemsa stain)

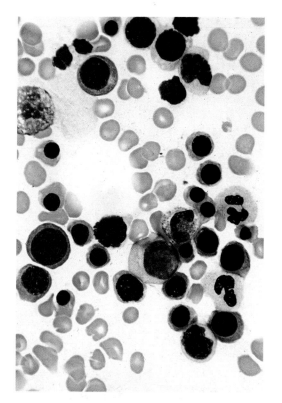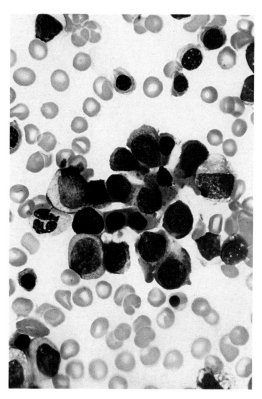

Figure 11
ERYTHROPOIESIS

Left: Bone marrow smear from a patient with erythroid hyperplasia. All stages of erythroid maturation are present. The large cell to the upper left of center is a proerythroblast. There are several basophilic, polychromatic, and orthochromatic normoblasts. (Wright-Giemsa stain)

Right: A group of basophilic and early polychromatic erythroblasts surrounding a macrophage containing phagocytosed erythrocytes and green granules interpreted as iron. A proerythroblast is at the upper right of the cell cluster. (Wright-Giemsa stain)

Erythroid maturation is marked by decreasing cell size and increasing hemoglobin synthesis; this is accompanied by decreasing cytoplasmic basophilia and extrusion of the nucleus at the orthochromatic stage of development (fig. 11). Early erythroid precursors occur in islands that appear randomly distributed in marrow biopsies but are generally related to vascular structures (fig. 12). These foci usually reflect the relative proportions of maturational stages as shown in Table 1. Biopsies from patients undergoing marrow engraftment or in the regenerative phase following chemotherapy may show large foci of erythropoiesis; some may contain a disproportionate number of early erythroid precursors (figs. 13, 14).

Megakaryocytes are usually randomly distributed throughout the bone marrow and in normal individuals occur singly (fig. 15). Megakaryocyte maturation contrasts with the maturation of the other myeloid cells by a progressive increase in size (see fig. 6). The mature megakaryocyte has a polylobulated nucleus and a finely granulated cytoplasm which gives rise to platelets.

Differentiation and maturation of normal lymphocytes, unlike the myeloid cells, occurs in several anatomic sites. The major portion of lymphocyte development is extramedullary, principally in the lymph nodes. In normal hematopoiesis the pluripotential hematopoietic stem cell in the bone marrow appears to be the precursor of the lymphoid stem cell which traffics to the various lymphoid sites. Unlike granulopoiesis where there is clear morphologic evidence of maturation from the myeloblast to immature granulocytes to mature granulocytes, there is no comparable morphologic developmental sequence that can be reliably identified in lymphocytopoiesis. The

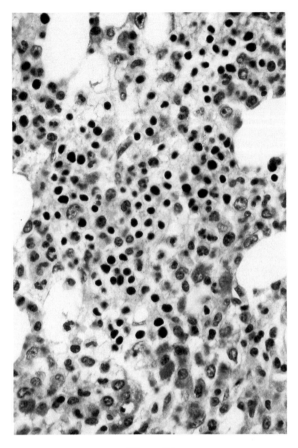

Figure 12
FOCUS OF ERYTHROPOIESIS
A focus of erythroid precursors. The majority of the precursors are at a late stage of maturation. (Hematoxylin and eosin stain)

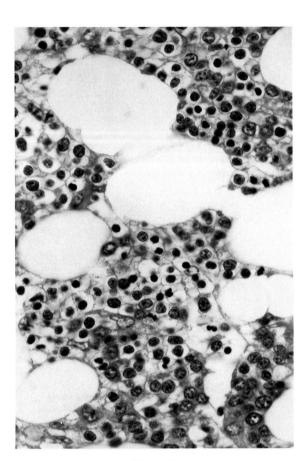

Figure 13
FOCUS OF ERYTHROPOIESIS FOLLOWING
BONE MARROW TRANSPLANTATION
Bone marrow biopsy obtained 21 days following autologous bone marrow transplantation. There is a large focus of erythroid precursors at all stages of maturation with a predominance of more mature cells. (Hematoxylin and eosin stain)

relationship of the lymphoblast of acute lymphoblastic leukemia to mature lymphocytes is unclear. The problem of depicting lymphocytogenesis morphologically is further complicated by the capacity of small lymphocytes to transform to large cells which have features morphologists generally associate with immaturity, including cytoplasmic basophilia, dispersed nuclear chromatin, and nucleoli. This capacity for transformation is reflected in some cases of B-cell chronic lymphocytic leukemia, which are complicated by prolymphocytoid transformation or Richter transformation.

The immunologic development of the lymphocyte system is marked by the presence of cytoplasmic and membrane antigens identifying lymphocytes as either B- or T-cell type. Membrane antigen composition varies with stages of maturation. A simplified schema of the immunologic development of the lymphoid system is shown in figure 16.

Approximately 10 percent of marrow cells in the normal adult are small lymphocytes. These lymphocytes are diffusely scattered throughout the interstitium. Lymphocytic aggregates are present in approximately 20 percent of marrow biopsies performed for a variety of reasons other than for malignant lymphoma or chronic lymphocytic leukemia (17). The incidence of this finding increases with age, being more frequent after the fourth decade, and is higher in females than males. These structures may result from a nonspecific immune response and whether they represent a normal finding is questionable.

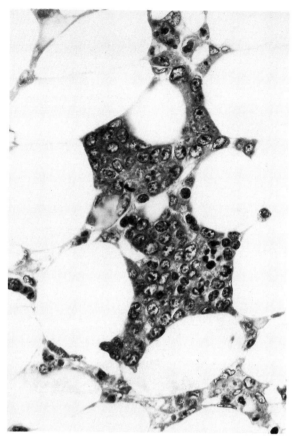

Figure 14
FOCUS OF ERYTHROPOIESIS IN
ENGRAFTING BONE MARROW
The same biopsy as illustrated in figure 13 showing a predominance of very early erythroid precursors. (Hematoxylin and eosin stain)

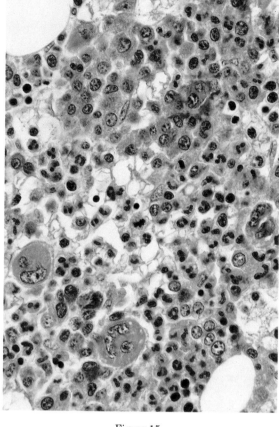

Figure 15
MEGAKARYOCYTES
Two normal-appearing megakaryocytes in a bone marrow biopsy from a young adult. To the upper right is a small perivascular focus of neutrophil myelocytes. The neutrophils show a normal maturation sequence. Scattered erythroid precursors are present. (Hematoxylin and eosin stain)

The number of plasma cells in the normal bone marrow is low, usually less than 1 percent. They are frequently present in perivascular locations and may appear increased in particle crush specimens of the bone marrow. They are frequently increased in the marrows from patients with acute and chronic immune reactions and are notably prominent in marrow specimens from patients with the acquired immune deficiency syndrome (AIDS).

Among the normal cellular constituents of the bone marrow is a small to medium sized cell resembling a lymphocyte, which has been referred to as a hematogone (12,16). The hematogone has a very high nuclear-cytoplasmic ratio, in some instances little or no discernable cytoplasm, smooth homogeneous clumped chromatin, and no evident nucleoli (fig. 17). The nuclear outline may be round or occasionally, markedly irregular with clefts and lobulation. The nature of this cell is indeterminate but it may be a type of marrow precursor cell. Hematogones are most numerous in bone marrows from very young children and decrease in number with increasing age. They may express CD19, CD10, and terminal deoxynucleotidyltransferase (12,16). In sections hematogones are diffusely scattered throughout the interstitium (fig. 17). These cells may be increased in a variety of benign hematologic disorders including iron deficiency anemia and idiopathic thrombocytopenic purpura and in the bone marrows of children with neuroblastoma,

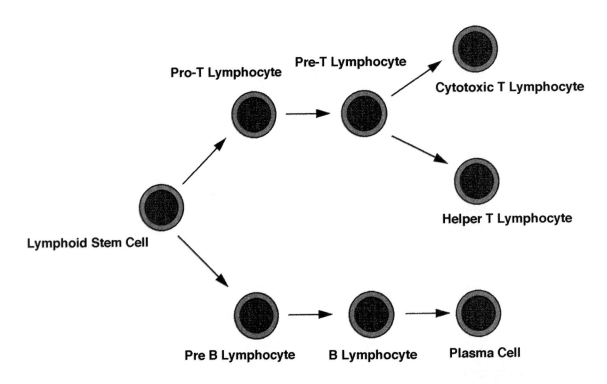

Figure 16
SCHEMATIC REPRESENTATION OF THE IMMUNOLOGIC DEVELOPMENT OF LYMPHOCYTES

with or without marrow metastasis (fig. 18). They may be numerous in regenerating marrows following chemotherapy.

Osteoblasts and osteoclasts occur along the endosteal surface of the bone structure in marrow sections and are frequently located along the margins in marrow smears. Although uncommon in normal marrow smears, these cells are frequently found in the marrow smears from patients with metastatic tumor or metabolic bone disease (figs. 19, 20). Osteoblasts may also be abundant in marrow specimens taken from healing biopsy sites.

Tissue mast cells are present in very low numbers in normal bone marrow; they are frequently associated with the periadventitia of the vascular structures (fig. 21). They may be increased in a variety of disorders including systemic mastocytosis, immune reactions, and lymphoproliferative disorders. These cells are part of the residual cell population in aplastic bone mar-

rows. Some histiocytes are found in virtually every marrow. The degree of phagocytic activity varies substantially; marked phagocytic activity is usually related to an inflammatory reaction.

Healing biopsy sites may have histologic features that may lead to misinterpretations and are therefore included in this section. Repeated marrow biopsies are frequently performed for assessment of the effects of chemotherapy or for determining the degree of engraftment following bone marrow transplantation and may be taken from sites from which recent biopsies were obtained. The histologic findings depend on the time interval separating the two biopsies; most repeat biopsies are obtained at 2 to 3 week intervals. At this time the healing site has abundant granulation tissue with beginning new bone formation and minimal deposition of adipose tissue (fig. 22). Subsequent biopsies show restructuring of bone trabeculae and deposition of adipose tissue followed by islands of hematopoietic cells.

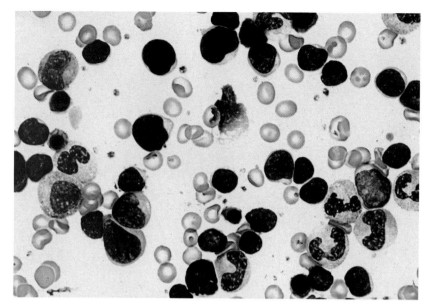

Figure 17
HEMATOGONES
Bone marrow smear from a child showing numerous hematogones which vary in size. The three large cells in the upper left have a sparse amount of lightly basophilic cytoplasm. (Wright-Giemsa stain)

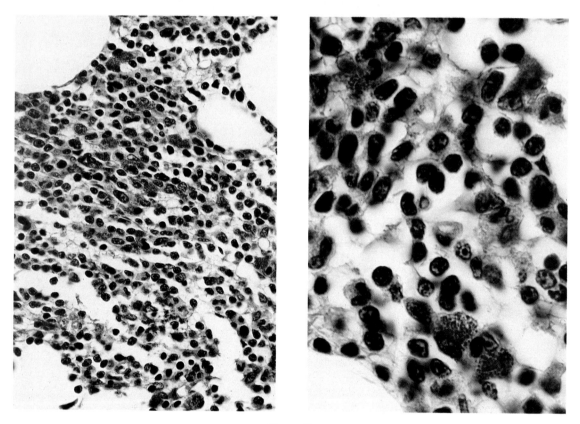

Figure 18
INCREASED HEMATOGONES IN A BONE MARROW SMEAR
FROM A 5-MONTH-OLD BOY WITH A NEUROBLASTOMA

Left: Bone marrow biopsy from the same patient as illustrated in figure 17 showing numerous small lymphocytes with coarse nuclear chromatin and no evident nucleoli. The cells are evenly distributed among the other hemopoietic cells. (Hematoxylin and eosin stain)

Right: High magnification of the specimen on the left showing hematogones with clumped nuclear chromatin and no evident nucleoli. There are no mitotic figures in these cells. (Hematoxylin and eosin stain)

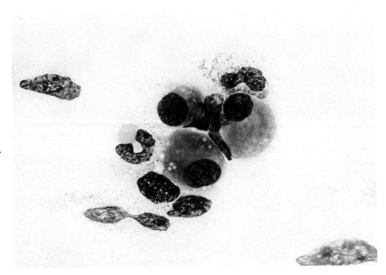

Figure 19
OSTEOBLASTS
Three osteoblasts in a bone marrow smear. These cells have abundant blue cytoplasm and an eccentrically located nucleus in which a single nucleolus can usually be identified. The cytoplasmic margins are frequently indistinct. These cells are approximately twice the size of plasma cells. (Wright-Giemsa stain)

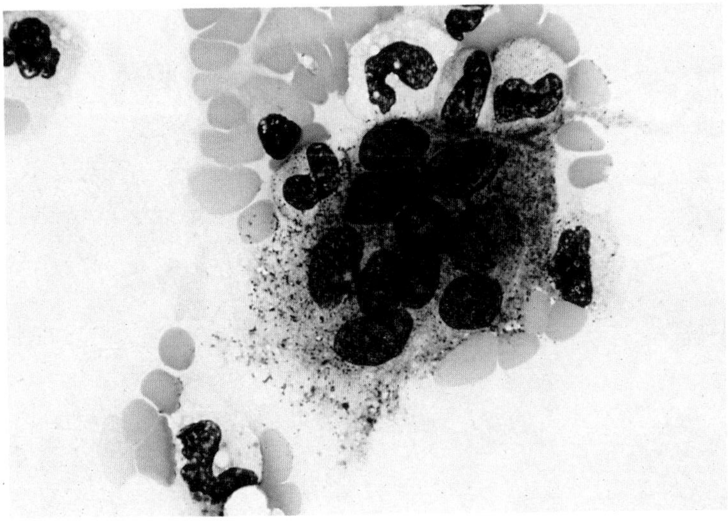

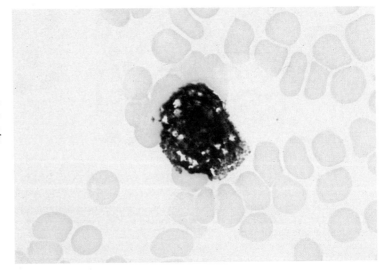

Figure 20
OSTEOCLAST
The osteoclast is a very large cell with multiple nuclei which have distinct nucleoli. The cytoplasm usually contains coarse, variably sized azurophilic granules. (Wright-Giemsa stain)

Figure 21
TISSUE MAST CELL
The tissue mast cell contains basophilic granules that are uniform in size. The nucleus is usually round and single; the nuclear margin may be obscured by the dense concentration of granules. (Wright-Giemsa stain)

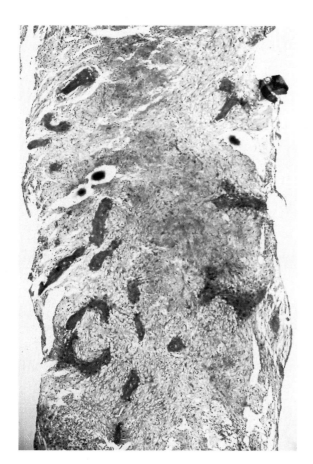 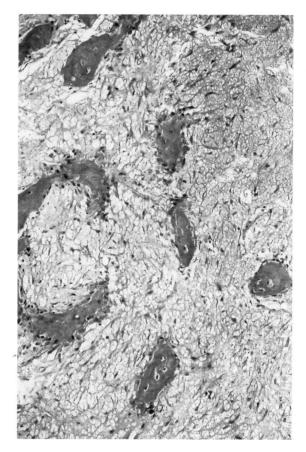

Figure 22
BONE MARROW BIOPSY SITE

Left: Bone marrow biopsy from a site biopsied 3 weeks previously. The biopsy consists of granulation tissue and new bone formation. (Hematoxylin and eosin stain)

Right: High magnification of the specimen on the left. The intertrabecular areas consist of granulation tissue with no evidence of adipose tissue or hematopoietic cells. Numerous osteoblasts are present along the endosteal surfaces of the new bone structures. (Hematoxylin and eosin stain)

REFERENCES

Introduction

1. Bennett JM, Catovsky D, Daniel MT, et al. Criteria for the diagnosis of acute leukemia of megakaryocytic lineage (M7). A report of the French-American-British Cooperative Group. Ann Intern Med 1985;103:460–2.

2. _____, Catovsky D, Daniel MT, et al. Proposals for the classification of the acute leukaemias. French-American-British (FAB) Cooperative Group. Br J Haematol 1976;33:451–8.

3. _____, Catovsky D, Daniel, MT, et al. Proposals for the classification of chronic (mature) B and T lymphoid leukaemias. French-American-British (FAB) Cooperative Group. J Clin Pathol 1989;42:567–84.

4. _____, Catovsky D, Daniel MT, et al. Proposals for the classification of the myelodysplastic syndromes. Br J Haematol 1982;51:189–99.

5. _____, Catovsky D, Daniel MT, et al. Proposed revised criteria for the classification of acute myeloid leukemia. A report of the French-American-British (FAB) Cooperative Group. Ann Intern Med 1985;103:620–5.

6. Berlin NI. Diagnosis and classification of the polycythemias. Semin Hematol 1975;12:339–51.

7. Cheson BD, Cassileth PA, Head D, et al. Report of the National Cancer Institute-sponsored workshop on definitions of diagnosis and response in acute myeloid leukemia. J Clin Oncol 1990;8:813–9.

8. Durie BG. Staging and kinetics of multiple myeloma. Semin Oncol 1986;13:300–9.
9. Murphy S, Iland H, Rosenthal D, Laszlo J. Essential thrombocythemia: an interim report from the Polycythemia Vera Study Group. Semin Hematol 1986;23:177–82.
10. National Cancer Institute sponsored study of classifications of non-Hodgkin's lymphomas: summary and description of a working formulation for clinical usage. The Non-Hodgkin's Lymphoma Pathologic Classification Project. Cancer 1982;49:2112–35.

Normal Bone Marrow

11. Bloom W, Fawcett DW. A textbook of histology. 10th ed. Philadelphia: WB Saunders, 1975:204–32.
12. Caldwell CW, Poje E, Helikson MA. B-cell precursors in normal pediatric bone marrow. Am J Clin Pathol 1991;98:816–23.
13. Campbell AD, Wicha MS. Extracellular matrix and the haematopoietic microenvironment. J Lab Clin Med 1988;112:140–6.
14. Hartsock RJ, Smith EB, Petty CS. Normal variations with aging of the amount of hematopoietic tissue in bone marrow from the anterior iliac crest. A study made from 177 cases of sudden death examined by necropsy. Am J Clin Pathol 1965;43:326–31.
15. Lambertsen RH, Weiss L. A model of intramedullary hematopoietic microenvironment based on stereologic study of the distribution of endocloned marrow colonies. Blood 1984;63:287–97.
16. Longacre TA, Foucar K, Crago S, et al. Hematogones: a multiparameter analysis of bone marrow precursor cells. Blood 1989;73:543–52.
17. Maeda K, Hyun BH, Rebuck JW. Lymphoid follicles in bone marrow aspirates. Am J Clin Pathol 1977;67:41–8.
18. Sundberg RD. Aspiration biopsy of bone marrow. Bull Univ Minn Hosp Minn Med Found 1950;21:471–505.
19. Weiss LP. Functional organization of the hematopoietic tissues. In: Hoffman R, Benz EJ Jr, Shattil SJ, Furie B, Cohen HJ, eds. Hematology: basic principles and practice. New York: Churchill Livingstone, 1991:82–96.
20. Wintrobe MM, Lee GR, Boggs DR, et al. Clinical hematology. 8th ed. Philadelphia: Lea & Febiger, 1981:41–50.

❖❖❖

ACUTE LEUKEMIAS

The acute leukemias are neoplasias of hematopoietic cell precursors manifest by a proliferative process involving primarily the bone marrow and blood. *Acute lymphoblastic leukemia (ALL) is* a proliferation of lymphoblasts that have their origin in a lymphocyte progenitor cell. *Acute myeloid leukemia (AML)* originates in the myeloid hematopoietic progenitor cell system which includes myeloblasts, monoblasts, erythroblasts, and megakaryoblasts; the proliferative process may involve one or more of these precursor cells. In the majority of cases of acute leukemia there is exclusive involvement of the myeloid or lymphocytic cells. In some instances, however, the leukemic process involves both the myeloid and lymphoid precursors; this is referred to as *mixed lineage acute leukemia* (7,9,14). Acute leukemia of either lymphoid or myeloid lineage may originate in an extramedullary site. This occurs more frequently in ALL which may arise in the thymus in T-cell ALL or in the small intestine or other sites in ALL-L3.

The reported incidence of leukemia in the white population in the United States in 1986 was 9.5 per 100,000 (8). The incidence of acute leukemia was 3.7 per 100,000: 2.1 cases of AML and 1.6 cases of ALL. The average annual incidence of acute leukemia per 100,000 population for all races and both sexes for the years 1982–1986 in the United States is seen in Table 2. As shown, ALL is more common in children and AML is more common in adults. Acute leukemia constitutes 30 percent of all neoplasms in individuals under the age of 15 years and is the most common tumor in that age group (11). The incidence of ALL in white children under 15 years of age is approximately twice that of black children (Table 3) (11).

The manifestations of acute leukemia in the blood and bone marrow vary. The leukocyte count may be increased, decreased, or normal. Approximately 70 percent of patients with AML present with leukocytosis while 10 to 20 percent present with leukopenia (13). Anemia, thrombocytopenia, and neutropenia occur in the majority of patients due to bone marrow replacement by the leukemic cells.

In acute leukemia the marrow is hypercellular in the majority of cases; a minority of patients, primarily older individuals, have hypocellular marrow that may resemble aplastic anemia. This is more frequently noted in AML than ALL.

The cytologic and histologic features of the acute leukemias are detailed in the discussions of the individual types of leukemia. The most common cytologic characteristics of AML and ALL are listed in Table 4. As a general rule, lymphoblasts are smaller than myeloblasts and have coarser nuclear chromatin, less prominent nucleoli, and less cytoplasm; cytoplasmic granules are usually not

Table 2

**AVERAGE ANNUAL INCIDENCE
OF ACUTE LEUKEMIA
PER 100,000 POPULATION***

Age	Acute Lymphoblastic Leukemia	Acute Myeloid Leukemia
Less than 5	5.2	0.4
5–9	2.8	0.3
10–14	1.8	0.5
15–19	1.3	0.6
20–24	0.6	0.6
25–29	0.5	0.8
30–34	0.3	0.8
35–39	0.5	1.5
40–44	0.5	1.3
45–49	0.7	1.9
50–54	0.6	2.8
55–59	0.5	3.7
60–64	0.6	5.4
65–69	1.0	8.0
70–74	0.9	11.2
75–79	1.4	15.1
80–84	2.5	19.4
85+	2.2	19.8

*All races, both sexes, in the United States, 1982–1986 (8).

Table 3

AGE-ADJUSTED ANNUAL INCIDENCE OF ACUTE LEUKEMIA
IN THE UNITED STATES FOR PERSONS UNDER 15 YEARS OF AGE: 1973–1982*

	Males		Incidence/Million Females		Both Sexes	
	White	Black	White	Black	White	Black
Acute lymphoblastic leukemia	35.9	14.4	29.7	15.3	32.9	14.8
Acute myeloid leukemia	5.6	4.3	6.5	6.2	6.1	5.2

*Data from reference 11.

Table 4

CYTOLOGIC FEATURES OF BLASTS IN ACUTE MYELOID
AND ACUTE LYMPHOBLASTIC LEUKEMIAS

	Acute Myeloid Leukemia	Acute Lymphoblastic Leukemia
Blast size	Medium to large, usually uniform	Variable, small to medium size
Cytoplasm	Fine granules may be present	Usually scant, coarse granules sometimes present
Auer rods	Present in 60 to 70 percent of cases	Not present
Nuclear chromatin	Usually finely dispersed	Fine to coarse
Nucleoli	2 to 4, often prominent	1 to 3, often indistinct
Other cell types	Often dysplastic changes in maturing myeloid cells	Myeloid cells not dysplastic

Table 5

CYTOCHEMICAL PROFILES OF ACUTE LEUKEMIAS

	MPO/SBB	CAE	NSE	PAS	Acid Phosphatase
Acute lymphoblastic leukemia	–	–	+/– (focal)	+ (75%)	+/– (focal T-cell ALL)
Acute myeloid leukemia	+	+	+ (monocytic, diffuse)	–/+	+

MPO = Myeloperoxidase, SBB = Sudan black B, CAE = Chloroacetate esterase, NSE = Nonspecific esterase, PAS = Periodic acid–Schiff.

present. In many cases of acute leukemia the blasts exhibit ambiguous morphologic features. In these instances cytochemical staining is an important supplement to the morphologic assessment. Table 5 lists the comparative cytochemical reactions for ALL and AML.

The classification of the acute leukemias used in this Fascicle is based on proposals introduced in 1976 by the French-American-British (FAB) Cooperative Group, with modifications proposed in 1982 and 1985 (1–4). Further refinements proposed by a United States National Cancer Institute panel are incorporated (5). The classification is based primarily on morphologic characteristics augmented by cytochemical reactivity patterns and immunophenotypic and ultrastructural studies.

Additional modifications based on the authors' experience and observations of other hematopathologists have been used primarily in the classification of the AMLs. These modifications are relatively minor but are noted to avoid misunderstanding. In a slight variance from the proposals of the FAB committee, the requisite minimum of blasts for a diagnosis of acute leukemia is 30 percent in the blood or bone marrow, as recommended by a National Cancer Institute (NCI) working committee on establishing guidelines for the definition of the diagnosis of AML and the evaluation of response following treatment (5).

The promonocyte, a monocytic cell intermediate in maturation to the monoblast and the monocyte, and most characteristically found in acute monocytic leukemia, differentiated (M5B), is considered equivalent to a blast for the purpose of arriving at a blast percentage for establishing a diagnosis of acute monocytic leukemia, differentiated (M5B) and acute myelomonocytic leukemia (M4). The acceptance of this cell as equivalent to a blast is not clearly stated in the FAB proposals. However, it is accepted as equivalent in the NCI proposed guidelines for AML-M5B. We have extended the acceptance of the promonocyte as a blast equivalent to AML-M4 as well in this Fascicle.

In accordance with the modified FAB proposals published in 1985, the diagnosis of erythroleukemia (AML-M6) is established when the number of erythroid precursors is 50 percent or more of the marrow cells and myeloblasts are 30 percent or more of the nonerythroid marrow cells. The diagnosis of erythroleukemia in this Fascicle is extended to those instances in which the erythroid precursors comprise 30 to 50 percent of the marrow cells and manifest marked morphologic abnormalities and the myeloblasts are 30 percent or more of the nonerythroid cells. The essentials of this extended definition of erythroleukemia were incorporated into a large national study of AML and myelodysplastic syndromes by the Groupe Francais de Morphologic Hematologique and were also part of the definition of erythroleukemia in the original FAB proposals in 1976 (2,6).

We also describe a very rare variant of erythroleukemia in which the marrow is virtually completely replaced by abnormal erythroblasts and for which we have retrieved the term *erythremic myelosis*. The number of identifiable myeloblasts in this disorder is too low to be significant and the criterion of 30 percent myeloblasts in the nonerythroid component is not applicable.

Another variance from the revised FAB proposals, which has virtually no impact on diagnosis or classification, is the form of the differential used in subclassifying AML-M1 to AML-M5. The FAB committee suggests that subclassification be based on a differential of the nonerythroid myeloid cells, whereas in this Fascicle subclassification is based on a differential of all marrow cells, including lymphocytes and plasma cells.

Although the AMLs should be classified as precisely as possible, in some cases there are overlapping morphologic features: AML with maturation (AML-M2) may show some cytomorphologic features of acute myelomonocytic leukemia (AML-M4). The use of cytochemical profiles resolves the problem in most instances but in some cases the classification may be arbitrary. Erythroleukemia by definition involves both the granulocytes and erythroid cells. In addition, a substantial number of cases of erythroleukemia involve the megakaryocytes and are basically acute panmyelopathies. Some of these processes are accompanied by marrow fibrosis and may be referred to as acute myelofibrosis. Similarly, cases of acute megakaryocytic leukemia may show substantial involvement of the erythroid cells and granulocytes.

The cytomorphologic findings in bone marrow and blood specimens at relapse may show some variance from the initial diagnostic specimen. This may be accompanied by changes in the immunophenotypic characteristics of the major blast population. These findings underscore the multipotential nature of the myeloid precursor cell.

The introduction of immunologic markers for distinguishing B and T lymphocytes has resulted in an immunologic classification of the ALLs. The role of immunologic markers in the AMLs relates primarily to the identification of blast cells that have no differentiating morphologic or cytochemical features and to the identification of mixed lineage acute leukemias. These points will be expanded in the sections on ALL and AML.

The impact of cytogenetic studies in the acute leukemias relates primarily to two factors: correlation of specific chromosomal abnormalities with morphologic and immunologic types, and prognosis (10,12,15). Several associations between specific chromosome abnormalities and

Table 6

ASSOCIATION OF NONRANDOM CHROMOSOME ABNORMALITIES WITH MORPHOLOGIC TYPES OF ACUTE MYELOID LEUKEMIA*

FAB Classification	Chromosome Abnormality	Frequency (percent)
M3	t(15;17)(q22;q11–12)	95–100
M4EO	inv(16)(p13q22) or t(16;16)(p13;q22)	100
M2	t(8;21)(q22;q22)	18–20
M1, M2	t(9;22)(q34;q11)	8
M1, M2, M4, M5, M6	+8	9
M1, M4, M5	t(v;11)(v;q23)**	9
M1, M2, M4	t(6;9)(p23;q34)	2
M1, M2, M4, M6	inv(3)(q21q26) or t(3;3)(q21;q26)	2
M1, M2, M4, M6, M7	-7	9
M1, M2, M4, M6, M7	-5 or del(5q)	6
M1, M2, M4, M5, M6, M7	complex defects	14

*Data compiled from references 12 and 15.
**v: The other chromosomes involved in translocations involving 11q23 vary and include chromosomes 9 and 19.

the morphologic or immunologic type of acute leukemia have been established (10,12). The most specific abnormality in AML is the t(15;17) chromosome rearrangement, which occurs in 95 to 100 percent of cases of acute promyelocytic leukemia (AML-M3). Other abnormalities, such as the t(8;21) found in approximately 20 percent of cases of acute myeloblastic leukemia with maturation (AML-M2), have a relatively high degree of specificity but lower incidence. Table 6 lists the most well-established relationships between karyotype and morphology in AML. For ALL, the highest association of karyotype to morphology and immunophenotype is the t(8;14)(q24;q32) chromosome abnormality, which is found in more than 90 percent of cases of ALL-L3 (12). Other cytogenetic associations in ALL are listed in Table 7.

The relevance of chromosome abnormalities to prognosis is recognized for both AML and ALL. Although other factors, such as leukocyte count and age are interactive, some cytogenetic abnormalities identify risk groups in both AML and ALL (10,15). Tables 8 and 9 show a prognostic stratification of cases of AML and ALL based on cytogenetic findings.

ACUTE MYELOID LEUKEMIAS

The classification of the acute myeloid leukemias (AMLs) is based on the morphologic characteristics and cytochemical reactivity pattern of the predominant leukemic cell population (20,22). In two types, AML with minimal differentiation (M0) and acute megakaryoblastic leukemia (M7), the morphology and cytochemical reactions are not definitive and immunologic markers or ultrastructural studies are necessary (19,40,63).

The basic requisite for a diagnosis of AML is the presence of 30 percent or more blasts in the blood or bone marrow (22,40). Two major types of blasts are recognized based on nuclear and cytoplasmic characteristics (21,40).

The *type I myeloblast* is a cell with fine nuclear chromatin, usually two to four distinct nucleoli, and a moderate rim of pale to basophilic cytoplasm without azurophilic granules (fig. 23-I).

The *type II myeloblast* is a cell with nuclear and cytoplasmic features similar to the type I myeloblast with the addition of up to 20 delicate azurophilic granules in the cytoplasm (fig. 23-II).

Table 7

ASSOCIATION OF NONRANDOM CHROMOSOME ABNORMALITIES AND MORPHOLOGIC AND IMMUNOLOGIC TYPES OF ACUTE LYMPHOBLASTIC LEUKEMIA*

Type of ALL	Chromosome Abnormality	Frequency (percent)
Morphologic type		
L3	t(8;14)(q24;q32); less common, t(2;8) or t(8;22)	>90
Immunologic type		
B-cell ALL (SIg+)	t(8;14)(q24;q32); less common, t(2;8) or t(8;22)	>90
Pre–B-cell ALL (CIg μ+)	t(1;19)(q23;p13)	25
T-cell ALL	Translocations of 14q11	25
	Normal chromosomes	40
Mixed lineage ALL	Translocations of 11q23; t(9;22)(q34;q11); translocations of 14q32	?

*Data compiled from references 10 and 12.

Table 8

PROGNOSTIC IMPLICATIONS OF CHROMOSOME FINDINGS IN ACUTE MYELOID LEUKEMIA*

Chromosome Findings	Prognostic Group
Inv(16) or t(16;16), single miscellaneous defects	Favorable
+8, t(15;17), t(6;9), t(8;21), t(9;11), t(9;22)	Intermediate
-7 or del(7q), complex defects	Unfavorable
Normal chromosomes, inv(3), del(5q), two to three miscellaneous defects	Undetermined

*Data from reference 15.

Table 9

PROGNOSTIC IMPLICATIONS OF CHROMOSOME FINDINGS IN ACUTE LYMPHOBLASTIC LEUKEMIA*

Chromosome Findings	Prognostic Group
Hyperdiploidy: >50 chromosomes	Favorable
Hyperdiploidy: 47–50 chromosomes Normal chromosomes	Intermediate
Hypodiploidy All translocations	Unfavorable

*Data from reference 10.

The promyelocyte is larger than the type I and II myeloblasts and has numerous azurophilic granules (fig. 23-pro).

Uncommonly, some cases of AML present with myeloblasts with numerous azurophilic granules. These myeloblasts have been referred to as *type III blasts* (fig. 24) (22,40). The type III myeloblast may be the predominant blast in occasional cases of AML-M2 (AML with maturation) and may be associated with a t(8;21) chromosome abnormality (24,40).

The diagnostic requisite of 30 percent type I and II myeloblasts in the bone marrow or blood cannot be applied uniformly to all types of AML. In acute promyelocytic leukemia (M3), the pre-

dominant leukemic cell is an abnormal promyelocyte; the myeloblasts are rarely 30 percent or higher (86). In acute monoblastic leukemia (M5A), the predominant proliferating cell is the monoblast, a cell with morphologic and cytochemical features distinct from type I and II myeloblasts. In acute monocytic leukemia, differentiated (M5B), the predominant cell is the promonocyte, which is intermediate in maturation to the monoblast and monocyte. The megakaryoblasts of acute megakaryoblastic leukemia vary in morphology but uniformly lack the cytochemical properties of myeloblasts. For purposes of determining the requisite 30 percent blasts for a diagnosis of AML, the abnormal promyelocytes in M3, the monoblasts in M5A, the monoblasts

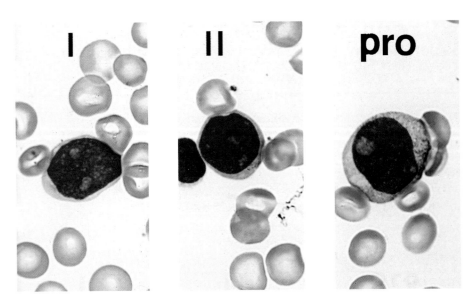

Figure 23

TYPE I AND II MYELOBLASTS AND PROMYELOCYTE

I: The type I myeloblast has basophilic cytoplasm and a nucleus with finely dispersed chromatin and distinct nucleoli. The cytoplasm is agranular. (Wright-Giemsa stain)

II: The type II myeloblast has the nuclear and cytoplasmic features of a type I blast and the additional finding of a few azurophilic granules in the cytoplasm. (Wright-Giemsa stain)

Pro: The promyelocyte is the largest cell in neutrophil development. It has a lower nuclear-cytoplasmic ratio than the type I and II myeloblasts, moderately basophilic cytoplasm, slightly coarse chromatin, and prominent nucleoli. There are numerous azurophilic granules scattered throughout the cytoplasm and overlying the nucleus. A focal, less basophilic area of the cytoplasm, corresponding to the Golgi region, may be present. (Wright-Giemsa stain)

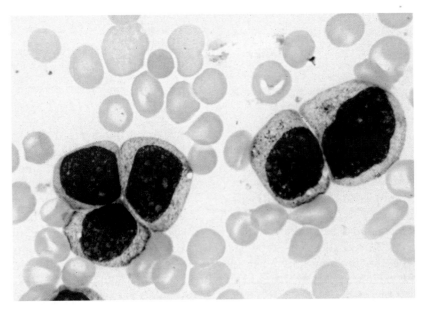

Figure 24

TYPE III MYELOBLASTS

Blood smear from a 72-year-old male with acute myeloblastic leukemia with maturation (AML-M2). The leukocyte count was 70×10^9/L and was comprised almost entirely of myeloblasts with numerous azurophilic granules. These are type III blasts. (Wright-Giemsa stain)

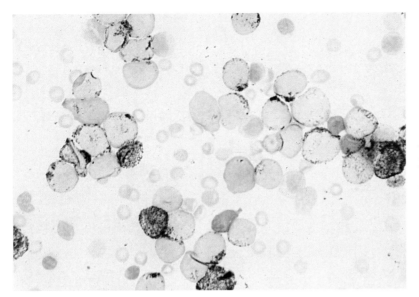

Figure 25
ACUTE MYELOBLASTIC
LEUKEMIA WITH
MATURATION (AML-M2):
MYELOPEROXIDASE REACTION
MPO reaction on a bone marrow
smear from a patient with acute myelo-
blastic leukemia with maturation.
Most of the myeloblasts have numerous
positive granules. The more mature
neutrophils are intensely positive.
(Myeloperoxidase stain)

and promonocytes in M5B and acute myelomonocytic leukemia (M4), and the megakaryoblasts in
acute megakaryoblastic leukemia (M7) are considered equivalent to myeloblasts.

Cytochemistry

An important basis for the classification of the
AMLs is the cytochemical reactivity pattern of the
proliferating cells (20,57,100). The most useful
cytochemical stains are myeloperoxidase (MPO),
Sudan black B (SBB), and nonspecific esterase
(NSE); chloroacetate esterase (CAE) is less sensitive than MPO and SBB and has utility only in
certain subtypes, most notably acute myelomonocytic leukemia with increased marrow eosinophils
(M4EO), in which the granules in the abnormal
eosinophils are CAE positive (27,28). Monoclonal
antibodies may be utilized in the demonstration of
MPO and have been reported to be more sensitive
than the cytochemical reaction (37).

MPO reacts with cells of neutrophil, eosinophil,
and monocyte lineage. The reaction in the neutrophils and eosinophils increases in intensity with
maturation. Myeloblasts generally have a few
MPO-positive granules; segmented neutrophils
react intensely (fig. 25). Promyelocyte reactivity is
usually intense. Normal monocytes contain a few
scattered MPO granules. The monoblasts and promonocytes of acute monocytic leukemia and acute
myelomonocytic leukemia may manifest no MPO
reactivity or may contain a few scattered granules.

Uncommonly, monoblasts and promonocytes are
intensely MPO positive. Reactivity with SBB
generally parallels the reactivity pattern of
MPO, with occasional discrepancies. Because of
this, it is advisable to perform both reactions in
all cases of poorly differentiated acute leukemia.
It is important, when assessing the results of
cytochemical reactivity in acute leukemias, that
the percent of positive cells be based only on the
blast population.

NSE is important in the recognition of those
types of AML with a monocytic component: acute
monoblastic leukemia (M5A), acute monocytic leukemia (M5B), and acute myelomonocytic leukemia
(M4). NSE is not present in significant amounts in
normal granulocytes when the method of Yam et
al. (100) is used. The abnormal promyelocytes in
approximately 25 percent of cases of acute promyelocytic leukemia are NSE positive (42). The
enzyme may be present in megakaryoblasts but
the intensity of the reaction is less than in monocytes and is usually focal, in contrast to the diffuse
reactivity in monocytes. The blasts and promyelocytes in occasional cases of AML-M2 (AML
with maturation) may react with NSE.

CAE reactivity is restricted to cells of neutrophil and mast cell lineage in normal bone marrows. It may also be positive in the abnormal
granules of the eosinophils in acute myelomonocytic leukemia associated with pericentric
inversion of chromosome 16 (27). It may also
manifest as a slight blush in the cytoplasm of

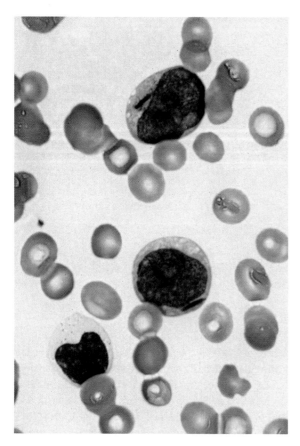

Figure 26
AUER RODS
Two myeloblasts with single, prominent Auer rods. (Wright-Giemsa stain)

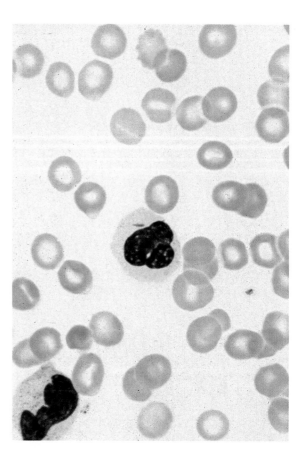

Figure 27
AUER ROD IN SEGMENTED NEUTROPHIL
A segmented neutrophil with an Auer rod in a blood smear from a patient with acute myeloblastic leukemia with maturation (AML-M2). (Wright-Giemsa stain)

monoblasts in M5A (66). Myeloblasts are frequently CAE negative. Promyelocytes and more mature cells of the neutrophil series react intensely with CAE, similar to reactions with MPO and SBB.

A staining technique combining NSE and CAE or MPO is used to identify a mixed population of neutrophils and monocytes, and leukemic cells with features of both neutrophils and monocytes (57,100). This combined stain has utility primarily in acute and chronic myelomonocytic leukemia. The combined stain should always be accompanied by separate staining for NSE and MPO since there may be diminished reactivity of both enzymes in the combined procedure.

An important morphologic finding, present in the leukemic cells of approximately 60 to 70 percent of cases of AML, is the Auer rod. The Auer rod is an azurophilic linear structure of varying length and width, that may be found in most

types of AML (fig. 26). Auer rods may be present in numerous blasts or only in rare cells; single or multiple Auer rods may be present. Auer rods may uncommonly be detected in more mature cells of the neutrophil series, including segmented forms (fig. 27). They are generally MPO, SBB, and CAE positive and these reactions may aid in their recognition. Ultrastructurally, the Auer rod is an alignment and crystallization of azurophilic granules. In the context of a blast proliferation of 30 percent or more, the presence of an Auer rod in one or more blasts is definitive evidence of AML. The finding is not specific for any one type of AML; it is rarely found in acute monoblastic leukemia. Auer rods do not occur in cells of erythroid or megakaryocyte lineage. Table 10 is a summary of the cytochemical reactivity and incidence of Auer rods for the subtypes of AML.

Table 10

CYTOCHEMICAL REACTIVITY PATTERNS AND
FREQUENCY OF AUER RODS IN ACUTE MYELOID LEUKEMIA*

		MPO/SBB	NSE	Auer Rods
AML	M0	–	–	0
	M1	+ (≥3% blasts)	–	50%
	M2	++	–	70%
	M3	++	+ **	95–100%
	M4	+ (neutrophils)	+ (monocytic cells)	60%
	M5	–	++[+]	M5A: 0% / M5B: 30%
	M6	+ (myeloblasts)	–	60% (myeloblasts)
	M7	–	–[‡]	0

MPO = Myeloperoxidase,   SBB = Sudan black B,   NSE = Nonspecific esterase
* From reference 86.
** Approximately 20 percent of cases of acute promyelocytic leukemia have a population of NSE-positive cells.
[+] Occasional cases of AML-M5A are NSE negative.
[‡] Megakaryocytes can show weak focal NSE positivity.

Table 11

IMMUNOPHENOTYPE OF ACUTE MYELOID LEUKEMIA*

Surface Antigens	FAB Subgroups					
	M0	M1/M2	M3	M4/M5	M6	M7
HLA-DR	+	+	–	++	–	+
CD11	+	+	+	++	–	–
CD13	+	+	+	++	–	–
CD14	+	+	–	++	–	–
CD33	+	++	+	++	+	+
CD41, CD61	–	–	–	–	–	++
Glycophorin A	–	–	–	–	++**	–

* Modified from Erber et al. (45), Koike (58), Lee et al. (63), and the Third MIC Cooperative Study Group (91).
** Reactivity of the erythroblasts only.

Monoclonal antibodies to membrane surface antigens and cytoplasmic constituents may be useful in the identification of cell lineage in cases of AML unclassifiable by routine morphology. The immunologic markers have particular utility in cases of AML with minimal differentiation (M0), acute megakaryoblastic leukemia (M7), and cases of mixed lineage acute leukemia (19,40,45, 55,58,69,71,76,99). The occasional cases of acute monoblastic leukemia in which the monoblasts are NSE negative may be identified with monoclonal antibodies to cells of monocytic lin- eage. Antibodies to erythroid cell membranes or to hemoglobin are useful in the identification of erythroid precursors (95). Table 11 summarizes the immunophenotype characteristics of the major cell components in the AML subtypes.

Classification

Eight major classifications of AML are recognized (Table 12). The major diagnostic criteria and immunophenotype of the predominant blasts for the various classes of AML are summarized in Table 13.

Table 12

CLASSIFICATION OF ACUTE MYELOID LEUKEMIA

Acute myeloblastic leukemia, minimally differentiated - M0 (AML-M0)
Acute myeloblastic leukemia without maturation - M1 (AML-M1)
Acute myeloblastic leukemia with maturation - M2 (AML-M2)
Acute promyelocytic leukemia - M3 (AML-M3)
    Hypergranular acute promyelocytic leukemia (APL)
    Microgranular (hypogranular) acute promyelocytic leukemia - M3V (APL-V)
Acute myelomonocytic leukemia - M4 (AML-M4)
    Acute myelomonocytic leukemia with increased marrow eosinophils (AML-M4EO)
Acute monocytic leukemia - M5 (AML-M5)
    Acute monoblastic leukemia (acute monocytic leukemia, poorly differentiated) - M5A (AML-M5A)
    Acute monocytic leukemia (acute monocytic leukemia, differentiated) - M5B (AML-M5B)
Erythroleukemia - M6 (AML-M6)
Acute megakaryoblastic leukemia - M7 (AML-M7)

Other entities that represent types of AML not included in the FAB classification or unusual manifestations of AML include acute basophilic leukemia, hypocellular AML, and acute myelofibrosis. Granulocytic sarcoma is an extramedullary tumor of myeloid cells, usually myeloblasts and promyelocytes. It may occur in both AML and the chronic myeloproliferative disorders. It may also be observed in the evolution of myelodysplastic syndromes.

Acute Myeloblastic Leukemia, Minimally Differentiated (AML-M0)

Definition. A type of AML in which less than 3 percent of the blasts react for MPO and SBB, and Auer rods are not found. The myeloid origin of the blasts is demonstrated by reactivity of more than 20 percent blasts with at least one myeloid lineage–specific antibody (CD13, CD14, CD33) or with ultrastructural studies. The blasts are nonreactive with lymphocyte-specific antibodies (40,63).

Incidence and Clinical Findings. AML-M0 has been estimated at 5 to 10 percent of cases of AML (63). There are no specific clinical features. AML-M0 has been reported to be more refractory to chemotherapy than other types of AML (63).

Laboratory Findings. Similar to other types of AML, the majority of patients present with thrombocytopenia and anemia. The leukocyte count varies from markedly elevated to decreased.

Blood and Bone Marrow Findings. The blasts generally comprise more than 90 percent of the marrow cells and are virtually all type I (fig. 28A). The nuclear chromatin varies from fine to slightly coarse; two to four variably prominent nucleoli may be present. The cytoplasm is pale to slightly basophilic. Some blasts may resemble lymphoblasts. Auer rods are not present. Maturing granulocytes with dysplastic features may be present.

Cytochemical Findings. Less than 3 percent of the blasts are positive for MPO and SBB; in most cases, no or only rare blasts are reactive (fig. 28B).

Histopathologic Findings. The bone marrow biopsy in the majority of patients is hypercellular and replaced by blasts (fig. 28C). In older individuals the marrow may be hypocellular.

Ultrastructural Findings. The blast cells may be uniformly agranular or show scattered granules (63). In specimens reacted for MPO, reactivity may be present in the granules, the nuclear envelope, and the endoplasmic reticulum (fig. 28D). The number of reactive cells varies, but is usually less than 50 percent of the blasts.

Immunologic Findings. Twenty percent or more blasts are reactive with one or more myeloid lineage–specific antibodies: CD13, CD14, and CD33; the blasts are negative with lymphocyte lineage–specific antibodies (40). The terminal deoxynucleotidyltransferase (TdT) reaction may be positive, but positivity may be less than the 90 to 95 percent found in most cases of ALL.

Table 13

SUMMARY OF DIAGNOSTIC FEATURES OF ACUTE MYELOID LEUKEMIAS

FAB Type	Bone Marrow Findings	Immunophenotype
AML-M0	≥30% blasts; <3% blasts reactive for MPO, SBB, or NSE	≥ 20% blasts express one or more myeloid antigens: CD13, CD14, CD33; may be TdT positive; blasts negative for lymphocyte antigens
AML-M1	≥30% blasts; ≥3% blasts reactive for MPO or SBB; <10% of marrow nucleated cells are promyelocytes or more mature neutrophils	Blasts express myeloid antigens: CD13, CD14, CD33
AML-M2	≥30% blasts; ≥3% blasts reactive for MPO or SBB; ≥10% of marrow nucleated cells are promyelocytes or more mature neutrophils	Blasts myeloid antigen positive; blasts in 40% to 80% of t(8;21)-associated cases are CD19 positive; blasts in approximately 20% of t(8;21)-associated cases are TdT positive
AML-M3	≥30% blasts and abnormal promyelocytes; intense MPO and SBB reactivity; promyelocytes and blasts with multiple Auer rods (faggot cells); t(15;17) cytogenetic abnormality	Blasts and promyelocytes express myeloid antigens; promyelocytes are HLA-DR negative in most cases
AML-M4	≥30% myeloblasts, monoblasts, and promonocytes; ≥20% monocytic cells in marrow; ≥5×10^9/L monocytic cells in blood; ≥20% neutrophils and precursors in marrow; monocytic cells reactive for NSE; abnormal eosinophils in M4 with associated inv(16) chromosome abnormality	Varying proportions of blasts and monocytic cells express CD13, CD14, CD15, CD33; monocyte cells express CD36
AML-M5A	≥80% monocytic cells; monoblasts ≥80% of monocytic cells; monoblasts and promonocytes NSE positive (approximately 10 to 20% of cases are negative or equivocally positive); monoblasts usually MPO and SBB negative (may be positive in a minority of cases)	Varying proportions of CD13, CD14, CD15, and CD33-positive cells; monoblasts express CD36 and may express CD4
AML-M5B	≥80% monocytic cells; monoblasts <80% of monocytic cells; promonocytes predominate; monoblasts and promonocytes NSE positive; promonocytes may have scattered MPO- and SBB-positive granules	Varying proportions of monoblasts and promonocytes express CD13, CD14, CD15, CD33; monoblasts and promonocytes express CD36
AML-M6	≥50% erythroid precursors; ≥30% of nonerythroid precursors are myeloblasts; Auer rods may be present in myeloblasts; dyserythropoiesis; erythroid precursors frequently PAS positive	Myeloblasts express myeloid antigens; erythroid precursors express glycophorin A, react with antibody to hemoglobin A, and express CD36
AML-M7	≥30% blasts; ≥50% megakaryocytic cells by morphology, immunophenotype studies, or electron microscopy	Megakaryocytic cells express pan-myeloid antigen CD33, and platelet glycoproteins (CD41 and CD61) and CD36

MPO: Myeloperoxidase
SBB: Sudan black B
NSE: Nonspecific esterase
PAS: Periodic acid–Schiff
TdT: Terminal deoxynucleotidyltransferase
CD: Cluster designation

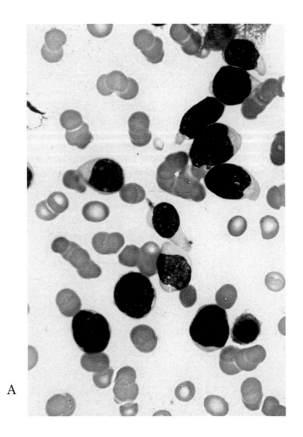

A

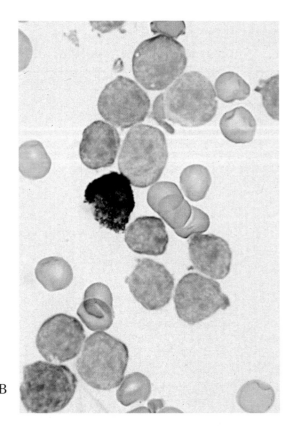

B

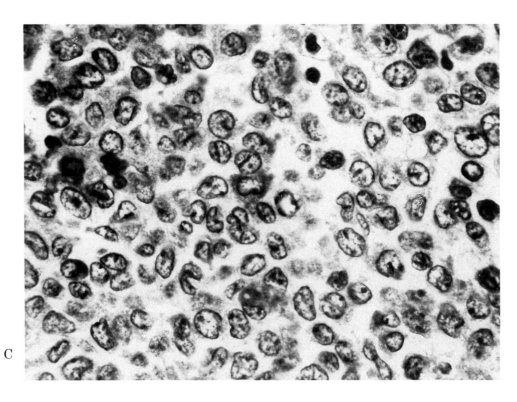

C

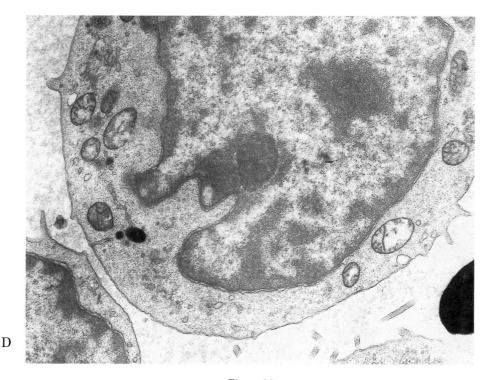

D

Figure 28
ACUTE MYELOBLASTIC LEUKEMIA, MINIMALLY DIFFERENTIATED (AML-M0)
A. The blasts in this bone marrow specimen lack differentiating features and are nonreactive for SBB and MPO. More than 20 percent of the blasts expressed CD13 and CD33. The blasts were TdT negative and nonreactive with antibodies to lymphocytes. (Wright-Giemsa stain)
B. The blasts are MPO negative. An intensely positive, more mature neutrophil is present. (Myeloperoxidase and Giemsa stains)
C. Bone marrow section showing complete replacement by blasts with no evidence of differentiation. (Hematoxylin and eosin stain)
D. Electron micrograph of a blast from the bone marrow specimen illustrated in A and B reacted for MPO. Two granules with dense reaction product are present. (Lead citrate stain only, X14,000)

Differential Diagnosis. The differential diagnosis of AML-M0 includes ALL, acute monoblastic leukemia (M5A), acute megakaryoblastic leukemia (M7), and acute basophilic leukemia.

ALL is distinguished from AML-M0 by the negative reactivity of lymphoblasts with the myeloid lineage–specific antibodies and positive reactivity with lymphocyte-specific antibodies. The blasts in the majority of cases of acute monoblastic leukemia are diffusely positive with NSE and show weak diffuse reactivity with CAE. Serum and urine lysozyme levels may also be elevated. The ultrastructural localization of peroxidase in megakaryoblasts is in the nuclear envelope and endoplasmic reticulum; the granules are negative. The reaction in megakaryoblasts is ablated by the fixation process used for myeloblasts. The diagnosis of acute basophilic leukemia is based on the specific ultrastructural characteristics of the basophil granules which have a speckled electron-dense structure (78).

Uncommonly, AML presents with blood and bone marrow findings resembling AML with maturation (AML-M2) in that the blasts are less than 90 percent of the marrow nucleated cells, possibly in the range of 30 to 50 percent, with substantial numbers of maturing granulocytes and erythroid cells. Less than 3 percent of blasts are reactive with MPO or SBB; in some cases none of the blasts are cytochemically reactive. The characterization of the blasts as myeloid is based on immunophenotyping or ultrastructural studies. Based on the negative cytochemical results the process could be classified as AML-M0. However, if dysplastic changes are present in the maturing granulocytes, AML-M2 is a more appropriate designation.

Acute Myeloblastic Leukemia without Maturation (AML-M1)

Definition. A type of AML characterized by a predominance of myeloblasts in the bone marrow; in the majority of cases the myeloblasts exceed 90 percent. At least 3 percent of the blasts are reactive for MPO or SBB. Less than 10 percent of the marrow cells manifest evidence of maturation to promyelocytes or more mature neutrophils.

Incidence and Clinical Findings. AML-M1 comprises approximately 10 to 20 percent of cases of AML (49,86). The disease affects individuals of all ages but is more common in adults than children; the median age is 46 years (86).

Patients frequently present with constitutional symptoms: fever, fatigue, and malaise. Hepatosplenomegaly and lymphadenopathy are present in approximately 30 percent of patients.

Laboratory Findings. Approximately 50 percent of patients with AML-M1 present with a leukocytosis and 25 percent present with leukopenia. The leukocytes exceed 100×10^9/L in approximately 30 percent of patients (86). Almost all patients are anemic and 75 percent are thrombocytopenic; half have platelet counts less than 50×10^9/L.

Blood and Bone Marrow Findings. The blasts in the majority of cases are type I. The myeloblasts may show considerable variability in size, amount of cytoplasm, and nuclear characteristics (figs. 29–35). Auer rods are found in a variable number of blasts in approximately 50 percent of cases and may be detected in myeloblasts in cases with less than 3 percent MPO- or SBB-positive blasts. The presence of Auer rods in these instances suffices for the diagnosis of AML-M1. Maturing neutrophils, if present, may show dysplastic features.

The blood may be characterized by a severe pancytopenia or there may be a marked leukocytosis consisting predominantly of blasts.

Cytochemical Findings. At least 3 percent of the blasts react with MPO or SBB (figs. 29, right and 31, right) and are nonreactive with NSE. In 10 to 15 percent of cases the blasts are TdT positive (30).

Histopathologic Findings. Bone marrow biopsies from patients with AML-M1 usually show complete replacement of normal marrow cells by blasts (fig. 36). Uncommonly, the marrow may be hypocellular (as in hypocellular acute leukemia).

The blasts are relatively uniform in appearance with round to oval, sometimes indented nuclei, two to four variably prominent nucleoli, and a moderate amount of cytoplasm. Mitotic activity is variable. There may be some increase in reticulin fibers but marked fibrosis is uncommon.

Ultrastructural Findings. The ultrastructural findings parallel the light microscopy features. The myeloblasts have round to indented nuclei with finely dispersed chromatin and prominent nucleoli (fig. 37). The cytoplasm contains profiles of rough endoplasmic reticulum, an active Golgi region and a variable number of electron-dense granules. The number of agranular blasts varies substantially.

Auer rods, when present, are elongated, electron-dense structures enclosed by a smooth membrane and have an internal, crystalline substructure with a periodicity of 8 to 12 mµ.

Ultrastructural peroxidase reactions show most myeloblasts to have activity in the nuclear envelope, rough endoplasmic reticulum, Golgi, and granules. Agranular blasts have reaction product in the nuclear envelope and endoplasmic reticulum; the Golgi may or may not be reactive.

Differential Diagnosis. Similar to AML-M0, the major types of leukemia from which AML-M1 must be distinguished include ALL-L2, acute monoblastic leukemia (M5A), acute megakaryoblastic leukemia (M7), and acute basophilic leukemia.

AML-M1 is distinguished from ALL-L2 by the reactivity of 3 percent or more blasts for MPO and SBB. The distinction of AML-M1 from acute monoblastic leukemia (M5A) is based primarily on the reaction patterns with MPO, SBB, and NSE. Three percent or more of the myeloblasts in AML-M1 react with MPO or SBB; myeloblasts are negative or only weakly reactive for NSE. The monoblasts in the majority of cases of acute monoblastic leukemia are negative for MPO and SBB and are moderately to strongly reactive for NSE. The megakaryoblasts of AML-M7 are MPO and SBB negative. Ultrastructural studies for platelet peroxidase or reactivity with immunologic markers to platelet glycoproteins are necessary to distinguish acute megakaryoblastic leukemia (M7) from AML-M1.

The blasts in acute basophilic leukemia may contain coarse azurophilic granules that may be MPO positive or negative. The definitive method for distinguishing this type of leukemia is ultrastructural examination (78,97).

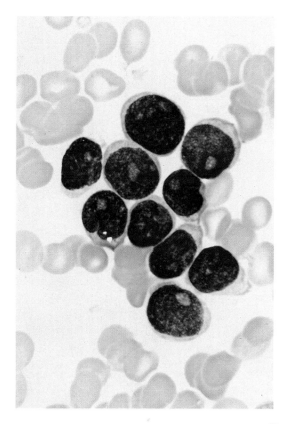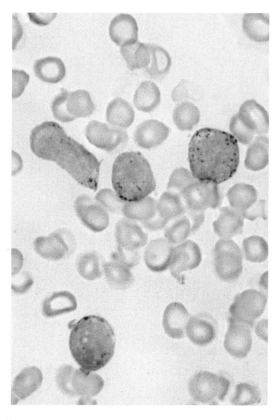

Figure 29
ACUTE MYELOBLASTIC LEUKEMIA WITHOUT MATURATION (AML-M1)

Left: Bone marrow specimen with several blasts that show slight variation in size. The majority of the cells have a rim of pale to slightly basophilic agranular cytoplasm and prominent nucleoli. The nuclei have finely dispersed chromatin and prominent nucleoli. (Wright-Giemsa stain)

Right: SBB reaction of the specimen illustrated on the left shows blasts with numerous positive granules. (Sudan black B and Giemsa stains)

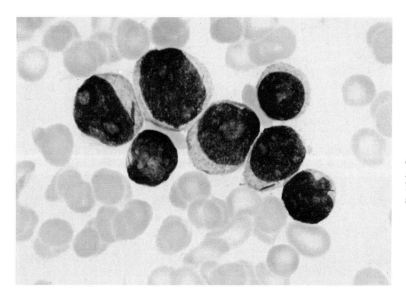

Figure 30
ACUTE MYELOBLASTIC
LEUKEMIA WITHOUT
MATURATION (AML-M1)

Bone marrow smear with several myeloblasts. The blasts vary in size, number, and prominence of nucleoli. Four of the blasts contain Auer rods. (Wright-Giemsa stain)

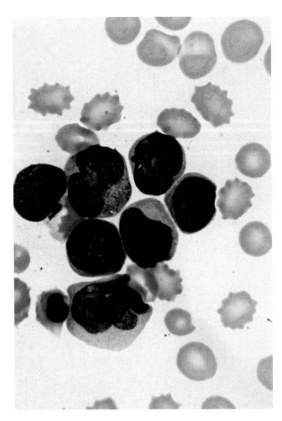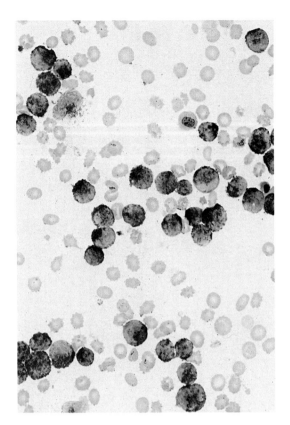

Figure 31
ACUTE MYELOBLASTIC LEUKEMIA WITHOUT MATURATION (AML-M1)
Left: Several of the myeloblasts in this bone marrow smear have nuclei with irregular folding and invagination, resulting in lighter areas partially or completely overlying the nucleus. These invaginations resemble nucleoli. One of the myeloblasts has numerous azurophilic granules. (Wright-Giemsa stain)
Right: A MPO reaction of the specimen illustrated on the left shows intense reactivity in the cytoplasm of the blasts. Reactivity partially overlying the nuclei corresponds to the lighter areas illustrated on the left. (Myeloperoxidase and Giemsa stains)

Figure 32
ACUTE MYELOBLASTIC
LEUKEMIA WITHOUT
MATURATION (AML-M1)
The myeloblasts in this blood smear vary in size, have markedly condensed nuclear chromatin, indistinct nucleoli, and irregularly shaped nuclei resembling poorly differentiated lymphoma cells. One blast contains a small, thin Auer rod. (Wright-Giemsa stain)

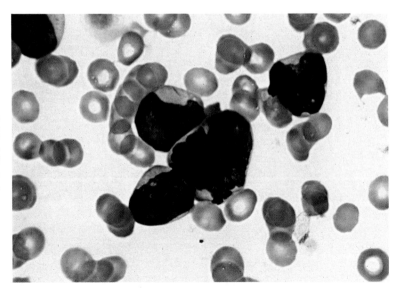

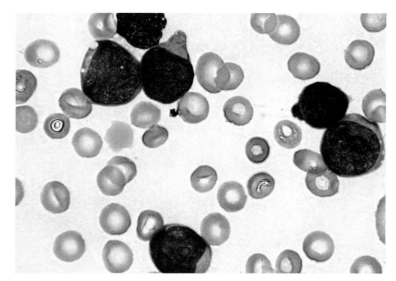

Figure 33
ACUTE MYELOBLASTIC LEUKEMIA
WITHOUT MATURATION (AML-M1)
The myeloblasts in this bone marrow
smear show some variability; two blasts
have more intensely basophilic cytoplasm
and coarse nuclear chromatin. Both types of
blasts reacted for MPO and SBB. (Wright-
Giemsa stain)

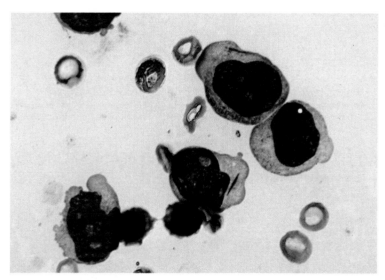

Figure 34
ACUTE MYELOBLASTIC LEUKEMIA
WITHOUT MATURATION (AML-M1)
The myeloblasts in this bone marrow
smear are large with abundant basophilic
cytoplasm. Two of the cells contain prominent
Auer rods; one cell contains numerous
azurophilic granules. Two postmitotic erythroblasts are present. (Wright-Giemsa stain)

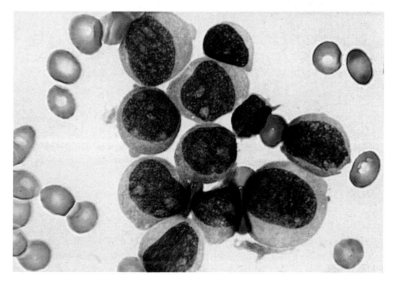

Figure 35
ACUTE MYELOBLASTIC LEUKEMIA
WITHOUT MATURATION (AML-M1)
Agranular myeloblasts in a bone marrow
smear from a patient with AML-M1 showing
variation in size, amount of cytoplasm, and
degree of cytoplasmic basophilia. (Wright-
Giemsa stain)

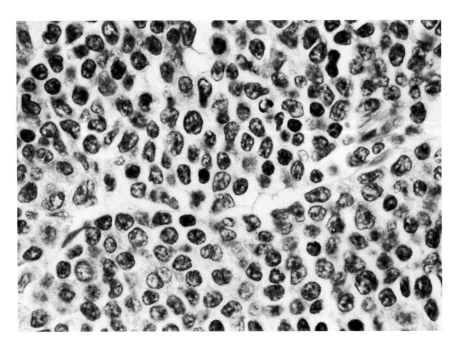

Figure 36
ACUTE MYELOBLASTIC LEUKEMIA WITHOUT MATURATION (AML-M1)
Bone marrow section from a case of acute myeloblastic leukemia without maturation. This marrow is completely replaced by a population of blasts. The predominant blasts have a round to oval nucleus; occasional nuclei are slightly irregular. Nucleoli are not prominent. The amount of cytoplasm varies from sparse to abundant. (Hematoxylin and eosin stain)

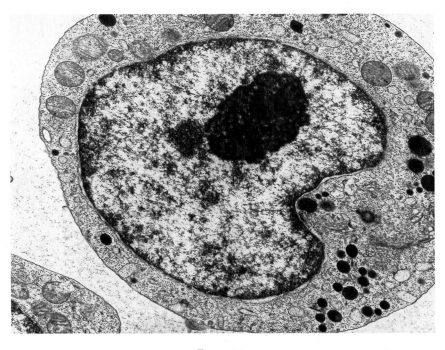

Figure 37
ACUTE MYELOBLASTIC LEUKEMIA WITHOUT MATURATION (AML-M1): ULTRASTRUCTURE
Electron micrograph of a myeloblast from the bone marrow specimen of a patient with AML-M1. There are numerous electron-dense granules in the Golgi region. Granules are scattered throughout the cytoplasm. A very prominent nucleolus is present. (Uranyl acetate–lead citrate stains, X19,000)

Acute Myeloblastic Leukemia with Maturation (AML-M2)

Definition. An AML subtype characterized by 30 percent or more blasts in the blood or bone marrow and evidence of maturation to promyelocytes and more mature neutrophils in 10 percent or more of the cells (20,22).

Incidence and Clinical Findings. AML-M2 comprises 30 to 45 percent of cases of AML (49,86). The disease occurs at all ages: 20 percent of patients are less than 25 years of age and 40 percent are 60 years of age or older (86).

The most common presenting symptoms are constitutional and hemorrhagic including epistaxis, gingival bleeding, ecchymoses, and melena. Approximately 25 percent of patients present with lymphadenopathy and 15 percent with hepatosplenomegaly (86).

Laboratory Findings. Almost all patients are anemic and thrombocytopenic. Leukocytosis is present in half of the patients and leukopenia in one fourth (86). Approximately 20 percent of patients have evidence of disseminated intravascular coagulation at diagnosis.

Blood and Bone Marrow Findings. Because the blast number ranges from 30 to 90 percent, there is considerable variation in the morphologic manifestations of AML-M2 in both the blood and bone marrow (see fig. 24 and figs. 38–43). Blasts may predominate or there may be a substantial population of maturing neutrophils which may manifest marked abnormalities of cytoplasmic and nuclear development. Abnormalities in cytoplasmic development primarily manifest as hypogranulation, hypergranulation, or abnormal clumping of granules resembling the Chediak-Higashi granulation anomaly (fig. 41). The abnormalities in nuclear development are characterized by hypolobulation, pseudo–Pelger-Huet changes, or hyperlobulation. In some cases, markedly bizarre nuclear configurations may be present.

The myeloblasts vary from medium sized cells, 10 to 12 µm, with relatively sparse, agranular cytoplasm to large cells with abundant cytoplasm and scattered azurophilic granules. Type II blasts frequently predominate. Auer rods are found in blasts in approximately 60 to 70 percent of cases. They may be present in many blasts or may be detected only after prolonged search. In most instances, a blast contains a single Auer rod, but two or more may be present. Rarely, blasts contain multiple Auer rods (fig. 41B). Auer rods may also be detected in more mature forms and, rarely, in segmented neutrophils (see fig. 27). In some cases, the Auer rods appear to be embedded in a coalesced mass of fused specific granules.

Approximately 20 to 25 percent of cases of AML-M2 are associated with a t(8;21) chromosome abnormality (fig. 40) (24,28,41,48,74,83–85). The blasts in these cases may contain numerous azurophilic granules which may coalesce (24). Auer rods are usually observed and are frequently thin and elongated; blasts with three or four Auer rods may be noted. In some cases of AML-M2 with the t(8;21) chromosome abnormality, the specific granules in the myelocytes and later stages appear unusually prominent and manifest a tendency to coalesce, giving a smudge-like appearance to the granules. Promyelocytes may show prominent azurophilic granulation. An increase in marrow eosinophils may be present (89). Five percent or more myeloblasts in approximately 55 percent of cases of AML-M2 with the t(8;21) chromosome abnormality are TdT positive (84). The myeloblasts in 80 percent of cases of t(8;21)-associated AML-M2 in children are CD19 positive (56). The association of marked leukocytosis and the t(8;21) chromosome abnormality in AML-M2 has been reported to confer a poor prognosis (74). An association of AML-M2 with the t(8;21) abnormality and granulocytic sarcoma has been reported (fig. 43) (90).

Infrequently, cases of AML-M2 present with a predominance of type III myeloblasts; the number of type I and II blasts in these cases may not exceed 10 percent. The type III blasts contain numerous fine azurophilic granules (see fig. 24). Evidence of maturation to promyelocytes may not be present but the cells are usually intensely MPO and SBB positive. The M2 designation is also used for cases of AML with a predominance of myeloblasts with no evidence of maturation if the number of type II blasts exceeds 10 percent (fig. 42).

Rarely, cases of AML present with less than 30 percent blasts and markedly increased promyelocytes. The blasts and promyelocytes have increased coarse azurophilic granules with evidence of maturation to more mature cells that show dysplastic changes (fig. 41). Auer rods may be found and, rarely, some cells may have multiple

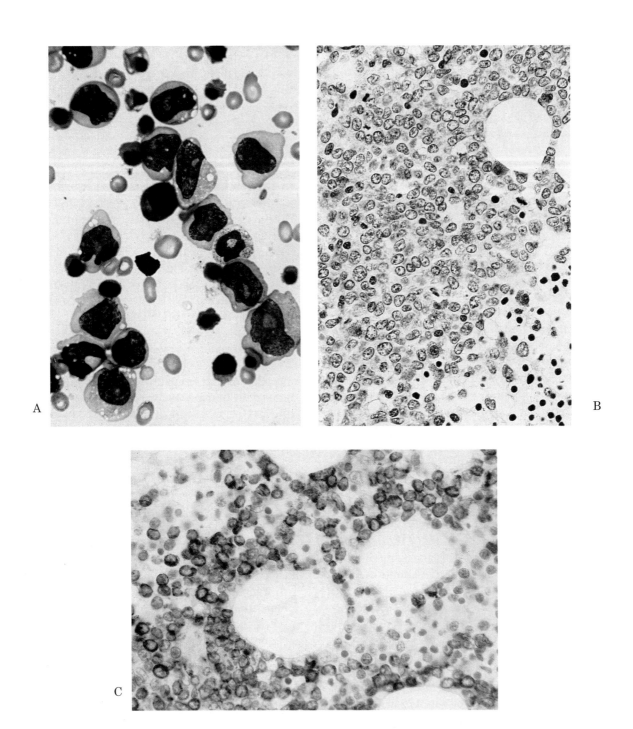

Figure 38
ACUTE MYELOBLASTIC LEUKEMIA WITH MATURATION (AML-M2)

A. This bone marrow smear shows several myeloblasts and evidence of maturation to promyelocytes, myelocytes, and segmented neutrophils. Several erythroblasts are present. (Wright-Giemsa stain)

B. A trephine biopsy from the specimen illustrated in A shows a markedly hypercellular marrow. A high percentage of the cells are blasts. Maturation to more mature neutrophils is less apparent than in the smears. Red blood cell precursors and scattered eosinophils are present. (Hematoxylin and eosin stain)

C. The specimen in B reacted with antibody to MPO. The blasts and immature neutrophils are intensely positive. The red blood cell precursors are negative. (Peroxidase-antiperoxidase stain)

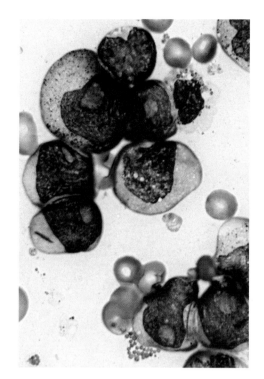
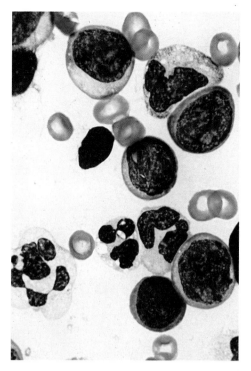

Figure 39
ACUTE MYELOBLASTIC LEUKEMIA WITH MATURATION (AML-M2)

Left: Bone marrow smear from a patient with acute myeloblastic leukemia with maturation showing several blasts with prominent nucleoli, a promyelocyte, and a myelocyte. Two of the blasts contain prominent Auer rods. (Wright-Giemsa stain)

Right: This bone marrow smear shows several myeloblasts and evidence of maturation to segmented neutrophils. The cytoplasm of the segmented neutrophils is hypogranular. (Wright-Giemsa stain)

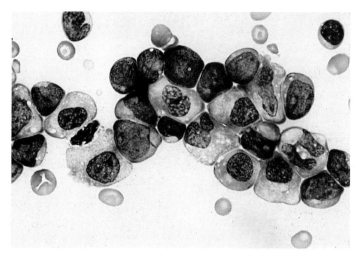
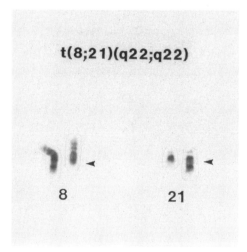

Figure 40
ACUTE MYELOBLASTIC LEUKEMIA WITH MATURATION (AML-M2)
ASSOCIATED WITH A t(8;21) CHROMOSOME ABNORMALITY

Left: Bone marrow smear from a 23-year-old female with acute myeloblastic leukemia with maturation associated with a t(8;21) chromosome abnormality. The numerous myelocytes have abundant cytoplasm with prominent specific granulation. One of the myeloblasts to the left of center contains a prominent Auer rod. (Wright-Giemsa stain)

Right: G-banded Wright-Giemsa stained partial karyotype showing the 8;21 chromosome translocation. The abnormal chromosomes are on the right, with breakpoints designated by arrowheads.

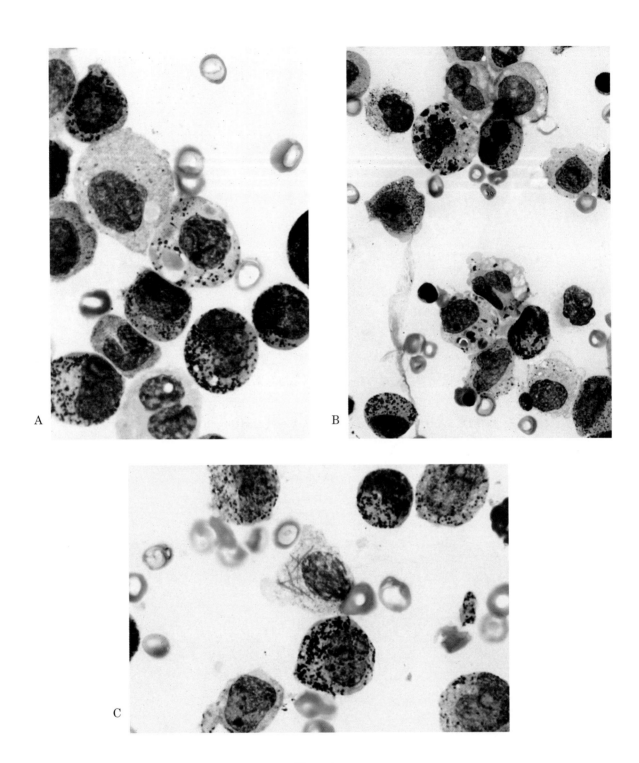

Figure 41
ACUTE MYELOBLASTIC LEUKEMIA WITH MATURATION (AML-M2)
Bone marrow smear from an adult male with an unusual morphologic variant of AML-M2. The leukemic cells have abundant coarse azurophilic granules similar to acute promyelocytic leukemia. There is clumping of azurophilic (A) and specific (B) granules resembling the Chediak-Higashi granulation anomaly. A rare cell with several long slender Auer rods similar to the faggot cells in APL was identified (C). Numerous promonocytes are also present. Chromosome analysis showed a +8 and no t(15;17) abnormality. There was no clinical or laboratory evidence of disseminated intravascular coagulation preceding or during therapy. (Wright-Giemsa stain)

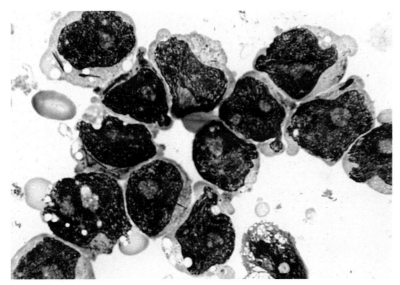

Figure 42
ACUTE MYELOBLASTIC
LEUKEMIA WITH
MATURATION (AML-M2)

The myeloblasts in this bone marrow smear are variable in size with some very large cells with pseudopod formation. The amount of cytoplasm varies but is generally abundant. Several blasts have prominent Auer rods. The number of promyelocytes and more mature neutrophils is less than 10 percent, but because the number of blasts with numerous azurophilic granules exceeds 10 percent, the case is appropriately classified as AML-M2. (Wright-Giemsa stain)

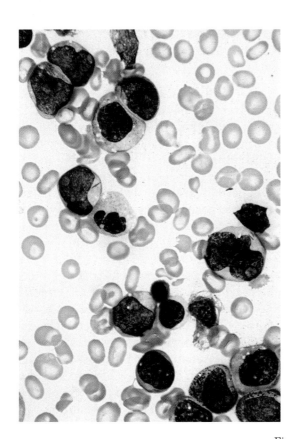

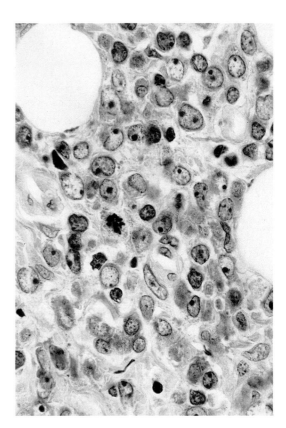

Figure 43
GRANULOCYTIC SARCOMA ASSOCIATED WITH ACUTE MYELOBLASTIC LEUKEMIA
WITH MATURATION (AML-M2) AND A t(8;21) CHROMOSOME ABNORMALITY

Left: Bone marrow smear from a 7-year-old boy presenting with bilateral proptosis. There were approximately 20 percent myeloblasts in the blood and 40 percent in the bone marrow. Several of the myeloblasts contained Auer rods as shown in the myeloblast at the left of center. There is maturation to promyelocytes and more mature cells. (Wright-Giemsa stain)

Right: Biopsy of one of the orbital lesions showing an infiltration of blast cells. Several immature eosinophils are present. Cytogenetic study of the cells in this lesion showed a t(8;21) chromosome abnormality. (Hematoxylin and eosin stain)

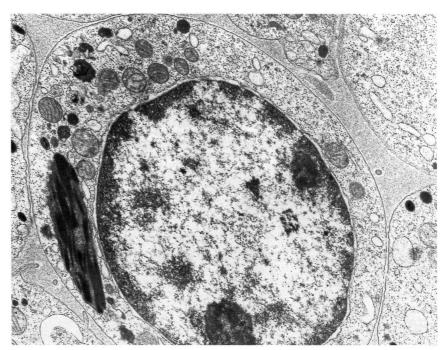

Figure 44
ACUTE MYELOBLASTIC
LEUKEMIA WITH
MATURATION (AML-M2):
ULTRASTRUCTURE
Electron micrograph of a neutrophil precursor in a bone marrow specimen from a patient with AML-M2. There are numerous primary granules and fusion of Auer rods. (Uranyl acetate–lead citrate stains, X15,000)

Auer rods (fig. 41). Some of these cases are associated with extramedullary granulocytic sarcomas. These cases may be difficult to distinguish from acute promyelocytic leukemia based on the morphologic findings; cytogenetic studies may be helpful in excluding the latter.

Because the percentage of blasts in AML-M2 may be relatively low (i.e., 30 percent), there may be a substantial number of erythroid precursors, monocytes and megakaryocytes. These cells may display nuclear and cytoplasmic abnormalities suggesting involvement of these cell lines in the neoplastic process. When changes in the erythroid series are marked, the findings may resemble those found in erythroleukemia (M6). The distinction of AML-M2 from erythroleukemia should be based on the percentage of erythroblasts. The FAB proposals recommend 50 percent erythroblasts as a minimum for a diagnosis of erythroleukemia (22). However, if the percent of erythroid precursors is 30 or more with marked abnormalities and the myeloblast percentage is 30 or higher, a diagnosis of erythroleukemia is more appropriate than AML-M2 (49,86).

Cytochemical Findings. Cytochemical studies are not usually necessary to establish a diagnosis of AML-M2. The myeloblasts and maturing neutrophils are usually MPO and SBB positive; the intensity of reactivity in the blasts is variable. The promyelocytes and more mature neutrophils may show normal MPO and SBB reactivity or decreased or absent reactivity due to abnormal granule development. In some cases, the promyelocytes and myelocytes may show dual reactivity with NSE and MPO.

Histopathologic Findings. The bone marrow is generally markedly hypercellular. The myeloblasts may be uniformly distributed throughout the interstitium or present in large focal aggregates (fig. 38B). Immunohistochemical reactions with antibodies to myeloid enzymes are helpful in identifying the myeloid nature of the blasts and immature granulocytes (fig. 38C). In those cases with a relatively low myeloblast percentage, there may be a near normal number of megakaryocytes and erythroid precursors.

Fibrosis is uncommon, although in a small number of cases reticulin fibrosis is present and may be prominent. If moderate to marked fibrosis is present, the diagnosis of acute myelofibrosis should be considered.

Ultrastructural Findings. The ultrastructural characteristics of the myeloblasts in AML-M2 are essentially the same as those observed in

AML-M1. In AML-M2 associated with the t(8;21) chromosome abnormality, the leukemic cells show prominent granulation (fig. 44) (36). Giant granules resulting from fusion of smaller granules are common; these structures are membrane bound and have dense crystalloid cores with distinct periodicities of 8 to 10 mμ. Occasional granules have crystalline arrays with a periodicity of 18 to 20 mμ. Auer rods with a periodicity of 8 to 10 mμ are usually found. Fusion of Auer rods may occur (fig. 44).

Differential Diagnosis. The major differential diagnoses in AML-M2 include AML without maturation (M1), acute myelomonocytic leukemia (M4), erythroleukemia (M6), and refractory anemia with an excess of blasts in transformation (RAEB-T). The distinction of AML-M2 from these entities is based on the criteria outlined for the specific type of leukemia and the less than 30 percent myeloblasts in RAEB-T.

The rare cases of AML-M2 presenting with a predominant population of type III myeloblasts are a particularly difficult diagnostic problem. These cases must be distinguished from acute promyelocytic leukemia, the "maturation arrest" at the promyelocyte stage that occurs in drug-related agranulocytosis and a leukemoid reaction. The presence of cells with multiple Auer rods and laboratory findings of disseminated intravascular coagulation are evidence for acute promyelocytic leukemia. In some instances, the distinction may depend on cytogenetic studies to exclude the presence of the t(15;17) chromosome abnormality which is specific for acute promyelocytic leukemia.

Clinical and hematologic findings are important in distinguishing the "hypergranular" variant of M2 from a leukemoid reaction and agranulocytosis. In both of the latter disorders, the platelet and hemoglobin values are usually normal; this is reflected in the bone marrow by preservation of the megakaryocytes and erythroid cells. In a leukemoid reaction, there is balanced maturation with a predominance of segmented neutrophils; the neutrophils show toxic alterations. The majority of patients with agranulocytosis usually have a relevant clinical history of drug administration. In equivocal cases, cytogenetic studies and a period of observation may be necessary before a diagnosis can be established.

Acute Promyelocytic Leukemia (APL)

Definition. A form of AML characterized primarily by a proliferation of abnormal promyelocytes. It is usually accompanied by disseminated intravascular coagulation and a t(15;17) chromosome rearrangement in the leukemic cells. The disease presents in two morphologic types: hypergranular APL in which the predominant cell is an abnormal promyelocyte with markedly increased and coarse azurophilic granules and microgranular or hypogranular APL in which the predominant cell is an abnormal promyelocyte with diminished or small azurophilic granules (47,67,87).

Incidence and Clinical Findings. Acute promyelocytic leukemia comprises 5 to 10 percent of cases of AML (49,86). The disease occurs in all age groups but is uncommon before 10 years of age; the median age is 38 years. The male to female ratio is 2 to 1.

The most common presenting symptoms, occurring in 90 percent of patients, relate to hemorrhagic manifestations and include easy bruisability, bleeding gums, hemoptysis, epistaxis, petechiae, and symptoms of gastrointestinal bleeding and intracranial hemorrhage. Hepatosplenomegaly and lymphadenopathy are present in less than 20 percent of patients.

Laboratory Findings. The leukocyte count varies from marked leukopenia to marked leukocytosis. Patients with hypergranular APL frequently present with leukopenia: the median white blood cell count is 1.8×10^9/L. Patients with the microgranular variant (M3V) more commonly present with leukocytosis: the median leukocyte count is 83×10^9/L (67). Eighty to 90 percent of patients are anemic: approximately half have hemoglobin levels of less than 10 g/dL. Ninety percent of patients are thrombocytopenic: 75 percent have platelet counts of less than 50×10^9/L. Eighty to 90 percent present with laboratory evidence of disseminated intravascular coagulation. The leukemic cells in 95 to 100 percent of cases have a t(15;17) chromosome abnormality (fig. 45, right) (83).

Blood and Bone Marrow Findings. Seventy-five to 80 percent of APL cases are hypergranular; 20 percent are the microgranular or hypogranular variant (M3V) (67). The primary distinction between these two types is the number

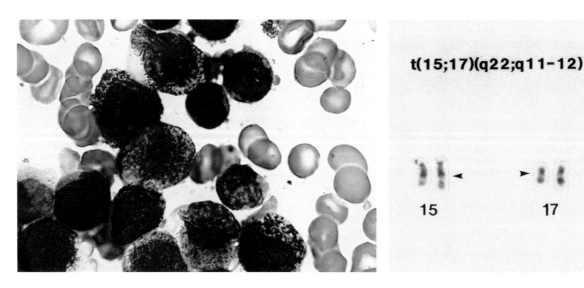

Figure 45
HYPERGRANULAR ACUTE PROMYELOCYTIC LEUKEMIA (AML-M3)
Left: Bone marrow aspirate from a patient with hypergranular acute promyelocytic leukemia. The cytoplasm of the majority of promyelocytes contains abundant azurophilic granulation. Two microgranular promyelocytes with lobulated nuclei and basophilic cytoplasm are present. (Wright-Giemsa stain)
Right: G-banded Wright-Giemsa stained partial karyotype showing the 15;17 chromosome translocation. The breakpoints on the abnormal chromosomes are designated by arrowheads.

and size of the azurophilic granules in the abnormal promyelocytes. The distinctive features of APL, disseminated intravascular coagulation and the t(15;17) chromosome abnormality are present in both types (47,67).

Hypergranular APL. The myeloblasts are less than 30 percent of the marrow cells in 90 to 95 percent of cases. The median blast percentage is 8 to 10 (86). The predominant cell is an abnormal promyelocyte that contains numerous coarse azurophilic granules; the density of the granules frequently obscures the nuclear outline (fig. 45, left). The granules are usually larger and darker staining than the azurophilic granules of normal promyelocytes. Promyelocytes with aggregates of very dark-staining granules several times larger than normal granules are frequently found. In most cases, there is a minor population of promyelocytes that contains abundant, unusually fine, rust colored cytoplasmic granules. The nuclei vary in size and shape. Nuclear-cytoplasmic asynchrony is frequently observed. The nucleus may have blast-like chromatin and one or more nucleoli, and may be folded or reniform resembling an immature monocyte. A variable number of the

leukemic cells with monocytoid nuclei contain relatively sparse granulation.

A population of promyelocytes with markedly basophilic cytoplasm containing sparse or indistinct azurophilic granules and unusually lobulated or bilobed nuclei may be present. Most of these cells are approximately half the size of a normal promyelocyte (fig. 45, left). These hyperbasophilic promyelocytes are usually present in small numbers, but in some instances may be the predominant cell in the blood, with typical hypergranular promyelocytes predominating in the bone marrow (67). The hyperbasophilic promyelocyte may resemble a micromegakaryocyte.

Promyelocytes containing multiple, delicate, needle-like Auer rods frequently intertwined are found in 90 to 95 percent of cases of APL; these cells have been referred to as "faggot" cells (figs. 46, 47) (20). In most cases of hypergranular APL, faggot cells are not difficult to find. In some instances, however, only one or two may be found after extensive examination. Frequently, these cells are damaged, with dispersal of the cytoplasmic contents. In some cases, faggot cells may be more easily found in understained smears than in well-stained preparations. Cells with single

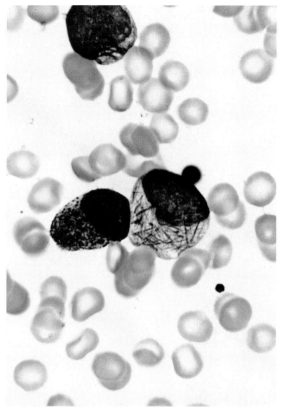

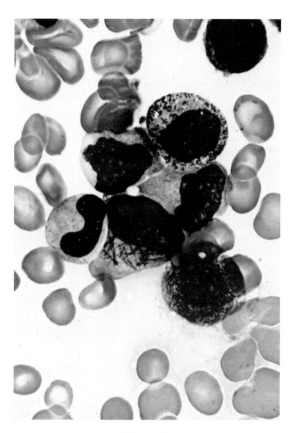

Figure 46
HYPERGRANULAR ACUTE PROMYELOCYTIC
LEUKEMIA (AML-M3)

Bone marrow aspirate from a patient with hypergranular acute promyelocytic leukemia showing a "faggot" cell with numerous intertwining Auer rods. (Wright-Giemsa stain) (Fig. 44.12 from Litz CE, Brunning RD. Acute myeloid leukemias. In: Knowles DM, ed. Neoplastic hematopathology. Baltimore: Williams & Wilkins, 1992:1315–49.)

Figure 47
HYPERGRANULAR ACUTE PROMYELOCYTIC
LEUKEMIA (AML-M3)

Postchemotherapy bone marrow smear from a patient with hypergranular acute promyelocytic leukemia. A single "faggot" cell with numerous Auer rods is present in a background of normal neutrophil precursors. (Wright-Giemsa stain)

Auer rods may also be observed. Large, round to oval or elliptical azurophilic cytoplasmic inclusions of Auer-like material resembling Chediak-Higashi granules are present in a variable, but usually low proportion of the leukemic promyelocytes in some cases. Myelodysplastic changes, including hypolobulation of nuclei and hypogranulation, may be observed in maturing neutrophils.

The number of abnormal promyelocytes in the blood is variable and may be very low; faggot cells may be present. The blood smear may show the findings of a microangiopathic hemolytic anemia including red blood cell fragments and occasional spherocytes. However, these morphologic findings may not be present in patients with laboratory and clinical evidence of disseminated intravascular coagulation.

Microgranular APL (M3V). In microgranular APL the promyelocytes are characterized by less abundant or finer azurophilic granulation than in the hypergranular type (47,67). Most of the leukemic cells exhibit marked nuclear irregularity with folding, lobulation, or convolution imparting a monocytoid appearance (fig. 48). Cells containing multiple Auer rods or large inclusions of Auer-like material are found in the vast majority of cases; this is similar to the findings in hypergranular APL. Small hyperbasophilic promyelocytes may be identified and even predominate, although this is uncommon (fig. 49). A minor population of hypergranular promyelocytes is usually present.

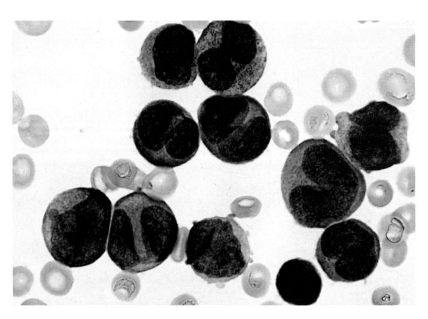

Figure 48
ACUTE PROMYELOCYTIC
LEUKEMIA,
MICROGRANULAR
VARIANT (AML-M3V)

Blood smear from a 47-year-old male with microgranular acute promyelocytic leukemia showing a marked leukocytosis with abnormal promyelocytes. The promyelocytes vary in size and degree of cytoplasmic basophilia. The cytoplasm contains abundant, fine, azurophilic granules. The nuclei are markedly lobulated and invaginated. (Wright-Giemsa stain)

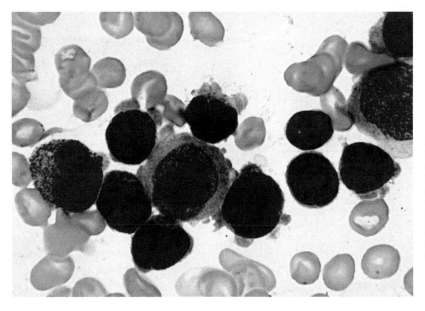

Figure 49
ACUTE PROMYELOCYTIC
LEUKEMIA,
MICROGRANULAR
VARIANT (AML-M3V)

Bone marrow smear from a patient with the microgranular variant of acute promyelocytic leukemia with a predominant population of small hyperbasophilic promyelocytes. Cytoplasmic budding is prominent. The nuclei are lobulated and the cytoplasm in the majority of cases is sparsely granular. The cells were intensely MPO positive. (Wright-Giemsa stain)

Cytochemical Findings. The leukemic promyelocytes in both the hypergranular and microgranular forms of APL react intensely for MPO, SBB, and CAE. There is no apparent difference between hypergranular and microgranular APL in the intensity of reaction or percentage of reacting cells. The Auer rods generally stain brilliantly but occasionally are identified by their negative-staining image imposed on a strongly positive cytoplasm. The leukemic promyelocytes manifest weak NSE reactivity in approximately 15 to 20 percent of cases (42).

Histopathologic Findings. Trephine biopsy sections of the bone marrow from most patients with hypergranular APL show marked hypercellularity with little evidence of residual normal hematopoiesis (fig. 50). Occasionally, islands of normoblasts and scattered megakaryocytes are present. The abnormal promyelocytes have abundant, deeply eosinophilic cytoplasm in hematoxylin and eosin stained sections. The cytoplasm has a distinctly granular appearance resembling mast cells or eosinophils and the nuclear border is frequently irregular or indented.

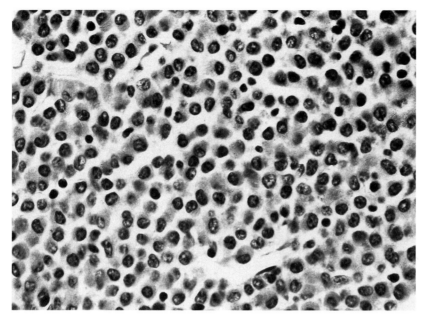

Figure 50
HYPERGRANULAR ACUTE
PROMYELOCYTIC
LEUKEMIA (AML-M3)
Trephine biopsy from a case of hypergranular acute promyelocytic leukemia. The bone marrow is almost completely replaced by promyelocytes with abundant cytoplasm and generally round to oval, frequently eccentrically located nuclei. Occasional nuclei are indented or clefted. The nuclear chromatin is somewhat condensed and nucleoli are indistinct in the majority of cells. (Hematoxylin and eosin stain)

Figure 51
HYPERGRANULAR ACUTE
PROMYELOCYTIC
LEUKEMIA (AML-M3)
Bone marrow trephine biopsy from a patient with hypergranular acute promyelocytic leukemia. The promyelocytes are relatively uniform appearing with abundant cytoplasm containing dense azurophilic granulation. The nuclei are round, oval, or lobulated. Two cells in the center of the field contain multiple Auer rods. (Hematoxylin and eosin stain)

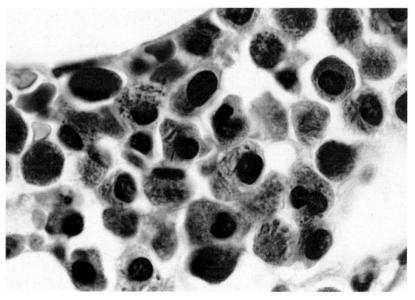

The cells may resemble plasma cells at low magnification. Faggot cells may occasionally be identified in well-processed sections (fig. 51). The promyelocytes in microgranular APL may be slightly smaller than in the hypergranular type and have less intensely eosinophilic cytoplasm. On occasion, the bone marrow biopsy in APL shows an increase in reticulin fibers. In trephine biopsy sections from patients in early relapse or following chemotherapy the distribution of the leukemic proliferation may have a distinctly focal character.

Ultrastructural Findings. The diagnostic ultrastructural features are confined to the promyelocyte cytoplasm, which typically contains numerous electron-dense granules. The differences between hypergranular APL and microgranular APL relate to the number and size of the granules (36). In hypergranular APL the granules range from 120 to 1000 mμ in diameter with a predominance of larger granules (fig. 52). In microgranular APL most leukemic cells contain unusually small granules, 100 to 400 mμ in diameter (fig. 53), and in many cases the granules are sparse (36,67).

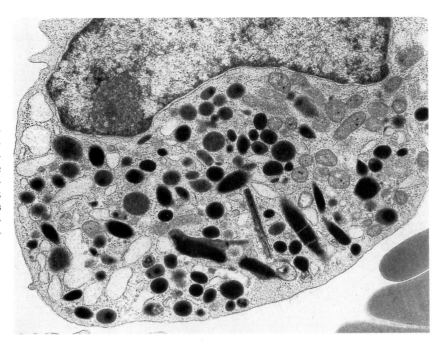

Figure 52
HYPERGRANULAR
ACUTE PROMYELOCYTIC
LEUKEMIA (AML-M3):
ULTRASTRUCTURE
Electron micrograph of a promyelocyte in a bone marrow specimen from a patient with hypergranular acute promyelocytic leukemia. The nucleus has dispersed chromatin and a prominent nucleolus. The cytoplasm contains numerous dense granules and several Auer rods. (Uranyl acetate–lead citrate stains, X22,000)

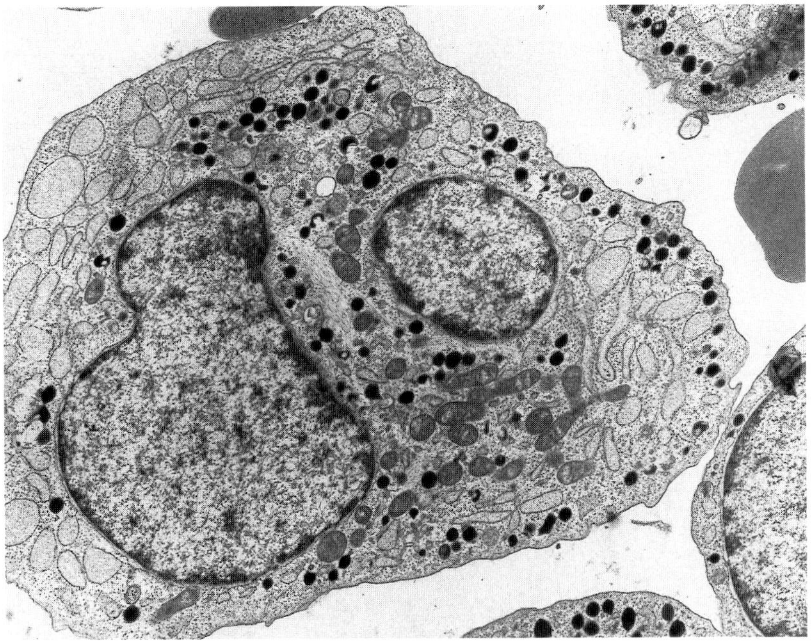

Figure 53
ACUTE PROMYELOCYTIC
LEUKEMIA, MICROGRANULAR
VARIANT (AML-M3V):
ULTRASTRUCTURE
Electron micrograph of an abnormal promyelocyte in a bone marrow specimen from a patient with acute promyelocytic leukemia, microgranular variant. In contrast to the cell illustrated in figure 52, the dense granules are much smaller and more uniform in size. The endoplasmic reticulum is prominent. (Uranyl acetate–lead citrate stains, X9,000)

The Auer rods in APL have ultrastructural characteristics that are different from other types of AML. The substructure consists of a hexagonal arrangement of tubular structures with a specific periodicity of approximately 250 mμ (fig. 54) (31). In other types of AML, the Auer rods have an internal laminar periodicity of 6 to 10 mμ and lack a tubular substructure.

The rough endoplasmic reticulum (RER) is typically markedly dilated and filled with dense amorphous material. Two distinct configurations of RER may be identified: a multilaminar endoplasmic reticulum consisting of at least two parallel cisternae of RER closely adherent over a variable distance and a complex structure with a central, dense, smooth, dilated cisterna of RER in

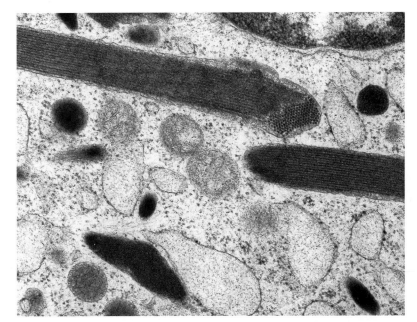

Electron micrograph of a promyelocyte in a bone marrow specimen from a patient with hypergranular acute promyelocytic leukemia. A cross section of an Auer rod shows the characteristic tubular structure. (Uranyl acetate–lead citrate stains, X47,000)

Figure 55
ACUTE PROMYELOCYTIC
LEUKEMIA, MICROGRANULAR
VARIANT (AML-M3V):
ULTRASTRUCTURE
Electron micrograph of a portion of an abnormal promyelocyte in a bone marrow specimen from a patient with acute promyelocytic leukemia, microgranular variant, showing a stellate array of endoplasmic reticulum. This finding is characteristic of this type of APL. (Uranyl acetate–lead citrate stains, X25,000)

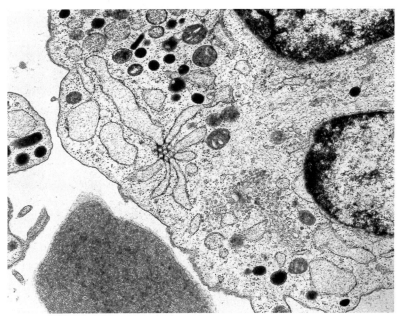

a stellate arrangement (fig. 55). The stellate complexes of RER appear to be specific for APL (36).

Differential Diagnosis. The most important aspect in the differential diagnosis of APL is distinguishing the microgranular variant from acute monocytic leukemia with differentiation (M5B) or acute myelomonocytic leukemia (M4). The sparse dust-like granulation and the striking nuclear irregularity in microgranular APL may resemble immature monocytes. The presence of some hypergranular promyelocytes, cells with multiple Auer rods, and inclusions of Auer-like material, in combination with the cytochemical findings of a weak or negative NSE reaction and intense MPO or SBB reactivity, are strong evidence for APL.

The small hyperbasophilic promyelocytes that may predominate in some cases of microgranular APL may resemble the micromegakaryocytes of acute megakaryoblastic leukemia.

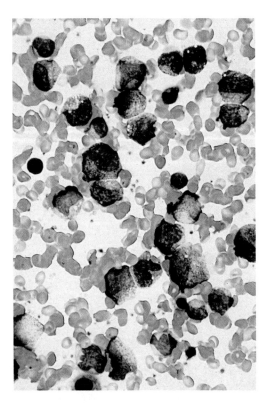 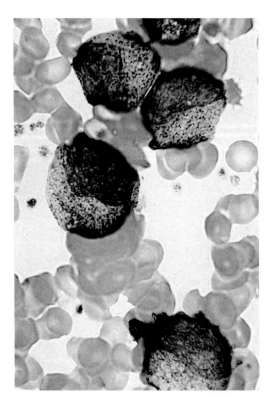

Figure 56
AGRANULOCYTOSIS
Left: Bone marrow smear from a patient with drug-related agranulocytosis. There are numerous promyelocytes and myelocytes with essentially no evidence of maturation to segmented neutrophils. (Wright-Giemsa stain)
Right: High magnification of the specimen illustrated on the left showing four promyelocytes with regular, round nuclei and numerous azurophilic granules. (Wright-Giemsa stain)

The promyelocytes are intensely MPO positive; megakaryocytes are invariably MPO negative.

Also included in the differential diagnosis of hypergranular APL are AML-M2 and agranulocytosis with a "promyelocyte arrest." AML-M2 has a well-defined population of type I and II myeloblasts that exceed 30 percent of the nucleated cells in the bone marrow or blood. The granulation in the promyelocytes and myelocytes is generally not as dense or as coarse as in hypergranular APL and characteristic faggot cells are not usually present, although cells with multiple Auer rods may be detected in rare cases of AML-M2. There may be occasional cases in which distinction between these two types of leukemia cannot be made by examination of routine bone marrow and blood smears and cytogenetic studies may be necessary for appropriate classification. The presence of the t(15;17) chromosome abnormality is definitive for APL (83).

In agranulocytosis, the percentage of promyelocytes is usually substantially less than in APL. In some instances, however, the promyelocytes may be moderately or markedly increased and manifest intense azurophilic granulation; they are otherwise morphologically normal (fig. 56). Cells with Auer rods or Auer-like inclusions are not present. In most patients with uncomplicated agranulocytosis, there is normal erythropoiesis and megakaryocytopoiesis with normal platelet counts and hemoglobin levels and no evidence of disseminated intravascular coagulation. The distinctive ultrastructural and cytogenetic abnormalities of APL are lacking.

Bone marrow specimens from patients treated with recombinant granulocyte growth factor may show a striking increase in promyelocytes and myelocytes. The cells frequently show intense azurophilic granulation. The therapeutic history and absence of Auer rods are distinguishing features.

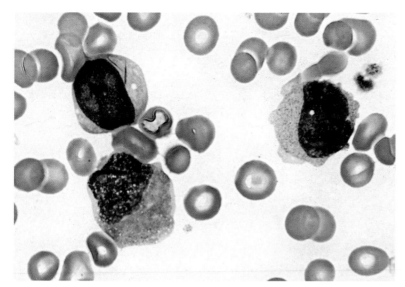

Figure 57
ACUTE MYELOMONOCYTIC
LEUKEMIA (AML-M4)
Blood smear from a patient with acute myelomonocytic leukemia. The cell in the upper left is a myeloblast with two long slender Auer rods. The cell below the myeloblast is a neutrophil myelocyte with smudged specific granules. The cell on the right is a promonocyte. The cytoplasm of this cell has abundant azurophilic granules and a nucleus with delicate folds and creases. (Wright-Giemsa stain)

Acute Myelomonocytic Leukemia (AML-M4)

Definition. A form of AML in which there is concurrent proliferation of both the neutrophil and monocyte cell lines. The number of monocytic cells in the blood, including monoblasts, promonocytes, and mature monocytes is 5×10^9/L or greater. The percentage of myeloblasts, promonocytes, and monoblasts in the bone marrow or blood is 30 percent or more. Twenty percent or more of the nucleated marrow cells are of monocytic lineage.

Incidence and Clinical Findings. AML-M4 comprises 15 to 25 percent of AML cases (49,86). This type of acute leukemia occurs in all age groups but is more common in older individuals; the median age of presentation is 50 years. There is a male to female ratio of 1.4 to 1 (86).

The most common signs and symptoms are fatigue, fever, bleeding disorders, and gingival hyperplasia; leukemia cutis may be present. Lymphadenopathy is present in approximately half of patients and hepatosplenomegaly in 30 to 35 percent. A soft tissue leukemic infiltrate occurs in 5 to 10 percent of cases (86).

Laboratory Findings. Approximately 85 percent of patients present with leukocytosis while 10 percent are leukopenic: the median leukocyte count at presentation is 46×10^9/L. Ninety percent of patients are anemic: 50 percent have a hemoglobin level of less than 10 g/dL.

Thrombocytopenia is seen in 80 percent of patients: 50 percent have platelet counts of less than 50×10^9/L (86). The serum lysozyme level is increased in the majority of patients.

Blood and Bone Marrow Findings. The requisite 30 percent blasts for a diagnosis of AML-M4 includes type I and type II myeloblasts, monoblasts, and promonocytes. The monoblasts, which are the predominant cells in acute monoblastic leukemia (M5A), are larger than myeloblasts, measuring up to 40 μm in diameter. These cells have abundant cytoplasm that may contain a variable number of scattered azurophilic granules. The nucleus is round to oval and the nuclear chromatin is finely dispersed. There may be a single prominent nucleolus or multiple nucleoli. The promonocyte is also large, measuring up to 35 μm. This cell has abundant light gray or lightly basophilic cytoplasm that in most instances contains scattered azurophilic granules (figs. 57–61). The nuclei show varying degrees of lobulation and there may be delicate folding or creasing of the nuclear membrane imparting a somewhat cerebriform appearance. The nuclear chromatin is finely stippled to lace-like. Nucleoli are present but not prominent. The promonocytes and monocytes may be remarkably heteromorphous in an individual case.

The myeloblasts and maturing neutrophils may manifest abnormalities similar to those observed in AML-M2 (fig. 60). Auer rods are identified in myeloblasts in approximately 60 percent

Figure 58
ACUTE MYELOMONOCYTIC
LEUKEMIA (AML-M4)
Bone marrow smear from a patient with acute myelomonocytic leukemia. Monocytes and neutrophils at different stages of maturation are intermixed. Several promonocytes with abundant cytoplasm containing fine azurophilic granules and delicately creased nuclei are present. (Wright-Giemsa stain)

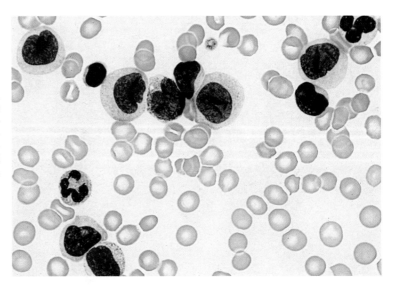

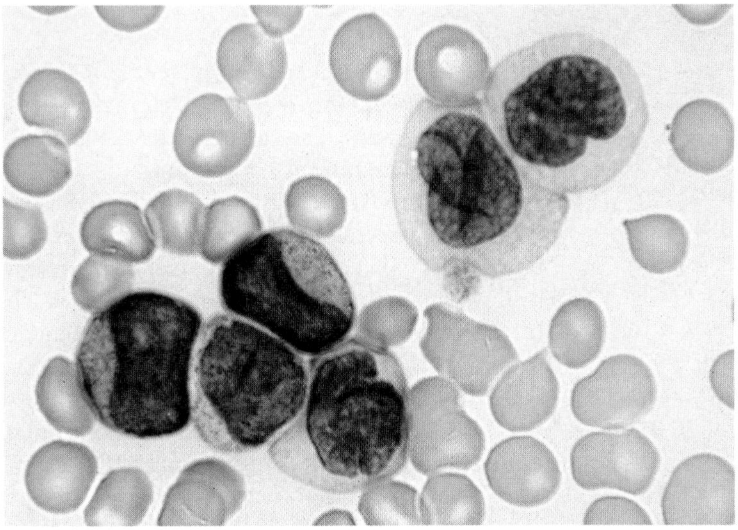

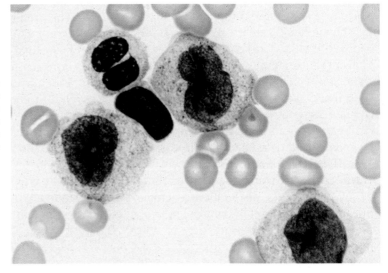

Figure 59
ACUTE MYELOMONOCYTIC
LEUKEMIA (AML-M4)
Bone marrow smear from a patient with AML-M4. The two promyelocytes on the left with basophilic cytoplasm containing coarse azurophilic granules contrast with the two promonocytes in the upper right which have abundant pale cytoplasm and delicate nuclear folds. (Wright-Giemsa stain)

Figure 60
ACUTE MYELOMONOCYTIC
LEUKEMIA (AML-M4)
Bone marrow smear from a case of AML-M4. There are three promonocytes, which are large cells with abundant cytoplasm containing numerous fine azurophilic granules. A dysplastic neutrophil with a pseudo–Pelger-Huet nucleus is in the upper left. (Wright-Giemsa stain)

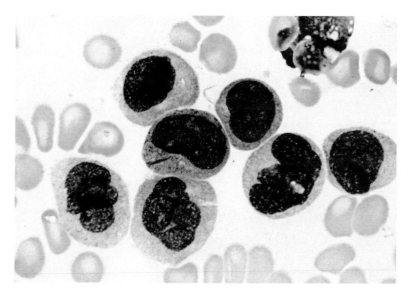

Figure 61
ACUTE MYELOMONOCYTIC
LEUKEMIA (AML-M4)
Bone marrow smear from a case of AML-M4 showing five promonocytes and two promyelocytes (center). One of the promyelocytes contains numerous azurophilic granules and a prominent Auer rod. (Wright-Giemsa stain)

of cases (figs. 57, 61) but are not seen in promonocytes or monoblasts. Dyserythropoiesis and dysplastic megakaryocytes are frequent findings.

The predominant cells in the blood smear are monocytes, promonocytes, and neutrophils and precursors. Myeloblasts may be few in number.

There are variants of AML-M4 in which the number of monocytic cells in the blood is less than 5×10^9/L or in which the monocytic cells in the bone marrow are less than 20 percent (22). In the first variant, although the number of monocytic cells in the blood is less than 5×10^9/L, the marrow has 20 percent or more monocytic cells. The diagnosis is established if the serum or urine lysozyme level exceeds the upper range of normal by threefold. In the second variant, the bone marrow findings are those of AML-M2 and the number of monocytic cells in the blood is 5×10^9/L or higher. The diagnosis of AML-M4 is appropriate if 20 percent or more cells in the marrow smear are positive with the NSE reaction or if the serum or urine lysozyme level exceeds three times the normal value.

Cytochemical Findings. The cytochemical reactivity pattern of the leukemic cells in the majority of cases of AML-M4 reflects the percentages of neutrophils and monocytes. The neutrophils and precursors react for MPO and SBB while the monocytes, promonocytes, and monoblasts react for NSE and are usually weakly positive or negative with MPO and SBB. In occasional cases, the monocytic cells are intensely MPO and SBB positive. In some cases of AML-

M4, there is a population of cells that react for both the neutrophil and monocyte enzymes, i.e., the cells stain for MPO, SBB, or CAE and NSE (57, 100). These cells appear to be a hybrid monocyte-granulocyte. A combined NSE and CAE stain shows the dual reacting populations of cells (fig. 62). In other cases, the neutrophil precursors have no or weak reactivity with MPO or SBB.

Histopathologic Findings. In the majority of cases the biopsy shows a hypercellular bone marrow with heteromorphic features reflecting the smear preparation (fig. 63). Erythroid cells and megakaryocytes are decreased. A slight increase in reticulin fibers may be present; uncommonly, there may be a moderate to marked increase in reticulin fibers.

Appropriate antibodies may be used to demonstrate the monocytic and neutrophilic pattern of the cells in the trephine biopsy. Antibody to MPO can be used to identify cells of the neutrophil series; the antilysozome antibody reacts with cells of both the neutrophil and monocyte series (70).

AML-M4 with Increased Marrow Eosinophils (AML-M4EO). Approximately 15 to 30 percent of cases of AML-M4 present with increased eosinophils in the marrow (greater than 3 percent) (16,27,28). In most cases the increase in marrow eosinophils is not reflected in the blood. In a variable proportion of eosinophils, some of the granules are large, misshapen, and basophilic (fig. 64, left). These abnormal granules

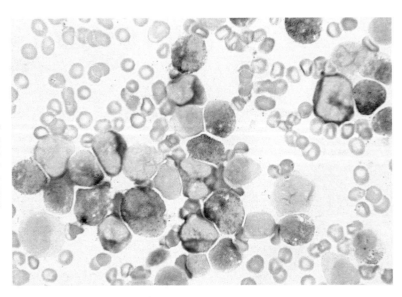

Figure 62
ACUTE MYELOMONOCYTIC
LEUKEMIA (AML-M4):
COMBINED ESTERASE
REACTION
Bone marrow smear from a case of acute myelomonocytic leukemia stained for both CAE (blue), which stains neutrophils and NSE (reddish brown), which stains monocytes. The staining pattern reflects approximately equal numbers of neutrophils and monocytes. (Chloroacetate esterase and nonspecific esterase stains)

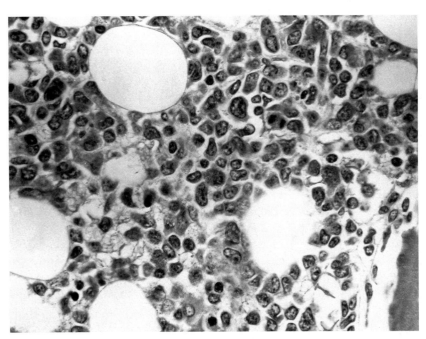

Figure 63
ACUTE MYELOMONOCYTIC
LEUKEMIA (AML-M4)
Bone marrow biopsy from a patient with AML-M4. The marrow is markedly hypercellular with a heteromorphous cell population. The predominant cells are immature monocytes and neutrophils. Many of the immature monocytes have irregularly shaped nuclei and prominent nucleoli. (Hematoxylin and eosin stain)

appear to be more common in immature eosinophils. They resemble basophil granules but are distinguished by reactivity with MPO. Unlike the granules in normal eosinophils, these granules react for CAE and periodic acid–Schiff (PAS) (27). AML-M4 with increased marrow eosinophils has been associated with abnormalities of chromosome 16, either an inv(16) (p13q22) or a t(16;16) (p13;q22) rearrangement (fig. 64, right) (27,60,62, 101). These findings are usually, but not invariably, associated with a favorable prognosis (16,60). The chromosome 16 abnormality associated with abnormal marrow eosinophils is not unique for AML-M4 and has been observed in other types of AML and myelodysplastic syndromes including AML-M2, AML-M5, refractory anemia with an excess of blasts, and refractory anemia with an excess of blasts in transformation (38).

There is an uncommon variant of AML that is associated with abnormalities of chromosome 16 (inv(16) or t(16;16)) that morphologically closely resembles microgranular acute promyelocytic

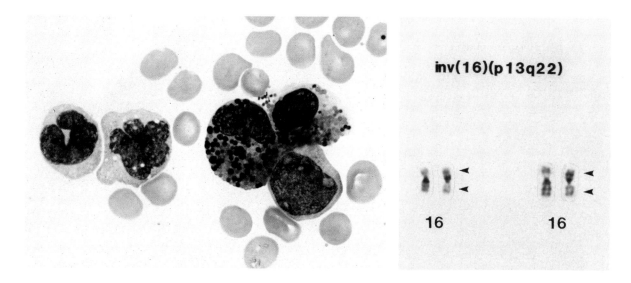

Figure 64
ACUTE MYELOMONOCYTIC LEUKEMIA WITH INCREASED MARROW EOSINOPHILS (AML-M4EO)
Left: Bone marrow smear from a 22-year-old male with AML-M4 with increased marrow eosinophils and an associated inv(16) chromosome abnormality. The eosinophil precursors in this field show prominent basophilic-staining granules. These granules react with CAE and MPO. (Wright-Giemsa stain)
Right: Two G-banded Wright-Giemsa stained chromosome 16 pairs showing the pericentric inversion commonly associated with the M4EO morphologic subtype. In each case, the abnormal chromosome 16 is on the right and the breakpoints are designated with arrowheads.

leukemia. The leukemic cells may show marked nuclear infolding (fig. 65). These cells are MPO positive and NSE negative. There are abnormal eosinophils in the marrow but the number may be low. Faggot cells are not observed and there is no evidence of disseminated intravascular coagulation. The serum lysozyme level may be increased. The morphologic features of these cells appear to be compatible with a diagnosis of AML-M2, but depending on the cytochemical reactivity pattern in an individual case, AML-M4 may be the appropriate classification.

Ultrastructural Findings. The ultrastructural findings in AML-M4 parallel the light microscopic observations: there is an admixture of granulocytes, primarily neutrophils, and monocytes. Two types of monocytes are observed in specimens reactive for MPO. In one type, the MPO reaction product is localized to the cytoplasmic granules, a characteristic of normal monocytes. In the second type, which appears to represent a cell with both monocytic and neutrophilic features, the reaction product is present in the nuclear envelope rough endoplasmic reticulum, Golgi region, and granules.

Ultrastructural studies of the abnormal eosinophils in AML-M4 with increased marrow eosinophils show large, pale, electron-lucent granules intermixed with smaller, more electron-dense granules. Typical eosinophil granule crystalloids are not present (fig. 65, right) (36).

Differential Diagnosis. The three major processes from which AML-M4 must be distinguished are AML-M2, AML-M5B, and chronic myelomonocytic leukemia in transformation to acute leukemia.

Although the findings in the blood and bone marrow in AML-M2 and AML-M4 may overlap to some extent, the number of monocytic cells in the blood in AML-M2 is less than 5×10^9/L and the percentage of monocytic cells in the marrow is less than 20.

In AML-M5B, there are 80 percent or more monocytic cells in the bone marrow, which precludes the necessary requisite of 20 percent or more neutrophils and precursors for a diagnosis of AML-M4.

The distinction between AML-M4 and chronic myelomonocytic leukemia in transformation to acute leukemia is based on the less than 30 percent blasts and promonocytes in the latter disorder.

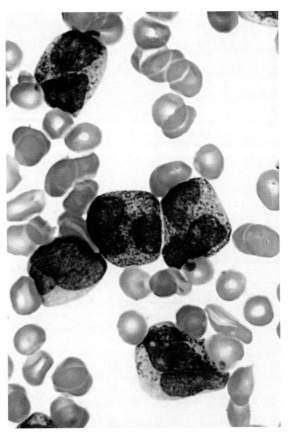
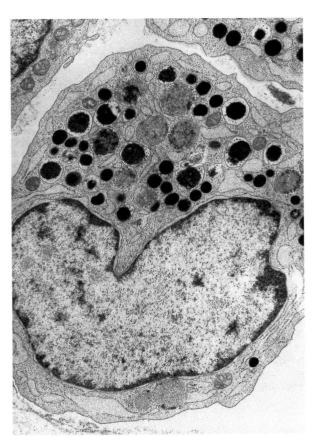

Figure 65

ACUTE MYELOID LEUKEMIA WITH INV(16) CHROMOSOME ABNORMALITY

Left: Blood smear from a 17-year-old boy with acute myeloid leukemia with an associated inv(16) chromosome abnormality and a leukocyte count of 90×10^9/L. The majority of cells have markedly lobulated nuclei similar to the blasts and abnormal promyelocytes in microgranular acute promyelocytic leukemia. These cells were intensely MPO and SBB positive; 4 to 5 percent were reactive for NSE. The marrow contained 2.2 percent eosinophils, some with abnormal, basophilic granules. Cells with single Auer rods were present; no faggot cells were identified. The serum lysozyme level was markedly elevated. There was no evidence of disseminated intravascular coagulation either prior to or during chemotherapy. The case was classified as AML-M2. Cytogenetic study showed an inv(16) (p13q22) chromosome abnormality. (Wright-Giemsa stain)

Right: Electron micrograph of an abnormal eosinophil in the bone marrow from the specimen illustrated on the left. There are numerous electron-dense and electron-lucent granules. Both types of granules lack crystalline cores. (Uranyl acetate–lead citrate stains, X17,000) (Fig. 44.26 from Litz CE, Brunning RD. Acute myeloid leukemias. In: Knowles DM, ed. Neoplastic hematopathology. Baltimore: Williams & Wilkins, 1992:1315–49.)

Acute Monocytic Leukemia (AML-M5)

Definition. A type of AML in which 80 percent or more of the marrow cells are of monocytic lineage: monoblasts, promonocytes, and monocytes. Two major morphologic types are recognized based on the percentage of monoblasts in the marrow or blood: acute monoblastic leukemia (M5A) in which 80 percent or more of the monocytic cells are monoblasts and acute monocytic leukemia, differentiated (M5B) in which less than 80 percent of the monocytic cells are monoblasts.

Acute Monoblastic Leukemia (AML-M5A)

Incidence and Clinical Findings. AML-M5A comprises 5 to 8 percent of all cases of AML (49,86). The disease occurs in all decades of life but is more common in younger individuals; the median age is 16 years and 75 percent of cases occur in individuals 25 years of age or less.

The primary symptoms are fatigue and weakness; bleeding disorders occur in approximately 20 percent of patients. Presenting physical findings include hepatosplenomegaly in approximately 50

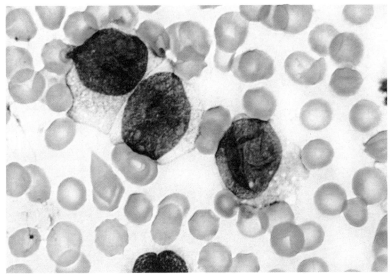

Figure 66
ACUTE MONOBLASTIC
LEUKEMIA (AML-M5A)
Blood smear from a patient with acute monoblastic leukemia showing two monoblasts and one promonocyte. The two monoblasts on the left have abundant cytoplasm with numerous azurophilic granules. The promonocyte on the right has abundant cytoplasm with fine azurophilic granules; the nuclear membrane has delicate folds and creases. (Wright-Giemsa stain)

Figure 67
ACUTE MONOBLASTIC
LEUKEMIA (AML-M5A)
Bone marrow smear from a 17-year-old female with acute monoblastic leukemia. The monoblasts are large cells with abundant cytoplasm containing numerous fine azurophilic granules. The nuclear chromatin is slightly coarse; two to three distinct nucleoli are present. (Wright-Giemsa stain)

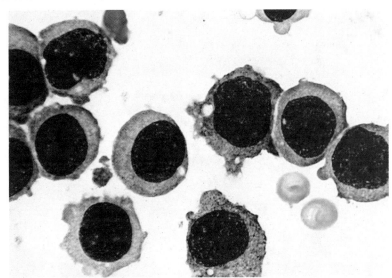

percent of patients and lymphadenopathy in 30 to 35 percent (86). Extramedullary tumor masses are relatively common. Sites of involvement include the orbit, skin, paraspinal tissue, and testes (77). The presenting symptoms may relate to the site of extramedullary involvement, such as neurologic syndromes secondary to a paraspinal mass.

Laboratory Findings. Approximately equal numbers of patients present with leukopenia, leukocytosis, and normal leukocyte counts. The median leukocyte count is 7.3×10^9/L; the count exceeds 100×10^9/L in about 10 percent of cases (86). Anemia is present in 80 percent of cases and thrombocytopenia in 70 percent.

The serum lysozyme level is increased in approximately half of the patients. Evidence of disseminated intravascular coagulation is documented in 50 percent of patients (66) and approximately 25 percent have an associated t(9;11)(p21–23;q23) chromosome abnormality (50,83).

Blood and Bone Marrow Findings. In the typical case of AML-M5A more than 80 percent of the marrow cells are monoblasts, which are characteristically large, measuring up to 40 to 50 mm in diameter. The abundant, variably basophilic cytoplasm may be irregularly distributed with prominent pseudopod formation (figs. 66–70) (66). Fine to coarse azurophilic granules dispersed throughout the cytoplasm are usually

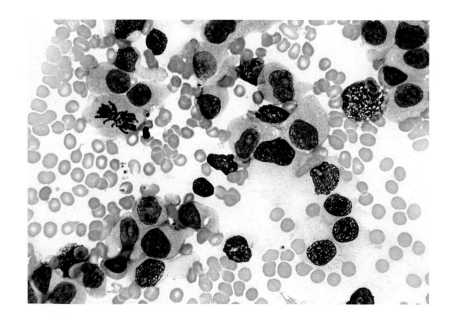

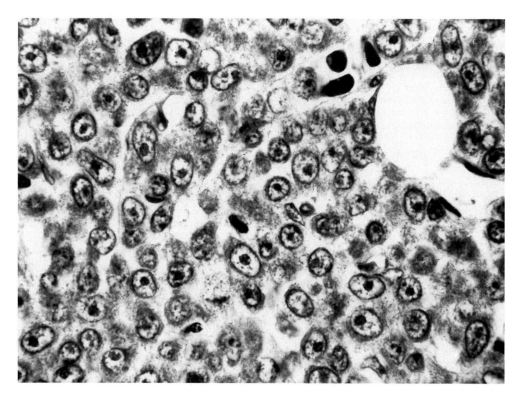

Figure 68
ACUTE MONOBLASTIC LEUKEMIA (AML-M5A)

Top: Bone marrow smear from a 17-year-old male with acute monoblastic leukemia. The monoblasts are large with very abundant cytoplasm that contains fine azurophilic granules. Several of the monoblasts show pseudopod formation. (Wright-Giemsa stain)

Bottom: Bone marrow biopsy from the specimen illustrated on the top. The marrow is completely replaced by monoblasts, which are large cells with abundant cytoplasm and round to oval nuclei. Nucleoli are prominent in many of the cells. (Hematoxylin and eosin stain)

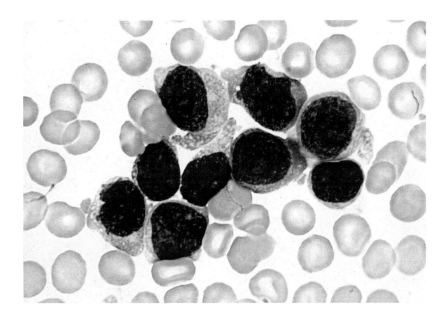

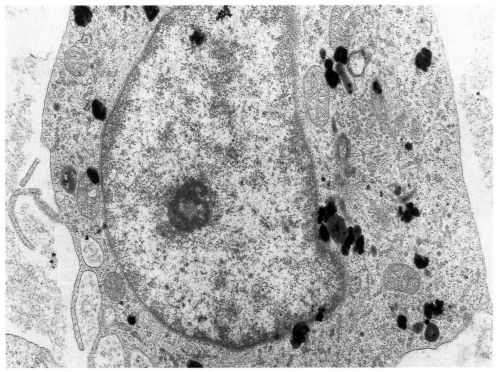

Figure 69
ACUTE MONOBLASTIC LEUKEMIA (AML-M5A)

Top: The monoblasts in this bone marrow smear from a 78-year-old male with marked splenomegaly vary from cells with a sparse amount of intensely basophilic cytoplasm to cells with abundant, slightly basophilic cytoplasm. The cytoplasm of some of the cells contains small vacuoles but is devoid of granules. The monoblasts in this case were NSE negative but manifested characteristic monoblast features and NSE reactivity on electron microscopy. The serum lysozyme level was markedly elevated. (Wright-Giemsa stain)

Bottom: Electron micrograph of a monoblast from the specimen illustrated on the top reacted for NSE. There are scattered electron-dense deposits indicating enzyme activity. (Lead citrate stain only, X20,000)

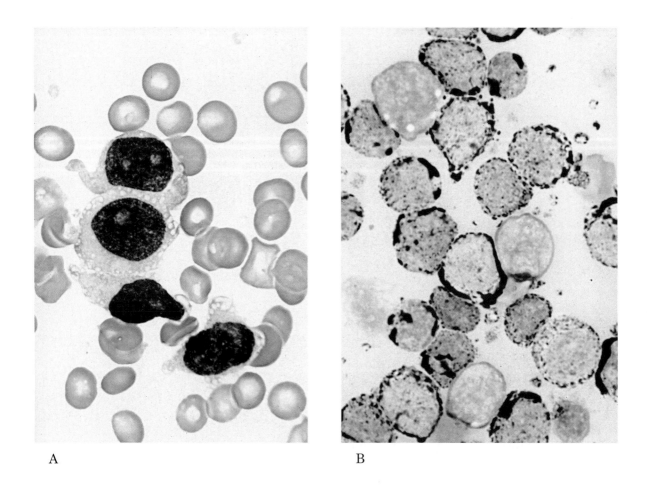

A

B

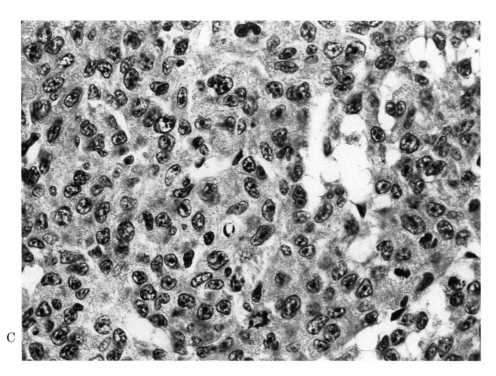

C

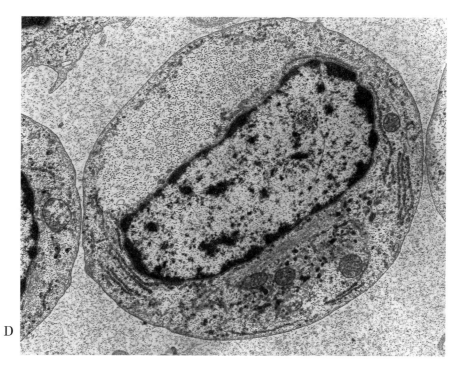

D

Figure 70
ACUTE MONOBLASTIC LEUKEMIA (AML-M5A)

A. The monoblasts in this bone marrow smear are large with abundant pale cytoplasm containing numerous vacuoles and prominent pseudopod formation. Nucleoli are distinct but not unusually prominent. (Wright-Giemsa stain)

B. Buffy coat smear reacted with PAS showing intense positivity in the vacuoles. (Periodic acid–Schiff stain)

C. Bone marrow section from the specimen illustrated in A and B. The monoblasts are large with abundant cytoplasm. The nuclear outlines vary from round to irregular. Many of the blasts have single prominent nucleoli. (Hematoxylin and eosin stain)

D. Electron micrograph of a monoblast from the specimen illustrated in A and B. A large portion of cytoplasm is replaced by a focal area of glycogen deposition. The remaining cytoplasm shows scattered dense granules and a paranuclear fibrillar array. (Uranyl acetate–lead citrate stains, X9,000)

present. Uncommonly, the cytoplasm may contain prominent vacuoles that are PAS positive (fig. 70B). The nuclei are round to oval with a single prominent nucleolus or multiple nucleoli. There may be limited evidence of maturation to promonocytes. A few mature monocytes may be present. Auer rods are not usually detected in typical monoblasts, but may be found in myeloblasts, which may be present in low numbers.

Variant forms of acute monoblastic leukemia occur in which the monoblasts lack the features described. In these cases the monoblasts are smaller, with a moderate amount of cytoplasm containing fine peroxidase-negative granules. These blasts may more closely resemble myeloblasts or lymphoblasts. The monoblastic nature is confirmed by intense NSE positivity or reactivity with monoclonal antibodies to monocytes.

In those instances in which the monoblastic proliferation has its inception as an extramedullary tumor, the bone marrow may show partial and, occasionally, minimal involvement. These cases should be considered as analogous to a granulocytic sarcoma with marrow involvement.

Cytochemical Findings. The monoblasts in acute monoblastic leukemia manifest variable degrees of reactivity with NSE, even within the same case. In some instances virtually every monoblast is intensely positive (fig. 71); in approximately 20 to 25 percent of cases, the monoblasts are only very weakly positive or nonreactive. Monoblasts are usually negative with MPO and SBB, although in a minority of cases some of the blasts show some degree of reactivity and, rarely, are intensely positive. The monoblasts in these instances react for both NSE and MPO. There is no relationship

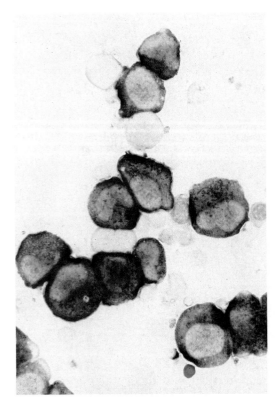

Figure 71
ACUTE MONOBLASTIC LEUKEMIA (AML-M5A):
NONSPECIFIC ESTERASE REACTION
Bone marrow smear from a case of acute monoblastic leukemia reacted for NSE. The monoblasts are intensely positive. (Alpha napthyl acetate and methyl green stains)

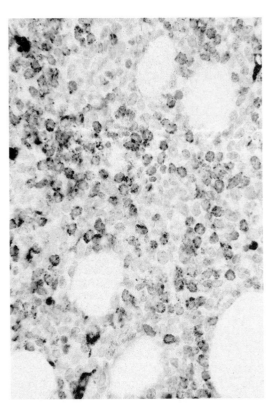

Figure 72
ACUTE MONOBLASTIC LEUKEMIA (AML-M5A)
WITH EXPRESSION OF CD68 (KP-1)
Bone marrow biopsy from a patient with acute monoblastic leukemia reacted with antibody to CD68 (KP-1). A high percentage of blasts are positive. The blasts did not react with antibodies to MPO or lysozyme in the sections and were NSE negative in smears. The blasts expressed CD33 and CD14. (Peroxidase-antiperoxidase stain)

between the number of azurophilic granules and MPO reactivity in monoblasts; monoblasts with abundant azurophilic granules are usually MPO negative. There is usually weak diffuse reactivity with CAE (66). PAS reactivity varies: in the majority of cases there is minimal or no PAS reactivity. In a rare case, the monoblasts contain large PAS-positive cytoplasmic globules (fig. 70B). The acid phosphatase reaction is positive in virtually all cases and may be intense. It is characterized by a diffuse granular pattern and is ablated following incubation with tartaric acid.

Histopathologic Findings. In the majority of cases of AML-M5A the normal marrow cells are virtually completely replaced by the leukemic cells. In a minority of cases, there is substantial sparing of normal myeloid cells and the monoblasts are interspersed throughout the interstitium. This partial involvement may be related to the inception of the process in an extramedullary site (77). As noted, these cases should be considered analogous to granulocytic sarcomas with marrow involvement.

The monoblasts in bone marrow sections are large with abundant amphophilic to lightly eosinophilic cytoplasm. The nucleus is round to oval. Nucleoli may be single or multiple, are usually eosinophilic, and may be unusually prominent (figs. 68, bottom and 70C). A minor population of leukemic cells may manifest nuclear lobulation.

Monoblasts may be positive with antibodies to cells of monocyte macrophage origin reactive in paraffin-embedded specimens such as antilysozyme and KP-1 which recognizes CD68 (fig. 72). The results of the reactions with these antibodies should be used in conjunction with other studies and should not be viewed as definitive for identifying cells of monocyte origin, since positive reactions may also occur in other types of myeloid leukemia.

Ultrastructural Findings. On ultrastructural examination, the monoblast cytoplasm contains abundant fine filaments, free ribosomes and polyribosomes, strands of rough endoplasmic reticulum, and variable numbers of electron-dense granules which have a dense core surrounded by a halo (66). Ribosome-lamella complex–like structures are present in 20 to 90 percent of the monoblasts in approximately one fourth of cases (36). Ultrastructural studies for NSE are usually positive, including those cases in which the blasts are negative by routine methods (fig. 69, bottom).

Differential Diagnosis. The major types of leukemia from which AML-M5A must be distinguished are AML-M1, AML-M0, and ALL-L2. The myeloblasts in AML-M1 and M0 are generally smaller and have less cytoplasm than monoblasts and are NSE negative. By definition, 3 percent or more of the myeloblasts in AML-M1 react for MPO or SBB; the monoblasts are usually MPO and SBB negative and NSE positive. AML-M0 is identified by ultrastructural and immunologic studies.

In ALL-L2, the blasts may be very poorly differentiated and occasionally resemble monoblasts. The diffuse, fine, granular NSE positivity characteristic of the monoblasts in most cases of M5A is not found in lymphoblasts. Lymphoblasts may occasionally show punctate esterase positivity but lack the diffuse cytoplasmic positivity characteristic of monoblasts. The lymphoblasts in 90 to 95 percent of cases of ALL show nuclear TdT positivity. The monoblasts are usually negative. Immunologic markers are definitive for diagnosis.

In 15 to 20 percent of cases of AML-M5A, the blasts are NSE negative. In these instances, the distinction from AML-M0 and ALL-L2 is made on the basis of immunologic or ultrastructural studies. An elevated serum or urine lysozyme level is suggestive evidence of monocytic differentiation.

The monoblasts in AML-M5A may resemble the prolymphocytes of prolymphocytic leukemia. Distinction is based on the NSE positivity of the monoblast and the reactivity of the prolymphocyte with lymphocyte antibodies.

Plasmablastic myeloma, because of the blastic features of the cells, may resemble the more poorly differentiated leukemias, particularly acute monoblastic leukemia. The problem is accentuated if the plasmablastic process presents with leukemic manifestations (fig. 73). Serum and urine protein studies and calcium levels are important in distinguishing plasmablastic myeloma from acute monoblastic leukemia. Immunophenotyping is definitive; the plasmablasts have intracytoplasmic light chain restricted immunoglobulin, are CD38 positive, and do not express the surface antigens found on monoblasts.

Acute Monocytic Leukemia (AML-M5B) (Acute Monocytic Leukemia, Differentiated)

Incidence and Clinical Findings. Acute monocytic leukemia, differentiated, is uncommon and comprises 3 to 6 percent of cases of AML (49,86). The male to female ratio is 1.8 to 1. The disease occurs in all decades of life but is more common in older individuals; the median age is 49 years (86).

The most common presenting symptoms relate to bleeding disorders. Hepatosplenomegaly and lymphadenopathy are present in approximately 50 percent of cases. Extramedullary lesions occur in 30 percent of cases (86); cutaneous and gingival infiltration are common extramedullary manifestations.

Laboratory Findings. Virtually all patients are anemic. Slightly more than half of the patients present with leukocytosis: approximately one third have leukocyte counts in excess of 100×10^9/L. Seventy-five to 80 percent of patients are thrombocytopenic (86).

Blood and Bone Marrow Findings. The number of myeloblasts and monoblasts in a typical case of acute monocytic leukemia may not exceed 10 to 15 percent of the bone marrow cells. The predominant cell type is the promonocyte, a cell intermediate in maturation to the monoblast and monocyte (figs. 74–76). The promonocyte is large with abundant, pale blue to slightly gray cytoplasm. The cytoplasm usually contains abundant fine to coarse azurophilic granules. The nucleus is slightly lobulated. The lobulation generally takes the form of delicate folds or creases in the nuclear membrane imparting a cerebriform appearance to the nucleus. In occasional

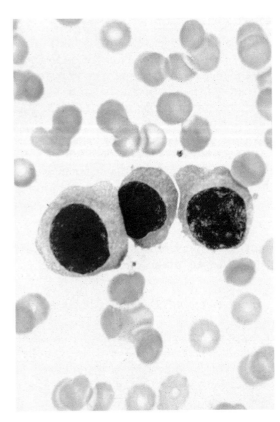
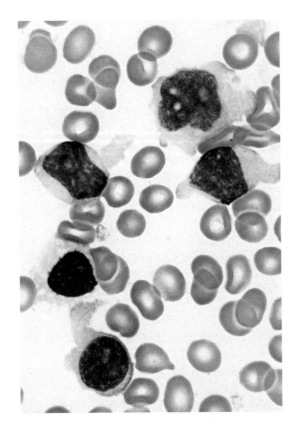

Figure 73
PLASMABLASTIC LEUKEMIA

Left: Blood smear from a 47-year-old male with a leukocyte count of 11×10^9/L and 30 percent blasts. The blasts were NSE and MPO negative. They contained intracytoplasmic IgG lambda, expressed CD38, and were negative for all myeloid and lymphoid antigens. Serum immunoelectrophoresis showed a 2.9 g IgG lambda monoclonal protein. Urine immunoelectrophoresis showed marked Bence Jones proteinuria. (Wright-Giemsa stain)

Right: Bone marrow smears showing blastic-appearing cells with abundant irregularly distributed cytoplasm. (Wright-Giemsa stain)

Figure 74
ACUTE MONOCYTIC
LEUKEMIA (AML-M5B)

Blood smear from a 55-year-old female with acute monocytic leukemia, differentiated. The leukocyte count was 77×10^9/L. The predominant promonocytes have abundant cytoplasm with scattered MPO-negative azurophilic granules. The nuclei are marked by delicate folds and creases. Nucleoli are inconspicuous. (Wright-Giemsa stain)

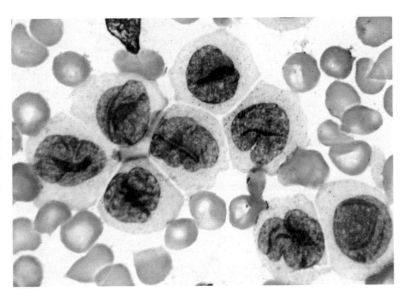

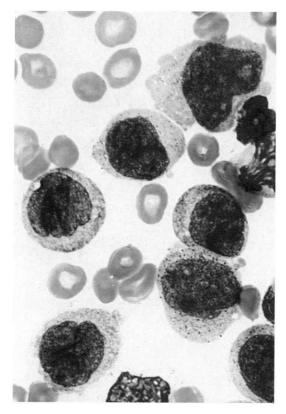

Figure 75
ACUTE MONOCYTIC LEUKEMIA (AML-M5B)
Bone marrow smear from an adult male with acute monocytic leukemia showing a range of maturation of monocytic cells. The cells with nuclei with delicate folds and creases are promonocytes. (Wright-Giemsa stain)

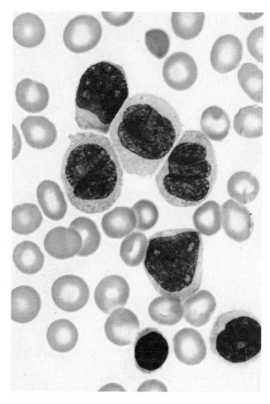

Figure 76
ACUTE MONOCYTIC LEUKEMIA (AML-M5B)
Bone marrow smear from an adult female with acute monocytic leukemia showing two myeloblasts and three promonocytes. The myeloblasts have a high nuclear-cytoplasmic ratio and round to oval nuclei. The promonocytes have abundant cytoplasm with delicate azurophilic granules. The nuclei are characterized by lobulation and delicate folds and creases in the nuclear membrane. (Wright-Giemsa stain)

cases the nuclear lobulation is more marked. The nuclear chromatin is finely dispersed; nucleoli are usually multiple and not unusually prominent. For purposes of classification as acute leukemia or myelodysplastic syndrome, the promonocyte is included in the blast percentage. Myeloblasts with Auer rods may be found. Dysgranulopoiesis, dyserythropoiesis, and dysplastic megakaryocytes may be present.

The blast percentage in the blood may be low. Similar to the bone marrow, the predominant cell is the promonocyte. Mature monocytes are usually present in low numbers.

Cytochemical Findings. The monocytic cells in AML-M5B are reactive for NSE in virtually all cases and the more mature cells are usually intensely positive (fig. 77). Monocytic cells at all stages of maturation are reactive for tartrate-sensitive acid phosphatase. Reactivity

with MPO and SBB is usually weak or absent although occasional cells are moderately positive. The reaction with PAS varies: the cells in the majority of cases show no or a minimal reaction that manifests as finely dispersed granules. In occasional cases the leukemic cells show coarse granules and globular inclusions.

Histopathologic Findings. In trephine biopsies, the bone marrow is usually markedly hypercellular with a marked decrease in normal marrow cells. The leukemic cells have a slight to moderate amount of amphophilic cytoplasm. The nuclear outline varies from round to oval to markedly convoluted (fig. 78). Nucleoli may be prominent in the cells with round or oval nuclei; they are generally indistinct in the cells with convoluted or contorted nuclei. Normal hematopoietic cells are markedly decreased.

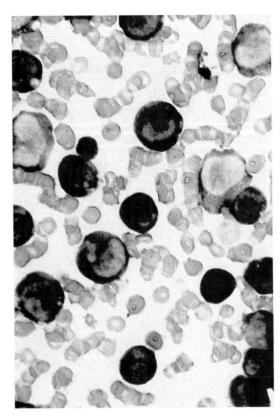

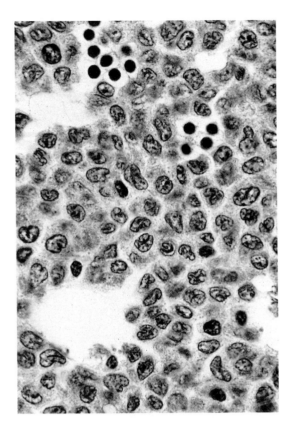

Figure 77
ACUTE MONOCYTIC LEUKEMIA (AML-M5B):
NONSPECIFIC ESTERASE REACTION
NSE stain of a bone marrow smear from an adult woman with AML-M5B. All of the monocytic cells are intensely positive; a single segmented neutrophil is negative. (Nonspecific esterase stain)

Figure 78
ACUTE MONOCYTIC LEUKEMIA (AML-M5B)
Bone marrow section from a patient with AML-M5B. Many of the leukemic cells have lobulated and indented nuclei corresponding to the nuclear characteristics in the smear preparation. Most of the cells have a moderate rim of granular cytoplasm. Nucleoli are not prominent. (Hematoxylin and eosin stain)

Ultrastructural Findings. The promonocytes are large cells with irregularly folded nuclei with dispersed chromatin (fig. 79). Nuclear lobes with bridging connections are frequently present. Nucleoli are present but not unusually prominent. The promonocyte has abundant cytoplasm that may have numerous pseudopods. Numerous small, round or irregularly shaped, dense, membrane-bound granules are scattered diffusely in the cytoplasm (36). Mitochondria are numerous. Cytoplasmic bundles of microfilaments, frequently in a perinuclear location, are usually present.

Differential Diagnosis. The two most important processes from which AML-M5B must be distinguished are APL, microgranular type, and AML-M4. As noted in the discussion of APL, the abnormal promyelocytes in the microgranular variant may have contorted or lobulated nuclei closely resembling the nucleus of the promonocyte and monocyte. The MPO or SBB and NSE reactivity patterns are virtually definitive in distinguishing the two cell types. The leukemic promyelocyte is intensely MPO and SBB positive and generally NSE negative. In approximately 20 percent of cases of APL, the leukemic promyelocytes are weakly to moderately NSE positive. A majority of the monocytes and promonocytes in AML-M5B are intensely NSE positive and MPO negative or weakly positive. Faggot cells, which are present in virtually all cases of APL, are not found in AML-M5B.

AML-M5B is distinguished from AML-M4 by the percentage of monocytic cells, which are 80 percent or more in M5B and less than 80 percent in AML-M4.

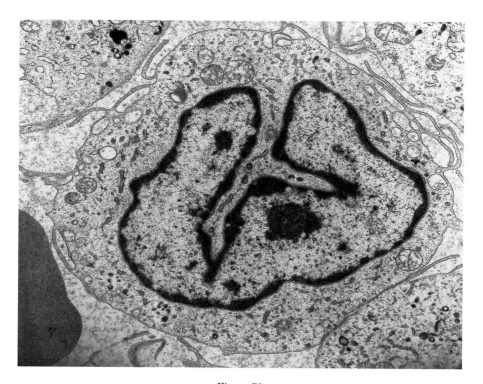

Figure 79
ACUTE MONOCYTIC LEUKEMIA (AML-M5B): ULTRASTRUCTURE
Electron micrograph of a promonocyte in a bone marrow specimen from a patient with AML-M5B. The nucleus is markedly lobulated; the chromatin is marginated at the nuclear membrane. The cytoplasm contains numerous small cisternae of rough endoplasmic reticulum and a few scattered dense granules. (Uranyl acetate–lead citrate stains, X19,000)

Erythroleukemia (AML-M6)

Definition. A type of AML characterized by a concurrent proliferation of granulocytes and abnormal erythroblasts. The erythroblasts are usually in excess of 50 percent of the marrow cells, and because of this the number of type I and II blasts may be less than the requisite 30 percent of all marrow cells. As a result, if the erythroid precursors in the marrow exceed 50 percent in a case with findings suggestive of erythroleukemia or myelodysplastic syndrome, the blast percentage is calculated on the basis of the nonerythroid nucleated marrow cells. The blast percentage includes type I and II myeloblasts; proerythroblasts are not included. If the erythroid precursors exceed 50 percent and the type I and II blasts are 30 percent or more of the nonerythroid cells, the diagnosis is erythroleukemia (22). If type I and II blasts are less than 30 percent the diagnosis is a myelodysplastic syndrome, if other findings are consistent with that diagnosis (fig. 80).

If a case of AML presents with a marrow erythroblast percentage between 30 and 50 with marked abnormalities of the erythroblasts and the type I and II blasts are 30 percent or more of the nonerythroid cells, the diagnosis of erythroleukemia is appropriate (49,86).

Incidence and Clinical Findings. Erythroleukemia is relatively uncommon and accounts for approximately 5 percent of cases of AML (49, 86). It occurs in all age groups but is more frequent in older individuals; the median age is 54 years. There is a slight male predominance (86).

The most common symptoms at presentation are constitutional: fatigue and malaise. Organomegaly is uncommon; hepatomegaly is present in 25 percent of patients. Splenomegaly and lymphadenopathy are present in less than 20 percent.

Laboratory Findings. Anemia and thrombocytopenia are present in virtually all patients. The white blood cell count varies and patients may present with a low, normal, or elevated leukocyte count (86).

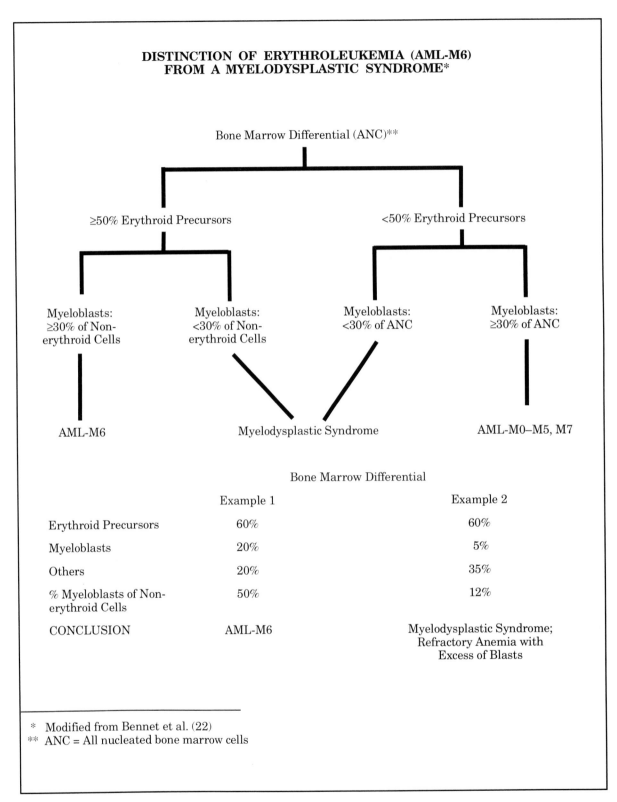

Figure 80
DISTINCTION OF ERYTHROLEUKEMIA (AML-M6) FROM A MYELODYSPLASTIC SYNDROME

De novo erythroleukemia is reported to have a high association with abnormalities of chromosomes 5 and 7, similar to the cytogenetic pattern in patients with therapy-related AML. Loss of part of the long arm of chromosomes 5 or 7 or both was observed in 65 percent of patients in one study (75). These abnormalities tended to occur in older patients and were associated with shorter median survival rates than observed in patients with erythroleukemia who did not have the abnormality.

Blood and Bone Marrow Findings. The blood and bone marrow findings in erythroleukemia are extraordinarily diverse because of the variable degrees of erythroid proliferation and dyserythropoiesis (figs. 81–84, 87). The proliferation of the erythroid cells may primarily involve the proerythroblasts and basophilic erythroblasts, or all maturation stages. The erythroid cells may be relatively uniform in size and nuclear and cytoplasmic characteristics or may show marked cytologic abnormalities with giant forms. Cytoplasmic vacuolation is common. The vacuoles occur primarily in the basophilic erythroblast and proerythroblast stages of maturation but may be present in polychromatic cells. The vacuoles have a tendency to coalesce forming large lacunae. The vacuoles are usually intensely positive with the PAS reaction. Nuclear abnormalities are characterized by lobulation, karyorrhexis, multinucleation, and a megaloblastoid nuclear chromatin. Multinucleation and multilobulation occur in cells at all stages of development (figs. 83, 84). Type III (ringed) sideroblasts may be numerous in iron stain preparations.

The myeloblasts are type I and II myeloblasts as in other types of AML and Auer rods are present in the myeloblasts in approximately 60 to 70 percent of cases (fig. 82, right). Dysgranulopoiesis may be prominent. Megakaryocyte proliferation with dysplastic megakaryocytes may be present. In some instances, the blood and bone marrow findings are those of a panmyelosis.

The blood findings are variable: anemia is frequently severe and thrombocytopenia is common. Immature granulocytes are usually present. Red blood cell precursors may be numerous and may include all stages of maturation with a predominance of polychromatic and orthochromatic cells (fig. 85). In cases in which the marrow erythroid cells are predominantly basophilic erythroblasts, these will be the predominant type in the blood. The abnormalities of the nucleus and cytoplasm present in the marrow cells will also be present in the erythroblasts in the blood.

Cytochemical Findings. The erythroblasts in a high percentage of cases stain positive for PAS; positivity ranges from less than 10 percent of cells with a slight degree of reactivity to cases in which virtually all of the erythroblasts are intensely positive (fig. 86). The type of reactivity varies with the stage of maturation. In proerythroblasts and basophilic erythroblasts the positivity usually occurs in the form of globules or granules. In the polychromatic and orthochromatic stages, the reactivity is diffuse. In some cases, the polychromatic and orthochromatic erythroblasts have cytoplasmic vacuoles. In these cells the PAS positivity is globular, granular, and diffuse. The myeloblasts in erythroleukemia react for MPO and SBB.

Histopathologic Findings. The appearance of the bone marrow sections varies depending on the percentage of erythroid cells and the degree of maturation. When proerythroblasts and basophilic erythroblasts predominate, the marrow may resemble AML-M1, ALL-L2, or an undifferentiated leukemia (fig. 87). The erythroblasts usually have abundant basophilic cytoplasm; the chromatin is slightly coarser than in myeloblasts or L2 lymphoblasts. Nucleoli are distinct and may be unusually prominent. Immunohistochemical reactions with antihemoglobin A antibody aid in recognizing the erythroid nature of the cells (fig. 87, bottom). Islands of erythroblasts may be present in the marrow sinuses, and in some instances, may appear to emanate from the sinusoidal lining cells. Mitotic figures may be numerous. In other cases there is clear evidence of differentiation of the proerythroblasts and basophilic erythroblasts to more mature stages of development (fig. 81C).

In those cases of erythroleukemia in which there is a substantial nonerythroid component, the marrow sections may contain a large number of myeloblasts and megakaryocytes. The megakaryocytes in these cases are frequently dysplastic; numerous micromegakaryocytes, frequently nonlobulated or hypolobulated, may be present. There may be an increase in reticulin fibers.

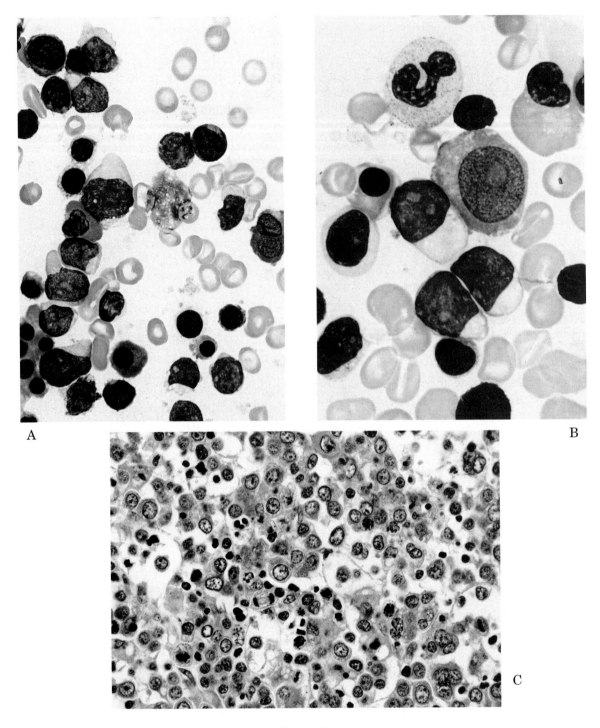

Figure 81
ERYTHROLEUKEMIA (AML-M6)

A. Bone marrow smear from a patient with AML-M6 showing numerous myeloblasts and erythroid precursors at all stages of maturation. (Wright-Giemsa stain)

B. High magnification of the specimen in A showing a megaloblastoid erythroblast and three myeloblasts. (Wright-Giemsa stain)

C. Bone marrow trephine biopsy from the specimen illustrated in A and B showing evidence of maturation of the early stage erythroblasts to late stage erythroblasts. Mature granulocytes are markedly reduced. Small megakaryocytes are present at the upper and lower margins. (Hematoxylin and eosin stain)

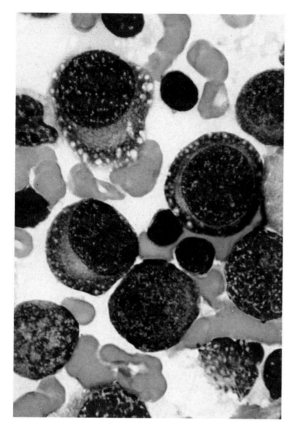 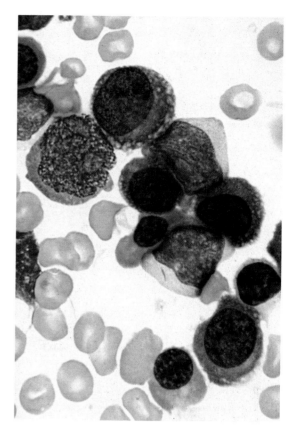

Figure 82
ERYTHROLEUKEMIA (AML-M6)

Left: Bone marrow smear from a patient with erythroleukemia containing several immature erythroid precursors with markedly basophilic cytoplasm with numerous poorly defined vacuoles primarily at the periphery of the cell. (Wright-Giemsa stain)

Right: The same specimen as on the left showing two myeloblasts, one of which contains an Auer rod. (Wright-Giemsa stain) (Fig. 44.27 from Litz CE, Brunning RD. Acute myeloid leukemias. In: Knowles DM, ed. Neoplastic hematopathology. Baltimore: Williams & Wilkins, 1992:1315–49.)

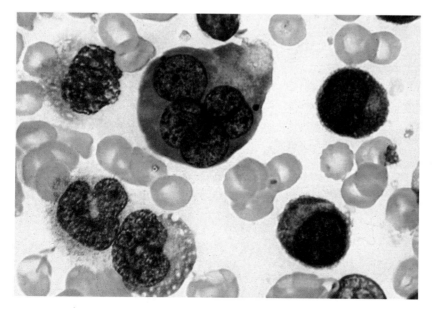

Figure 83
ERYTHROLEUKEMIA (AML-M6)
Bone marrow smear from a case of erythroleukemia showing a multi-nucleated erythroblast with megaloblastoid nuclear chromatin. (Wright-Giemsa stain)

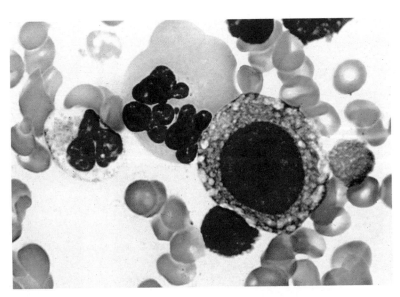

Figure 84
ERYTHROLEUKEMIA (AML-M6)
Two abnormal erythroblasts at different stages of maturation. The very large proerythroblast has a very prominent nucleolus and vacuolated cytoplasm; the late polychromatic erythroblast has a markedly lobulated nucleus and several Pappenheimer bodies near the nucleus. (Wright-Giemsa stain) (Fig. 44.28 from Litz CE, Brunning RD. Acute myeloid leukemias. In: Knowles DM, ed. Neoplastic hematopathology. Baltimore: Williams & Wilkins, 1992:1315–49.)

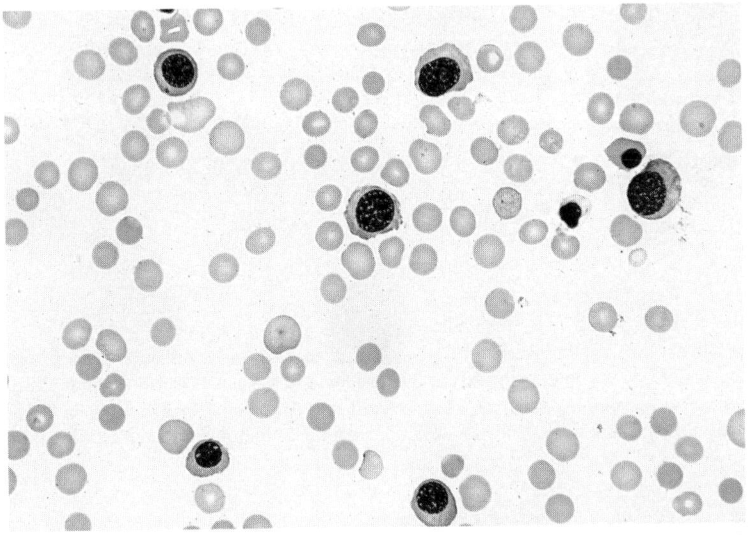

Figure 85
ERYTHROLEUKEMIA: BLOOD
Blood smear from a patient with erythroleukemia (AML-M6) and a history of post-trauma splenectomy. There were approximately 2000 erythroid precursors per 100 leukocytes in the smear. A majority of the erythroid precursors are at the polychromatic and basophilic stages of maturation. The marked normoblastemia may be related to both the leukemia and the asplenic state. (Wright-Giemsa stain)

Figure 86
ERYTHROLEUKEMIA (AML-M6): PERIODIC ACID–SCHIFF STAIN
PAS reaction in a bone marrow smear from a patient with erythroleukemia. The vacuoles in the immature erythroid precursors are intensely positive. The cytoplasm of the more mature erythroid precursors is diffusely PAS positive. (Periodic acid–Schiff stain) (Fig. 44.30 from Litz CE, Brunning RD. Acute myeloid leukemias. In: Knowles DM, ed. Neoplastic hematopathology. Baltimore: Williams & Wilkins, 1992:1315–49.)

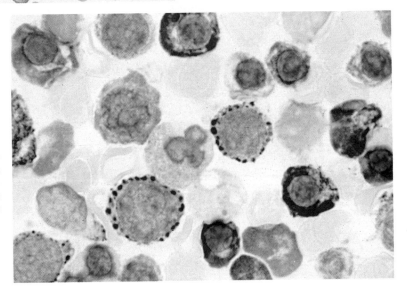

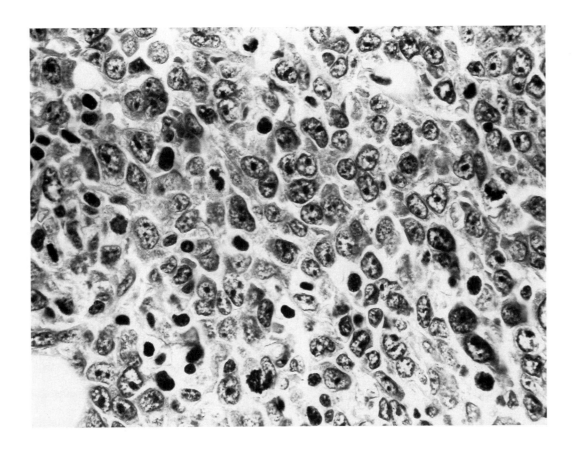

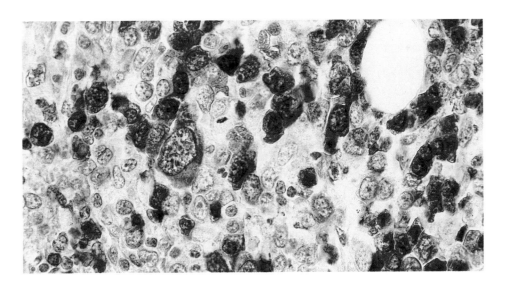

Figure 87
ERYTHROLEUKEMIA (AML-M6)

Top: Bone marrow trephine biopsy showing replacement by blasts of considerable size variation and minimal evidence of differentiation to more mature erythroid precursors. The more immature erythroblasts have dispersed nuclear chromatin and prominent nucleoli. (Hematoxylin and eosin stain)

Bottom: Specimen from the case illustrated on the top reacted with antibody to hemoglobin A. Several of the cells are positive including one very large abnormal cell. (Alkaline phosphatase–antialkaline phosphatase stain)

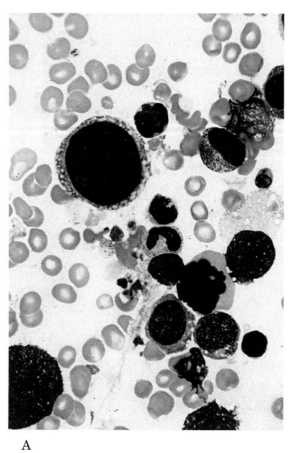

A

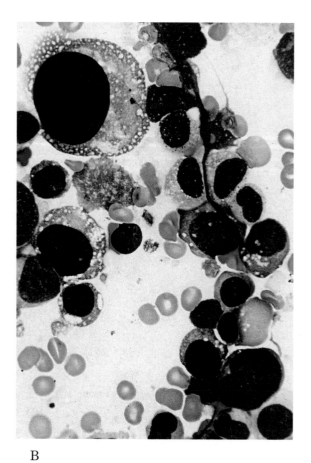

B

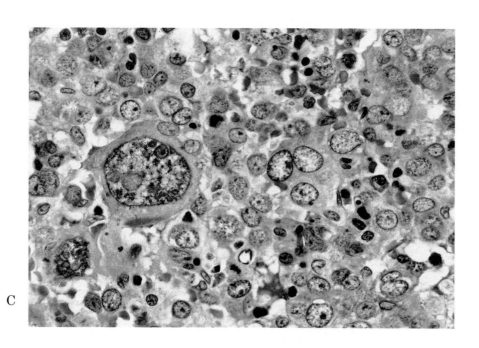

C

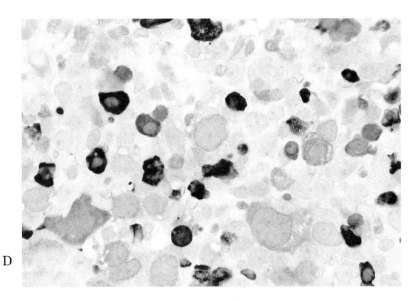

D

Figure 88
ERYTHREMIC MYELOSIS

A. Bone marrow smear from an 8-year-old boy 2 1/2 years following treatment and remission of CD19, CD10, TdT-positive B-cell precursor acute lymphoblastic leukemia. This marrow biopsy was performed because of pancytopenia. The predominant marrow population consists of abnormal erythroid precursors at all stages of maturation. The neutrophils and precursors appeared morphologically normal. (Wright-Giemsa stain)

B. The same bone marrow smear showing very large abnormal erythroid precursors. (Wright-Giemsa stain)

C. Bone marrow section with extensive replacement by immature erythroid precursors. There are scattered very large abnormal cells. (Hematoxylin and eosin stain)

D. The bone marrow in C reacted with antihemoglobin A antibody, showing a positive reaction in several cells including large abnormal cells, supporting an erythroid origin. Cytogenetic studies of this marrow specimen documented several clonal chromosome abnormalities including 5q-, 7q-, and 11q-. (Alkaline phosphatase–antialkaline phosphatase stain)

Ultrastructural Findings. Ultrastructurally, the erythroblasts in erythroleukemia show abnormalities of both cytoplasmic and nuclear structures. The nuclear features reflect the light microscopy findings including binucleation and lobulation of the nuclei. There may be duplication of the nuclear envelope, greatly enlarged nuclear pores, and hypercondensed chromatin with a spongy appearance (36). The cytoplasm may contain large siderosomes, iron-containing mitochondria, annulate lamellae, cytoplasmic vacuoles, and increased amounts of glycogen.

Erythremic Myelosis. A rare variant of erythroid neoplasia is the process referred to as erythremic myelosis, a neoplastic disorder appearing to involve only red blood cell precursors (figs. 88–90). The erythroblasts, primarily proerythroblasts and basophilic erythroblasts, may constitute 90 percent or more of the marrow cells (fig. 89). The myeloblasts are not significantly increased, less than 5 percent in most cases, and are difficult to distinguish from the proerythroblasts. The erythroid precursors show abnormalities of nuclear and cytoplasmic development including megaloblastoid nuclear chromatin, nuclear lobulation, and karyorrhexis. Giant erythroblasts with multilobulated nuclei may be prominent. Cytoplasmic vacuoles, which have a tendency to coalesce and form large lacunae and which are usually positive with the PAS stain, may be prominent (fig. 90).

Patients with this type of leukemia usually present with very low hemoglobin levels. The red blood cells in the blood may be normochromic normocytic or normochromic macrocytic; aniso-poikilocytosis may be prominent. Erythroid precursors at all stages of maturation may be present in the blood and are sometimes numerous. Despite the low myeloblast percentage, these cases are appropriately classified as leukemia.

Cases presenting as erythremic myelosis may relapse as a more typical erythroleukemia following chemotherapy-induced remission.

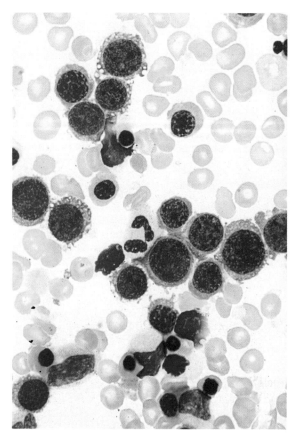

Figure 89
ERYTHREMIC MYELOSIS
Bone marrow smear from a patient with erythremic myelosis. Proerythroblasts and basophilic erythroblasts predominate. Many of these cells have numerous cytoplasmic vacuoles. (Wright-Giemsa stain)

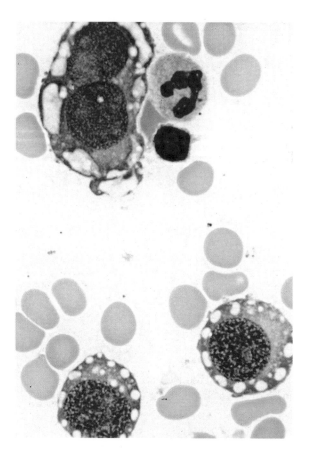

Figure 90
ERYTHREMIC MYELOSIS
Three immature erythroblasts in a bone marrow smear from a patient with erythremic myelosis. The cytoplasm of these cells contains large clear vacuoles. The larger vacuoles result from coalescence of smaller vacuoles and are usually intensely PAS positive. (Wright-Giemsa stain)

Differential Diagnosis. The two types of acute leukemia from which erythroleukemia must be distinguished are AML-M2 and AML-M4 when these processes are accompanied by some degree of erythroid hyperplasia and dyserythropoiesis. As noted, if the erythroid precursors are greater than 30 percent and there is a marked degree of dyserythropoiesis, the diagnosis of erythroleukemia more accurately reflects the type of leukemic process than acute myeloblastic leukemia M2 or M4.

Distinction of erythroleukemia from a myelodysplastic syndrome is based on the percentage of type I and II myeloblasts: these must be 30 percent or more of the nonerythroid cells for a diagnosis of erythroleukemia. Proerythroblasts are not included in the blast percentage.

Cases of erythremic myelosis in which there is no or minimal involvement of the nonerythroid myeloid cell lines can present difficult diagnostic problems. If the proliferation consists principally of cells at the proerythroblast and basophilic erythroblast stages of development, the distinction from AML-M1, AML-M7, ALL-L2, ALL-L3, or marrow involvement by malignant lymphoma may be difficult. As noted previously, 3 percent or more of the blasts in acute myeloblastic leukemia without maturation are MPO or SBB positive. Distinguishing between AML-M7 and erythremic myelosis usually necessitates immunologic and ultrastructural studies. The lymphoblasts in ALL-L2 are TdT positive. The vacuoles in the lymphoblasts of ALL-L3 are PAS negative and oil red O positive in contrast to the vacuoles in the erythroblasts of erythroleukemia or erythremic myelosis which are PAS positive and oil red O negative. Antihemoglobin A antibodies may be used in paraffin-embedded tissues to demonstrate the erythroid nature of a proliferative process (fig. 87, bottom). Antiglycophorin A and anticarbonic anhydrase I antibodies may be used in immunocytochemical stains of smears or in flow cytometry as markers of erythroid cells (95).

Acute Megakaryoblastic Leukemia (AML-M7)

Definition. A type of acute myeloid leukemia in which the predominant blast population is of megakaryocytic lineage. Similar to other forms of AML, the number of blasts in the blood or bone marrow is 30 percent or more, of which 50 percent or more should be of megakaryocytic lineage as demonstrated by ultrastructural studies or immunologic markers (19,32,45,55,58,99). The term should be restricted to processes in which there is no history of a chronic myeloproliferative disorder.

Incidence and Clinical Findings. The incidence of AML-M7 is reported as 8 to 10 percent of AML cases (55,99). The disease occurs in all age groups.

Hepatosplenomegaly and lymphadenopathy may be prominent. Radiographic evidence of discrete lytic bone lesions has been reported in children (99). An association of AML-M7 with mediastinal germ cell tumors has been reported in young adult males (44,73).

Laboratory Findings. Anemia is present in virtually all patients. The leukocyte and platelet counts may be normal, decreased, or increased.

Blood and Bone Marrow Findings. The morphologic spectrum of AML-M7 ranges from cases with a proliferation of blasts that appear essentially undifferentiated in routinely stained smears to processes that show clear evidence of maturation of the blasts to mature megakaryocytes (figs. 91–93). In the poorly differentiated type, the blasts vary from lymphoid appearing with sparse cytoplasm, dense nuclear chromatin, and inconspicuous nucleoli, to larger cells with a moderate rim of cytoplasm, dispersed nuclear chromatin, and distinct nucleoli. The larger blasts with more abundant cytoplasm usually contain very fine azurophilic granules frequently localized

to the perinuclear zone. In the more differentiated cases there is a clear maturational sequence from blasts to promegakaryocytes to megakaryocytes. The promegakaryocyte is intermediate in maturation to the megakaryoblast and megakaryocyte; it has more abundant cytoplasm than the megakaryoblast and an irregular paranuclear distribution of fine azurophilic granules. There is usually an accentuation of cytoplasmic basophilia in the area of granule formation. The distribution of granules gives the appearance of a zoning phenomenon with a paranuclear granular zone and a clear marginal zone. The cytoplasm may be irregularly distributed around the nucleus and show pseudopod formation. The nuclear chromatin is dispersed and nucleoli are usually distinct.

Mature megakaryocytes in AML-M7 are frequently smaller than normal megakaryocytes, approximately 7 to 10 μm, with nonlobulated nuclei. These are usually referred to as micromegakaryocytes or dwarf megakaryocytes. The nucleus of the micromegakaryocyte is usually hyperchromatic with attached strands of finely granulated cytoplasm that give the appearance of budding platelets. Megakaryoblasts and promegakaryocytes usually occur singly but may occasionally cluster, mimicking clumps of metastatic tumor (fig. 92) (80). The association of AML-M7 with morphologic features resembling metastatic tumor and a t(1;22)(p13;q13) chromosome abnormality has been reported in infants (39). Some of the leukemias associated with this chromosome abnormality have features of a panmyelosis (fig. 94).

As in other forms of AML, AML-M7 may show evidence of involvement of other cells of myeloid lineage and abnormalities of erythroid precursors may be prominent.

The blood smear may have a monomorphous blast population with little or no differentiating features, or there may be a spectrum from undifferentiated blasts to promegakaryocytes to mature megakaryocytes. The mature megakaryocytes may be predominantly small. In patients with elevated platelet counts there may be numerous atypical platelets which characteristically are large, irregular in outline, and completely or partially devoid of granules. Immature cells of the neutrophil and erythroid series may be present.

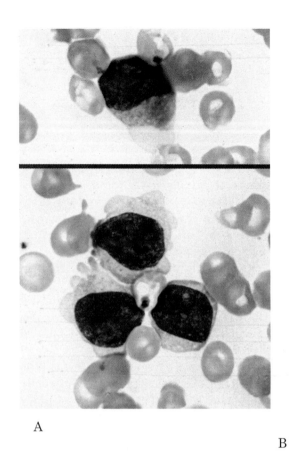

A

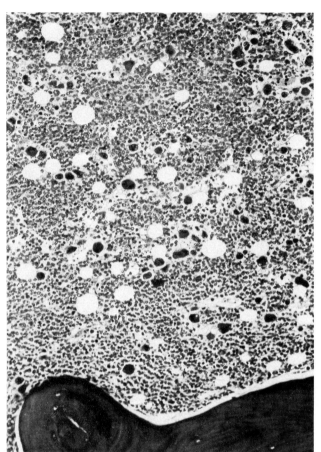

B

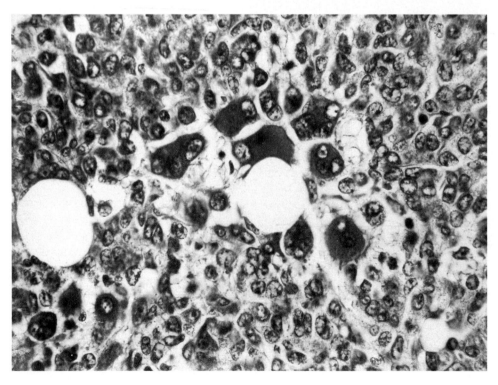

C

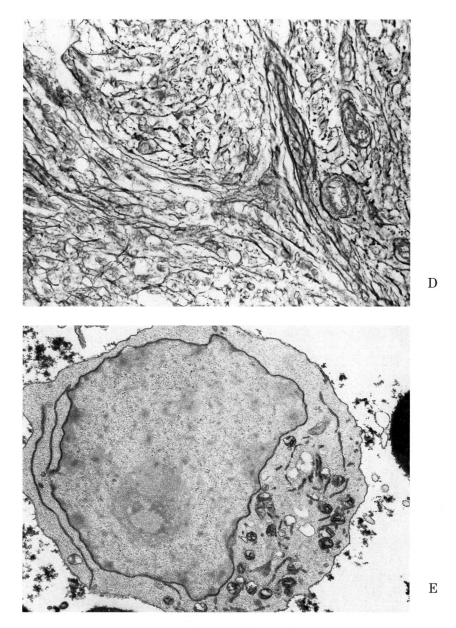

Figure 91
ACUTE MEGAKARYOBLASTIC LEUKEMIA (AML-M7)

A. Blood smear from a 7-month-old male with hepatomegaly. The predominant population is blasts. The cells have abundant cytoplasm. (Wright-Giemsa stain)

B. Bone marrow biopsy from the specimen illustrated in A. The marrow is hypercellular with a predominant population of blasts with numerous scattered mature megakaryocytes. The section was stained with PAS to accentuate positive-reacting megakaryocytes. (Periodic acid–Schiff stain) (Fig. 44.33A from Litz CE, Brunning RD. Acute myeloid leukemias. In: Knowles DM, ed. Neoplastic hematopathology. Baltimore: Williams & Wilkins, 1992:1315–49.)

C. High magnification of the biopsy illustrated in B. The blast nuclei are predominantly round or oval with dispersed chromatin. Nucleoli are distinct but not unusually prominent. The mature megakaryocytes have abundant eosinophilic cytoplasm. There are scattered micromegakaryocytes. (Periodic acid–Schiff stain) (Fig. 44.33B from Litz CE, Brunning RD. Acute myeloid leukemias. In: Knowles DM, ed. Neoplastic hematopathology. Baltimore: Williams & Wilkins, 1992:1315–49.)

D. A reticulin stain of the specimen in B and C shows a marked increase in reticulin fibers. (Wilder reticulin stain)

E. Electron micrograph of a blast from the bone marrow specimen illustrated in B–D reacted for platelet peroxidase. The dense reaction product is localized to the nuclear envelope and rough endoplasmic reticulum; the granules and Golgi region are negative. (Lead citrate stain only, X20,000)

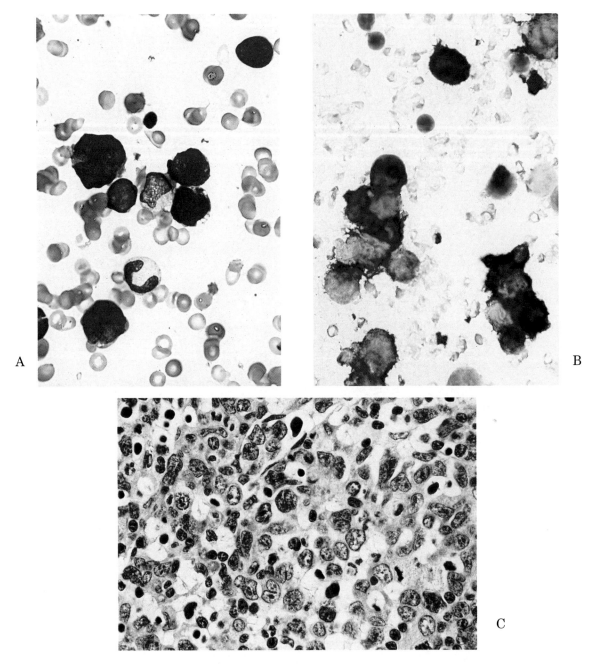

Figure 92

ACUTE MEGAKARYOBLASTIC LEUKEMIA (AML-M7)

A. Bone marrow smear from a 14-month-old child containing large blasts and promegakaryocytes. The promegakaryocytes are larger than the blasts and have a coarse nuclear chromatin and irregularly shaped nuclei; cytoplasmic budding is present. Neutrophil precursors are present. (Wright-Giemsa stain)

B. A bone marrow smear from the case illustrated in A reacted with monoclonal antibody to CD61 (platelet glycoprotein IIIa). A very high percentage of the blasts and promegakaryocytes are positive. The blasts and promegakaryocytes show a tendency to cluster, mimicking metastatic tumor. (Alkaline phosphatase–antialkaline phosphatase stain) (Fig. 44.31 (right) from Litz CE, Brunning RD. Acute myeloid leukemias. In: Knowles DM, ed. Neoplastic hematopathology. Baltimore: Williams & Wilkins, 1992:1315–49.)

C. Trephine biopsy from the case illustrated in A and B. There is extensive infiltration by blasts, which have a sparse amount of cytoplasm and frequently cleft or convoluted nuclei. The nuclear chromatin is finely dispersed and nucleoli are distinct, but not unusually prominent. A small number of erythroblasts and granulocytes are scattered among the leukemic cells. (Hematoxylin and eosin stain)

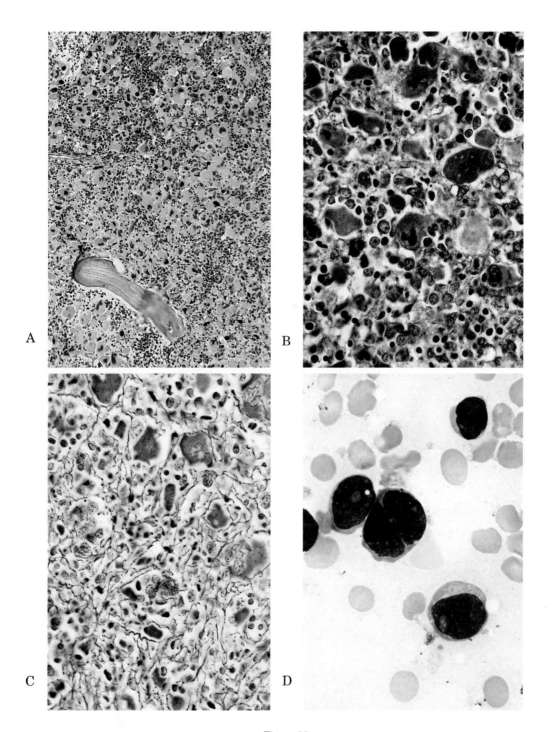

Figure 93
ACUTE MEGAKARYOBLASTIC LEUKEMIA (AML-M7)

A. Bone marrow sections from a 64-year-old male with pancytopenia. There is a marked proliferation of megakaryocytes that show considerable variation in size and nuclear characteristics. (Hematoxylin and eosin stain)

B. High magnification of the specimen in A showing both large megakaryocytes and micromegakaryocytes. Many immature cells and erythrocyte precursors are interspersed among the megakaryocytes. (Periodic acid–Schiff stain)

C. A reticulin stain of the specimen illustrated in A and B showing increased reticulin fibers. (Wilder reticulin stain)

D. A touch preparation of the trephine biopsy illustrated in A–C showing three blasts with basophilic cytoplasm, coarse nuclear chromatin, and distinct nucleoli. (Wright-Giemsa stain)

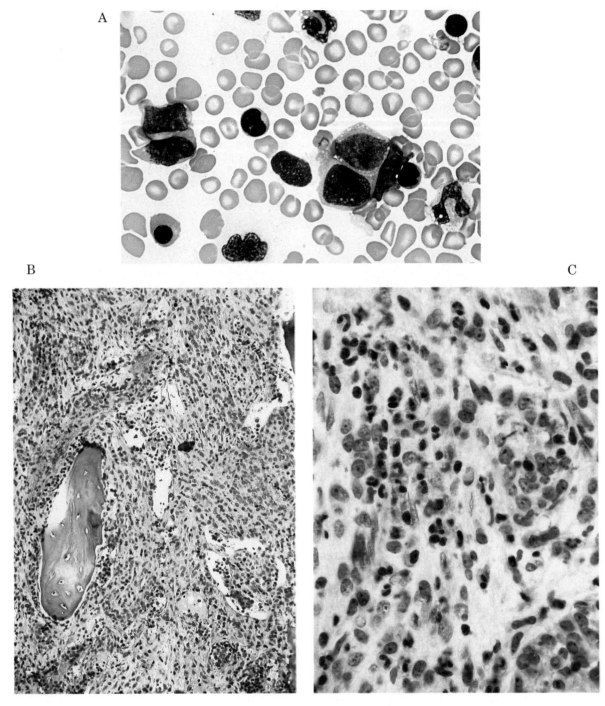

Figure 94
ACUTE PANMYELOSIS ASSOCIATED WITH A t(1;22) CHROMOSOME ABNORMALITY

A. Bone marrow smear from a 5-month-old child with acute myeloid leukemia associated with a t(1;22) chromosome abnormality. There are numerous blasts, some of which expressed CD61. The erythroid and granulocyte cells were also abnormal and the findings were consistent with an acute leukemia involving all myeloid cell lines. (Wright-Giemsa stain)

B. Bone marrow biopsy from the child whose blood smear is illustrated in A. There is partial replacement of normal marrow cells by blasts and an associated increase in fibrous tissue. (Hematoxylin and eosin stain)

C. High magnification of the specimen in B showing numerous blasts, which in this area show a slight tendency to cluster. (Hematoxylin and eosin stain)

Cytochemical and Immunologic Findings. The megakaryoblasts are MPO and SBB negative. They may react with NSE in a focal paranuclear distribution. The acid phosphate reaction may be positive with scattered granules; the pattern is nonspecific. Megakaryoblasts may react with PAS with diffusely scattered positive granules. Promegakaryocytes and mature megakaryocytes are more intensely positive.

Several monoclonal antibodies to platelet glycoproteins are used to identify megakaryoblasts. Antibodies to platelet glycoproteins Ib, IIb/IIIa, and IIIa are the most widely used (32,45). Reactivity of the blasts with one or more of these antibodies may be demonstrated by flow cytometry or immunocytochemistry on smears, imprints, or cytospin preparations. Immunocytochemical methods allow visualization of the cells giving the positive reaction (fig. 92B). Antibodies to CD61 (platelet glycoprotein IIIa) have a high degree of sensitivity for cells of megakaryocyte lineage and are relatively specific; however, cross reactivity of antibodies to platelet glycoproteins with erythroblasts and monocytes has been reported (33). Weak reactivity of rhabdomyosarcoma cells with antibodies to platelet glycoproteins has been observed by the authors. Antibodies to factor VIII–related antigen are less sensitive in the identification of megakaryoblasts. Megakaryoblasts may react with antibodies to HLA-DR, CD33, and CD34 (58). Mature megakaryocytes are negative with these antibodies. Reactivity of megakaryoblasts with antibodies to CD2, the sheep red blood cell receptor normally found in T lymphocytes, has been reported (45).

Immunohistochemical identification of megakaryocyte lineage cells in paraffin-embedded routinely processed marrow biopsies has been reported with the use of antibodies to factor VIII–related antigen and *Ulex europaeus*. However, these antibodies lack the sensitivity and specificity of the monoclonal antibodies to platelet glycoproteins (92).

Histopathologic Findings. The histopathologic findings of AML-M7 in bone marrow biopsies vary from cases with a predominant population of poorly differentiated blasts to cases in which there is clear evidence of differentiation of blasts to megakaryocytes (figs. 91–93). Abnormal megakaryocytic differentiation may be particularly prominent. Micromegakaryocytes, occurring singly, in small clusters, or in broad sheets,

may be numerous. The micromegakaryocytes are characteristically small with a rim of uniform, intensely eosinophilic cytoplasm. Nuclear cytoplasmic asynchrony, characterized by fine nuclear chromatin and a rim of eosinophilic cytoplasm, is common. The nuclei are usually nonlobulated but may be markedly irregular. An important distinguishing feature of the mature megakaryocyte is the smooth, uniformly eosinophilic cytoplasm that varies substantially in amount from cell to cell. The megakaryocytes, including the micromegakaryocytes, are usually accentuated in sections stained with PAS, although there may be substantial variability in reactivity in an individual case: some megakaryocytes react intensely while others show minimal or no staining. Granulocyte and erythroid precursors may be present but are not usually numerous.

AML-M7 may be accompanied by a substantial increase in reticulin fibers (figs. 91D, 93C). Frank collagenous fibrosis is uncommon. The reticulin fiber increase may be relatively uniform or may be focally more marked in perivascular or paratrabecular locations. Bands of reticulin fibers are frequently associated with sheets of maturing megakaryocytes. Marrow fibrosis is not an invariable finding in AML-M7 and cases with a predominance of megakaryoblasts and little or no evidence of maturation may show no significant increase in reticulin fibers.

Blast proliferation, with or without evidence of differentiation to micromegakaryocytes, may be present in extramedullary sites such as lymph nodes (fig. 95).

Ultrastructural Findings. Ultrastructural studies should include the demonstration of platelet peroxidase in the leukemic blasts. Characteristically, the platelet peroxidase reaction product is deposited in the perinuclear envelope and endoplasmic reticulum but not in the Golgi region or small granules (fig. 91E) (32). In contrast in the myeloblast, MPO reaction product is present in the nuclear envelope, endoplasmic reticulum, Golgi region, and granules.

Studies of the specificity and sensitivity of immunophenotyping and ultrastructural demonstration of platelet peroxidase in AML-M7 have shown that platelet peroxidase is present at an earlier stage of development than the platelet glycoproteins (58). In occasional cases there may be a deficiency of platelet peroxidase. Immature erythroid cells from cases of erythroleukemia have

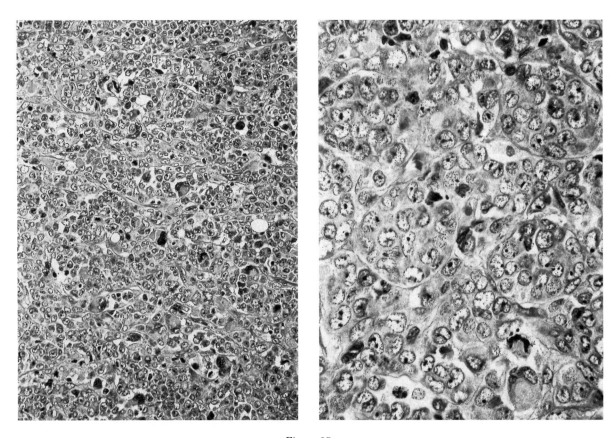

Figure 95
ACUTE MEGAKARYOBLASTIC LEUKEMIA (AML-M7) INFILTRATING A LYMPH NODE

Left: Lymph node biopsy from a 3-year-old child with Down syndrome and acute megakaryoblastic leukemia. There is total effacement of the lymph node by a predominant population of blasts. Scattered megakaryocytes at various stages of maturation are present. (Hematoxylin and eosin stain)

Right: The blasts have finely dispersed nuclear chromatin and small but distinct nucleoli. Occasional nuclei are lobulated. Mitotic figures are present. (Hematoxylin and eosin stain)

been shown to contain a peroxidase reaction similar to that observed in megakaryoblasts; the specificity of the reaction is, thus, uncertain (34).

Differential Diagnosis. The acute leukemias from which AML-M7 must be distinguished include AML-M1, acute monoblastic leukemia (M5A), acute basophilic leukemia, ALL-L1, ALL-L2, AML-M0, and erythremic myelosis. The use of cytochemistry and appropriate immunologic markers distinguish these various types of acute leukemia. In occasional instances, such as in acute basophilic leukemia, electron microscopy may be necessary. Because megakaryoblasts may occur in clusters in marrow smears, metastatic tumor may be included in the differential diagnosis. This clustering effect may be a particular problem in very young children because the clusters may resemble metastatic neuroblastoma or rhabdomyosarcoma.

Distinguishing AML-M7 from acute myelofibrosis may be difficult because of the nature of the immature cell population in a fibrotic bone marrow (17,54). In both disorders the marrow sections may show a blast proliferation with evidence of abnormal megakaryocytic differentiation. Acute myelofibrosis or acute myelosclerosis as described by Bearman et al. (18) is a panmyelopathy with involvement of erythroid cells, granulocytes, and megakaryocytes; increased immature cells of all three lineages and varying degrees of fibrosis are present. AML-M7, in contrast, is primarily a proliferation of one cell line, the megakaryocyte. However, there are cases of AML-M7 which have minor erythroid and granulocytic components. If the marrow is characterized by a proliferation of relatively uniform-appearing blasts with clear evidence of differentiation to megakaryocytes by morphology, immunocytochemistry, or ultrastructural studies, and fibrosis is present, the diagnosis is AML-M7. If the findings are those of blastic panmyeloid hyperplasia with approximately equal proliferations of megakaryocytes, granulocytes, and erythroid precursors with fibrosis, the term *acute myelofibrosis* is more appropriate. In some cases, because of overlapping features, distinction between these two disorders is not always possible and whether it is clinically relevant is unclear.

Acute Myeloid Leukemia Associated with Chromosome Abnormality 3(q21;q26)

An association between AML or myelodysplastic syndromes presenting with normal platelet counts or thrombocytosis, and abnormalities of the long arm of chromosome 3, has been reported (25,29). The platelet count can exceed $1000×10^9$/L. Chromosome 3 abnormalities include structural rearrangements involving bands 3q21 and 3q26.

AMLs associated with these abnormalities are difficult to classify morphologically; AML-M1, AML-M4, and AML-M6 have been reported. These cases generally have associated abnormalities of megakaryocytopoiesis including increased megakaryocytes and micromegakaryocytes. These findings have been associated with an unfavorable prognosis. Figures 96 and 97 illustrate blood and bone marrow findings in AML associated with an inv(3)(q21q26) chromosome abnormality.

The t(3;5) (q25.1;q34) chromosome abnormality has been associated with AML with involvement of the granulocytes, megakaryocytes, and erythroid precursors (fig. 98).

Acute Basophilic Leukemia

Definition. A type of AML in which the predominant differentiation of the blasts is to basophils (78,97).

Incidence and Clinical Findings. Acute basophilic leukemia is a rare form of AML. There are no distinctive clinical features. The majority of patients have some degree of organomegaly and lymphadenopathy. Clinical signs of hyperhistaminemia have been reported (97).

Laboratory Findings. The leukocyte count varies and may exceed $100×10^9$/L. Most patients have anemia and thrombocytopenia.

In some patients there is an associated t(9;22) chromosome abnormality (61,78). Trisomy 21 and deletion 7q- have also been reported (78).

Blood and Bone Marrow Findings. The predominant cells in the blood and bone marrow are agranular blasts that may resemble myeloblasts or lymphoblasts. The cytoplasm may be intensely basophilic. Immature blast-like cells with basophil granules may be present (fig. 99). An increase in mature basophils occurs in a minority of cases. Dysplastic neutrophils may be present.

Cytochemical Findings. In the majority of cases, the blasts are negative for MPO and SBB. The blasts are generally negative with the toluidine blue reaction; granules in the mature basophils are reactive (fig. 100). TdT-positive blasts have been reported (78).

Histopathologic Findings. The bone marrow is generally hypercellular. A moderate increase in reticulin fibers may be present. The blasts have no specific differentiating features (fig. 101). The nuclei may be indented or lobulated and nucleoli may be prominent.

Ultrastructural Findings. The blasts show considerable variability. The amount of cytoplasm varies, the nuclear chromatin is fine to coarse, and nucleoli are usually prominent (fig. 102). The number of blast-like cells with basophil granules varies from 1 to 90 percent. Blasts with mast cell granules may also be present (78).

Differential Diagnosis. The acute leukemias from which acute basophilic leukemia must be distinguished are AML-M1, AML-M0, and ALL. Distinction may not be possible by routine cytochemical stains and immunologic markers. Any evidence of basophil maturation in a poorly differentiated leukemia which is MPO, SBB, NSE, and TdT negative should suggest acute basophilic leukemia. The definitive evidence is ultrastructural.

Myelodysplastic syndromes and AML-M2 may present with increased basophils associated with the t(6;9) chromosome abnormality (52). In these cases the increased basophils are one component of a more generalized myeloid proliferation.

A marked increase in basophils is not uncommon in the accelerated phase or blast crisis of chronic myeloid leukemia; the initial manifestation of chronic myeloid leukemia may be a blast

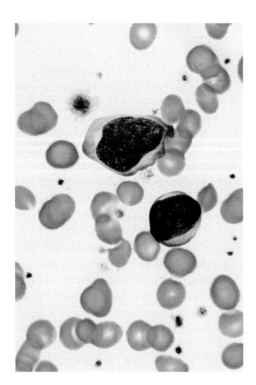 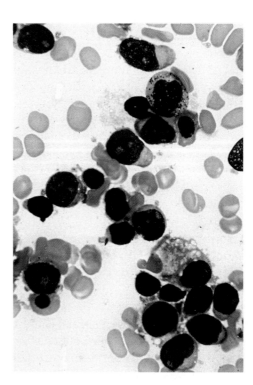

Figure 96
ACUTE MYELOBLASTIC LEUKEMIA WITHOUT MATURATION (AML-M1)
ASSOCIATED WITH INV(3)(q21q26)

Left: Blood smear from an adult male with acute myeloblastic leukemia without maturation and a platelet count of 800×10^9/L. The larger blast is approximately twice the size of the smaller blast. There are numerous platelets that are predominantly small and normal appearing. Cytogenetic studies showed an inv(3)(q21q26) chromosome abnormality. (Wright-Giemsa stain)

Right: Bone marrow smear from the case illustrated on the left. The numerous blasts have prominent nucleoli. A small megakaryocyte with granular cytoplasm is in the lower right quadrant. Two normoblasts and a neutrophil myelocyte are also present. The blasts were MPO and SBB negative. No immunologic or ultrastructural studies were performed and the case was classified as AML-M1. This case was classified as myeloid based on the morphologic evidence of abnormal megakaryocytes. (Wright-Giemsa stain)

Figure 97
ACUTE MYELOBLASTIC
LEUKEMIA WITH
MATURATION ASSOCIATED
WITH INV(3)(q21q26)
AND MONOSOMY 7

Bone marrow biopsy from a 37-year-old woman with AML-M2 associated with inv(3)(q21q26) and monosomy 7. The marrow smear contained approximately 30 percent blasts and numerous small nonlobulated and hypolobulated megakaryocytes. As illustrated, the biopsy shows a marked increase in small megakaryocytes with nonlobulated and hypolobulated nuclei. (Hematoxylin and eosin stain)

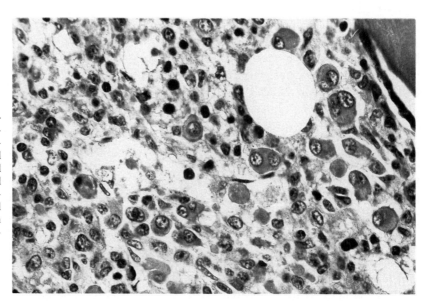

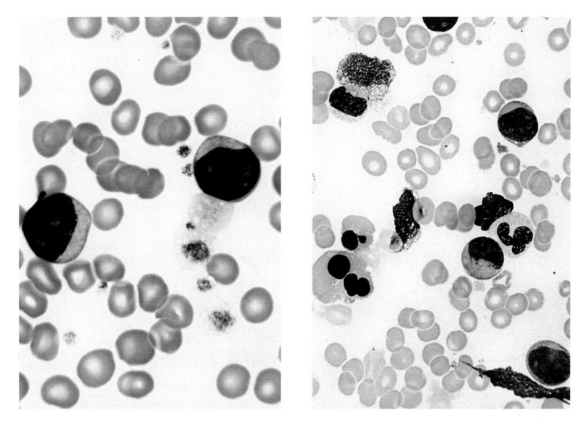

Figure 98
ACUTE MYELOBLASTIC LEUKEMIA WITH MATURATION ASSOCIATED WITH
A t(3;5) CHROMOSOME ABNORMALITY

Left: Blood smear from a 37-year-old man with AML-M2 associated with a t(3;5)(q25.1;q34) chromosome abnormality. The platelet count was 221×10^9/L; an atypical platelet is juxtaposed to a blast. (Wright-Giemsa stain)

Right: Bone marrow smear showing evidence of maturation of the myeloblasts to more mature neutrophils. Dyserythropoietic changes are present. (Wright-Giemsa stain)

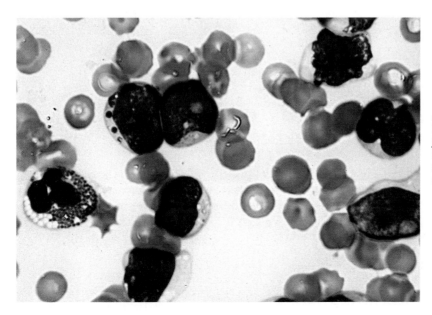

Figure 99
ACUTE BASOPHILIC
LEUKEMIA

Bone marrow smear from an adult male with acute leukemia with basophilic differentiation. The majority of blasts show no differentiating features. One blast contains coarse azurophilic granules. (Wright-Giemsa stain)

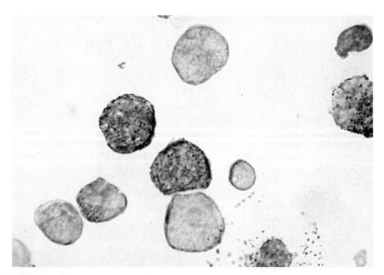

Figure 100
ACUTE BASOPHILIC LEUKEMIA:
TOLUIDINE BLUE REACTION
Bone marrow smear from a patient with acute basophilic leukemia reacted with toluidine blue. Several maturing basophils contain metachromatic granules. (Toluidine blue O stain)

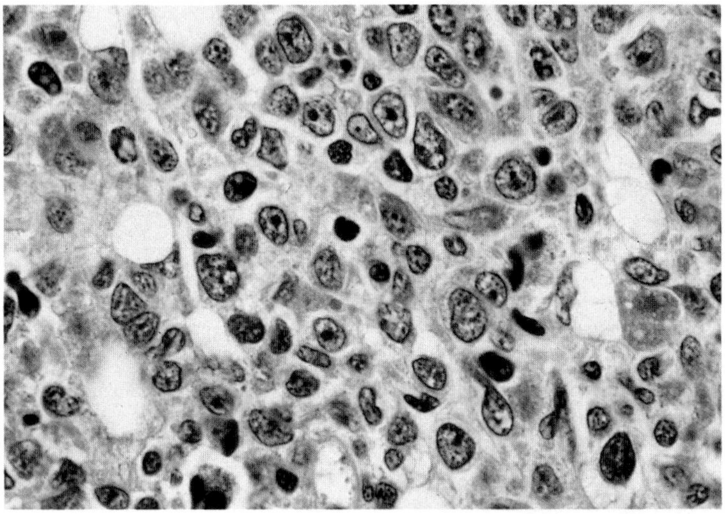

Figure 101
ACUTE BASOPHILIC LEUKEMIA
Bone marrow trephine biopsy from a patient with acute basophilic leukemia in relapse. The blasts and immature basophils show variation in nuclear size and prominence of nucleoli. Scattered plasma cells, endothelial cells, and macrophages with hemosiderin are present. A reticulin stain showed increased reticulin fibers. (Hematoxylin and eosin stain)

Figure 102
ACUTE BASOPHILIC
LEUKEMIA:
ULTRASTRUCTURE
Electron micrograph of an immature basophil in a blood specimen from a patient with acute basophilic leukemia. The granules contain a characteristic speckled amorphous substance. One granule contains a myelin figure. (Uranyl acetate–lead citrate stains, X39,000).

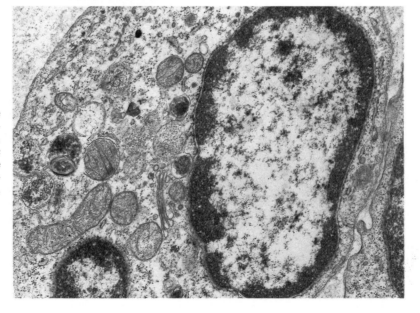

crisis with a marked increase in basophils. These processes are usually characterized by involvement of several myeloid cell lines in contrast to acute basophilic leukemia in which the immature cells are primarily of basophilic lineage.

Hypocellular Acute Myeloid Leukemia

Definition. A type of AML in which the bone marrow cellularity is less than 30 percent (23,40,53). The term does not define a specific cytologic type although the majority of cases are AML-M0, AML-M1, or AML-M2.

Incidence and Clinical Findings. Approximately 5 percent of adult patients presenting with AML have hypocellular bone marrow biopsies. This finding is more common in older individuals; it occurs only rarely in childhood. There is no predominance of either sex.

The presenting clinical findings relate to marrow failure: fatigue and dyspnea due to anemia and infections and hemorrhagic manifestations due to neutropenia and thrombocytopenia.

Laboratory Findings. The majority of patients are markedly pancytopenic.

Blood and Bone Marrow Findings. The blast percentage in the marrow and/or blood is 30 percent or more. The classification is usually AML-M0, AML-M1, or AML-M2. There may be clear evidence of differentiation of the blasts to more mature granulocytes that may manifest dysplastic features. In other instances, the non-blast population consists almost exclusively of mature lymphocytes and plasma cells with few or no granulocyte precursors. Occasional blasts may be present in the blood.

Cytochemical Findings. Blast reactivity for MPO and SBB varies and is often less than 3 percent, similar to the findings in AML-M0. In these instances, the evidence for myeloid differentiation is based on immunologic or ultrastructural studies.

Histopathologic Findings. The bone marrow, by definition, is less than 30 percent cellular. In some cases the cellularity is 10 to 15 percent and resembles aplastic anemia (fig. 103). The predominant cells have the features of blasts: a high nuclear-cytoplasmic ratio, fine chromatin, and one to three variably prominent nucleoli. Maturing granulocytes, erythroid cells, and scattered megakaryocytes may be present.

Ultrastructural Findings. The blasts have the features of the blasts observed in AML-M0 and AML-M1. In occasional cases they have the characteristics of monoblasts.

Differential Diagnosis. The major disorder from which hypoplastic AML must be distinguished is hypoplastic or aplastic anemia. The similarity relates both to the hypoplastic marrow sections and the marked pancytopenia. The cytologic characteristics of the predominant cells distinguish the two. In aplastic or hypoplastic anemia, the erythroid cells, granulocytes, and megakaryocytes are markedly reduced in the marrow and the predominant cell is a well-differentiated lymphocyte. Plasma cells and mast cells may also be present. Blasts are not increased and are usually difficult to find.

Acute Myeloid Leukemia and Transient Myeloproliferative Disorder in Down Syndrome

Individuals with Down syndrome have an incidence of acute leukemia estimated at 18 to 21 times that of normal individuals (46,82). The leukemia may be of myeloid or lymphocytic type. In children less than 1 year of age, the leukemia is predominantly myeloid, usually with distinctive morphologic features. There may be prominent extramedullary manifestations with extensive lymphadenopathy and hepatosplenomegaly.

The major differential diagnosis of AML in individuals with Down syndrome is a transient myeloproliferative disorder (TMD) that occurs primarily in the neonatal period. TMD is morphologically indistinguishable from AML (26, 43,46,51). The leukocyte count ranges up to 100×10^9/L and there may be a severe thrombocytopenia. The hemoglobin level is generally normal or slightly decreased. The blast count in the blood varies but is usually in excess of 30 percent. The blasts have stippled chromatin, prominent nucleoli, and a scant to moderate amount of basophilic cytoplasm (figs. 104, 105). In a majority of cases, the blasts contain coarse azurophilic granules which on ultrastructural study are theta granules (fig. 106). These structures have been reported in cells of both basophil and erythroid origin (33,36). Numerous promyelocytes and micromegakaryocytes are usually present. The neutrophils may show no abnormalities or slight myelodysplastic changes.

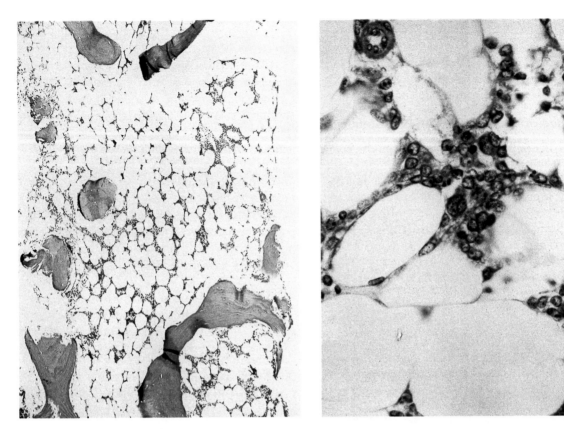

Figure 103
HYPOCELLULAR ACUTE MYELOID LEUKEMIA
Left: Bone marrow biopsy from a 57-year-old male with severe pancytopenia and rare blasts in the blood. The marrow is markedly hypocellular for the age of the patient. (Hematoxylin and eosin stain)

Right: High magnification of the specimen illustrated on the left. The cells in the interstitium consist predominantly of blasts. (Hematoxylin and eosin stain)

Figure 104
TRANSIENT MYELOPROLIFERATIVE DISORDER IN DOWN SYNDROME

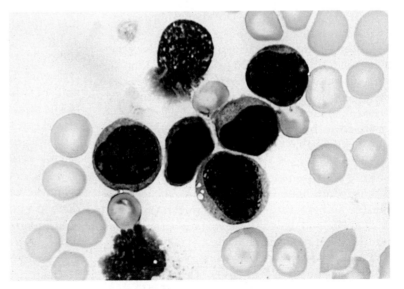

Blood smear from a 3-day-old female with Down syndrome. The leukocyte count was 62×10^9/L, the hemoglobin level was 16.2 g/dL, the platelet count was 28×10^9/L. The smear contained 50 to 55 percent blasts as illustrated. A similar percentage of blasts was present in the bone marrow. The blasts have basophilic cytoplasm, dispersed nuclear chromatin, and several distinct nucleoli. Azurophilic granules are present in one of the blasts. The leukocyte count increased to 77×10^9/L on day 5 and gradually diminished over 8 weeks at which time the blood smear was normal. There was no recurrence with a 5-year follow-up. (Wright-Giemsa stain)

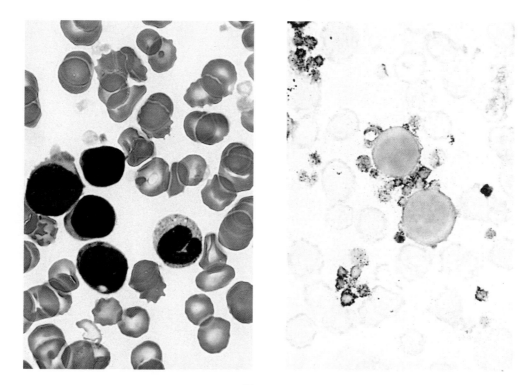

Figure 105
TRANSIENT MYELOPROLIFERATIVE DISORDER IN DOWN SYNDROME

Left: Blood smear from a 20-day-old female with Down syndrome. The leukocyte count was 54×10^9/L, hemoglobin level 16.4 g/dL, and the platelet count within normal limits. Approximately 50 percent of the leukocytes were blasts. The platelets are very large; occasional platelets are poorly granulated. The leukocyte count returned to normal within 3 weeks. Three months later the leukocyte count increased following a bacterial infection; blast cells were numerous. The process spontaneously regressed but relapsed 2 months later, at which time the child was treated for acute leukemia. (Wright-Giemsa stain)

Right: Blood smear from the patient described on the left reacted with monoclonal antibody to CD61 (platelet glycoprotein IIIa). The micromegakaryocytes, promegakaryocytes, and platelets are positive; the blasts were nonreactive. (Alkaline phosphatase–antialkaline phosphatase stain)

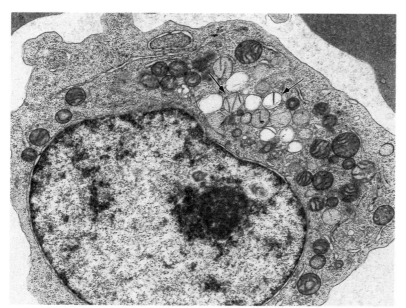

Figure 106
TRANSIENT MYELOPROLIFERATIVE DISORDER IN A NEONATE WITH DOWN SYNDROME: ULTRASTRUCTURE

Electron micrograph of an immature cell from a blood specimen from a 10-day-old patient with Down syndrome and transient myeloproliferative disorder. The cell has abundant cytoplasm and a nucleus with finely dispersed chromatin and a prominent nucleolus. The cytoplasm contains numerous mitochondria and theta granules (arrows). The theta granules have a central bisecting membrane. (Uranyl acetate–lead citrate stains, X25,000).

The blasts are negative for MPO, SBB, CAE, NSE, and TdT; usually express CD7, CD34, and CD36; and show variable expression of CD13, CD14, and CD33. The promegakaryocytes, micro-megakaryocytes, and megakaryocytes are reactive with antibodies to the platelet glycoproteins CD41a and CD61 (fig. 105, right). The bone marrow sections are hypercellular with increased immature cells; some cells may show evidence of megakaryocytic differentiation.

Because TMD is morphologically indistinguishable from AML, the diagnosis of AML in Down syndrome individuals in the first year of life and particularly in the neonatal period should be made with extreme caution (43). TMD usually undergoes spontaneous remission in 2 to 14 weeks; it may recur following a bacterial or viral infection. Persistence or recurrence of the process, deteriorating hematologic findings, and specific cytogenetic abnormalities are evidence for a leukemic process (fig. 107).

Leukemoid proliferation identical to the TMD in Down individuals may occur in rare instances in phenotypically normal individuals during the neonatal period (fig. 108) (35). The hematopoietic cells may show a trisomy 21. As with TMD, the hematologic abnormalities are transient and with regression of the process there is loss of the trisomy 21 in the hematopoietic cells.

Acute Myelofibrosis

Definition. An acute panmyeloid proliferation with accompanying bone marrow fibrosis (54). Other terms for this disorder include *acute myelosclerosis* and *acute myelodysplasia with myelofibrosis* (18,64,88). This disorder may occur in patients previously treated with chemotherapy and radiation (88).

Incidence and Clinical Findings. This form of myeloproliferative disorder is distinctly uncommon. It is primarily a disease of adults and occurs rarely in children.

Patients present with constitutional symptoms including weakness and fatigue; easy bruisability is a frequent complaint. In contrast to chronic idiopathic myelofibrosis (agnogenic myeloid metaplasia), there is no or minimal splenomegaly. The clinical course is generally rapidly progressive, similar to AML.

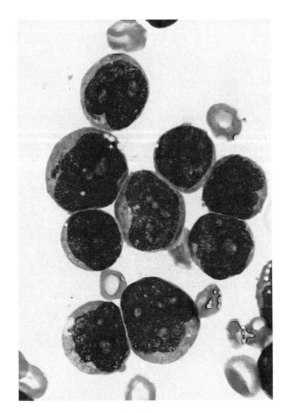

Figure 107
ACUTE MYELOID LEUKEMIA
IN DOWN SYNDROME

Bone marrow smear from a child with Down syndrome and acute myeloblastic leukemia with maturation (M2). This patient was observed for 5 months before the diagnosis of acute leukemia was established. During this period there was a gradual increase in the marrow blasts and progressive marrow failure. Several of the blasts have coarse basophilic granules, similar to the blasts in the transient myeloproliferative syndrome associated with trisomy 21. The blasts were nonreactive with MPO and SBB but expressed CD13 and CD33. (Wright-Giemsa stain) (Fig. 44.39 from Litz CE, Brunning RD. Acute myeloid leukemias. In: Knowles DM, ed. Neoplastic hematopathology. Baltimore: Williams & Wilkins, 1992:1315–49.)

Laboratory Findings. The majority of patients present with a pancytopenia that is frequently marked.

Blood and Bone Marrow Findings. Bone marrow aspiration is usually unsuccessful and the major findings are in the trephine biopsies. The marrow biopsy is hypercellular with varying degrees of hyperplasia of the erythroid precursors, granulocytes, and megakaryocytes. Foci of immature cells, including blasts, are scattered throughout (fig. 109). Clusters of late stage erythroid

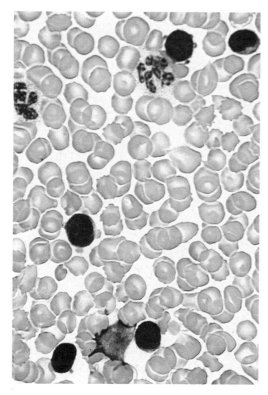

Figure 108
TRANSIENT MYELOPROLIFERATIVE DISORDER
IN A PHENOTYPICALLY NORMAL NEWBORN
WITH TRISOMY 21 IN MYELOID CELLS

Blood smear from a phenotypically normal newborn with a leukocyte count of 30×10^9/L, a hemoglobin level of 17.5 g/dL, and a platelet count of 40×10^9/L. Approximately 60 percent of the cells in the blood were blasts, some of which had pseudopod formation. Hypersegmented neutrophils are present. Chromosome analysis of a blood specimen obtained at the time of this blood smear showed a trisomy 21 in the hematopoietic cells; analysis of epithelial cells showed a normal karyotype. Chromosome analysis of a bone marrow specimen at 12 weeks of age, when the bone marrow and blood appeared normal, showed a normal karyotype. There was no recurrence of the proliferative process within a 9-year follow-up. (Wright-Giemsa stain)

precursors may be prominent. Abnormal megakaryocytes may be particularly conspicuous; small to large megakaryocytes with dysplastic features are usually present and micromegakaryocytes may be numerous. The nuclei of the micromegakaryocytes are frequently nonlobulated with dispersed chromatin. The cytoplasm is uniformly eosinophilic. The megakaryocytes are accentuated in sections reactive with PAS.

The degree of fibrosis varies. In most patients there is a marked increase in reticulin fibers (fig. 109C). Frank collagenous fibrosis is less common.

The blood is usually characterized by severe pancytopenia. The red blood cells show no or minimal poikilocytosis. Occasional immature cells of the neutrophil cell line, including blasts, may be identified. Variations of this pattern occur and there may be substantial differences in the morphologic findings in the blood.

Differential Diagnosis. The differential diagnosis of acute myelofibrosis includes acute leukemia with associated bone marrow fibrosis, metastatic tumor with a desmoplastic reaction, and chronic idiopathic myelofibrosis.

Acute leukemia with associated fibrosis is distinguished by the predominance of one cell line. Acute myelofibrosis is basically a panmyelosis with proliferation of granulocytes, erythroid precursors, and megakaryocytes; the proportion of these cells varies. The distinction between these two processes may not always be histologically possible and whether it is clinically relevant is questionable (17). Acute myelofibrosis is distinguished from chronic idiopathic myelofibrosis by the predominance of more immature cells in the acute process and the characteristics of the megakaryocytes. In chronic idiopathic myelofibrosis the majority of the megakaryocytes have condensed nuclear chromatin in contrast to the dispersed, stippled chromatin in the acute process. Physical findings in the chronic disorder invariably include splenomegaly, which may be marked. Splenomegaly is absent or minimal in the acute process. Metastatic tumor is excluded by studies with appropriate antibodies to both hematopoietic and nonhematopoietic cells.

Treatment and Prognosis. The published clinical data on this entity are based on a small number of cases. In addition, there is some overlap in the data between cases of what is defined as acute myelofibrosis and AML with fibrosis. In general, acute myelofibrosis follows an aggressive clinical course similar to AML and the therapy is essentially the same. In some instances the clinical course may be inexplicably prolonged.

Granulocytic Sarcoma

Definition. A tumor mass of immature myeloid cells occurring in an extramedullary site (81).

Incidence and Clinical Findings. Granulocytic sarcomas are uncommon and the exact incidence is not determined. They appear to be more

A

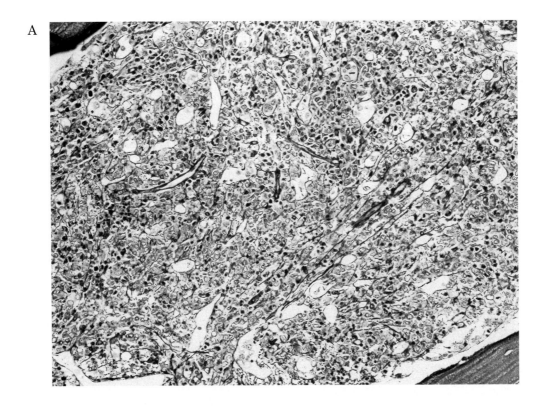

B

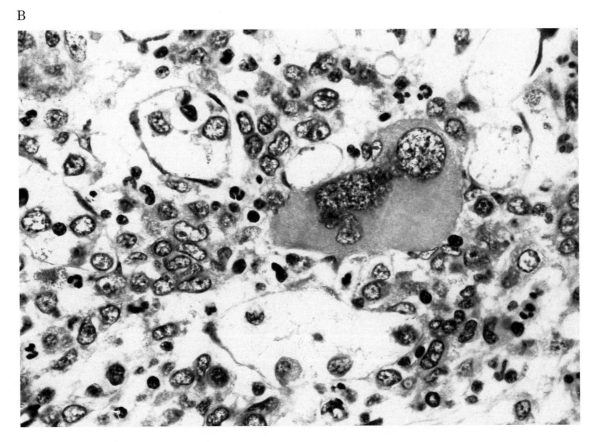

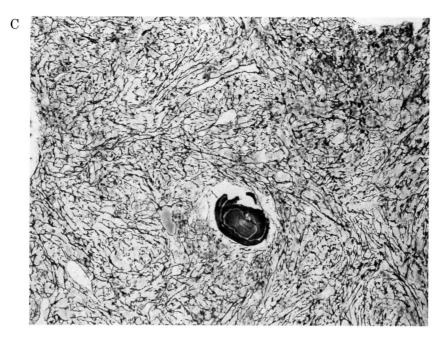

Figure 109
ACUTE MYELOFIBROSIS
A. Reticulin stained bone marrow biopsy from a patient with pancytopenia and occasional blasts in the blood. The marrow is markedly hypercellular with a proliferation of blasts and maturing cells. Increased coarse reticulin fibers are present. (Wilder reticulin stain)

B. High magnification of a hematoxylin and eosin stained section of the specimen illustrated in A. The predominant cells are blasts with evidence of maturation to more mature granulocytes. Occasional scattered segmented neutrophils and late stage erythroblasts are noted. A large megakaryocyte with a poorly lobulated nucleus and dispersed chromatin contrasts with the blasts. (Hematoxylin and eosin stain)

C. High magnification of a reticulin stain of the specimen illustrated in A and B shows an increase in coarse reticulin fibers. (Wilder reticulin stain)

common in children than in adults (81). These lesions may occur as isolated tumor masses without blood or bone marrow evidence of myeloid leukemia or in association with AML, chronic myeloid leukemia, chronic idiopathic myelofibrosis, hypereosinophilic syndrome, or polycythemia vera (68,72,98). The most frequent association is with AML and chronic myeloid leukemia; granulocytic sarcoma should be suspected whenever a tumor mass occurs in a patient with a myeloproliferative disorder. When a granulocytic sarcoma arises outside the context of a myeloproliferative disorder, as an isolated finding, the possibility of an incorrect diagnosis is increased because of the similarity of these lesions to poorly differentiated lymphoma (68).

The most common sites of occurrence are subperiostial bone structures of the skull, paranasal sinuses, sternum, ribs, vertebrae, and pelvis. Lymph nodes and skin are also frequent sites of involvement. The lesions may present in the orbit or spinal canal and lead to proptosis or neurologic deficits. The lesions may also present as mediastinal masses. An isolated granulocytic sarcoma may precede blood and bone marrow manifestations of leukemia by months or years. In occasional instances, there is no progression beyond the extramedullary site (68).

A very careful blood and bone marrow examination should be performed for every patient with a granulocytic sarcoma. In some instances, the blood or marrow involvement is characterized by only a rare blast with an Auer rod.

Laboratory Findings. The hemoglobin level, leukocyte count, and platelet count may be normal in those patients in whom a granulocytic sarcoma is an isolated lesion unrelated to a myeloproliferative process. If the granulocytic sarcoma occurs in the context of a myeloproliferative process such as chronic myeloid leukemia,

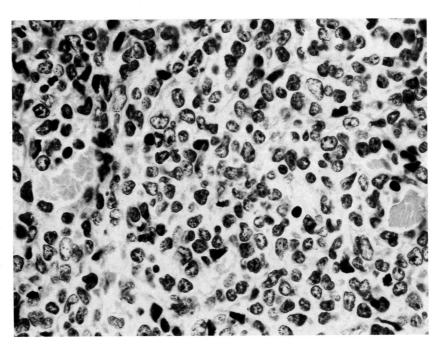

Figure 110
GRANULOCYTIC SARCOMA
Sections of a mediastinal mass from a 19-year-old male with back pain and dyspnea. The immature cells have stippled chromatin and small nucleoli. The CAE stain was negative. The blasts were CD7 and CD33 positive on flow cytometry. Rare blasts were detected in the blood smear. The blast percentage in the marrow smear was in the normal range but occasional blasts contained Auer rods. The patient achieved remission following chemotherapy for AML and, subsequently, received an allogeneic bone marrow transplant. (Hematoxylin and eosin stain)

chronic myeloid leukemia in blast crisis, or acute myeloid leukemia, the findings in the blood are those of the primary process.

An association of granulocytic sarcoma and AML-M2 with the t(8;21) chromosome abnormality has been reported (fig. 43) (90).

Pathologic Findings. Because of the high MPO content of some granulocytic sarcomas, there may be a greenish appearance on cut surface and the descriptive term chloroma was used for these lesions in earlier literature. Tumors composed of poorly differentiated myeloblasts may contain minimal amounts of MPO and lack a green appearance.

Histopathologic Findings. Granulocytic sarcoma can be classified histologically according to the degree of differentiation: blastic, immature, or differentiated (68). The blastic type is composed of myeloblasts with little or no evidence of differentiation to promyelocytes (fig. 110). The myeloblasts have a slight to moderate rim of basophilic cytoplasm and fine nuclear chromatin. Two to four distinct nucleoli are present. The nuclear outline may show some degree of irregularity. The immature type contains principally myeloblasts and promyelocytes; eosinophils and neutrophil myelocytes may also be present (fig. 111). The differentiated type is composed primarily of promyelocytes and more mature neutrophils and eosinophils (fig. 112).

The blastic type is the most difficult to recognize, particularly in the absence of a leukemic process. The CAE reaction, which stains neutrophils and precursors, is positive if promyelocytes and more mature stages are present (fig. 111B). However, myeloblasts at an early stage of development may not react for CAE. The blasts in the more undifferentiated lesions may be identified with immunohistologic techniques utilizing antibodies to myeloid cells, such as antimyeloperoxidase, antilysozyme, antileukocyte elastase, and anti-Cathepsin G (fig. 111C) (70,79,92,96). Antimyeloperoxidase and antilysozyme antibodies are particularly useful (79). Touch preparations stained with a Romanowsky stain are superior to section preparations for the recognition of the granulocytic nature of a tumor mass. Auer rods may be found and the MPO and SBB stains are usually definitive.

A variant of granulocytic sarcoma that may be a particular diagnostic problem is a monoblastic tumor mass (77). Monoblastic tumors may be concurrent with or precede blood and bone marrow findings of acute monoblastic leukemia. Because of the large size of some monoblasts, these lesions may be mistaken for a large cell lymphoma. The CAE reaction, which may react weakly with monoblasts in smears and imprints, is not readily detected in monoblasts in tissue

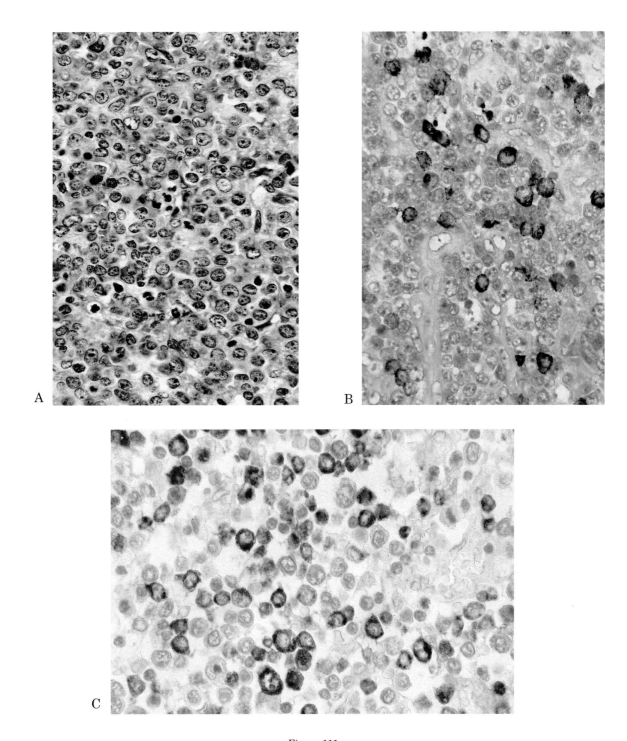

Figure 111
GRANULOCYTIC SARCOMA

A. Lymph node–associated mass from the anterior cervical region of a 7-year-old male. Most of the cells are immature, with round to oval nuclei with distinct, relatively prominent, eosinophilic nucleoli. The majority of cells have moderate to abundant cytoplasm. Several immature eosinophils are present. (Hematoxylin and eosin stain)

B. CAE stain of the specimen illustrated in A showing numerous positive-reacting cells. The intensity of the reaction varies.

C. Antimyeloperoxidase reaction on the specimen illustrated in A and B. Numerous positive-reacting cells are present. (Alkaline phosphatase–antialkaline phosphatase stain)

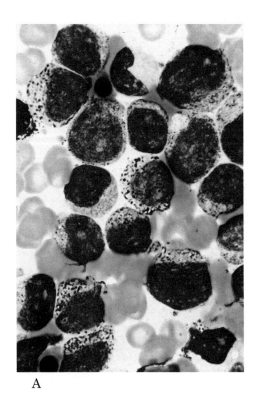

A

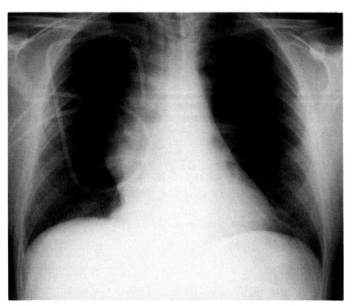

B

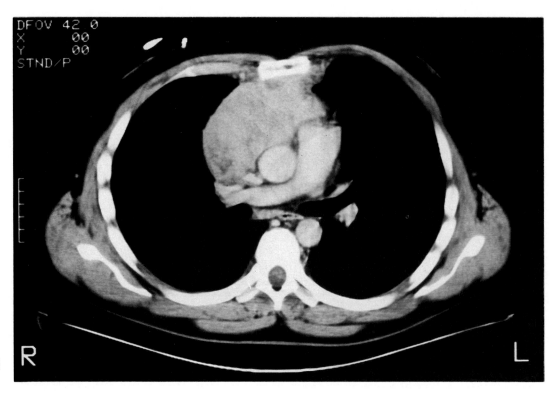

C

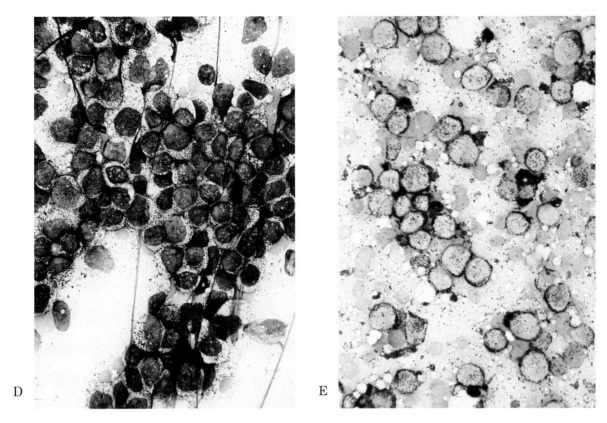

Figure 112
GRANULOCYTIC SARCOMA ASSOCIATED WITH AML-M2

A. Bone marrow aspirate from a 47-year-old male with an anterior mediastinal mass. The cells have numerous azurophilic granules and are type III blasts and promyelocytes. The process was classified as AML-M2 and the patient was treated with adriamycin, cytosine arabinoside, and 6-thioguanine. A complete bone marrow remission was attained, but the size of the mediastinal mass did not change. (Wright-Giemsa stain)

B. Chest X ray of patient described in A showing widening of the anterior superior mediastinum.

C. CT scan of the chest showing a very large anterior superior mediastinal mass.

D. Fine-needle aspiration specimen from the mediastinal mass illustrated in B and C. The specimen was obtained following chemotherapy for AML at which time the bone marrow was in remission. The cell population is identical to the cell population in the marrow aspirate illustrated in A. (Wright-Giemsa stain)

E. MPO reaction of the fine-needle aspiration specimen. The mediastinal mass was subsequently treated with radiotherapy. A suboptimal response was obtained. The patient died 4 months following diagnosis from bone marrow relapse.

sections. Reaction with antibodies to lysozyme and CD68 is usually positive; the reaction with anti-Cathepsin G may be negative or weakly positive (70).

Differential Diagnosis. The major lesions from which a granulocytic sarcoma must be distinguished are non-Hodgkin lymphoma and poorly differentiated carcinoma. The more poorly differentiated granulocytic sarcomas may be particularly problematic because of the lack of distinguishing features. The presence of immature eosinophils and more mature cells of the neutrophil series should suggest the possibility of a granulocytic lesion. CAE stains and immunoperoxidase reactions utilizing antibodies to neutrophils and monocytes will frequently be diagnostic. Panels of monoclonal antibodies in immunoperoxidase studies of poorly differentiated lymphomas should always include neutrophil and monocyte antibodies.

Treatment. Granulocytic sarcomas occurring in the absence of blood and bone marrow involvement may respond to local radiation therapy. The process in the majority of patients evolves to a form of AML. In some patients the evolution will be manifest as tumor masses at additional sites (68). In some instances, local irradiation appears to be curative.

Treatment and Prognosis of AML

The initial treatment of AML is uniform for all the subtypes and is generally based on combination chemotherapy. The most efficacious regimen employed in front-line protocols for newly diagnosed untreated adults with AML consists of a combination of an anthracycline (daunorubicin or doxorubicin) and cytosine arabinoside, with or without 6-thioguanine. Remission rates in the range of 65 to 70 percent are achieved with these drug combinations (65). Uncontrolled trials using high dose cytosine arabinoside as a single agent or in combination with L-asparaginase and prednisone have resulted in response rates ranging from 41 to 65 percent (65). The response with either regimen is influenced considerably by the age of the patient: approximately 75 percent of patients less than 60 years of age have a complete response to an anthracycline and cytosine arabinoside; approximately 50 percent of patients over the age of 60 achieve remission (65).

The duration of the remission in AML is prolonged by the administration of postremission chemotherapy employing the same agents used in the initial induction. Maintenance chemotherapy has also been reported to prolong remission in some patients (93,94). The duration of median remission for adult patients receiving postinduction therapy was 30 months compared to 12 months for patients not receiving such therapy.

In children, the combination of an anthracycline, cytosine arabinoside, and 5-azacytidine plus consolidation therapy results in a remission rate of approximately 70 percent, comparable to the results in adults less than 60 years of age (59). The median duration of remission is approximately 1 year in most studies.

Several prognostic factors are interactive in AML. Individuals over the age of 60 do less well than younger individuals and patients with marked leukocytosis are at higher risk than patients with lower white blood cell counts. The complications of disseminated intravascular coagulation, which occurs in a high percentage of patients with acute promyelocytic leukemia,

places this group of patients at greater risk during the initial phase of the disease. Chromosome changes appear to be one of the more important factors in predicting survival and, as noted in Table 9, certain chromosome alterations have been associated with either a favorable or unfavorable prognosis (101).

ACUTE LYMPHOBLASTIC LEUKEMIAS

The acute lymphoblastic leukemias (ALLs) are systemic neoplastic proliferations of lymphoblasts that have their origin in a bone marrow lymphocyte progenitor cell.

ALL is the most common type of leukemia in children, accounting for approximately 80 to 85 percent of cases, whereas in adults only approximately 20 percent of cases of acute leukemia are ALL. Overall, 70 percent of cases of ALL occur in patients less than 17 years of age. Males are affected more often than females by a ratio of 1.4 to 1 (165). In pediatric patients, 80 to 88 percent of cases of ALL are classified as FAB-L1, 8 to 18 percent are L2, and 1 to 3 percent are L3 (106, 155,156,160,161,194). In adults 35 to 40 percent of cases are L1, approximately 60 percent are L2, and 1 to 3 percent are L3 (106,110).

Onset of clinical manifestations may be acute or insidious. The presenting signs and symptoms are similar to those of AML and are usually related to blood cytopenias. Lethargy, malaise, fever, and infection are the most common. In children extremity and joint pain are common early complaints. Symptoms related to bleeding occur in approximately 25 percent of cases. The most frequent physical findings are pallor, organomegaly, ecchymoses or petechia, and lymphadenopathy. In a minority of patients the presenting clinical manifestations are caused by extramedullary leukemic infiltrates. Central nervous system, testicular, renal, and bone and joint involvement are the most common but any organ system can be affected.

Blood counts are abnormal in more than 90 percent of cases; there is usually bicytopenia or pancytopenia. Anemia is the most common abnormality and may be mild to severe. The red cell indices are generally normochromic and normocytic and the reticulocyte count is decreased. Approximately 75 percent of patients have platelet counts below 100×10^9/L; 15 percent have

Table 14

FAB CLASSIFICATION OF ACUTE LYMPHOBLASTIC LEUKEMIAS*

Cytologic Features	L1	L2	L3
Cell size	Small cells predominate	Large, heterogeneous in size	Medium to large and homogeneous
Amount of cytoplasm	Scant	Variable, often moderately abundant	Moderately abundant
Nucleoli	Not visible, or small and inconspicuous	One or more present, often large	One or more present, often prominent
Nuclear shape	Regular, occasional clefting or indentation	Irregular, clefting and indentation common	Regular, oval to round
Nuclear chromatin	Homogeneous in any one case	Variable, heterogeneous in any one case	Finely stippled and homogeneous
Basophilia of cytoplasm	Variable, usually moderate	Variable, occasionally intense	Intensely basophilic
Cytoplasmic vacuolation	Variable	Variable	Prominent

* Data from reference 105.

less than 10×10^9/L. Bleeding manifestations are generally found in patients with severely depressed platelet counts.

Approximately one fourth of patients present with leukopenia or leukocyte counts in the low normal range. Half of the patients have leukocyte counts between 5 and 25×10^9/L and 10 percent have more than 100×10^9/L. Lymphoblasts are present in blood smears in the majority of cases, including most of the patients that present with leukopenia. The neutrophil count is usually reduced. The rate of infections increases with the severity of neutropenia.

Classification

The French-American-British (FAB) Cooperative Group classification separates the lymphoblastic leukemias into three morphologic types: L1, L2, and L3, defined by the cytologic features of the lymphoblasts in Romanowsky stained bone marrow smears (105). The criteria for the FAB classification are listed in Table 14. Cell size, amount of cytoplasm, and prominence of nucleoli are the most important criteria for distinguishing L1 from L2. Cytoplasmic basophilia and vacuolation are important defining characteristics of ALL-L3.

A scoring system was introduced by the FAB group to facilitate distinguishing ALL-L1 and L2 (106). The system includes four cytologic criteria: nuclear-cytoplasmic ratio, nucleoli, nuclear membrane irregularity, and lymphoblast size. Other modifications of the FAB classification have also been proposed (160). The nuclear-cytoplasmic ratio and the presence of nucleoli appear to be the most significant morphologic features separating L1 and L2 and defining clinical groups (155). In the recent past, a designation as L1 or L2 was an independent indicator of prognosis, with cases of L2 having an earlier relapse and shorter median survival period. With present day treatment protocols, the distinction between these two groups appears to be of decreasing importance (136,145,155,160,161,194).

Acute Lymphoblastic Leukemia, L1 (ALL-L1)

Blood and Bone Marrow Findings. The majority of the lymphoblasts in ALL-L1 are small, approximately twice the size of normal small lymphocytes, with sparse cytoplasm and a high nuclear-cytoplasmic ratio. The nucleus is generally round or oval but some cells have an indented or convoluted nuclear outline. In some

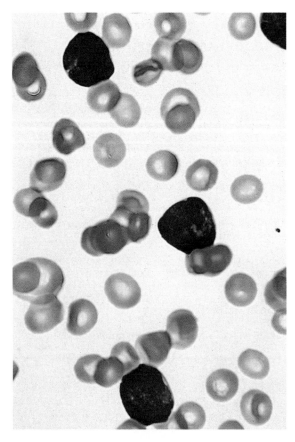

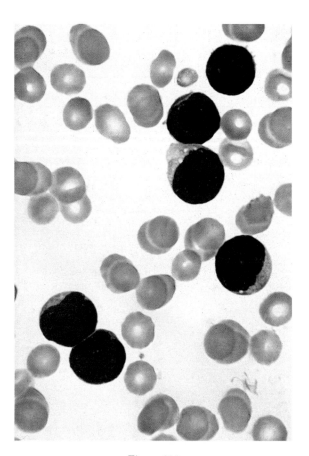

Figure 113
ACUTE LYMPHOBLASTIC LEUKEMIA, L1 (ALL-L1)
A blood smear from a 3-year-old female with ALL-L1 with an early B-cell precursor immunophenotype. The blasts are relatively small with minimal cytoplasm, coarse nuclear chromatin, and no visible nucleoli. The nuclei have a moderately irregular contour. The blast on the top is cleaved. The erythrocyte and platelet counts are reduced. (Wright-Giemsa stain)

Figure 114
ACUTE LYMPHOBLASTIC LEUKEMIA, L1 (ALL-L1)
The lymphoblasts on this blood smear from a 10-year-old male with T-cell ALL have coarse nuclear chromatin and more cytoplasm than those in figure 113. Some of the cells have small indistinct nucleoli. The cytoplasm is variably basophilic. (Wright-Giemsa stain)

cases lymphoblasts with convoluted nuclei predominate. The chromatin is usually uniformly homogeneous in an individual case but may be more finely dispersed in larger lymphoblasts and more condensed in small blasts. Nucleoli are small and indistinct or not visualized. The sparse cytoplasm is variably basophilic. Vacuoles are often present but only rarely are they as abundant or distinctive as in ALL-L3. A minority of the lymphoblasts may exhibit variant morphology, with features more typical of L2 lymphoblasts (figs. 113–116).

Cytochemical Findings. The cytochemical characteristics of the lymphoblasts in ALL are listed in Table 15. They are always MPO negative but may be SBB positive in rare cases. The PAS

stain is positive in 70 to 75 percent of cases; the stain is distributed in coarse granules or clumps in the cytoplasm and generally corresponds to glycogen deposits (fig. 117) (158).

Histopathologic Findings. In trephine biopsy sections, the bone marrow is usually markedly hypercellular (fig. 118). Normal hematopoietic cells are replaced by a uniform, diffuse proliferation of lymphoblasts. Scattered megakaryocytes and small collections of normoblasts may be observed (fig. 119). The lymphoblasts are relatively uniform cytologically. The cytoplasm is barely discernable in the majority of cells. The nuclei are mostly medium sized with evenly dispersed chromatin and small inconspicuous nucleoli. Nuclear contour is often heterogeneous; convoluted cells

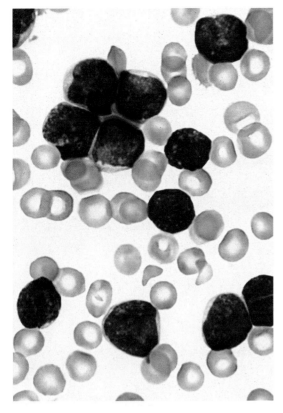

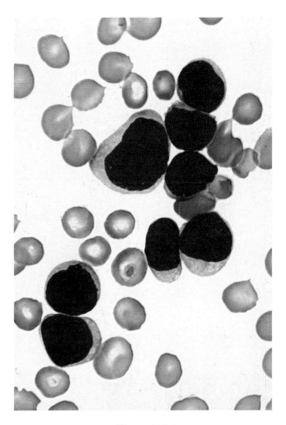

Figure 115
ACUTE LYMPHOBLASTIC LEUKEMIA, L1 (ALL-L1)
The lymphoblasts in this bone marrow smear from a 3-year-old male with ALL-L1 show moderate variation in size and density of nuclear chromatin. There is minimal cytoplasm. The nuclear contour is irregular. Some of the blasts have small nucleoli. (Wright-Giemsa stain)

Figure 116
ACUTE LYMPHOBLASTIC LEUKEMIA, L1 (ALL-L1)
A bone marrow smear from a 22-year-old female. The blasts in this case show a spectrum of size and moderate variation in chromatin density. Most of the blasts have a moderate amount of cytoplasm, round nuclei, and relatively coarse chromatin. Some resemble mature lymphocytes. (Wright-Giemsa stain)

Table 15

CYTOCHEMICAL REACTIONS IN ACUTE LYMPHOBLASTIC LEUKEMIA

| | ALL | | | |
	L1	L2	L3	AML
Myeloperoxidase and Sudan black B	−	−	−	+
Nonspecific esterase	+/− (focal)	+/−	−	+ (monocytic)
Periodic acid–Schiff	+ ($\approx$75%)	+	−	+/−
Acid phosphatase	+ (T cell)	+	−	+/−
Oil red O	−	−	+ (vacuoles)	−
Methyl green pyronine	+/−	+/−	+	+/−

103

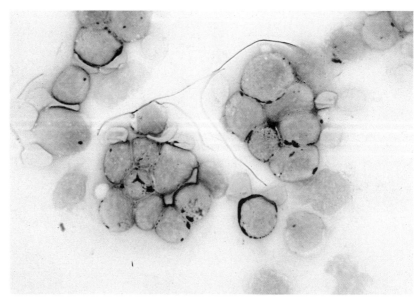

Figure 117
ACUTE LYMPHOBLASTIC
LEUKEMIA: PAS STAIN
Bone marrow lymphoblasts show
block and coarse granular staining.
Lymphoblasts in approximately 75
percent of cases of ALL are PAS positive and manifest the characteristic
pattern illustrated. The percentage
of positive-staining blasts is variable. (Periodic acid–Schiff stain)

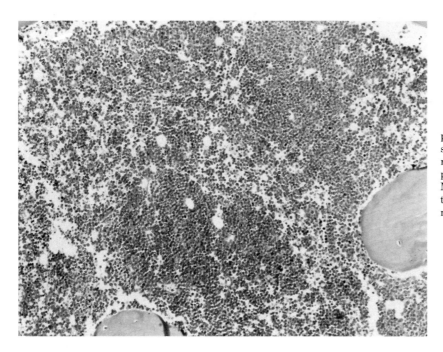

Figure 118
ACUTE LYMPHOBLASTIC
LEUKEMIA, L1 (ALL-L1)
This low magnification of a trephine biopsy from a 7-year-old
shows marked hypercellularity and
replacement of the normal hematopoietic cells with lymphoblasts.
Marked hypercellularity is characteristic of ALL at presentation. (Hematoxylin and eosin stain)

are usually present and may be abundant (figs. 120, 121). Mitotic activity is variable but mitoses are always easily identified.

Ultrastructural Findings. Ultrastructural studies are occasionally important in distinguishing ALL from AML-M0, AML-M5A, and AML-M7 (114,124,130,131). They may also be useful in the differential diagnosis of ALL and metastatic small cell tumors, most notably neuroblastomas and rhabdomyosarcomas.

The most common lymphoblasts in ALL-L1 are small, with a high nuclear-cytoplasmic ratio. The cytoplasm is sparse and contains scattered small mitochondria, a moderate sized Golgi region with associated small vesicles, scattered polyribosomes, and rare strands of rough endoplasmic reticulum. Occasional cells contain lipid inclusions, clusters of glycogen-like material, and scattered small electron-dense granules. Nuclear shape is variable, ranging from round to

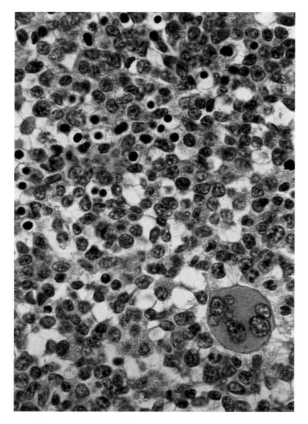

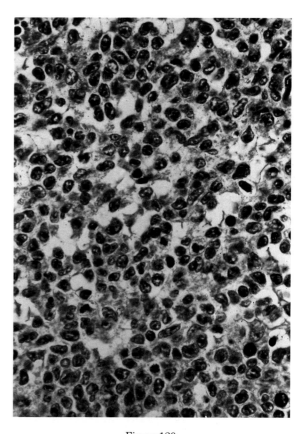

Figure 119
ACUTE LYMPHOBLASTIC LEUKEMIA, L1 (ALL-L1)

A high magnification of a trephine biopsy section shows predominantly lymphoblasts. A megakaryocyte is present on the lower right and normoblasts are dispersed in the top half of the field. Numerous eosinophils and eosinophil precursors are scattered throughout the field. (Hematoxylin and eosin stain)

Figure 120
ACUTE LYMPHOBLASTIC LEUKEMIA, L1 (ALL-L1)

A bone marrow trephine biopsy section from a 2-year-old male. The marrow is replaced by lymphoblasts. The nuclei have convoluted and angulated borders. Nucleoli are visible in some of the blasts. There is minimal cytoplasm and indistinct cell margins. (Hematoxylin and eosin stain)

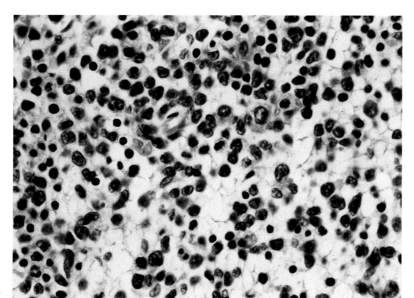

Figure 121
ACUTE LYMPHOBLASTIC
LEUKEMIA, L1 (ALL-L1)

The lymphoblasts in the trephine biopsy section are smaller and have more condensed nuclear chromatin than those in figure 120. (Hematoxylin and eosin stain)

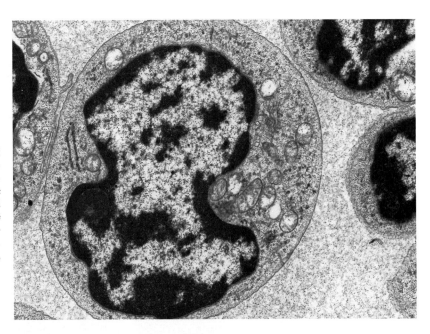

Figure 122
ELECTRON MICROGRAPH OF A LYMPHOBLAST FROM A CHILD WITH ACUTE LYMPHOBLASTIC LEUKEMIA, L1 (ALL-L1)

The cytoplasm contains scattered small mitochondria, a small Golgi region, scattered polyribosomes, and occasional strands of rough endoplasmic reticulum. The nucleus is indented and contains a small nucleolus. The chromatin is condensed and concentrated at the periphery of the nucleus. (Uranyl acetate–lead citrate stains, X19,000)

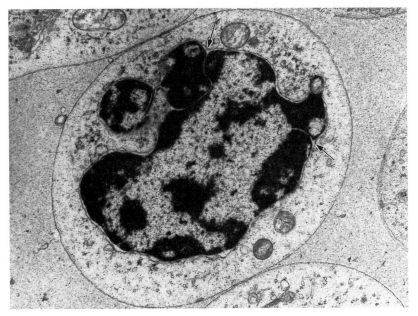

Figure 123
ELECTRON MICROGRAPH OF A LYMPHOBLAST FROM A PATIENT WITH T-CELL ACUTE LYMPHOBLASTIC LEUKEMIA, L1 (ALL-L1)

There is heavily condensed chromatin, prominent irregularity of the nuclear border, and nuclear splits and clefts (arrows) which appear to internally partition the nucleus. This cell appears to correspond to the small cells with hyperchromatic convoluted nuclei often observed by light microscopy on blood smears from patients with T-cell ALL. (Uranyl acetate–lead citrate stains, X21,000) (Fig. 4 from McKenna RW, Parkin J, Brunning RD. Morphologic and ultrastructural characteristics of T-cell acute lymphoblastic leukemia. Cancer 1979;44:1290–7.)

markedly irregular with indentations, clefting, and nuclear splits. The nuclear splits appear to represent duplications of the nuclear envelope. These are particularly prominent in the smallest blasts in some cases of T-cell ALL (159). Nuclear chromatin is typically characterized by peripheral condensation and moderate clumping but cells with heavily condensed chromatin may be present and nucleoli are usually identified (figs. 122, 123) (114,124,130,131).

Acute Lymphoblastic Leukemia, L2 (ALL-L2)

Blood and Bone Marrow Findings. The majority of the lymphoblasts in ALL-L2 are larger than those in L1. There is often considerable heterogeneity in cell size but most exceed twice the size of a normal small lymphocyte. The blasts have moderately abundant cytoplasm and a lower nuclear-cytoplasmic ratio than the lymphoblasts in L1. The nuclear outline is frequently irregular. The

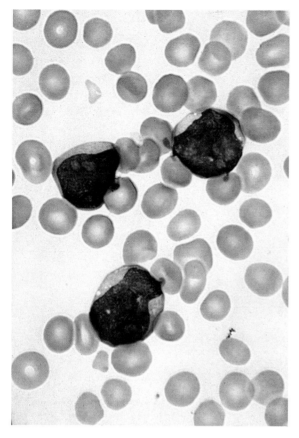

Figure 124
ACUTE LYMPHOBLASTIC LEUKEMIA, L2 (ALL-L2)

A blood smear from a 21-year-old male shows three large lymphoblasts with a moderate amount of cytoplasm and large nuclei. The nuclear chromatin is coarsely reticular. One to three prominent nucleoli are present. (Wright-Giemsa stain)

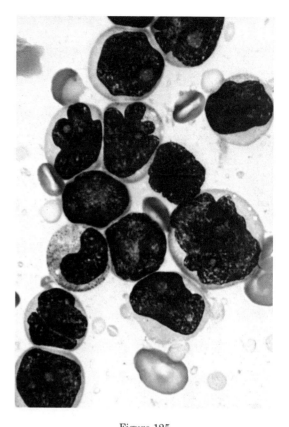

Figure 125
ACUTE LYMPHOBLASTIC LEUKEMIA, L2 (ALL-L2)

A bone marrow smear from a 2-year-old female. The lymphoblasts vary in size and show considerable nuclear irregularity. There is a moderate amount of cytoplasm. The nuclei have coarse chromatin and contain distinct nucleoli. (Wright-Giemsa stain)

chromatin varies from finely dispersed to coarse and may differ considerably among blasts in the same case. Nucleoli are often prominent and vary from one to four in number. The cytoplasm is variably basophilic and may contain vacuoles (figs. 124–126). A low nuclear-cytoplasmic ratio and prominent nucleoli are the most useful features in distinguishing L2 from L1.

Cytochemical Findings. The cytochemical profile of the lymphoblasts in L2 is similar to L1 and is listed in Table 15 (158).

Histopathologic Findings. In trephine biopsy sections, the bone marrow is hypercellular with diffuse replacement of normal hematopoietic cells by lymphoblasts. The pattern is similar to ALL-L1, however the lymphoblasts are larger with more abundant cytoplasm, show more nu-

clear irregularity, have dispersed or vesicular chromatin, and more prominent nucleoli than L1 lymphoblasts (fig. 127). Mitotic figures are easily found and may be abundant.

Ultrastructural Findings. The same diagnostic applications of electron microscopy in ALL-L1 apply to L2. The lymphoblasts in ALL-L2 show considerable nuclear heterogeneity and variation in size. They are generally larger and contain more cytoplasm than L1 blasts but the organelle content is similar. The nuclei vary in shape and degree of chromatin condensation. Nucleoli are large and may be multiple (fig. 128). Nuclear blebs and splits similar to those in L1 blasts may be observed (114,159).

In a low percentage of cases of both ALL-L1 and L2, granules are present that appear to correspond to azurophilic granules observed by light

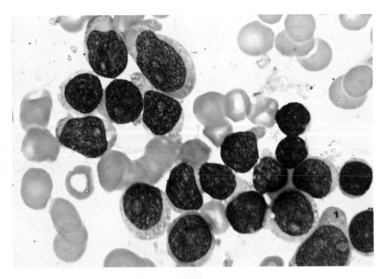

Figure 126
ACUTE LYMPHOBLASTIC
LEUKEMIA, L2 (ALL-L2)
The lymphoblasts in this bone marrow smear from a 12-year-old male vary in size, have reticular chromatin, prominent nucleoli, and lack the nuclear irregularity of the blasts in figure 125. A minority of the lymphoblasts have the cytologic features of ALL-L1. (Wright-Giemsa stain)

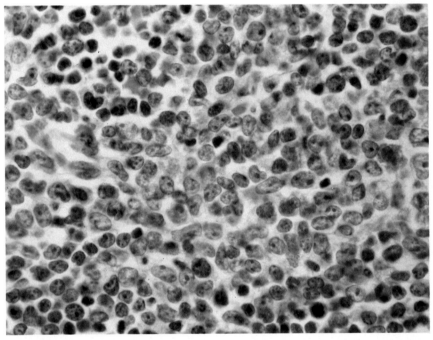

Figure 127
ACUTE LYMPHOBLASTIC
LEUKEMIA, L2 (ALL-L2)
A bone marrow section from a 24-year-old male. The lymphoblasts are relatively large and have dispersed chromatin. Nucleoli are prominent in many of the blasts. Nuclear shape varies from round or oval to mildly irregular or angulated. (Hematoxylin and eosin stain)

microscopy. In some cases they are electron-dense structures varying in size from 0.2 to 1.5 µm in diameter clustered near the Golgi region. They contain small vesicles, electron-dense glycogen-like particles, and occasional membranous lamellae and scrolls. Ultrastructural peroxidase positivity has been demonstrated in some (fig. 129) (114,169,189). These granules resemble immature mast cell–basophil granules (114,169). Their significance and the relationship of the cells containing them to mast cells and basophils is not clear. Despite this suggestive evidence for mast cell–basophil lineage, cases with cells containing granules of this type should be considered ALL in the presence of a lymphoblast immunophenotype. In other cases of ALL with granules identifiable by light microscopy, large cytoplasmic inclusions ranging from 1.5 to 2.5 µm in diameter have been observed. These are single membrane bound, and contain slightly electron-dense, amorphous material (fig. 130) (114). Cytoplasmic granules have also been attributed to abnormal mitochondria or fusion of cytoplasmic organelles (128,203).

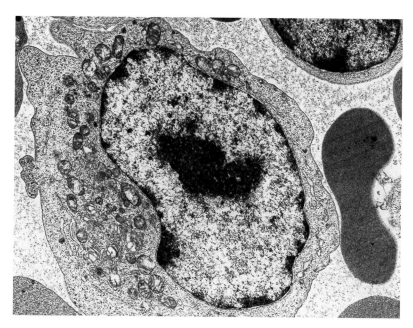

Figure 128
ELECTRON MICROGRAPH OF A LYMPHOBLAST FROM A PATIENT
WITH ACUTE LYMPHOBLASTIC LEUKEMIA, L2 (ALL-L2)

The cell is relatively large with moderately abundant cytoplasm, dispersed chromatin with moderate peripheral condensation, and a large prominent nucleolus. (Uranyl acetate–lead citrate stains, X11,000)

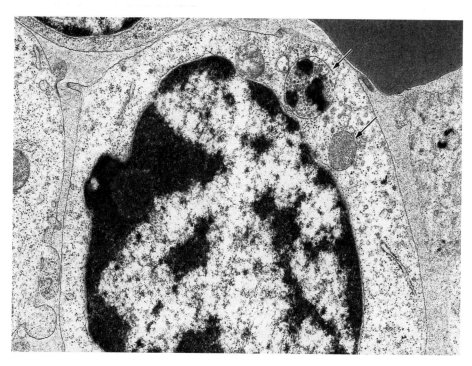

Figure 129
ELECTRON MICROGRAPH OF A LYMPHOBLAST FROM A PATIENT WITH DOWN SYNDROME (TRISOMY 21)

The cell contains cytoplasmic granules that are membrane bound and contain small vesicles, glycogen-like particles, and membranous lamellae and scrolls (arrows). These granules resemble immature mast cell–basophil granules. (Uranyl acetate–lead citrate stains, X23,000).

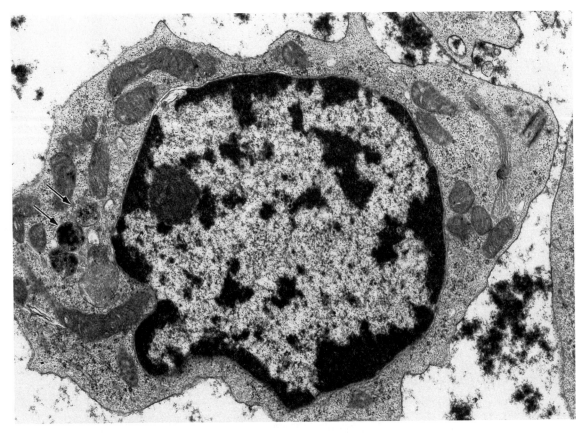

Figure 130
ELECTRON MICROGRAPH OF A LYMPHOBLAST FROM A PATIENT
WITH A t(9;22)(q34;q11) PHILADELPHIA CHROMOSOME–POSITIVE ALL
A group of cytoplasmic granules are characterized by dense limiting membranes (arrows). They contain amorphous material, small vesicles, and glycogen-like particles. (Uranyl acetate–lead citrate stains, X21,000)

Acute Lymphoblastic Leukemia, L3 (ALL-L3)

Blood and Bone Marrow Findings. The lymphoblasts in ALL-L3 are medium to large and morphologically homogeneous. They have the same cytologic features as small noncleaved cell lymphomas, Burkitt or non-Burkitt type (105,106, 113). The nucleus is round to slightly oval and nuclear irregularities are uncommon. The chromatin is stippled and homogeneous. Two to four nucleoli are usually observed. The cytoplasm is moderately abundant, deeply basophilic, and usually contains sharply defined clear vacuoles. The prominence of vacuolization varies from several vacuoles in nearly every blast to only a few in a minority of the cells (fig. 131). In most cases the vacuoles are abundant and the most striking cytologic characteristic.

Vacuoles similar to those observed in ALL-L3 may be found in lymphoblasts in cases of L1 or L2 (156). The distinction of L3 from these cases is based on the size and homogeneity of the lymphoblasts, amount of cytoplasm, degree of cytoplasmic basophilia, and nuclear characteristics (fig. 132). Rare cases of L3 lack some of the distinctive morphologic features (non-Burkitt type). In these cases there may be few or no cytoplasmic vacuoles, more variation in nuclear shape, and finer chromatin (fig. 133).

Cytochemical Findings. The vacuoles in cases of ALL-L3 stain positively with the oil red O stain and the cytoplasm is strongly positive with a methyl green pyronine (MGP) stain (fig. 134). The blasts are PAS negative, except in rare cases. Other cytochemical characteristics are shown in Table 15.

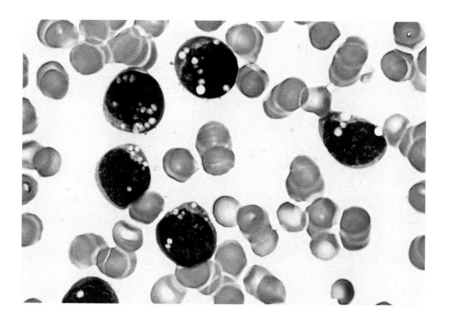

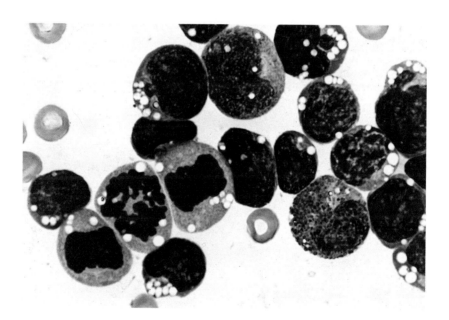

Figure 131
ACUTE LYMPHOBLASTIC LEUKEMIA, L3 (ALL-L3)

Top: A blood smear from a young man with an elevated leukocyte count. The leukemic cells are relatively uniform with a moderate amount of deeply basophilic cytoplasm and round nuclei. The chromatin is coarsely reticular; indistinct nucleoli can be identified in some of the blasts. The cytoplasm contains several sharply defined clear vacuoles. Some of the vacuoles overlie the nucleus. The blood contained an unusually large number of blasts in this case. (Wright-Giemsa stain)

Bottom: A bone marrow smear from a 19-year-old male who presented with a paraspinal mass. The marrow was heavily infiltrated with the characteristic cells of ALL-L3. There is variation in size of the blasts but all have round or oval nuclei with coarsely reticular chromatin and deeply basophilic cytoplasm containing the characteristic vacuoles. Nucleoli are prominent in some of the cells. Three cells on the lower left of this field are in mitosis. An eosinophil myelocyte and neutrophil promyelocyte are also present in this field. A tissue mass commonly accompanies ALL-L3, frequently in the ileocecal region. The morphologic features of L3 are identical to those of small noncleaved cell lymphomas. (Wright-Giemsa stain) (Fig. 37.23 (right) from McKenna RW. The bone marrow manifestations of Hodgkin's disease, the non-Hodgkin's lymphomas, and lymphoma-like disorders. In Knowles DM, ed. Neoplastic hematopathology. Baltimore: Williams & Wilkins, 1992:1135–80.)

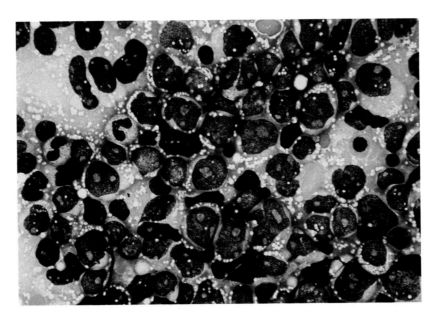

Figure 132
ACUTE LYMPHOBLASTIC LEUKEMIA, L2 (ALL-L2), WITH MARKED CYTOPLASMIC VACUOLATION
A bone marrow smear from a 71-year-old man with an unusual variant of ALL-L2. The blasts were TdT positive and expressed CD10 (CALLA) and CD19 (early B-cell precursor immunophenotype). The lymphoblasts are large with reticular chromatin and prominent nucleoli. The cytoplasm contains numerous sharply defined clear vacuoles similar to those observed in L3. The other cytologic features of the blasts, e.g., chromatin pattern, prominence of nucleoli, cell size, and nuclear shape are distinct from L3. Vacuolation of lymphoblasts is not restricted to L3 and may be a prominent feature in some cases of ALL-L1 or L2. (Wright-Giemsa stain)

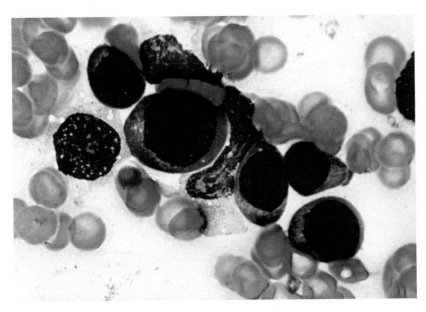

Figure 133
ACUTE LYMPHOBLASTIC LEUKEMIA, L3 (ALL-L3) (NON-BURKITT)
A bone marrow aspirate smear from a 70-year-old man with a radiographic gastric mass. The bone marrow was diffusely replaced by cells like those depicted in the illustration. Similar cells were present in the blood. The cells expressed monoclonal kappa surface immunoglobulin. A diagnosis of ALL-L3 non-Burkitt (small noncleaved cell lymphoma) was made. The cells have dispersed chromatin and more obvious nucleoli than usually observed in ALL-L3. They lack prominent vacuolization. (Wright-Giemsa stain)

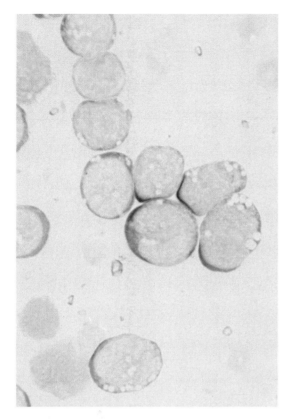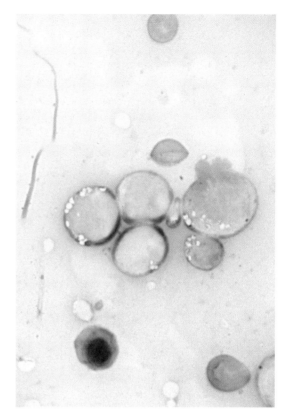

Figure 134
ACUTE LYMPHOBLASTIC LEUKEMIA, L3 (ALL-L3)
Bone marrow smear from an 8-year-old male. A methyl green pyronine (MGP) stain on the left shows strong uniform staining of the cytoplasm. On the right the cytoplasmic vacuoles stain with oil red 0.

Histopathologic Findings. The bone marrow on trephine biopsy sections is usually diffusely and extensively replaced by leukemic cells. In a minority of cases there is considerable marrow sparing, with normal hematopoietic cells evenly dispersed among leukemic blasts; rarely, focal concentrations of blasts are observed. Bone marrow necrosis is often present and occasionally the entire trephine biopsy consists of necrotic tumor (fig. 135) (113).

The lymphoblasts are morphologically uniform with only minimal variation in size. There is a moderate amount of cytoplasm and a distinctive cytoplasmic membrane. The vacuoles that are prominent in smear preparations may be difficult to appreciate in sections. Nuclei are round to oval; occasional cells may show slight nuclear indentation. Nucleoli are small, distinct, and vary from one to four in number. Mitotic figures are numerous (fig. 136). The "starry-sky"

appearance often observed in lymph node biopsies is usually lacking in the trephine sections (113).

Ultrastructural Findings. The lymphoblasts are large with abundant cytoplasm that contains numerous free polyribosomes, large mitochondria, rare strands of rough endoplasmic reticulum, and prominent lipid-like vacuoles. The lipid vacuoles correspond to the oil red 0–positive vacuoles observed by light microscopy. The nuclei are round or oval with finely dispersed chromatin, one or more prominent nucleoli, and frequent nuclear pockets and blebs (fig. 137) (113,114,154).

Variant Morphologic Features of ALL

There are several variant morphologic features occasionally found in ALL-L1 or L2 that warrant discussion because of the difficulty they present in diagnosis, classification, and assessment of post-therapy bone marrow.

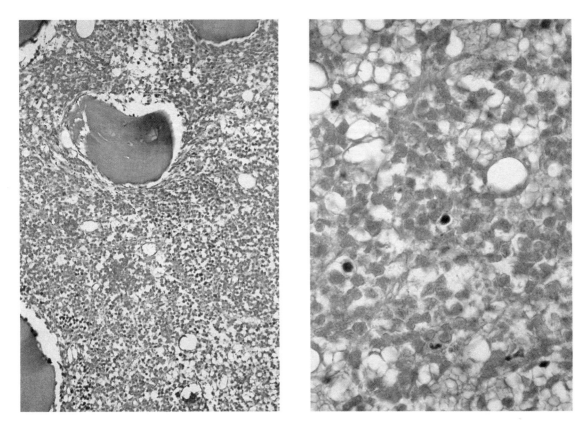

Figure 135

NECROTIC BONE MARROW BIOPSY FROM A PATIENT WITH ACUTE LYMPHOBLASTIC LEUKEMIA, L3 (ALL-L3)

Left: A bone marrow section from a patient with newly diagnosed ALL-L3. The section illustrates extensive necrosis. Necrotic areas are commonly observed in marrow sections of L3. In some instances the entire section consists of necrotic tissue.

Right: A higher magnification of the section shows a uniform population of leukemic cells showing advanced karyolysis. (Hematoxylin and eosin stain)

Figure 136
ACUTE LYMPHOBLASTIC
LEUKEMIA, L3 (ALL-L3)

A high magnification of a bone marrow section from a 19-year-old man. The cells are uniform with round or oval nuclei and one to three small nucleoli. The borders of many of the cells are well defined. There are numerous mitotic figures in this field. (Hematoxylin and eosin stain) (Fig. 37.23 (left) from McKenna RW. The bone marrow manifestations of Hodgkin's disease, the non-Hodgkin's lymphomas, and lymphoma-like disorders. In Knowles DM, ed. Neoplastic hematopathology. Baltimore: Williams & Wilkins, 1992:1135–80.)

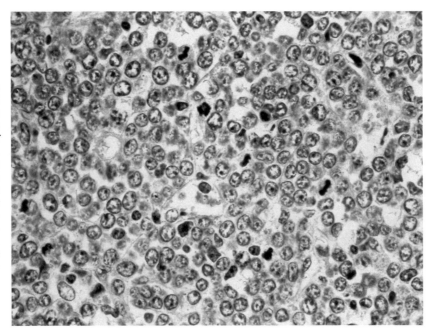

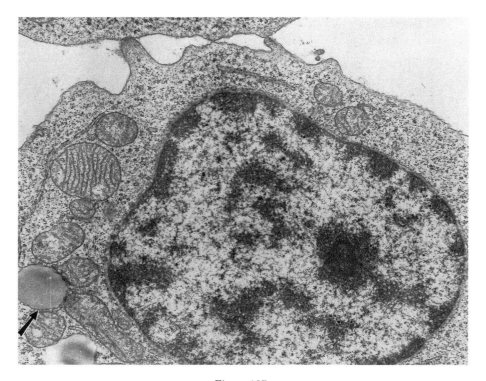

Figure 137
ELECTRON MICROGRAPH OF A BONE MARROW BLAST
FROM A PATIENT WITH ACUTE LYMPHOBLASTIC LEUKEMIA, L3 (ALL-L3)
The blasts in ALL-L3 are characterized by abundant cytoplasm, which contains numerous polyribosomes and large lipid vacuoles (arrow). The nuclei have peripherally condensed chromatin and one or more prominent nucleoli. (Uranyl acetate–lead citrate stains, X22,000)

ALL with Cytoplasmic Granules. Azurophilic granules may be observed in the cytoplasm in approximately 4.5 to 7 percent of cases of ALL (104, 117,123,128,135,137,189). The granules vary in size but are often larger than the azurophilic granules in myeloblasts. Some stain weakly and appear slightly pink or orange in Romanowsky stained smears. Occasionally, the granules appear to coalesce or aggregate in one area of the cytoplasm. These granules are negative for MPO but have been reported to be faintly PAS positive in some instances and SBB positive in rare cases (fig. 138) (189). The ultrastructure of the granules was described in the section on ultrastructural findings of ALL-L2 (see figs. 129, 130).

ALL with cytoplasmic granules is usually of B-cell precursor immunophenotype (123,137, 189). There have been no consistent cytogenetic associations, but several cases have been in children with Down syndrome and a number of oth-

ers have been associated with the Philadelphia chromosome, t(9;22)(q34;q11) (111,114,169). The presence of cytoplasmic granules in lymphoblasts is mainly important because of the potential for confusion with myeloblasts but has also been reported to convey a poor prognosis in children with ALL-L2 of B-cell precursor type (117).

Aplastic Presentation of ALL. Rarely, patients with ALL present with pancytopenia and a hypoplastic bone marrow (195). Leukemic blasts may not be identified initially. This hypocellular phase is typically followed by apparent bone marrow recovery and later by overt leukemia in a matter of weeks or a few months (195). Unlike the myelodysplastic syndromes that may precede AML, dysplastic changes are not observed in the hypoplastic phase preceding ALL (195). There are no distinctive morphologic, immunophenotypic, or cytogenetic characteristics associated with the overt leukemic phase.

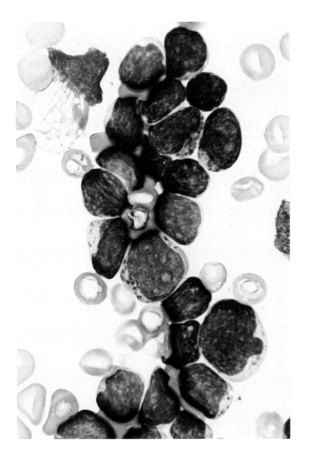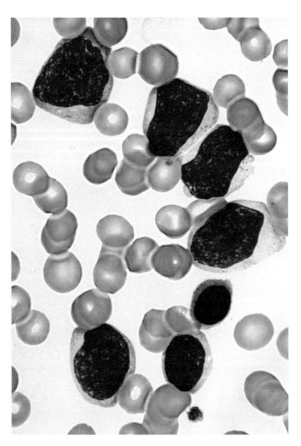

Figure 138

ACUTE LYMPHOBLASTIC LEUKEMIA WITH CYTOPLASMIC GRANULES

Left: A bone marrow smear from a patient with ALL-L1. Most of the blasts contain large azurophilic granules in the cytoplasm. The MPO and SBB stains were negative. Immunologic marker studies showed an early B-cell precursor immunophenotype. Note the large size and light azurophilia of the granules. Four to 7 percent of cases of ALL manifest a variable degree of cytoplasmic granulation in the lymphoblasts. (Wright-Giemsa stain)

Right: A blood smear from a patient with a high leukocyte count ALL-L2. Cytogenetic studies revealed a t(9;22)(q31;q11) chromosome abnormality (Philadelphia chromosome). Note the azurophilic granules in the cytoplasm of the blasts. The granules are smaller and less abundant than in the case illustrated on the left. (Wright-Giemsa stain).

Bone Marrow Necrosis. Patients with ALL may present with extensive bone marrow necrosis (see fig. 135) (166,167). The entire marrow specimen is necrotic in some instances and a definitive diagnosis may not be possible. A repeat bone marrow biopsy at another site may be helpful, but in some cases the marrow necrosis is generalized and a diagnosis can only be made by waiting a few days and repeating the biopsy.

ALL with Eosinophilia. Mild to marked eosinophilia is occasionally noted at diagnosis (104). Cases in which eosinophilia was so profound that the diagnosis of ALL was obscured have been reported. In these cases the process may be confused with a myeloproliferative disorder. Some patients have clinical manifestations of the hypereosinophilic syndrome. Eosinophilia generally resolves if a complete remission is achieved but may return with, or just prior to, relapse of ALL. Eosinophilia has been reported in both ALL-L1 and L2. There is no apparent correlation with immunophenotype. The lymphoblasts in some patients with marked eosinophilia have a t(5;14) chromosome rearrangement (138).

Hand-Mirror Cell Variant Leukemia. Cases of ALL in which most of the lymphoblasts in the bone marrow smears have a cytoplasmic uropod-like projection are referred to as hand-mirror cell variants (181,188). There has been no association of this finding with morphologic

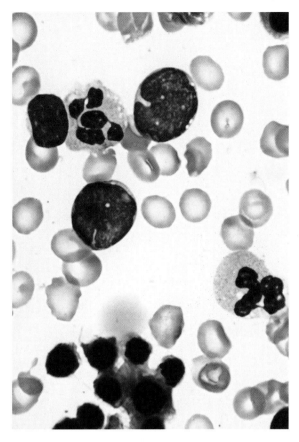

Figure 139
RELAPSE OF ACUTE LYMPHOBLASTIC LEUKEMIA
Two lymphoblasts are illustrated in the bone marrow from a patient with early relapse of ALL. The percentage of blasts was low. The marrow was composed mostly of normal hematopoietic cells. The lymphoblasts in patients with relapse of ALL are generally morphologically similar to those in the initial diagnostic marrow. In a minority of cases, the blast morphology changes from L1 to L2. When a small number of residual leukemic lymphoblasts are present following therapy or in early relapse, they may be difficult to distinguish from normal lymphocyte progenitor cells (hematogones). (Wright-Giemsa stain)

class, immunophenotype, cytogenetic change, or prognosis. The significance and mechanism of this morphologic variation is unclear.

Relapse of Lymphoblastic Leukemia. In most cases, the morphology of the lymphoblasts at relapse is similar to the initial diagnostic bone marrow (fig. 139). In a minority of patients there is evolution from ALL-L1 to L2; the reverse is rare (153). Immunophenotypic and karyotypic changes may also be observed at relapse. A summary of the alterations in lymphoblasts at relapse of ALL is shown in Table 16.

Table 16

CHANGES AT RELAPSE OF ALL

Morphologic
L1 $\Rightarrow$ L2 (in a minority of cases)

Terminal deoxynucleotidyltransferase (TdT)
Positive $\Rightarrow$ negative ($\approx 25\%$)

Immunologic
Major phenotype change (rare)
Gain or loss of an antigen (more common)
e.g., CD10+ $\Rightarrow$ CD10-

Cytogenetic
Clonal evolution common ($\approx 75\%$)
One or more new structural abnormalities

**Evolution to myeloid leukemia
(lineage switch)**
Therapy related in most cases
Often associated with a 11q23 chromosome abnormality

Secondary AML. Secondary AML (therapy related) has been reported in approximately 2 percent of patients treated for ALL (176). It appears to be more common in cases with a T-cell immunophenotype. This may reflect differences in therapy protocols for T-cell ALL and non–T-cell ALL. The secondary leukemia is presumed to result from effects of chemotherapy on myeloid stem cells. A rearrangement of chromosome 11 at band q23 is commonly found in the AML clone (172,176,202). There appears to be an association with epipodophyllotoxin chemotherapy (fig. 140) (172,176,202).

Immunology

Terminal deoxynucleotidyltransferase (TdT) is a unique DNA polymerase found in the nuclei of cortical lymphocytes of the normal human thymus and in a very small number of bone marrow lymphoid cells. It can be measured biochemically in cell suspensions but is most commonly assayed by immunofluorescent or enzyme immunocytochemical microscopy techniques, or by flow cytometry using anti-TdT antibodies (fig. 141).

The lymphoblasts in more than 90 percent of cases of T-cell and B-cell precursor ALL and lymphoblastic lymphoma are TdT-positive (142,196). Only rare cases of TdT-positive B-cell ALL (L3)

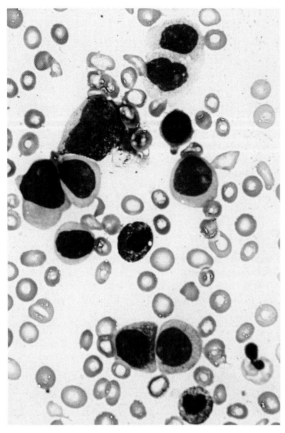

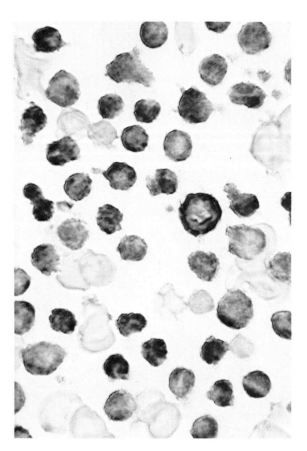

Figure 140
SECONDARY (THERAPY-RELATED)
ACUTE MYELOID LEUKEMIA
IN A PATIENT TREATED FOR
ACUTE LYMPHOBLASTIC LEUKEMIA

A bone marrow smear from a 6-year-old female with ALL diagnosed 3 years earlier. The patient was in a continuous complete remission and taken off all therapy 6 months before this marrow aspirate was obtained to evaluate pancytopenia. There were 40 percent blasts in the bone marrow. The blasts were MPO positive and lacked expression of any lymphocyte antigens. Epipodophyllotoxin drugs have been implicated in most cases of secondary (therapy-related) AML following treatment for ALL. (Wright-Giemsa stain)

Figure 141
IMMUNOPEROXIDASE STAIN FOR TdT ON A
BONE MARROW SMEAR FROM A PATIENT
WITH ACUTE LYMPHOBLASTIC LEUKEMIA

The nuclear distribution of the stain corresponds to the location of TdT in the lymphoblasts. (Immunoperoxidase–anti-TdT reaction)

have been reported. The chronic lympho-proliferative disorders and lymphomas other than lymphoblastic lymphoma are TdT negative.

TdT studies are useful in the distinction of ALL from AML and from other lymphoprolifera-tive disorders, especially the rare cases of adult T-cell leukemia that cytologically resemble T-cell ALL. Approximately 5 to 10 percent of cases of AML will manifest TdT-positive blasts; often the intensity of the reaction and the percentage of

positive blasts are significantly less in AML. The blasts in approximately 30 percent of cases of chronic myeloid leukemia in the blastic phase are TdT positive. These cases generally correspond to those with lymphoblastic morphology and im-munophenotype. The proliferative cells in chronic phase chronic myeloid leukemia are TdT negative.

Up to 10 percent of TdT-positive cells may be found in bone marrow from patients without hematologic malignancies and in normal indi-viduals, particularly young children. The pres-ence of a small percentage of TdT-positive cells in post-therapy bone marrow specimens should not be interpreted as evidence of residual disease or relapse of ALL without supportive morpho-logic criteria (163,185).

Table 17

IMMUNOLOGIC CLASSIFICATION OF ALL

	FAB Class	TdT	T-Cell Restricted Antigens	B-Cell Restricted Antigens	CIg	SIg
T-cell ALL	L1, L2	+	+	−	−	−
B-cell precursor ALL:						
Early B-cell precursor ALL	L1, L2	+	−	+	−	−
Pre–B-cell ALL	L1, L2	+	−	+	+	−
B-cell ALL	L3	−	−	+	−	+

The TdT assay applied to spinal fluid cytospins may be useful in identifying central nervous system leukemia in cases with low spinal fluid cell counts and equivocal morphology (139).

Immunologic Classes of ALL

The development of an array of lineage-restricted or -associated monoclonal antibodies (MoAbs) applicable to immunophenotyping of hematopoietic cells has advanced the understanding of the biology of ALL and provided important diagnostic and prognostic information (108,112,126, 127,150,164). Immunophenotyping may be essential in the distinction of ALL and AML when the leukemic blasts are morphologically and cytochemically undifferentiated (143). The use of a TdT assay, anti–pan-T-cell MoAbs, and anti–pan-B-cell MoAbs will identify the majority of cases of ALL (127,133). Anti–pan-myeloid MoAbs react with blasts in the majority of cases of AML. It is important to use panels of MoAbs that include all of the major cell lineages to avoid misinterpretations and to recognize phenotypic aberrancy and cases of mixed phenotype leukemia (148,179).

Several variations of immunologic classification of ALL have been published (108,127,133, 150). The classification shown in Table 17 is basic and has clinical relevance.

T-Cell ALL. Approximately 15 percent of cases of ALL are of T-cell type. The lymphoblasts in these cases react with one or more pan-T-cell MoAbs such as CD2, CD5, and CD7 (108,109, 178). CD3, which is highly specific for T cells, is commonly lacking on the cell surface in T-cell ALL, but a high percentage of cases express

cytoplasmic CD3 (162,193). Demonstration of clonal T-cell receptor gene rearrangements has provided additional evidence of T-cell origin in cases of early thymocyte ALL.

T-cell ALL can be subclassified into various stages corresponding to thymocyte development by using a panel of MoAbs (122,178). Studies have shown a fairly uniform distribution of T-cell ALL at early, intermediate, and mature thymocyte stages, but phenotypic aberrancy is relatively common. Remission rates for cases of T-cell ALL with an early thymocyte phenotype appear to be worse than for the intermediate and mature immunophenotypic subgroups (122). The lymphoblasts in T-cell lymphoblastic lymphoma are less likely to express an early thymocyte immunophenotype than those in T-cell ALL (122,196).

T-cell ALL may be either FAB-L1 or L2. Some studies have shown a higher proportion of cases of L2 than for non–T-cell ALLs. There are distinctive morphologic and cytochemical features that suggest T-cell ALL (159): in the majority of cases a variable number of distinct small cells with little or no cytoplasm and markedly hyperchromatic nuclei, often with prominent nuclear convolution, are found in blood and bone marrow smears (figs. 123, 142). These cells always occur with a predominant population of larger leukemic blasts; only a small percentage of patients with non–T-cell ALL have a similar cytologic pattern (159). Numerous mitotic figures are usually observed in both smears and trephine biopsy sections (fig. 143). The leukemic cells in most cases of T-cell ALL exhibit strong, focal paranuclear acid phosphatase activity in the cytoplasm (figs. 144,

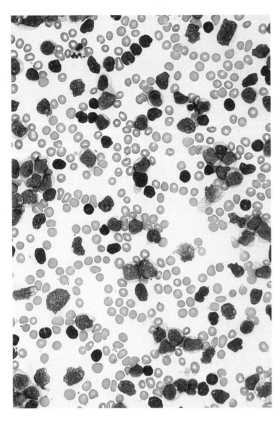 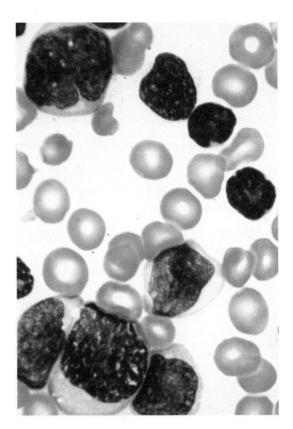

Figure 142
T-CELL ACUTE LYMPHOBLASTIC LEUKEMIA

Left: A low magnification of a blood smear from an 11-year-old male with T-cell ALL and a mediastinal mass. The leukocyte count is markedly elevated and there is striking heterogeneity of lymphoblast size and density of chromatin. Markedly elevated leukocyte counts are commonly encountered in cases of T-cell ALL. (Wright-Giemsa stain)

Right: Blood smear from a patient with high leukocyte count T-cell ALL-L2. A minor population of leukemic cells are small with little cytoplasm, markedly hyperchromatic nuclei, and prominent nuclear convolution. These cytologic features are highly suggestive of T-cell ALL. (Wright-Giemsa stain)

145) (116,159). The clinical and prognostic features of T-cell ALL are summarized in Table 18.

B-Cell Precursor ALL. Studies utilizing MoAbs and molecular probes have demonstrated that the lymphoblasts in nearly all non–T-cell ALLs are of B-cell lineage (108,164). Cases previously classified as non–T, non–B-cell ALL are now designated B-cell precursor ALL (108,118, 126,164). These cases are divided into subtypes based on expression of various B-associated or -restricted surface antigens, cytoplasmic μ, and surface immunoglobulin (108,164).

The characterization of B-cell precursor subtypes began in the mid 1970s with the development of an antisera that reacted with an antigen on the blasts from most cases of non–T-cell ALL but not with the lymphoblasts from T-cell ALL

Table 18

**CLINICAL CHARACTERISTICS
OF T-CELL ALL**

Older median age than average for ALL

Predominantly males

50% incidence of mediastinal mass

High blood leukocyte counts

Often chromosome rearrangements involving 14q11

Earlier relapse than non–T-cell ALL

High incidence of CNS relapse

Shorter survival than for non–T-cell ALL

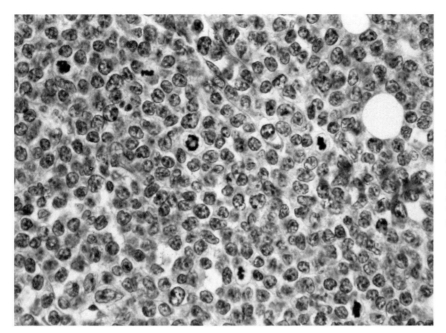

Figure 143
T-CELL ACUTE
LYMPHOBLASTIC
LEUKEMIA

Trephine biopsy section from a 21-year-old male. The lymphoblasts vary in size and show moderate nuclear irregularity. There are several mitotic figures in this field. T-cell ALL characteristically has a higher mitotic rate than B-cell precursor ALL. (Hematoxylin and eosin stain)

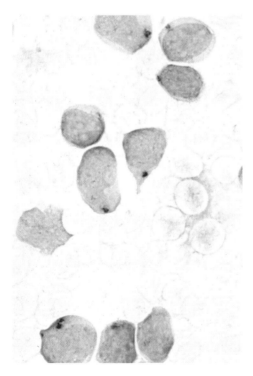

Figure 144
T-CELL ACUTE LYMPHOBLASTIC
LEUKEMIA: ACID PHOSPHATASE STAIN

The focal paranuclear acid phosphatase-staining reaction in the lymphoblasts in this blood smear is found in more than 90 percent of cases of T-cell ALL. Approximately 5 percent of non–T-cell ALL cases show a comparable reaction. (Acid phosphatase–pararosaniline stain)

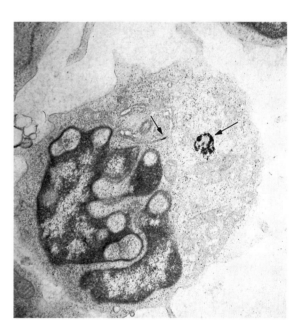

Figure 145
ELECTRON MICROGRAPH OF AN
ULTRACYTOCHEMICAL ACID
PHOSPHATASE REACTION IN A
LYMPHOBLAST FROM A PATIENT
WITH T-CELL ALL

The nucleus is markedly convoluted. Acid phosphatase activity is localized in the Golgi cisterna and in a large lysosome near the Golgi region (arrows). (Lead citrate stain, X24,000) (Fig. 2 from McKenna RW, Byrnes RK, Nesbit ME, et al. Cytochemical profiles in acute lymphoblastic leukemia. Am J Pediatr Hematol Oncol 1979;1:263–75.)

(132). The antigen to which the antisera reacted was designated *common acute lymphoblastic leukemia antigen* or *CALLA*. The lymphoblastic leukemias that reacted were referred to as common acute lymphoblastic leukemias (132). Monoclonal antibodies to CALLA (CD10) were subsequently introduced. The lymphoblasts in 80 to 90 percent of cases of B-cell precursor ALL express CALLA. The incidence of CALLA positivity is lower in children under 1 year of age (about 50 percent) and adults (121).

Cytoplasmic μ Chains (CIg). These are identified in the lymphoblasts in 20 to 25 percent of cases of CALLA-positive ALL. These cases are designated as *pre–B-cell ALL (CIg+)*. Studies using B-associated and -restricted MoAbs including HLA-DR, CD10, CD19, CD20, CD22, CD24, and molecular probes to identify immunoglobulin gene rearrangements have demonstrated that the large majority of the remaining (CIg-) cases of non–T-cell ALL are also of B-cell lineage. These are often designated *early B-cell precursor ALL*.

Cases with the earliest B-cell precursor immunophenotype may express only TdT and HLA-DR. Since this immunophenotype is not specific for B-cell lineage, these cases are often designated as *unclassified* or *presumed B-cell precursor ALL*. The absence of expression of myeloid or T-lymphocyte antigens in these cases is strong evidence for an early B-cell precursor lineage. Demonstration of immunoglobulin gene rearrangements in many of these cases further supports a B-cell lineage.

B-Cell ALL. The lymphoblasts in 1 to 3 percent of cases of ALL express monoclonal surface immunoglobulin (SIg) and pan–B-cell antigens. These cases are designated B-cell ALL. They are virtually always FAB-L3 and TdT negative (see fig. 131). The presence of SIg distinguishes B-cell ALL from other B-cell lineage ALLs (Table 17). The high incidence of mass disease, often in the ileocecal region, is clinical evidence that a relatively high percentage of cases of B-cell ALL represent blood and bone marrow involvement by small noncleaved cell lymphoma. Table 19 lists the distinctive clinical features of B-cell ALL.

Asynchronous and Mixed Phenotype Acute Leukemia. More than half of the cases of B-cell precursor ALL manifest simultaneous expression of combinations of early and late antigens not present on normal lymphoid cells

Table 19

CLINICAL CHARACTERISTICS OF SURFACE IMMUNOGLOBULIN (SIg)-POSITIVE ALL (B-CELL ALL)

Older median age than average for ALL

High incidence of abdominal mass - usually ileocecal

High incidence of CNS disease

Chromosome translocations involving 8q24

Poor response to therapy

Early relapse

(140,141,152,179). Asynchronous antigen expression is also found in T-cell ALL (133,179).

In approximately 15 to 20 percent of children with ALL, the lymphoblasts express one or more myeloid-associated antigens (152,170). This finding appears to be even more common in adults (184). A mixed phenotype may result from a mixed lineage leukemia in which the leukemic blasts coexpress both lymphoid and myeloid characteristics or from bilineal leukemia with individual leukemic cells expressing lymphoid or myeloid characteristics but not both (141). In addition to mixed immunophenotypes there may be a mixture of morphologic, cytochemical, and ultrastructural features in these cases (figs. 146–152) (141,147,168). Bilineal leukemias may be synchronous, with simultaneous, distinct populations of leukemic cells of more than one lineage, or metachronous (lineage switch) in which one lineage is expressed following the other (figs. 148, 149) (141,186,187). In the latter case, reappearance of the original clone must be demonstrated to distinguish from the emergence of a secondary (therapy-related) leukemia (see fig. 140).

In adults with ALL, the presence of myeloid antigen–positive blasts is an indicator of poor prognosis (184). Prognostic studies in children have been inconclusive; some investigators have reported mixed phenotype ALL as a poor prognostic factor while others have found no independent affect on prognosis (152,170,197). In children with ALL there appears to be a significant association of myeloid antigen expression with FAB-L2 morphology (197). There is an increased

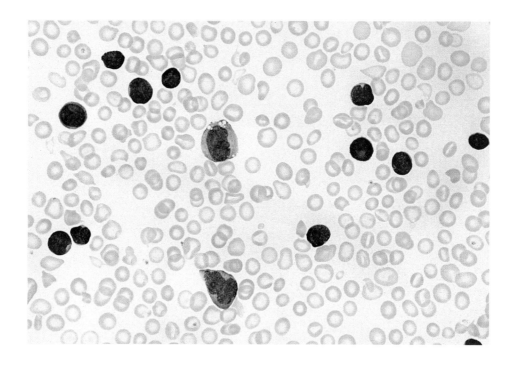

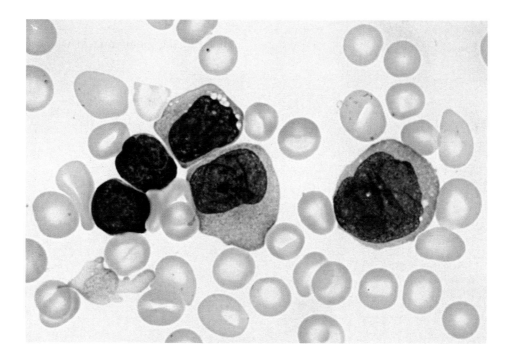

Figure 146
MIXED PHENOTYPE ACUTE LEUKEMIA (BILINEAL)

Top: Low magnification of a bone marrow smear from a 2-week-old female with mixed (bilineal) leukemia consisting of lymphoblasts and monoblasts.

Bottom: High magnification of the same case as illustrated above. The smaller cells with coarse chromatin and little or no cytoplasm are lymphoblasts by morphologic and immunophenotypic criteria. The large cells are monoblasts and promonocytes. Bone marrow cytogenetic studies revealed a t(4;11)(q21;q23) chromosome rearrangement. (Wright-Giemsa stain)

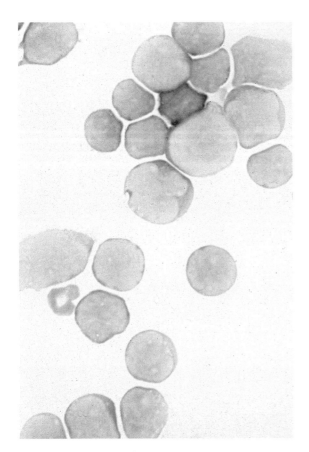
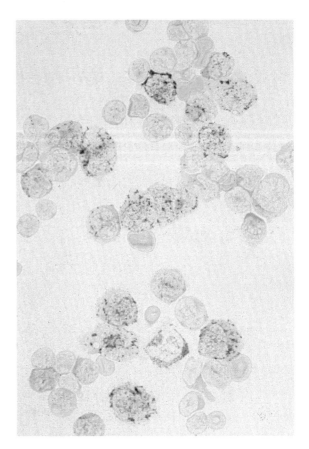

Figure 147
MIXED PHENOTYPE ACUTE LEUKEMIA (BILINEAL)

Left: A MPO stain on the bone marrow of the same case illustrated in figure 146. Both the lymphoblasts and monoblasts-promonocytes are MPO negative. (Myeloperoxidase stain)

Right: An immunoalkaline phosphatase reaction with an anti-CD68 antibody on the bone marrow smear. The larger cells (monoblasts) show a positive reaction in the cytoplasm. The smaller cells, lymphoblasts, are negative. (Alkaline phosphatase–antialkaline phosphatase CD68)

Figure 148
ACUTE LYMPHOBLASTIC
LEUKEMIA WITH A t(4;11)
CHROMOSOME REARRANGEMENT

A blood smear from a 3-week-old female with ALL-L1 and a leukocyte count of 180×10^9/L. The immunophenotype of the lymphoblasts was that of CD10 (CALLA)-negative B-cell precursor ALL. Only 30 percent of the blasts were TdT positive. Cytogenetic studies revealed a t(4;11)(q21;q23) chromosome abnormality. (Wright-Giemsa stain)

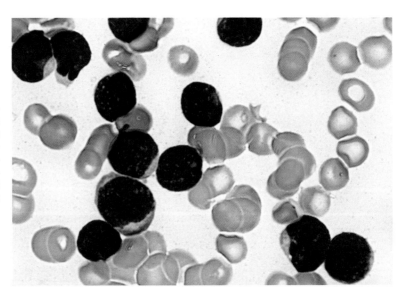

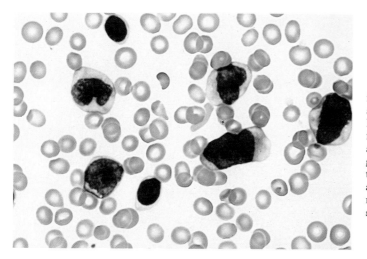

Figure 149
METACHRONOUS (LINEAGE SWITCH)
BILINEAL ACUTE LEUKEMIA

A blood smear taken 3 months after diagnosis from the same patient as in figure 148. The patient achieved a brief remission. At relapse the blasts were larger with more abundant cytoplasm. They manifested alpha naphthyl butyrate esterase activity and a myeloid immunophenotype. The same clonal cytogenetic abnormality, t(4;11)(q21;q23), was present in the diagnostic and relapse bone marrows. This case appears to represent a metachronous bilineal leukemia, lymphoblastic to monoblastic. (Wright-Giemsa stain)

Figure 150
MIXED PHENOTYPE ACUTE LEUKEMIA
(BILINEAL)

A blood smear from a 4-year-old female with acute mixed lineage (bilineal) leukemia. The small blasts express the immunophenotype of CD10 (CALLA)-negative early B-cell precursors. The large blasts marked immunophenotypically as monocyte precursors and were alpha naphthyl butyrate esterase positive. The child had a t(4;11) (q21;q23) bone marrow cytogenetic rearrangement. (Wright-Giemsa stain).

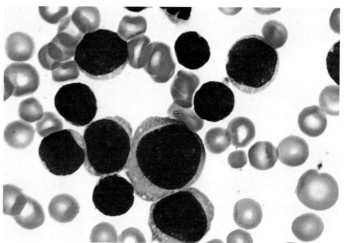

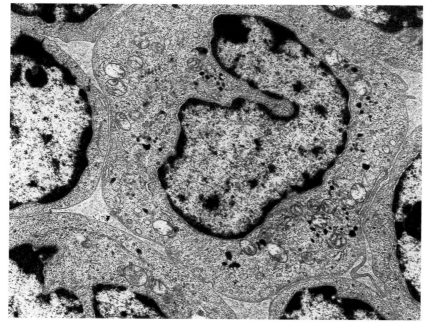

Figure 151
MIXED PHENOTYPE ACUTE
LEUKEMIA (BILINEAL)

Electron micrograph of a blast from the same patient as illustrated in figure 150. The cell manifests features of monocytic differentiation including a folded nucleus and scattered small electron-dense granules. Approximately 70 percent of the leukemic cells manifested morphologic and immunophenotypic features of lymphoblasts and 30 percent manifested features of monocytes. (Uranyl acetate–lead citrate stains, X15,000)

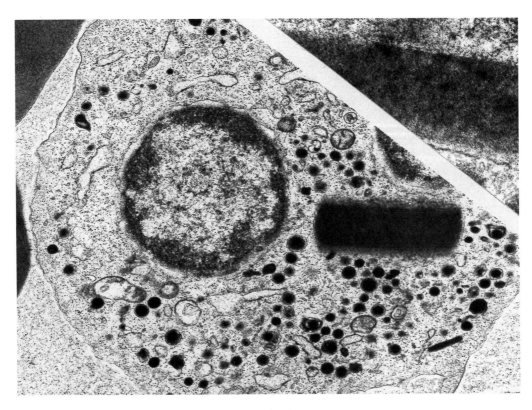

Figure 152
MIXED PHENOTYPE ACUTE LEUKEMIA (BILINEAL)

An electron micrograph of a neutrophil precursor from the bone marrow of a 40-year-old female with a t(4;11) (q21;q23)-associated acute leukemia. The majority of the blasts in this case manifested morphologic and immunophenotypic characteristics of lymphoblasts. The cell depicted contains an Auer rod. (Uranyl acetate–lead citrate stains, X21,000)

Inset. At higher magnification the Auer rod displays a 6 mµ periodicity characteristic of the Auer rods found in AML. (Uranyl acetate–lead citrate stains, X78,000) (Fig. 10-26 from Brunning RD, Parkin JL, McKenna RW. Acute lymphoblastic leukemia. In: Polliack A, ed. Human leukemias: cytochemical and ultrastructural techniques in diagnosis and research. Boston: Martinus Nijoff, 1984:173–218.)

incidence of chromosome translocations involving 11q23, 14q32, or t(9;22) in mixed phenotype ALL (172). Translocations involving these chromosomes are associated with a poor prognosis in all age groups.

Phenotypic Changes at Relapse. Patients that relapse with ALL generally express the same major immunophenotype on their lymphoblasts as was present at diagnosis. Rare cases of changes from a T-cell to B-cell precursor phenotype or vice versa have been reported. More commonly, there are losses or gains of individual antigens at relapse without a major evolution of immunophenotype. Loss, or less commonly, gain of TdT, CALLA (CD10), or HLA-DR expression are the most frequently reported alterations (134,174) (see Table 16).

Cytogenetics

Bone marrow cytogenetic studies supplement the morphologic and immunophenotypic classifications of ALL. Their greatest value is in identifying prognostic groups (107,198,201). Tables 7 and 9 in the introduction section on acute leukemias summarize the relationship of bone marrow karyotype findings to prognostic groups and FAB and immunologic classifications (107,172,175, 190,191,198,201).

When studied with refined cytogenetic techniques, at least 80 to 90 percent of cases of ALL have demonstrable chromosome abnormalities (200). Structural abnormalities are most common either alone or in combination with numerical changes (172,190,198).

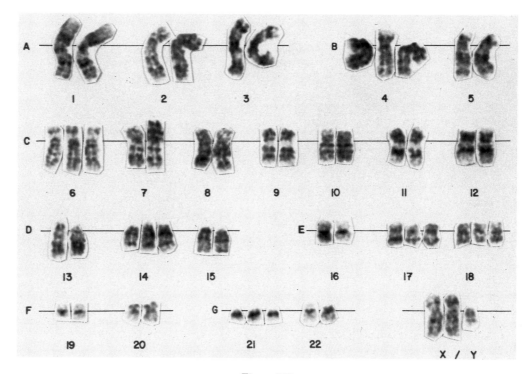

Figure 153
HYPERDIPLOID LYMPHOBLAST KARYOTYPE
This bone marrow karyotype is from a 5-year-old female with ALL. There is hyperdiploidy with 55 chromosomes. Hyperdiploidy with greater than 50 chromosomes is found in approximately 25 percent of children with ALL and is associated with a good prognosis. (Giemsa-trypsin banding) (Courtesy of Dr. Nancy Schneider, Dallas, Texas.)

Chromosome Numerical Groups in ALL. *Hyperdiploidy with More than 50 Chromosomes.* This is found in approximately 25 percent of cases of childhood ALL; it is less common in adults (fig. 153). It is associated with favorable clinical features including lower leukocyte counts, white race, and patients 2 to 10 years of age. Five-year survival rates for children with hyperdiploidy of more than 50 chromosomes is approximately 80 percent. A small number of patients (about 1 percent) in this group have a near tetraploid number of chromosomes. These are patients likely to have L2 morphology, a T-cell immunophenotype, an older age, and a poor prognosis (171). Patients that have structural changes, particularly translocations, in addition to more than 50 chromosomes, have a less favorable prognosis (175).

Hyperdiploidy with 47 to 50 Chromosomes. This is found in approximately 15 percent of cases. Structural abnormalities are present in roughly half of these, translocations in one third.

There are no specific presenting clinical features associated with this group. The prognosis is considered intermediate (172).

Normal Diploidy. This is found in 10 to 20 percent of cases (172). Approximately half of the patients with normal chromosomes have a T-cell immunophenotype. This group is associated with an intermediate prognosis.

Hypodiploidy. This is present in 3 to 9 percent of cases (172). Most of these have 45 chromosomes; chromosome 20 is commonly lost (172). No specific presenting clinical or phenotypic features are associated with this group. Hypodiploidy is considered an intermediate to poor prognostic factor, owing largely to a high percentage of cases with translocations.

Pseudodiploidy (46 Chromosomes but with Structural Abnormalities). Pseudodiploidy is found in approximately 40 percent of children with ALL and in a higher percentage of adults. Patients in this group often have high presenting leukocyte counts and less often express an early

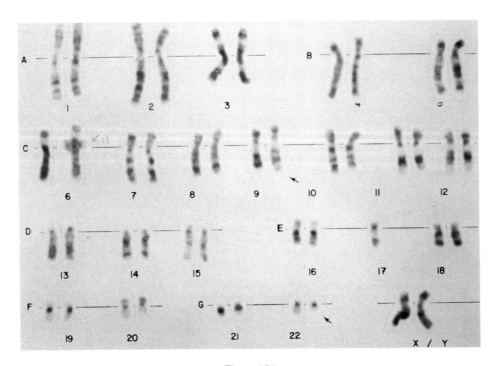

Figure 154

A t(9;22)(q34;q11) (PHILADELPHIA CHROMOSOME) LYMPHOBLAST KARYOTYPE

This karyotype is from the bone marrow of a 28-year-old man with ALL. Material from the long arm (q) of chromosome 22 is translocated to the long arm of chromosome 9 (arrows). This translocation is found in approximately 20 to 25 percent of adults and approximately 2 percent of children with ALL. It is associated with a poor prognosis. (Giemsa-trypsin banding) (Courtesy of Dr. Nancy Schneider, Dallas, Texas.)

B-cell precursor immunophenotype (172). Pseudodiploidy is associated with a poor prognosis because of the high percentage of cases with chromosome translocations.

Chromosome Structural Changes in ALL. Structural changes are always present in pseudodiploid ALL and may be found in the other numerical groups except the diploid group. Translocations are important because of their association with poor prognosis (198).

Philadelphia (Ph) Chromosome, t(9;22) (q34;q11). This is found in the lymphoblasts of approximately 2 percent of children and 20 to 25 percent of adults with ALL (fig. 154) (111,120,172, 183). Ph-positive ALL is characterized by an older age, high presenting leukocyte counts, L2 morphology, and central nervous system (CNS) involvement (figs. 130, 138, 155) (120). There is a spectrum of immunophenotypes but the majority are of the B-cell precursor type. The prognosis is unfavorable in both children and adults (107,120,125,183).

Translocation (1;19)(q23;p13). This chromosome abnormality is found in 25 percent of cases of pre–B-cell (CIg+) ALL and in approximately 1 percent of cases of early B-cell precursor (CIg-) ALL (115,177). It is the most common translocation in childhood ALL, with an incidence of 5 to 6 percent (172,177). High risk features are often associated with t(1;19) including increased leukocyte counts and black race. The poor prognosis ascribed to pre–B-cell ALL (CIg+) is strongly associated with the t(1;19) chromosome abnormality (119,177).

Reciprocal Translocations Involving Chromosome 8q24. Reciprocal translocations involving chromosome 8q24, L3 morphology, and B-cell phenotype (SIg+) are found in 1 to 3 percent of cases of ALL (see fig. 131). The most common translocation is t(8;14) (p24;q32.3). Two variant translocations involving the same locus in chromosome 8, t(2;8) and t(8;22), have been reported. In all of these translocations, the *myc* proto-oncogene on chromosome 8 assumes a position

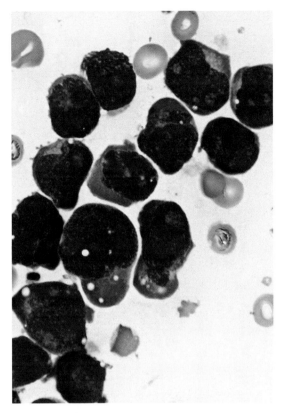

Figure 155
PHILADELPHIA CHROMOSOME
[t(9;22)(q34;q11)]-POSITIVE ACUTE
LYMPHOBLASTIC LEUKEMIA

The blasts from this bone marrow had the immunophenotype of B-cell precursors. The leukemic cells resemble early erythroblasts. This uncommon variant of Philadelphia chromosome-positive ALL has been referred to as pseudoerythroid ALL. (Wright-Giemsa stain)

adjacent to the immunoglobulin heavy chain gene or one of the light chain genes (172). A large malignant cell burden, CNS disease, and a poor prognosis are common in these cases. They are often designated leukemia-lymphoma.

Translocation (11;14)(p13;q11). Forty to 50 percent of cases of T-cell ALL have translocations. In approximately half of them breakpoints are in the locations of the T-cell receptor (TCR) genes (172). Translocation t(11;14)(p13;q11) is the most common; 14q11-q13 is the region of the α and γ TCR genes (199). The presence of these chromosome abnormalities has been found to correlate with poor prognosis (172,198).

Translocation (4;11)(p21;q23). Rearrangement of chromosome 11q23 is found in less than 5 percent of childhood ALL. Translocation (4;11)(q21;q23) is the most common rearrangement (fig. 156). It is associated with very young children, black race, markedly elevated leukocyte counts, splenomegaly, and a very poor prognosis (103,146,149,173). The majority of cases have an early B-cell precursor phenotype, usually CD10 (CALLA) negative (149,173). However, many have either features of myeloid leukemias, most often monocytic, or are mixed phenotype leukemias defined by cytochemical, immunophenotypic, or ultrastructural studies (see figs. 146, 147) (149, 168,173). Undifferentiated and, rarely, T-cell or B-cell cases with t(4;11) have been reported. It is likely that 11q23 rearrangement leukemias arise from multipotential stem cells (149,172).

Cytogenetic Evolution. Cytogenetic evolution from diagnosis to relapse is a frequent occurrence in ALL (Table 16) (172,174,182). The karyotype change at relapse is most commonly related to that at diagnosis. New structural abnormalities are most frequently observed.

Differential Diagnosis of ALL

Several reactive processes and other neoplastic disorders may manifest clinical or morphologic similarity to ALL. These include reactive lymphocytoses, hypoplastic anemia, increased bone marrow lymphoid progenitor cells (hematogones), acute myeloid leukemia, chronic lymphocytic leukemia, prolymphocytic leukemia, non-Hodgkin lymphoma, and metastatic small cell tumors.

Reactive Lymphocytoses. Several disorders associated with reactive lymphocytoses may present with clinical manifestations similar to ALL. Infectious mononucleosis (IM) is the most common. Children with infectious mononucleosis may present with atypical clinical manifestations and have a negative heterophile antibody study. A diagnosis of acute leukemia may be considered if these atypical clinical features are combined with unusual lymphocyte morphology or blood cytopenias. Reactive lymphocytes are generally easily recognized and have cytologic features distinct from lymphoblasts. They are morphologically heteromorphous with coarse nuclear chromatin, generally lack a nucleolus, and have moderately abundant cytoplasm. Many have distinctive cytoplasmic basophilia characterized by a radial distribution and accentuation at the cytoplasmic margin (fig. 157). Lymphoblasts have a more delicate chromatin and sparse cytoplasm

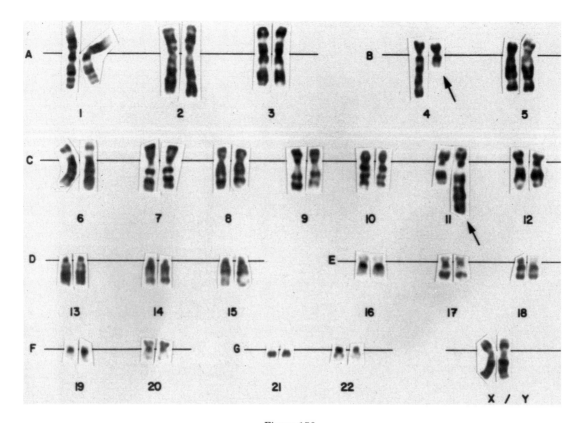

Figure 156

LYMPHOBLAST KARYOTYPE FROM A PATIENT WITH MIXED PHENOTYPE ACUTE LEUKEMIA (BILINEAL)

A karyotype from bone marrow cells of the patient whose blood smear is depicted in figure 146. There is a translocation of material from the long arm of chromosome 4 to the long arm of chromosome 11, t(4;11) (q21;q23). This translocation is found in less than 5 percent of cases of childhood ALL. It is associated with markedly elevated leukocyte counts and poor prognosis. Approximately 20 percent of patients are less than 1 month of age at diagnosis (congenital leukemia). (Giemsa-trypsin banding) (Courtesy of Dr. Nancy Schneider, Dallas, Texas.)

Figure 157
REACTIVE (ATYPICAL)
LYMPHOCYTES

This blood smear is from a 19-year-old male college student with infectious mononucleosis. The two reactive (atypical) lymphocytes are large, with abundant cytoplasm and coarse nuclear chromatin, and lack a nucleolus. Cytoplasmic basophilia is radial in distribution and accentuated at the cell margin. In contrast, lymphoblasts are generally smaller, have less cytoplasm with uniform basophilia and more dispersed nuclear chromatin, and may contain a nucleolus. (Wright-Giemsa stain)

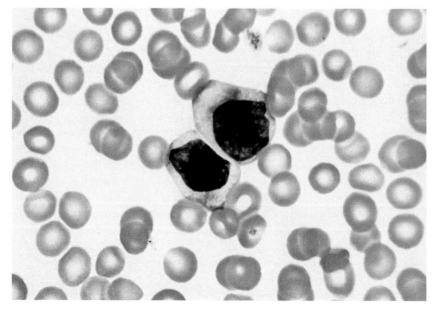

that is uniformly basophilic. In equivocal cases, serologic studies for Epstein-Barr virus (EBV) and other virus infections, such as cytomegalovirus (CMV), will often be diagnostic. It is rarely necessary to perform a bone marrow biopsy for diagnosis. If a marrow specimen is obtained, preservation of normal hematopoietic cells and, possibly, reactive changes will be found.

Children with pertussis or infectious lymphocytosis may present with profound lymphocytosis. The proliferative lymphocytes in these disorders are usually small with coarsely clumped chromatin. The nucleus of some of the lymphocytes may be cleaved or convoluted; nucleoli are lacking (fig. 158). The mature morphologic features of the lymphocytes, normal blood counts, and clinical manifestations of pertussis should exclude a diagnosis of ALL. The proliferative lymphocytes in pertussis have been shown to consist of a heterogeneous population of B cells and T-cell helper and suppressor subsets (151). Most of the cleaved and convoluted cells have a helper T-lymphocyte immunophenotype.

Hypoplastic Anemia. The usual clinical manifestations of both hypoplastic anemia and acute leukemia are related to blood cytopenias. Blood smears in cases of hypoplastic anemia may be similar to those of ALL in which lymphoblasts are absent or rare in the peripheral blood. A bone marrow trephine biopsy distinguishes the two disorders. In hypoplastic anemia, the marrow adipose tissue is increased with a corresponding decrease in hematopoietic cells. In contrast, the marrow in ALL is hypercellular with predominantly lymphoblasts (fig. 159).

Increased Bone Marrow Lymphocyte Progenitor Cells (Hematogones). Bone marrow aspirate specimens from young children contain increased numbers of bone marrow lymphocyte progenitor cells. Many of these are small lymphoid-appearing cells with morphologic features in common with the lymphoblasts of ALL or lymphoblastic lymphoma. These cells have been referred to as hematogones in the literature (157,163). They range in size from 10 to 20 μm and have a smudged homogeneous nuclear chromatin. The nucleus is frequently indented but usually lacks a nucleolus. Cytoplasm is sparse or lacking; when visible it is deeply basophilic and devoid of granules or vacuoles (figs. 160–162). In trephine biopsy sections, these cells are diffusely scattered

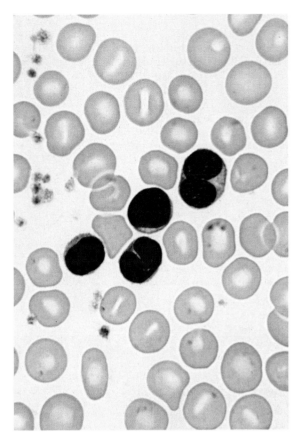

Figure 158
BLOOD LYMPHOCYTOSIS
IN A PATIENT WITH PERTUSSIS

The lymphocytes in this blood smear from an 18-month-old child with a *Bordetella pertussis* infection have lobulated nuclei. Lymphocytosis is characteristic of this disorder and the lymphocyte morphology is often atypical. The cytology of the cells could be mistaken for neoplastic lymphocytes. (Wright-Giemsa stain)

in the marrow and resemble small or medium sized lymphocytes but with a more homogeneous nuclear chromatin (fig. 163). They are occasionally found in blood smears from neonates.

Lymphocyte progenitor cells are found in bone marrow smears in large numbers in normal infants and older children with a number of diverse disease processes including iron deficiency anemia, congenital neutropenia, congenital red blood cell aplasia, neuroblastoma, retinoblastoma, and idiopathic thrombocytopenic purpura (ITP) (163). When present in increased numbers in the bone marrow of children being evaluated for cytopenias or organomegaly, a diagnosis of lymphoblastic leukemia or lymphoma may be

Figure 159
ACUTE LYMPHOBLASTIC
LEUKEMIA WITH RETICULIN
FIBROSIS CONTRASTED WITH
APLASTIC ANEMIA

Left: A trephine biopsy section from a 5-year-old male with ALL-L1 and reticulin fibrosis. A marrow aspirate was not obtainable from this patient and lymphoblasts were not present on the blood smear.

Right: This trephine biopsy section is from a patient with aplastic anemia. It is devoid of hematopoietic marrow. Lymphoblastic leukemia and aplastic anemia may present with similar clinical manifestations. The two processes are readily distinguished on the bone marrow trephine biopsy sections. (Hematoxylin and eosin stain)

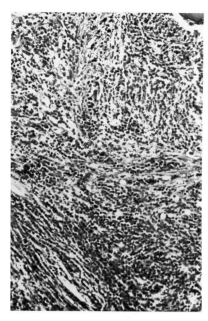 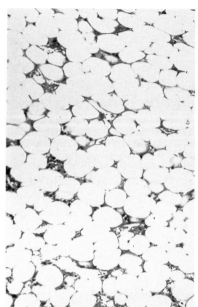

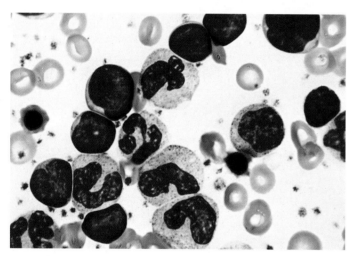

Figure 160
INCREASED BONE MARROW
LYMPHOCYTE PROGENITOR CELLS
(HEMATOGONES)

The bone marrow smear is from a 2-year-old male bone marrow transplant donor for a sibling with aplastic anemia. This normal bone marrow contains numerous lymphocyte progenitor cells (hematogones), some of which are cytologically similar to lymphoblasts. These cells could be erroneously interpreted as leukemic lymphoblasts in a patient presenting with cytopenias. The pathologist must be familiar with these cells and the conditions in which they may be increased in the bone marrow of young children. (Wright-Giemsa stain)

Figure 161
INCREASED BONE MARROW
LYMPHOCYTE PROGENITOR CELLS
(HEMATOGONES)

This bone marrow smear is from a 3-year-old male with anemia and mediastinal "widening" on chest X ray. A bone marrow examination was performed on the suspicion of lymphoblastic leukemia-lymphoma. The predominant cells in this field are lymphocyte progenitor cells (hematogones). They resemble lymphoblasts. A thoracotomy was performed and a pulmonary plasma cell pseudotumor was excised. The patient was treated for iron deficiency anemia. (Wright-Giemsa stain)

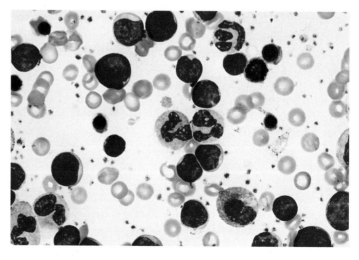

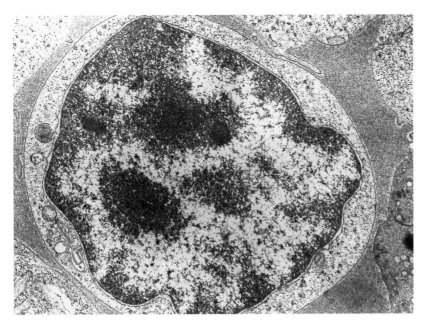

Figure 162
ELECTRON MICROGRAPH
OF A LYMPHOCYTE
PROGENITOR CELL
(HEMATOGONE)
The cell shows a small amount of cytoplasm with no distinctive features. The nucleus contains dispersed chromatin with some concentration at the margin. A small nucleolus is present. (Uranyl acetate–lead citrate stains, X19,000)

Figure 163
INCREASED BONE MARROW
LYMPHOCYTE
PROGENITOR CELLS
(HEMATOGONES)
This trephine biopsy section is from a normal 2-year-old bone marrow transplant donor (the same case as depicted in figure 160). The marrow contained approximately 50 percent immature lymphocytes (hematogones) which on this section resemble a lymphoblastic leukemia-lymphoma. (Hematoxylin and eosin stain) (Fig. 33 (bottom) from McKenna RW. Disorders of bone marrow. In Sternberg SS, ed. Diagnostic surgical pathology. 2nd ed. New York: Raven Press, 1994:623–72.)

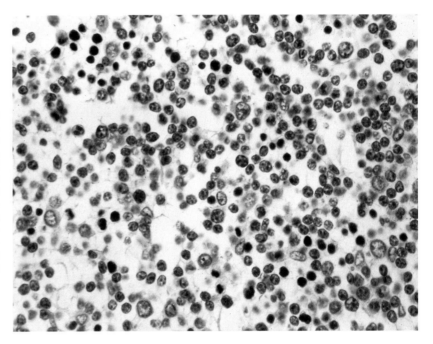

entertained. Increased lymphoid progenitor cells are commonly encountered in the regenerative bone marrow following chemotherapy for ALL (192). In this context there is potential for misinterpreting these cells as residual or recurrent lymphoblasts.

Many of these cells are TdT positive and express the common acute lymphoblastic leukemia antigen (CALLA) (CD10) and other pan–B-cell antigens (157,163,185,192). Immunophenotyping,

therefore, may not be helpful in distinguishing them from lymphoblasts of B-cell precursor ALL. However, DNA content is normal in these cells and clonality is not demonstrable by either cytogenetic or immunogenotypic analysis (157). Awareness of the conditions in which these normal lymphoid progenitor cells may be increased is essential to avoid an erroneous diagnosis of lymphoblastic leukemia or lymphoma.

Acute Myeloid Leukemia. The classes of AML that may be considered in the differential diagnosis of ALL are M0, M1, M5A, and M7. In cases of M0 in which there are no MPO-positive blasts, immunophenotyping using a combination of lymphoid and myeloid monoclonal antibodies is usually diagnostic. M1 is distinguished by the presence of MPO activity in 3 percent or more of the leukemic blasts (105).

M5A may be distinguished from ALL-L2 by the characteristic NSE reaction observed in most cases. In cases of esterase-negative M5A, immunophenotyping or electron microscopy are usually definitive.

M7 should be suspected in cases that morphologically resemble ALL-L1 or L2 in which there is myelofibrosis. Other morphologic features often found in M7 include atypical platelets on the blood smears, platelet-like material on the surface of some of the leukemic cells, and clusters of small megakaryocytes in the trephine biopsy sections. Studies for reactivity of the blasts with MoAbs to glycoprotein IIIa or IIb–IIIa complex may be confirmatory. The ultrastructural cytochemical reaction for platelet peroxidase is also a distinguishing diagnostic feature (see section on Acute Myeloid Leukemias).

Chronic Lymphocytic Leukemia (CLL). This is rarely a diagnostic consideration in cases of ALL. The cytologic features of lymphoblasts in ALL and the small lymphocytes of CLL are usually distinctive (fig. 164). Immunophenotyping will resolve cases in which an unusual clinical presentation or variant morphology results in a differential diagnosis problem.

Prolymphocytic Leukemia (PLL). PLL and L2 are rarely confused. PLL is predominantly a disease of individuals of advanced age. There are distinctive cytologic features of the leukemic cells including coarsely clumped nuclear chromatin and a single prominent vesicular nucleolus that usually distinguish PLL from ALL. In morphologically atypical cases, immunophenotyping can distinguish the two processes. The leukemic cells in PLL strongly express monoclonal surface immunoglobulin by immunofluorescence and lack TdT and CD10 (CALLA). T-cell PLL lacks TdT and expresses a peripheral T-cell immunophenotype.

Malignant Lymphoma. Two classes of malignant lymphoma are cytologically and immunologically identical to ALL: lymphoblastic lymphoma and small noncleaved cell lymphoma. The distinction of lymphoblastic lymphoma from leu-

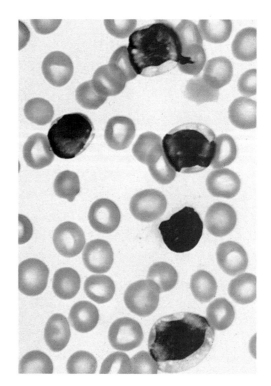

Figure 164
CHRONIC LYMPHOCYTIC LEUKEMIA
This blood smear is from a 53-year-old woman with chronic lymphocytic leukemia (CLL). The lymphocytes appear more mature than lymphoblasts. There is generally no difficulty in distinguishing ALL and CLL in blood and bone marrow smears but in this case the chromatin is less condensed than usual. (Wright-Giemsa stain)

kemia is somewhat arbitrary, usually based on the extent of bone marrow disease and extramedullary tissue masses. If a lymphoblast count is less than 25 percent in the marrow at the time of presentation, lymphoblastic lymphoma is the preferred diagnosis. In cases with greater than 25 percent bone marrow blasts and extensive extramedullary disease, the designation lymphoblastic leukemia-lymphoma is often used. Most of the cases in which the bone marrow is initially spared or minimally involved have a T-cell immunophenotype.

Small noncleaved cell lymphomas correspond cytologically to B-cell (SIg+) ALL-L3. The designation L3 leukemia is usually reserved for those cases with extensive bone marrow and blood involvement at presentation and relatively minimal extramedullary disease (see section on Bone Marrow Lymphomas).

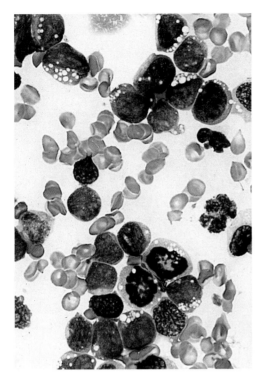

Figure 165
METASTATIC MEDULLOBLASTOMA

The medulloblastoma cells in this bone marrow resemble lymphoblasts of the type found in ALL-L2 or L3. In most cases, metastatic tumor cells are found in clumps. In this instance the marrow aspirate smears showed heavy infiltration with scattered individual cells. (Wright-Giemsa stain) (Figures 165 and 508, right are from the same patient.)

Metastatic Small Cell Tumors. Several metastatic tumors may present with extensive diffuse marrow involvement. The cytologic features of some of these may resemble lymphoblasts. In children, neuroblastoma is the most common nonhematopoietic tumor to involve the bone marrow and potentially cause problems in differential diagnosis. Embryonal rhabdomyosarcoma, retinoblastoma, Ewing sarcoma, and medulloblastoma in children, and rarely, small cell carcinoma in adults may also resemble ALL.

The necessity to distinguish one of these tumors from acute leukemia usually arises when a primary tissue mass is not identified and the patient is initially evaluated for blood cytopenias or a leukemoid reaction. Distinguishing metastatic disease from ALL in trephine biopsy sections is usually not difficult. In marrow aspirate smears, metastatic tumor cells will generally be found in clumps or clusters; large numbers of damaged tumor cells and bare nuclei may be observed throughout the smear. Occasionally, the tumor cells in rhabdomyosarcoma, neuroblastoma, retinoblastoma or medulloblastoma are spread evenly on the smear as single cells with few or no clumps (figs. 165, 166). When this occurs, the morphologic distinction from leukemia may be problematic. In equivocal cases, TdT assays, immunophenotyping, electron microscopy, and enzyme immunocytochemistry using appropriate antibodies for the characterization of small cell tumors will distinguish metastases from ALL (see section, Metastatic Tumors Involving the Bone Marrow).

Treatment and Prognosis of ALL

Advances in treatment over the past three decades have dramatically improved the prognosis for children with ALL. For B-cell precursor ALL, standard induction therapy with vincristine, prednisone, L-asparaginase, and daunorubicin produces remission in more than 95 percent of cases (129). With CNS prophylaxis and maintenance therapy with 6-mercaptopurine (6-MP), methotrexate, and vincristine, more than 50 percent of children achieve long-term disease-free survival and presumably a cure. Additional postinduction intensive chemotherapy may push cure rates to 70 percent (129).

For T-cell ALL and other high-risk types, treatment results have been less favorable with standard chemotherapy (102). By employing more aggressive therapy with high doses of rotating chemotherapeutic agents and adding drugs to the regimen, long-term disease-free survival has been achieved in 40 to 50 percent of children with T-cell ALL in some studies (102).

Allogeneic bone marrow transplantation is used following the first remission in children with high risk ALL and for patients who relapse following standard chemotherapy (144). Bone marrow transplant is the only treatment that offers a substantial chance of cure following relapse. Unfortunately this therapy is restricted to patients with a suitable donor.

Adults with ALL fair less well than children. This is at least in part because of a much greater incidence of high-risk types of ALL.

Numerous parameters have been studied for prognostic significance in ALL. They may be divided into clinical, morphologic, immunophenotypic, and cytogenetic indicators (103,107,108,115,

Figure 166
METASTATIC
NEUROBLASTOMA

The neoplastic cells in this bone marrow smear lack the usual cohesiveness of a metastatic tumor. They resemble lymphoblasts and have a distribution on the smear similar to leukemia. (Wright-Giemsa stain) (Fig. 37.46 (left) from McKenna RW. The bone marrow manifestations of Hodgkin's disease, the non-Hodgkin's lymphomas, and lymphoma-like disorders. In: Knowles DM, ed. Neoplastic hematopathology. Baltimore: Williams & Wilkins, 1992: 1135–80.)

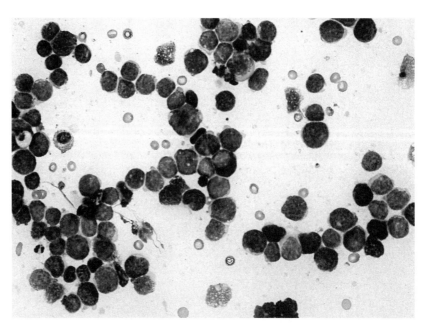

Table 20

PROGNOSTIC INDICATORS IN ALL

	Favorable	Less Favorable
Clinical		
Age	1 to 10 years	<1 and >10 years
Sex	Female	Male
Race	White	Black
WBC	<10×10^9/L	>50×10^9/L
Rapidity of cytoreduction	Bone marrow free of disease by day 14	Residual disease at day 14
Relapse	No relapse	Relapse
Morphologic	L1	L2, L3
Immunophenotypic	Early B-cell precursor CD10+ (CALLA positive)	Pre–B-cell (CIg+) CD10- (CALLA negative) T-cell ALL B-cell ALL
Cytogenetic	Hyperdiploidy >50 chromosomes	Translocations, especially t(9;22) and t(4;11)

118–122,125,133,136,156,160,172,177,180,190, 197,198). The most commonly considered prognostic factors are summarized in Table 20. The significance of these varies in different studies.

Several of the criteria that are indicators of poor prognosis by univariate analysis lose or have decreased significance by multivariate analysis (118,121,136,180). These include sex, age, FAB classification (L1, L2), and immunophenotype (T cell). Some of these criteria have lost prognostic significance for length of disease-free survival because of improved treatment regimens for high-risk ALL (156).

Cytogenetic findings that impart a favorable and unfavorable prognosis are summarized in Table 9. Recent studies suggest that chromosome translocations per se, with the exceptions of t(9;22) and t(4;11), may not decrease median survival in patients treated by present day protocols (180).

REFERENCES

1. Bennett JM, Catovsky D, Daniel MT, et al. Criteria for the diagnosis of acute leukemia of megakaryocytic lineage (M7). A report of the French-American-British Cooperative Group. Ann Intern Med 1985;103:460–2.

2. _____, Catovsky D, Daniel MT, et al. Proposals for the classification of the acute leukaemias. French-American-British (FAB) Cooperative Group. Br J Haematol 1976;33:451–8.

3. _____, Catovsky D, Daniel MT, et al. Proposals for the classification of the myelodysplastic syndromes. Br J Haematol 1982;51:189–99.

4. _____, Catovsky D, Daniel MT et al. Proposed revised criteria for the classification of acute myeloid leukemia. A report of the French-American-British Cooperative Group. Ann Intern Med 1985;103:620–5.

5. Cheson BD, Cassileth PA, Head D, et al. Report of the National Cancer Institute-sponsored workshop on definitions of diagnosis and response in acute myeloid leukemia. J Clin Oncol 1990;8:813–9.

6. Groupe Francaise de Morphologie Hematologique. French registry of acute leukemia and myelodysplastic syndromes. Age distribution and hemogram analysis of the 4496 cases recorded during 1982–1983 and classified according to FAB criteria. Cancer 1987;60:1385–94.

7. Mirro J, Zipf TF, Pui CH, et al. Acute mixed lineage leukemia: clinicopathologic correlations and prognostic significance. Blood 1985;66:1115–23.

8. National Cancer Institute. Division of Cancer Prevention and Control Surveillance Program. Cancer statistics review, 1973–1986. Bethesda, Maryland: USDHHS, 1989; NIH publication no. 89–2789.

9. Perentesis J, Ramsay NK, Brunning R, et al. Biphenotypic leukemia: immunologic and morphologic evidence for a common lymphoid-myeloid progenitor in humans. J Pediatr 1983;102:63–7

10. Pui CH, Crist WM, Look AT. Biology and clinical significance of cytogenetic abnormalities in childhood acute lymphoblastic leukemia. Blood 1990;76:1449–63.

11. Robison LL, Mertens A, Neglia JP. Epidemiology and etiology of childhood cancer. In: Fernbach DJ, Vietti TJ, eds. Clinical pediatric oncology. St Louis: Mosby Year Book, 1991:11–28.

12. Rowley JD. Recurring chromosome abnormalities in leukemia and lymphoma. Semin Hematol 1990;27:122–36.

13. Stanley M, McKenna RW, Ellinger G, Brunning RD. Classification of 358 cases of acute myeloid leukemia by FAB criteria: analysis of clinical and morphologic features. In: Bloomfield CD, ed. Chronic and acute leukemias in adults. Boston: Martinus Nijhoff, 1985:147–74.

14. Stass SA, Mirro J Jr. Lineage heterogeneity in acute leukaemia: acute mixed-lineage leukaemia and lineage switch. Clin Haematol 1986;15:811–27.

15. Yunis JJ, Brunning RD. Prognostic significance of chromosomal abnormalities in acute leukaemias and myelodysplastic syndromes. Clin Haematol 1986;15:597–620.

Acute Myeloid Leukemias

16. Arthur DC, Bloomfield CD. Partial deletion of the long arm of chromosome 16 and bone marrow eosinophilia in acute nonlymphocytic leukemia: a new association. Blood 1983;61:994–8.

17. Bain BJ, Catovsky D, O'Brien M, et al. Megakaryoblastic leukemia presenting as acute myelofibrosis—a study of four cases with the platelet-peroxidase reaction. Blood 1981;58:206–13.

18. Bearman RM, Pangalis GA, Rappaport H. Acute ("malignant") myelosclerosis. Cancer 1979;43:279–93.

19. Bennett JM, Catovsky D, Daniel MT, et al. Criteria for the diagnosis of acute leukemia of megakaryocytic lineage (M7). A report of the French-American-British Cooperative Group. Ann Intern Med 1985;103:460–2.

20. _____, Catovsky D, Daniel MT, et al. Proposals for the classification of the acute leukaemias. French-American-British (FAB) Cooperative Group. Br J Haematol 1976;33:451–8.

21. _____, Catovsky D, Daniel MT, et al. Proposals for the classification of the myelodysplastic syndromes. Br J Haematol 1982;51:189–99.

22. _____, Catovsky D, Daniel MT, et al. Proposed revised criteria for the classification of acute myeloid leukemia. A report of the French-American-British Cooperative Group. Ann Intern Med 1985;103:626–9.

23. Berdeaux DH, Glasser L, Serokmann R, Moon T, Durie BG. Hypoplastic acute leukemia: review of 70 cases with multivariate regression analysis. Hematol Oncol 1986;4:291–305.

24. Berger R, Bernheim A, Daniel MT, et al. Cytologic characterization and significance of normal karyotypes in t(8;21) acute myeloblastic leukemia. Blood 1982;59:171–8.

25. Bernstein R, Pinto MR, Behr A, Mendelow B. Chromosome 3 abnormalities in acute nonlymphocytic leukemia (ANLL) with abnormal thrombopoiesis: report of three patients with a "new" inversion anomaly and a further case of homologous translocation. Blood 1982;60:613–7.

26. Bessho F, Hayashi Y, Hayashi Y, Ohga K. Ultrastructural studies of peripheral blood of neonates with Down's syndrome and transient abnormal myelopoiesis. Am J Clin Pathol 1988;89:627–33.

27. Bitter MA, Le Beau MM, Larson RA, et al. A morphologic and cytochemical study of acute myelomonocytic leukemia with abnormal marrow eosinophils associated with inv(16)(p13q22). Am J Clin Pathol 1984;81:733–41.

28. _____, Le Beau MM, Rowley JD, et al. Associations between morphology, karyotype, and clinical features in myeloid leukemias. Hum Pathol 1987;18:211–25.

29. _____, Neilly ME, Le Beau MM, Pearson MG, Rowley JD. Rearrangements of chromosome 3 involving bands 3q21 and 3q26 are associated with normal or elevated platelet counts in acute nonlymphocytic leukemia. Blood 1985;66:1362–70.

30. Bradstock KF, Hoffbrand AV, Ganeshaguru K, et al. Terminal deoxynucleotidyl transferase expression in acute non-lymphoid leukaemia: an analysis by immunofluorescence. Br J Haematol 1981;47:133–43.

31. Breton-Gorius J, Houssay D. Auer bodies in acute promyelocytic leukemia. Demonstration of their fine structure and peroxidase localization. Lab Invest 1973;28:135–41.

32. _____, Vanhaeke D, Pryzwansky KB, et al. Simultaneous detection of membrane markers with monoclonal antibodies and peroxidatic activities in leukaemia: ultrastructural analysis using a new method of fixation preserving the platelet peroxidase. Br J Haematol 1984;58:447–58.

33. _____, Villeval JL, Kieffer N, Mitjavila MT, Guichard J, Vainchenker W. Limits of phenotypic markers for the diagnosis of megakaryoblastic leukemia. Blood Cells 1989;15:259–77.

34. _____, Villeval JL, Mitjavila MT, et al. Ultrastructural and cytochemical characterization of blasts from early erythroblastic leukemias. Leukemia 1987;1:173–81.

35. Brodeur GM, Dahl GV, Williams DL, Tipton RE, Kalwinsky DK. Transient leukemoid reaction and trisomy 21 mosaicism in a phenotypically normal newborn. Blood 1980;55:691–3.

36. Brunning RD, Parkin JL, Hanson CA. Hematopoietic and lymphoreticular neoplasms. In: Azar HA, ed. Pathology of human neoplasms: an atlas of diagnostic electron microscopy and immunohistochemistry. New York: Raven Press, 1988:221–303.

37. Buccheri V, Shetty V, Yoshida N, Morilla R, Matutes E, Catovsky D. The role of an anti-myeloperoxidase antibody in the diagnosis and classification of acute leukaemia: a comparison with light and electron microscopy cytochemistry. Br J Haematol 1992;80:62–8.

38. Campbell LJ, Challis J, Fok T, Garson OM. Chromosome 16 abnormalities associated with myeloid malignancies. Genes Chromosom Cancer 1991;3:55–61.

39. Chan WC, Carroll A, Alvarado CS, et al. Acute megakaryoblastic leukemia in infants with t(1;22) (p13;q13) abnormality. Am J Clin Pathol 1992;98:214–21.

40. Cheson BD, Cassileth PA, Head DR, et al. Report of the National Cancer Institute-sponsored workshop on definitions of diagnosis and response in acute myeloid leukemia. J Clin Oncol 1990;8:813–9.

41. Davey DD, Patil SR, Echternacht H, Fatemi C, Dick FR. 8;21 translocation in acute nonlymphocytic leukemia. Occurrence in M1 and M2 FAB subtypes. Am J Clin Pathol 1989;92:172–6.

42. Davey FR, Davis RB, MacCallum JM, et al. Morphologic and cytochemical characteristics of acute promyelocytic leukemia. Am J Hematol 1989;30:221–7.

43. de Alarcon PA, Patil S, Goldberg J, Allen JB, Shaw S. Infants with Down's syndrome. Use of cytogenetic studies and in vitro colony assay for granulocyte progenitor to distinguish acute nonlymphocytic leukemia from a transient myeloproliferative disorder. Cancer 1987;60:987–93.

44. deMent SH. Association between mediastinal germ cell tumors and hematologic malignancies: an update. Hum Pathol 1990;21:699–703.

45. Erber WN, Breton-Gorius J, Villeval JL, Oscier DG, Bai Y, Mason DY. Detection of cells of megakaryocytic lineage in haematological malignancies by immuno-alkaline phosphatase labelling cell smears with a panel of monoclonal antibodies. Br J Haematol 1987;65:87–94.

46. Fong C, Brodeur GM. Down's syndrome and leukemia: epidemiology, genetics, cytogenetics and mechanisms of leukemogenesis. Cancer Genet Cytogenet 1987;28:55–76.

47. Golomb HM, Rowley JD, Vardiman JW, Testa JR, Butler A. "Microgranular" acute promyelocytic leukemia: a distinct clinical, ultrastructural and cytogenetic entity. Blood 1980;55:253–9.

48. Groupe Francais de Cytogenetique Hematologique. Acute myelogenous leukemia with an -8;21 translocation. A report on 148 cases from the Groupe Francais de Cytogenetique Hematologique. Cancer Genet Cytogenet 1990;44:169–79.

49. Groupe Francais de Morphologie Hematologique. French registry of acute leukemia and myelodysplastic syndromes. Age distribution and hemogram analysis of the 4496 cases recorded during 1982–1983 and classified according to FAB criteria. Cancer 1987;60:1385–94.

50. Hagemeijer A, Hählen K, Sizoo W, Abels J. Translocation (9;11)(p21;q23) in three cases of acute monoblastic leukemia. Cancer Genet Cytogenet 1982;5:95–105.

51. Hayashi Y, Eguchi M, Sugita K, et al. Cytogenetic findings and clinical features in acute leukemia and transient myeloproliferative disorder in Down's syndrome. Blood 1988;72:15–23.

52. Heim S, Kristoffersson U, Mandahl N, et al. High resolution banding analysis of the reciprocal translocation t(6;9) in acute nonlymphocytic leukemia. Cancer Genet Cytogenet 1986;22:195–201.

53. Howe RB, Bloomfield CD, McKenna RW. Hypocellular acute leukemia. Am J Med 1982;72:391–5.

54. Hruban RH, Kuhajda FP, Mann RB. Acute myelofibrosis. Immunohistochemical study of four cases and comparison with acute megakaryoblastic leukemia. Am J Clin Pathol 1987;88:578–88.

55. Huang MJ, Li CY, Nichols WL, Young JH, Katzman JA. Acute leukemia with megakaryocytic differentiation: a study of 12 cases identified immunocytochemically. Blood 1984;64:427–39.

56. Hurwitz CA, Raimondi SC, Head D, et al. Distinctive immunophenotypic features of t(8; 21) (q22; q22) acute myeloblastic leukemia in children. Blood 1992;80:3182–8.

57. International Committee for Standardization in Haematology (ICSH). Recommended methods for cytological procedures in haematology. Clin Lab Haematol 1985;7:55–74.

58. Koike T. Megakaryoblastic leukemia: the characterization and identification of megakaryoblasts. Blood 1984;64:683–92.

59. Lampkin BC, Masterson M, Sambrono JE, Heckel JL, Jones G. Current chemotherapeutic treatment strategies in childhood acute nonlymphocytic leukemia. Semin Oncol 1987;14:397–406.

60. Larson RA, Williams SF, Le Beau MM, Bitter MA, Vardiman JW, Rowley JD. Acute myelomonocytic leukemia with abnormal eosinophils and inv(16) or t(16;16) has a favorable prognosis. Blood 1986;68:1242–9.

61. Lawlor E, McCann SR, Willoughby R, Dunne J, Temperley IJ. Basophil differentiation in Ph-positive blast cell leukaemia [Letter]. Br J Haematol 1983;54:157–60.

62. Le Beau MM, Larson RA, Bitter MA, Vardiman JW, Golomb HM, Rowley JD. Association of an inversion of chromosome 16 with abnormal marrow eosinophils in acute myelomonocytic leukemia. A unique cytogenetic-clinicopathological association. N Engl J Med 1983;309:630–6.

63. Lee EJ, Pollak A, Leavitt RD, Testa JR, Schiffer CA. Minimally differentiated acute nonlymphocytic leukemia: a distinct entity. Blood 1987;70:1400–6.

64. Lewis SM, Szur L. Malignant myelosclerosis. Br Med J 1963;2:472–7.
65. Mayer RJ. Current chemotherapeutic treatment approaches to the management of previously untreated adults with de novo acute myelogenous leukemia. Semin Oncol 1987;14:384–96.
66. McKenna RW, Bloomfield CD, Dick F, Nesbit ME, Brunning RD. Acute monoblastic leukemia: diagnosis and treatment of ten cases. Blood 1975;46:481–94.
67. _____, Parkin J, Bloomfield CD, Sundberg RD, Brunning RD. Acute promyelocytic leukaemia: a study of 39 cases with identification of a hyperbasophilic microgranular variant. Br J Haematol 1982;50:201–14.
68. Meis JM, Butler JJ, Osborne BM, Manning JT. Granulocytic sarcoma in nonleukemic patients. Cancer 1986;58:2697–709.
69. Mirro J, Zipf TF, Pui CH, et al. Acute mixed lineage leukemia: clinicopathologic correlations and prognostic significance. Blood 1985;66:1115–23.
70. Muller S, Sangster G, Crocker J, et al. An immunohistochemical and clinicopathological study of granulocytic sarcoma ("chloroma"). Hematol Oncol 1986;4:101–12.
71. Nagasaka M, Maeda S, Maeda H, et al. Four cases of t(4;11) acute leukemia and its myelomonocytic nature in infants. Blood 1983;61:1174–81.
72. Neiman RS, Barcos M, Berard C, et al. Granulocytic sarcoma: a clinicopathologic study of 61 biopsied cases. Cancer 1981;48:1426–37.
73. Nichols CR, Hoffman R, Einhorn LH, Williams SD, Wheeler LA, Garnick MB. Hematologic malignancies associated with primary mediastinal germ-cell tumors. Ann Intern Med 1985;102:603–9.
74. O'Brien S, Kantarjian HM, Keating M, et al. Association of granulocytosis with poor prognosis in patients with acute myelogenous leukemia and translocation of chromosomes 8 and 21. J Clin Oncol 1989;7:1081–6.
75. Olopade OI, Thangavelu M, Larson RA, et al. Clinical, morphologic, and cytogenetic characteristics of 26 patients with acute erythroblastic leukemia. Blood 1992;80:2873–82.
76. Perentesis J, Ramsay NK, Brunning R, Kersey JH, Filipovich AH. Biphenotypic leukemia: immunologic and morphologic evidence for a common lymphoid-myeloid progenitor in humans. J Pediatr 1983;102:63–7.
77. Peterson L, Dehner LP, Brunning RD. Extramedullary masses as presenting features of acute monoblastic leukemia. Am J Clin Pathol 1981;75:140–8.
78. Peterson LC, Parkin JL, Arthur DC, Brunning RD. Acute basophilic leukemia. A clinical, morphologic and cytogenetic study of eight cases. Am J Clin Pathol 1991;96:160–70.
79. Pinkus GS, Pinkus JL. Myeloperoxidase: a specific marker for myeloid cells in paraffin sections. Mod Pathol 1991;4:733–41.
80. Pui CH, Rivera G, Mirro J, Stass S, Peiper S, Murphy SB. Acute megakaryoblastic leukemia: blast cell aggregates simulating metastatic tumor. Arch Pathol Lab Med 1985;109:1033–5.
81. Rappaport H. Tumors of the hematopoietic system. Atlas of Tumor Pathology, 1st Series, Fascicle 8. Washington, D.C.: Armed Forces Institute of Pathology, 1966.
82. Robison LL, Nesbit ME Jr, Sather HN, et al. Down syndrome and acute leukemia in children: a 10-year retrospective survey from Children's Cancer Study Group. J Pediatr 1984;105:235–42.
83. Rowley JD. Recurring chromosome abnormalities in leukemia and lymphoma. Semin Hematol 1990;27:122–36.
84. Schachner J, Kantarjian H, Dalton W, McCredie K, Keating M, Freireich EJ. Cytogenetic association and prognostic significance of bone marrow blast cell terminal transferase in patients with acute myeloblastic leukemia. Leukemia 1988;2:667–71.
85. Second International Workshop on Chromosomes in Leukemia. Cytogenetic, morphologic, and clinical correlations in acute nonlymphocytic leukemia with t(8q-; 21q+). Cancer Genet Cytogenet 1980;2:99–102.
86. Stanley M, McKenna RW, Ellinger G, Brunning RD. Classification of 358 cases of acute myeloid leukemia by FAB criteria: analysis of clinical and morphologic features. In: Bloomfield CD, ed. Chronic and acute leukemias in adults. Boston: Martinus Nijhoff, 1985:147–74.
87. Stone RM, Mayer RJ. The unique aspects of acute promyelocytic leukemia. J Clin Oncol 1990;8:1913–21.
88. Sultan C, Sigaux F, Imbert M, Reyes F. Acute myelodysplasia with myelofibrosis. A report of eight cases. Br J Haematol 1981;49:11–6.
89. Swirsky DM, Li YS, Matthews JG, Flemans RJ, Rees JK, Hayhoe FG. 8;21 translocation in acute granulocytic leukaemia: cytological, cytochemical and clinical features. Br J Haematol 1984;56:199–213.
90. Tallman MS, Hakimian D, Shaw JM, Lissner GS, Russell EJ, Variakojis D. Granulocytic sarcoma is associated with the 8;21 translocation in acute myeloid leukemia. J Clin Oncol 1993;11:690–7.
91. Third MIC Cooperative Study Group. Recommendations for a morphologic, immunologic, and cytogenetic (MIC) working classification of the primary and therapy-related myelodysplastic disorders. Cancer Genet Cytogenet 1988;32:1–10.
92. van der Valk P, Mullink H, Huijgens PC, Tadema TM, Vos W, Meijer CJ. Immunohistochemistry in bone marrow diagnosis. Value of a panel of monoclonal antibodies on routinely processed bone marrow biopsies. Am J Surg Pathol 1989;13:97–106.
93. Vaughan WP, Karp JE, Burke PJ. Long chemotherapy-free remissions after single-cycle timed-sequential chemotherapy for acute myelocytic leukemia. Cancer 1980;45:859–65.
94. _____, Karp JE, Burke PJ. Two-cycle timed-sequential chemotherapy for adult acute nonlymphocytic leukemia. Blood 1984;64:975–80.
95. Villeval JL, Cramer P, Lemoine F, et al. Phenotype of early erythroblastic leukemias. Blood 1986;68:1167–74.
96. West KP, Warford A, Fray L, Allen M, Cambell AC, Lauder I. The demonstration of B-cell, T-cell and myeloid antigens in paraffin sections. J Pathol 1986;150:89–101.
97. Wick MR, Li CY, Pierre RV. Acute nonlymphocytic leukemia with basophilic differentiation. Blood 1982;60:38–45.
98. Wiernik PH, Serpick AA. Granulocytic sarcoma (chloroma). Blood 1970;35:361–9.
99. Windebank KP, Tefferi A, Smithson WA, et al. Acute megakaryocytic leukemia (M7) in children. Mayo Clin Proc 1989;64:1339–51.
100. Yam LT, Li CY, Crosby WH. Cytochemical identification of monocytes and granulocytes. Am J Clin Pathol 1971;55:283–90.
101. Yunis JJ, Brunning RD. Prognostic significance of chromosomal abnormalities in acute leukaemias and myelodysplastic syndromes. Clin Haematol 1986;15:597–620.

Acute Lymphoblastic Leukemias

102. Amylon MD. Treatment of T-lineage acute lymphoblastic leukemia. Hematol Oncol Clin North Am 1990;4:937–49.

103. Arthur DC, Bloomfield CD, Lindquist LL, Nesbit ME Jr. Translocation 4;11 in acute lymphoblastic leukemia: clinical characteristics and prognostic significance. Blood 1982;59:96–9.

104. Behm FG. Morphologic and cytochemical characteristics of childhood lymphoblastic leukemia. Hematol Oncol Clin North Am 1990;4:715–41.

105. Bennett JM, Catovsky D, Daniel MT, et al. Proposals for the classification of the acute leukemias. French-American-British (FAB) Cooperative Group. Br J Haematol 1976;33:451–8.

106. _____, Catovsky D, Daniel MT, et al. The morphological classification of acute lymphoblastic leukemia: concordance among observers and clinical correlations. Br J Haematol 1981;47:553–61.

107. Bloomfield CD, Goldman AI, Alimena G, et al. Chromosomal abnormalities identify high-risk and low-risk patients with acute lymphoblastic leukemia. Blood 1986;67:415–20.

108. Borowitz MJ. Immunological markers in childhood acute lymphoblastic leukemia. Hematol Oncol Clin North Am 1990;4:743–65.

109. _____, Dowell BL, Boyett JM, et al. Monoclonal antibody definition of T cell acute leukemia: a Pediatric Oncology Group study. Blood 1985;65:785–8.

110. Brearley RL, Johnson SA, Lister TA. Acute lymphoblastic leukemia in adults: clinicopathological correlation with the French-American-British (FAB) cooperative group classification. Eur J Cancer 1979;15:909–14.

111. Brunning RD. Philadelphia chromosome positive leukemia. Hum Pathol 1980;11:307–9.

112. _____, McKenna RW. Immunologic markers for acute leukemia: a morphologist's perspective. In: Berard C, Dorfman R, Kaufman N, eds. Malignant lymphoma. Baltimore: Williams & Wilkins, 1986:124–60. (IAP Monograph, No. 29).

113. _____, McKenna RW, Bloomfield CD, Coccia P, Gajl-Peczalska KJ. Bone marrow involvement in Burkitt's lymphoma. Cancer 1977;40:1771–9.

114. _____, Parkin JL, McKenna RW. Acute lymphoblastic leukemia. In: Polliack A, ed. Human leukemias: cytochemical and ultrastructural techniques in diagnosis and research. Boston: Martinus Nijoff, 1984:173–218.

115. Carroll AJ, Crist WM, Parmley RT, Roper M, Cooper MD, Finley WH. Pre-B cell leukemia associated with chromosome translocation 1;19. Blood 1984;63:721–4.

116. Catovsky D, Cherchi M, Greaves MF, Janossy G, Pain C, Kay HE. Acid-phosphatase reaction in acute lymphoblastic leukemia. Lancet 1978;1:749–51.

117. Cerezo L, Shuster JJ, Pullen DJ, et al. Laboratory correlates and prognostic significance of granular acute lymphoblastic leukemia in children. A Pediatric Oncology Group study. Am J Clin Pathol 1991;95:526–31.

118. Crist W, Boyett J, Pullen J, van Eys J, Viotti T. Clinical and biological features predict poor prognosis in acute lymphoid leukemias in children and adolescents: a Pediatric Oncology Group review. Med Pediatr Oncol 1986;14:135–9.

119. _____, Boyett J, Roper M, et al. Pre-B cell leukemia responds poorly to treatment: a pediatric oncology group study. Blood 1984;63:407–14.

120. _____, Carroll A, Shuster J, et al. Philadelphia chromosome positive childhood acute lymphoblastic leukemia: clinical and cytogenetic characteristics and treatment outcome. A Pediatric Oncology Group study. Blood 1990;76:489–94.

121. _____, Pullen J, Boyett J, et al. Clinical and biologic features predict a poor prognosis in acute lymphoid leukemias in infants: a Pediatric Oncology Group study. Blood 1986;67:135–40.

122. Crist WM, Shuster JJ, Falletta J, et al. Clinical features and outcome in childhood T-cell leukemia-lymphoma according to stage of thymocyte differentiation: a Pediatric Oncology Group study. Blood 1988;72:1891–7.

123. Darbyshire, PJ, Lilleyman JS. Granular acute lymphoblastic leukemia of childhood: a morphologic phenomenon. J Clin Pathol 1987;40:251–3.

124. Dvorak AM, Monahan RA, Dickersin GR. Diagnostic electron microscopy. I. Hematology: differential diagnosis of acute lymphoblastic and acute myeloblastic leukemia. Use of ultrastructural peroxidase cytochemistry and routine electron microscopic technology. Pathol Annu 1981;16(Pt 1):101–37.

125. Fletcher JA, Lynch EA, Kimball VM, Donnelly M, Tantravahi R, Sallan SE. Translocation (9;22) is associated with extremely poor prognosis in intensively treated children with acute lymphoblastic leukemia. Blood 1991;77:435–9.

126. Flug F, Dodson L, Wolff J, et al. B-lymphocyte associated differentiation antigen expression by "non-B, non-T" acute lymphoblastic leukemia. Leuk Res 1985;9:1051–8.

127. Foon KA, Todd RF III. Immunologic classification of leukemia and lymphoma. Blood 1986;68:1–31.

128. Fradera J, Vélez-García E, White JG. Acute lymphoblastic leukemia with unusual cytoplasmic granulation: a morphologic, cytochemical and ultrastructural study. Blood 1986;68:406–11.

129. Gaynon PS. Primary treatment of childhood acute lymphoblastic leukemia of non-T cell lineage (including infants). Hematol Oncol Clin North Am 1990;4:915–36.

130. Glick AD. Acute leukemia: electron microscopic diagnosis. Semin Oncol 1976;3:229–41.

131. _____, Paniker K, Flexner JM, Graber SE, Collins RD. Acute leukemia of adults. Ultrastructural, cytochemical and histologic observations in 100 cases. Am J Clin Pathol 1980;73:459–70.

132. Greaves MF, Brown G, Rapson NT, Lister TA. Antisera to acute lymphoblastic leukemia cells. Clin Immunol Immunopathol 1975;4:67–84.

133. _____, Janossy G, Peto J, Kay H. Immunologically defined subclasses of acute lymphoblastic leukemia in children: their relationship to presentation features and prognosis. Br J Haematol 1981;48:179–97.

134. _____, Paxton A, Janossy G, Lister TA, Pain C, Johnson S. Acute lymphoblastic leukemia associated antigen. III. Alterations in expression during treatment and relapse. Leuk Res 1980;4:1–14.

135. Grogan TM, Insalaco SJ, Savage RA, Vail ML. Acute lymphocytic leukemia with prominent azurophilic granulation and punctate acidic nonspecific esterase and phosphatase activity. Am J Clin Pathol 1981;75:716–22.

136. Hammond D, Sather H, Nesbit M, et al. Analysis of prognostic factors in acute lymphoblastic leukemia. Med Pediatr Oncol 1986;14:124–34.

137. Hay CR, Barnett D, James V, Woodcock BW, Brown MJ, Lawrence AC. Granular common acute lymphoblastic leukemia in adults: a morphologic study. Eur J Haematol 1987;39:299–305.

138. Hogan TF, Koss W, Murgo AJ, Amato RS, Fontana JA, VanScoy FL. Acute lymphoblastic leukemia with chromosomal 5;14 translocation and hypereosinophilia: case report and literature review. J Clin Oncol 1987;5:382–90.

139. Homans AC, Barker BE, Forman EN, Cornell CJ Jr, Dickerman JP, Truman JT. Immunophenotypic characteristics of cerebral spinal fluid cells in children with acute lymphoblastic leukemia at diagnosis. Blood 1990;76:1807–11.

140. Hurwitz CA, Loken MR, Graham ML, et al. Asynchronous antigen expression in B lineage acute lymphoblastic leukemia. Blood 1988;72:299–307.

141. _____, Mirro J Jr. Mixed-lineage leukemia and asynchronous antigen expression. Hematol Oncol Clin North Am 1990;4:767–94.

142. Hutton JJ, Coleman MS, Moffitt S, et al. Prognostic significance of terminal transferase activity in childhood acute lymphoblastic leukemia: a prospective analysis of 164 patients. Blood 1982;60:1267–76.

143. Imamura N, Tanaka R, Kajihara H, Kuramoto A. Analysis of peroxidase-negative acute unclassifiable leukemias by monoclonal antibodies. 1. Acute myelogenous leukemia and acute myelomonocytic leukemia. Eur J Haematol 1988;41:420–8.

144. Johnson FL. Role of bone marrow transplantation in childhood lymphoblastic leukemia. Hematol Oncol Clin North Am 1990;4:997–1008.

145. Kalwinsky DK, Roberson P, Dahl G, et al. Clinical relevance of lymphoblast biological features in children with acute lymphoblastic leukemia. J Clin Oncol 1985;3:477–84.

146. Kaneko Y, Maseki N, Takasaki N, et al. Clinical and hematologic characteristics in acute leukemia with 11q23 translocations. Blood 1986;67:484–91.

147. Kantarjian HM, Hirsch-Ginsberg C, Yee G, Huh Y, Freireich EJ, Stass S. Mixed-lineage leukemia revisited: acute lymphocytic leukemia with myeloperoxidase-positive blasts by electron microscopy. Blood 1990;76:808–13.

148. Kaplan SS, Penchansky L, Stolc V, Contis L, Krause JR. Immunophenotyping in the classification of acute leukemia in adults. Interpretation of multiple lineage reactivity. Cancer 1989;63:1520–7.

149. Katz F, Malcolm S, Gibbons B, et al. Cellular and molecular studies on infant null acute lymphoblastic leukemia. Blood 1988;71:1438–47.

150. Kersey J, Goldman A, Abramson C, et al. Clinical usefulness of monoclonal antibody phenotyping in childhood acute lymphoblastic leukemia. Lancet 1982;2:1419–23.

151. Kubic VL, Kubic PT, Brunning RD. The morphologic and immunophenotypic assessment of the lymphocytosis accompanying Bordetella pertussis infection. Am J Clin Pathol 1991;95:809–15.

152. Kurec AS, Belair P, Stefanu C, Barrett DM, Dubowy RL, Davey FR. Significance of aberrant lymphophenotypes in childhood acute lymphoid leukemia. Cancer 1991;67:3081–6.

153. Lanham GR, Rivera G, Weiss K, Stass SA. Comparison of morphology in ALL at presentation and relapse. Med Pediatr Oncol 1985;13:1–3.

154. Lewinski UH, Gafter U, Klein B, Djaldetti M. Transmission and scanning electron microscopy study on Burkitt-like leukemia. Arch Pathol Lab Med 1979;103:558–60.

155. Lilleyman JS, Hann IM, Stevens RF, Eden OB, Richards SM. French American British (FAB) morphological classification of childhood lymphoblastic leukaemia and its clinical importance. J Clin Pathol 1986;39:998–1002.

156. _____, Hann IM, Stevens RF, et al. Cytomorphology of childhood lymphoblastic leukaemia: a prospective study of 2000 patients. United Kingdom Medical Research Council's Working Party on Childhood Leukaemia. Br J Haematol 1992;81:52–7.

157. Longacre TA, Foucar K, Crago S, et al. Hematogones: a multiparameter analysis of bone marrow precursor cells. Blood 1989;73:543–52.

158. McKenna RW, Byrnes RK, Nesbit ME, et al. Cytochemical profiles in acute lymphoblastic leukemia. Am J Pediatr Hematol Oncol 1979;1:263–75.

159. _____, Parkin J, Brunning RD. Morphologic and ultrastructural characteristics of T-cell acute lymphoblastic leukemia. Cancer 1979;44:1290–7.

160. Miller DR, Krailo M, Bleyer WA, et al. Prognostic implications of blast cell morphology in childhood acute lymphoblastic leukemia: a report from the Children's Cancer Study Group. Cancer Treat Rep 1985;69:1211–21.

161. _____, Leikin S, Albo V, Sather H, Hammond D. Prognostic importance of morphology (FAB classification) in childhood acute lymphoblastic leukaemia (ALL). Br J Haematol 1981;48:199–206.

162. Mirro J Jr, Kitchingman G, Behm FG, Murphy SB, Goorha RM. T cell differentiation stages identified by molecular and immunologic analysis of the T cell receptor complex in childhood lymphoblastic leukemia. Blood 1987;69:908–12.

163. Muehleck SD, McKenna RW, Gale PF, Brunning RD. Terminal deoxynucleotidyl transferase (TdT)-positive cells in bone marrow in the absence of hematologic malignancy. Am J Clin Pathol 1983;97:277–84.

164. Nadler LM, Korsmeyer SJ, Anderson KC, et al. B cell origin on non T-cell acute lymphoblastic leukemia. A model for discrete stages of neoplastic and normal pre-B cell differentiation. J Clin Invest 1984;74:332–40.

165. National Cancer Institute. Division of Cancer Prevention and Control Surveillance Program. Cancer statistics review, 1973–1986. Bethesda, Maryland: USDHHS, 1989; NIH publication no. 89–2789.

166. Navari RM, Carter J, Hillmon RS. Bone marrow necrosis in acute leukemia. Acta Haematol 1983;69:158–63.

167. Niebrugge DJ, Benjamin DR. Bone marrow necrosis preceding acute lymphoblastic leukemia in childhood. Cancer 1983;52:2162–4.

168. Parkin JL, Arthur DC, Abramson CS, et al. Acute leukemia associated with the t(4;11) chromosome rearrangement: ultrastructural and immunologic characteristics. Blood 1982;60:1321–31.

169. _____, McKenna RW, Brunning RD. Ultrastructural features of basophil and mast cell granulopoiesis in blastic phase Philadelphia chromosome-positive leukemia. JNCI 1980;65:535–46.

170. Pui CH, Behm FG, Singh B, et al. Myeloid-associated antigen expression lacks prognostic value in childhood acute lymphoblastic leukemia treated with intensive multiagent chemotherapy. Blood 1990;75:198–202.

171. _____, Carroll AJ, Head D, et al. Near-triploid and near-tetraploid acute lymphoblastic leukemia of childhood. Blood 1990;76:590–6.

172. _____, Crist WM, Look AT. Biology and clinical significance of cytogenetic abnormalities in childhood acute lymphoblastic leukemia. Blood 1990;76:1449–63.

173. _____, Frankel LS, Carroll AJ, et al. Clinical characteristics and treatment outcome of childhood acute lymphoblastic leukemia with the t(4;11)(q21;q23): a collaborative study of 40 cases. Blood 1991;77:440–7.

174. _____, Raimondi SC, Behm FG, et al. Shifts in blast phenotype and karyotype at relapse of childhood lymphoblastic leukemia. Blood 1986;68:1306–10.

175. _____, Raimondi SC, Dodge RK, et al. Prognostic importance of structural chromosomal abnormalities in children with hyperdiploidy (>50 chromosomes) acute lymphoblastic leukemia. Blood 1989;73:1963–7.

176. _____, Ribeiro PC, Hancock ML, et al. Acute myeloid leukemia in children treated with epipodophyllotoxins for acute lymphoblastic leukemia. N Engl J Med 1991;325:1682–7.

177. _____, Williams DL, Kalwinsky DK, et al. Cytogenetic features and serum LDH level predict a poor treatment outcome for children with pre B-cell leukemia. Blood 1986;67:1688–92.

178. Roper M, Crist WM, Metzgar R, et al. Monoclonal antibody characterization of surface antigens in childhood T-cell lymphoid malignancies. Blood 1983;61:830–7.

179. Ross CW, Stoolman LM, Schnitzer B, Schlegelmilch JA, Hanson CA. Immunophenotypic aberrancy in adult acute lymphoblastic leukemia. Am J Clin Pathol 1990;94:590–9.

180. Rubin CM, Le Beau MM, Mick R, et al. Impact of chromosomal translocations on prognosis in childhood acute lymphoblastic leukemia. J Clin Oncol 1991;9:2183–92.

181. Schumacher HR, Perlin E, Klos JR, Holloway ML, Miller WM, Sanford SA. Hand-mirror cell leukemia: a new clinical and morphological variant. Am J Clin Pathol 1977;68:531–4.

182. Secker-Walker LM, Alimena G, Bloomfield CD, et al. Cytogenetic studies of 21 patients with acute lymphoblastic leukemia in relapse. Cancer Genet Cytogenet 1989;40:163–9.

183. _____, Craig JM, Hawkins JM, Hoffbrand AV. Philadelphia positive acute lymphoblastic leukemia in adults: age distribution, BCR breakpoint and prognostic significance. Leukemia 1991;5:196–9.

184. Sobol RE, Mick R, Royston I, et al. Clinical importance of myeloid antigen expression in adult acute lymphoblastic leukemia. N Eng J Med 1987;316:1111–7.

185. Stass SA, McGraw TP, Folds JD, Odle B, Bollum FJ. Terminal transferase in acute lymphoblastic leukemia in remission. Am J Clin Pathol 1981;75:838–40.

186. _____, Mirro J. Unexpected heterogeneity in acute leukemia: mixed lineages and lineage switch. Hum Pathol 1985;16:864–6.

187. _____, Mirro J, Melvin S, Pui CH, Murphy SB, Williams D. Lineage switch in acute leukemia. Blood 1984;64:701–6.

188. _____, Phillips TM, Weislow OS, Perlin E, Schumacher HR. Antigen-antibody complexes related to the baboon endogenous virus in humans with acute lymphoblastic leukemia—hand mirror variant (ALL-HMC). Blood 1980;56:661–6.

189. Stein P, Peiper S, Butler D, Melvin S, Williams D, Stass S. Granular acute lymphoblastic leukemia. Am J Clin Pathol 1983;79:426–30.

190. Third International Workshop on Chromosomes in Leukemia—Lund, Sweden, July 21–25, 1980. Cancer Genet Cytogenet 1981;4:96.

191. Uckun FM, Gajl-Peczalska KJ, Provisor AJ, Heerema NA. Immunophenotype-karyotype associations in human acute lymphoblastic leukemia. Blood 1989;73:271–80.

192. van den Doel LJ, Pieters R, Huisman DR, et al. Immunological phenotype of lymphoid cells in regenerating bone marrow of children after treatment for acute lymphoblastic leukemia. Eur J Haematol 1988;41:170–5.

193. van Dongen JJM, Krissansen GW, Wolvers-Tettero IL, et al. Cytoplasmic expression of the CD3 antigen as a diagnostic marker for immature T-cell malignancies. Blood 1988;71:603–12.

194. van Eys J, Pullen J, Head D, et al. The FAB classification of leukemia: the Pediatric Oncology Group experience with lymphoblastic leukemia. Cancer 1986;57:1046–51.

195. Wegelius R. Preleukemic states in children. Scand J Haematol 1986;45:133–9.

196. Weiss LM, Bindl JM, Picozzi VJ, Link MP, Warnke RA. Lymphoblastic lymphoma: an immunophenotype study of 26 cases with comparison of T cell acute lymphoblastic leukemia. Blood 1986;67:474–8.

197. Wiersma SR, Ortega J, Sobel E, Weinberg KI. Clinical importance of myeloid-antigen expression in acute lymphoblastic leukemia of childhood. N Engl J Med 1991;324:800–8.

198. Williams DL, Harber J, Murphy SB, et al. Chromosomal translocations play a unique role in influencing prognosis in childhood acute lymphoblastic leukemia. Blood 1986;68:205–12.

199. _____, Look AT, Melvin SL, et al. New chromosomal translocations correlate with specific immunophenotypes of childhood acute lymphoblastic leukemia. Cell 1984;36:101–9.

200. _____, Raimondi S, Rivera G, George S, Berard CW, Murphy SB. Presence of cloned chromosome abnormalities in virtually all cases of acute lymphoblastic leukemia. N Engl J Med 1985;313:640–1.

201. _____, Tsiatis A, Brodeur GM, et al. Prognostic importance of chromosome number in 136 untreated children with acute lymphoblastic leukemia. Blood 1982;60:864–71.

202. Winick NJ, McKenna RW, Shuster JJ, et al. Secondary acute myeloid leukemia in children with acute lymphoblastic leukemia treated with etoposide. J Clin Oncol 1993;11:209–17.

203. Yanagihara ET, Naeim F, Gale RP, Austin G, Waisman J. Acute lymphoblastic leukemia with giant intracytoplasmic inclusions. Am J Clin Pathol 1980;74:345–9.

MYELODYSPLASTIC SYNDROMES

The myelodysplastic syndromes (MDSs) are a group of bone marrow disorders characterized by dysplastic changes in the cells of the myeloid series, with or without a concurrent increase in myeloblasts. When the myeloblasts are increased, the number is less than the 30 percent requisite for a diagnosis of acute myeloid leukemia (AML) (2,3,4,10). MDSs occur as primary diseases and as secondary or therapy-related disorders. Therapy-related MDSs occur in patients who have been exposed to chemotherapeutic agents and radiotherapy (14,24,25,30,36).

PRIMARY MYELODYSPLASTIC SYNDROMES

Classification. Primary MDSs are classified as follows:
    Refractory anemia (RA)
    Refractory anemia with ringed sideroblasts
        (RARS)
    Refractory anemia with excess of blasts
        (RAEB)
    Refractory anemia with excess of blasts in
        transformation (RAEB-T)
    Chronic myelomonocytic leukemia (CMML)
    Chronic myelomonocytic leukemia in
        transformation (CMML-T)
    Myelodysplastic syndrome, unclassified
        (MDS-U)

The first five entities were proposed by the French-American-British (FAB) cooperative group in 1982 (3). Chronic myelomonocytic leukemia in transformation (CMML-T) and myelodysplastic syndrome, unclassified (MDS-U), are additional categories used by many observers.

Refractory anemia is used here for those disorders presenting with anemia refractory to hematinic therapy with no or only minimal abnormalities of granulocytes or megakaryocytes. The term is used by other observers to include MDSs that cannot be classified into one of the other types. As a result the term might be used for cases with marked dysplasia of the granulocytes and megakaryocytes but without an increase in blasts. In the classification presented here, MDS with dysplastic changes in two or more myeloid cell lines but without other specific diagnostic criteria are placed in the unclassified group.

Incidence and Clinical Findings. De novo or primary MDSs occur most commonly in individuals over the age of 50 years. Statistics on incidence are not available. In 1983, the French Registry of Acute Leukemia, which accesses the vast majority of cases of AML and MDS in France, recorded 579 cases of MDS and 1030 cases of de novo AML (16). MDSs are uncommon in the pediatric population and in this age group are frequently associated with specific cytogenetic abnormalities, such as an isolated monosomy 7 (11,51).

Patients with MDS generally present with some manifestation of bone marrow failure, most commonly fatigue due to anemia (13,16,22,42). Bleeding problems related to thrombocytopenia or infections resulting from a decreased number of neutrophils or neutrophil dysfunction are frequent presenting features. Organomegaly and lymphadenopathy are not usually present but may be detected in some patients (3).

Laboratory Findings. The MDSs comprise a somewhat heterogeneous group of disorders, and as a result the presenting laboratory findings vary. Anemia is present in virtually all patients (22). Macrocytic red blood cell indices may be present in all the types of MDS. Occasional patients may present with neutropenia or thrombocytopenia as the major abnormality (35).

Refractory anemia, if strictly defined, is not usually accompanied by other cytopenias. In refractory anemia with ringed sideroblasts (RARS), a decreased hemoglobin level is usually the only finding; the platelet and neutrophil counts are normal. Occasional patients with RARS or other types of MDS have a thrombocytosis (7). Patients with refractory anemia with excess of blasts (RAEB) usually have some degree of neutropenia and thrombocytopenia in addition to anemia. Chronic myelomonocytic leukemia (CMML) by definition has 1.0×10^9/L or more monocytes in the blood. Anemia and thrombocytopenia are frequently present. Refractory anemia with excess of blasts in transformation (RAEB-T) and CMML-T have variable leukocyte counts; anemia and thrombocytopenia are usually present.

MDS associated with the de novo 5q- syndrome or abnormalities of chromosome 3 at bands q21 and q26 may present with a thrombocytosis (26,45).

The diagnosis of MDS is based on quantitative and qualitative alterations in the immature and mature myeloid cells: granulocytes, monocytes, erythroid cells, and megakaryocytes. The quantitative changes relate to an increase in type I and II blasts in the bone marrow and blood. In three of the myelodysplastic syndromes, refractory anemia, RARS, and MDS-U, the findings are usually limited to cytologic abnormalities without an increase in blasts. In CMML the blast count may be normal or increased.

Dysplastic changes in the red blood cells are manifest as increased anisopoikilocytosis; macrocytosis is common (fig. 167). Abnormalities of the erythroid precursors include asynchronous nuclear cytoplasmic development, megaloblastic nuclei, nuclear lobulation, karyorrhexis and fragmentation, internuclear chromatin bridging, and multinucleation (fig. 168). Ringed sideroblasts, although the primary finding in sideroblastic anemia, may be present in all types of MDS.

Dysplastic changes in the neutrophil series are characterized by deficient or aberrant granule production, retarded nuclear segmentation manifested as nuclear hyposegmentation, pseudo–Pelger-Huet changes, and hypersegmentation. Abnormally small forms may be present (figs. 169, 170). Megakaryocytic dysplasia is frequently characterized by abnormally small megakaryocytes with nonlobulated or bilobed nuclei (fig. 171).

Refractory Anemia (RA). Anemia refractory to hematinic therapy is the major finding. The red blood cells are usually normochromic macrocytic or normochromic normocytic (fig. 172). The platelet and neutrophil counts are normal in the majority of patients but occasional patients may have bicytopenia or pancytopenia. The number of erythroid precursors varies from marked erythroid hypoplasia to hyperplasia. Some degree of dyserythropoiesis is usually present and megaloblastoid features may be prominent (fig. 173). Ringed sideroblasts may be present but are less than 15 percent of the nucleated red blood cells. Although morphologic abnormalities are usually restricted to the erythroid series, a slight degree of dysplastic change may be present in the granulocytes and megakaryocytes. The marrow blasts are less than 5 percent and blasts should not be observed in the blood.

The bone marrow sections in the majority of cases are hypercellular, usually with an increase in ery-

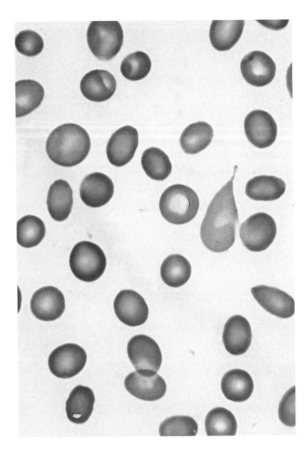

Figure 167
RED BLOOD CELL ABNORMALITIES
IN A MYELODYSPLASTIC SYNDROME
Blood smear from a 72-year-old man with RAEB-T. The red blood cells show moderate anisopoikilocytosis with macrocytes and dacryocytes. (Wright-Giemsa stain)

throid cells; in some instances there is marked erythroid hypoplasia. Neutrophils and megakaryocytes are normal in number (fig. 174). In a minority of patients the marrow is hypocellular; this finding is more common in older individuals.

Occasional patients present with anemia refractory to hematinic therapy, with or without thrombocytopenia or leukopenia, and minimal or no dysplastic changes and cytogenetic abnormalities associated with MDS, such as 20q- (70). These cases are appropriately classified as refractory anemia based on the cytogenetic findings.

Refractory Anemia with Ringed Sideroblasts (RARS). The defining criterion of RARS is the presence of 15 percent or more ringed sideroblasts in the bone marrow. Anemia is always present and the hemoglobin level is generally in the range

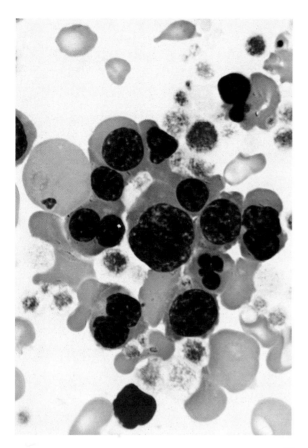
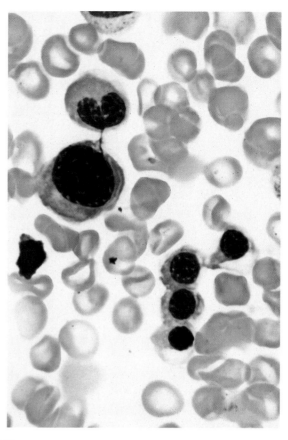

Figure 168
RED BLOOD CELL ABNORMALITIES IN A MYELODYSPLASTIC SYNDROME
Left: Bone marrow smear from an adult woman with a therapy-related MDS. Some of the red blood cell precursors are very large; the nuclei show lobulation and karyorrhexis. (Wright-Giemsa stain)
Right: Bone marrow smear from a 46-year-old male with refractory anemia. Two post-mitotic red blood cell precursors of dissimilar size and nuclear and cytoplasmic characteristics show internuclear chromatin bridging. (Wright-Giemsa stain)

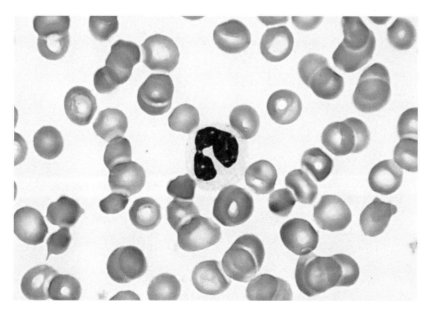

Figure 169
ABNORMAL NEUTROPHIL
IN A MYELODYSPLASTIC
SYNDROME
Neutrophil in the blood smear of an adult woman with RAEB. The cytoplasm is hypogranular. (Wright-Giemsa stain)

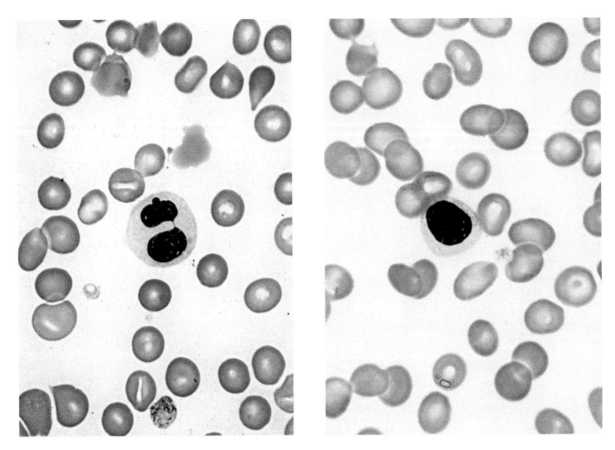

Figure 170
ABNORMAL NEUTROPHILS IN A MYELODYSPLASTIC SYNDROME

Left: Neutrophil with a bilobed, pseudo–Pelger-Huet nucleus and hypogranular cytoplasm in a blood smear from an adult man with RAEB. (Wright-Giemsa stain)

Right: Mature neutrophil with a nonlobulated nucleus in a blood smear from an adult man with RAEB-T. In addition to the nonlobulated nucleus, the cell is approximately half the size of a normal neutrophil. Cytoplasmic granulation is sparse. (Wright-Giemsa stain)

Figure 171
ABNORMAL MEGAKARYOCYTES
IN A MYELODYSPLASTIC
SYNDROME

Bone marrow smear from a patient with RAEB and an isolated 5q- chromosome abnormality showing two small megakaryocytes with nonlobulated nuclei. The cytoplasm is well granulated. (Wright-Giemsa stain)

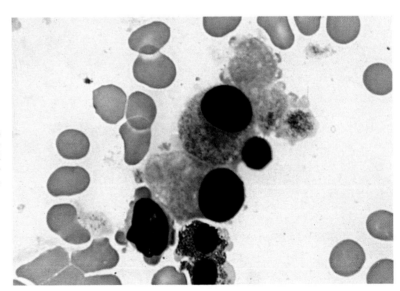

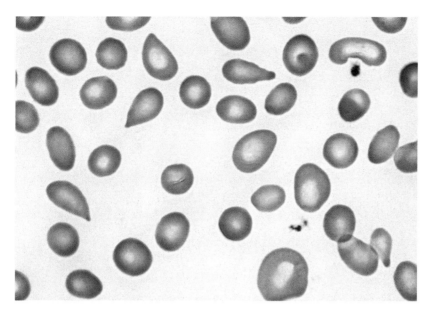

Figure 172
REFRACTORY ANEMIA
Blood smear from a patient with refractory anemia. The red blood cells show moderate to marked anisopoikilocytosis with several dacryocytes. A few normal-appearing platelets are present. (Wright-Giemsa stain) (Fig. 46.9A from Brunning RD. Myelodysplastic syndromes. In: Knowles DM, ed. Neoplastic hematopathology. Baltimore: Williams & Wilkins, 1992:1367–404.)

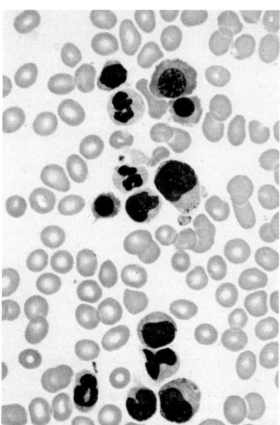

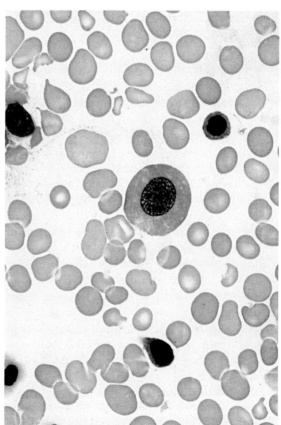

Figure 173
REFRACTORY ANEMIA

Left: Bone marrow smear from a patient with refractory anemia showing an erythroid precursor with a megaloblastoid nucleus. The granulocytes appear essentially normal. (Wright-Giemsa stain)

Right: High magnification of the specimen on the left showing a megaloblastic red blood cell precursor. (Wright-Giemsa stain) (Fig. 46.9B from Brunning RD. Myelodysplastic syndromes. In: Knowles DM, ed. Neoplastic hematopathology. Baltimore: Williams & Wilkins, 1992:1367–404.)

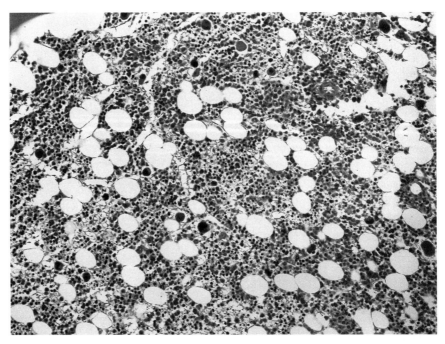

Figure 174
REFRACTORY ANEMIA
Bone marrow biopsy from a 53-year-old male with refractory anemia. The marrow is slightly hypercellular for the age of the patient. There is marked hyperplasia of erythroid precursors. The megakaryocytes are prominent but are proportionally normal in number. (Hematoxylin and eosin stain)

of 9 to 12 g/dL although lower levels may be present. The red blood cells may be normochromic macrocytic, normochromic normocytic, or dimorphic with populations of both hypochromic and normochromic cells (fig. 175). The platelets and granulocytes are usually normal in number and appearance. Some patients with RARS present with a thrombocytosis (7). The bone marrow aspirate shows erythroid hyperplasia, sometimes marked, with varying but usually minor degrees of dyserythropoiesis. In occasional cases prominent dyserythropoiesis with megaloblastoid features is present. In smears stained for iron, 15 percent or more of the erythroid precursors are ringed (type III) sideroblasts, erythroblasts in which the nucleus is completely or partially encircled by iron granules (fig. 175). On ultrastructural examination, perinuclear iron is present in the mitochondria (fig. 176). Granulopoiesis and megakaryocytopoiesis are essentially normal in most patients.

The marrow biopsy shows an overall hypercellularity with prominent erythroid hyperplasia. Megakaryocytes and granulocytes are morphologically and numerically normal in most cases. Sections stained for iron show numerous iron-laden macrophages. Ringed sideroblasts may be identified, but this finding is less apparent than in smear or imprint preparations.

RARS probably exists in two forms: a true MDS with potential to evolve to acute leukemia and a metabolically related disorder that has no increased risk for leukemic evolution. The latter group comprises the majority of cases (15). The distinction between these two types may not be readily apparent on initial evaluation. However, cases of RARS with changes limited to minor alterations in the red blood cells are more likely to be in the latter group. RARS accompanied by dysplastic changes in the megakaryocytes and granulocytes should be viewed with caution and the increased potential for leukemic evolution recognized. These cases should be carefully examined for the presence of Auer rods in the blasts even when there is less than 5 percent blasts. Regardless of the percentage of ringed sideroblasts, the presence of Auer rods, a blast count in excess of 5 percent in the bone marrow, or blasts in the blood categorizes the case into a higher grade of MDS, either RAEB or RAEB-T (23).

Cytogenetic studies may be of considerable aid in distinguishing the two types of RARS. The presence of one or more clonal chromosome abnormalities is evidence for the myelodysplastic type.

Refractory Anemia with Excess of Blasts (RAEB). The defining criterion of RAEB is 5 to 19 percent type I and type II blasts in the bone marrow; the number of blasts in the blood is less than 5

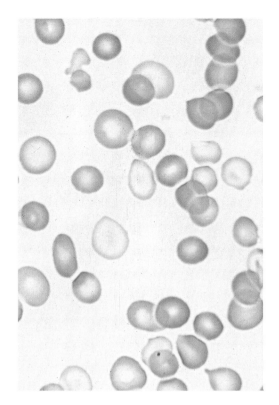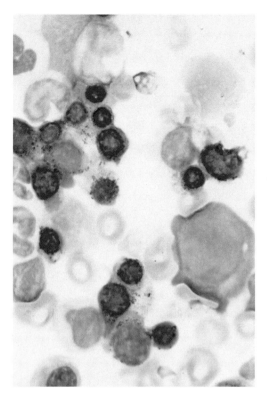

Figure 175

REFRACTORY ANEMIA WITH RINGED SIDEROBLASTS

Left: Blood smear from a 67-year-old man with refractory anemia with ringed sideroblasts. The red blood cells show a dimorphic pattern with populations of normochromic and markedly hypochromic cells. (Wright-Giemsa stain)

Right: Iron stain of a bone marrow smear from the patient illustrated on the left. The nuclei of a majority of the red blood cell precursors are encircled by small granules of iron. (Prussian blue followed by safranin O stain)

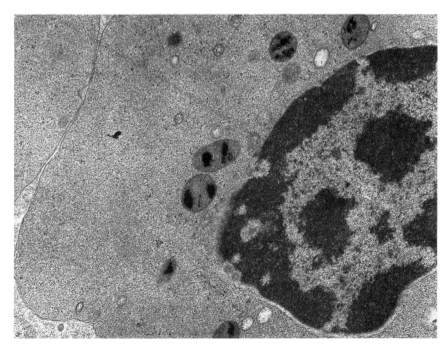

Figure 176

REFRACTORY ANEMIA WITH RINGED SIDEROBLASTS: ULTRASTRUCTURE

Electron micrograph of a red blood cell precursor in a bone marrow specimen from a patient with sideroblastic anemia. Iron deposits are present in the cristae of the mitochondria. (Uranyl acetate–lead citrate stains, X38,000)

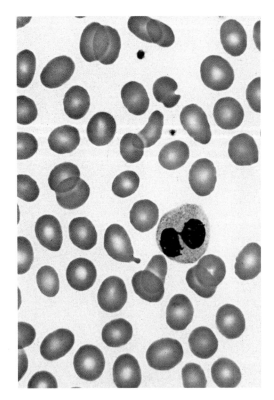

Figure 177
REFRACTORY ANEMIA
WITH EXCESS OF BLASTS

Blood smear from a patient with RAEB showing a mature neutrophil with a bilobed nucleus. The red blood cells show slight anisopoikilocytosis with occasional dacryocytes. (Wright-Giemsa stain) (Fig. 46.14B from Brunning RD. Myelodysplastic syndromes. In: Knowles DM, ed. Neoplastic hematopathology. Baltimore: Williams & Wilkins, 1992:1367–404.)

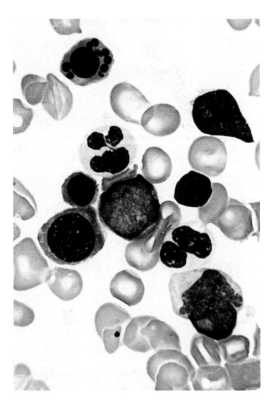

Figure 178
REFRACTORY ANEMIA
WITH EXCESS OF BLASTS

Bone marrow smear from a patient with RAEB. A blast is present in the center. Two hypogranular neutrophils are adjacent to the blast. A red blood cell precursor with multiple nuclear fragments is at the upper left. (Wright-Giemsa stain)

percent. The morphologic changes in the developing and mature granulocytes, erythroid cells, and megakaryocytes can vary markedly, ranging from minimal nuclear and cytoplasmic abnormalities to striking dysplastic changes in all myeloid cells.

Anemia is virtually always present; the red blood cells are normochromic normocytic or normochromic macrocytic. Increased anisopoikilocytosis is usually noted: dacryocytes and ovalocytes, including macro-ovalocytes, may be numerous (fig. 177). The majority of patients present with neutropenia and thrombocytopenia in addition to anemia. Neutrophil abnormalities such as nuclear hyposegmentation, pseudo–Pelger-Huet nuclei, and abnormalities of granulation such as hypogranulation are generally present and are frequently marked (fig. 177). Aggregates of granules resembling the Chediak-Higashi abnormality may be present but are much less frequent. Immature granulocytes are usually found in the blood; nucleated red blood cells occur less frequently. Small megakaryocytes and macrothrombocytes with diminished or absent granulation may be noted.

In many cases, the increase in blasts in the bone marrow is accompanied by an increase in promyelocytes. Auer rods are not found. Abnormalities of nuclear and cytoplasmic development are usually present in all of the myeloid cell lines (figs. 178, 179). Erythroid abnormalities include megaloblastoid nuclei, multinucleation, and nuclear lobulation and karyorrhexis. Ringed sideroblasts may be present and may occasionally exceed 15 percent of the nucleated red blood cells (23). Small megakaryocytes with hypolobulated nuclei may be present (see fig. 171).

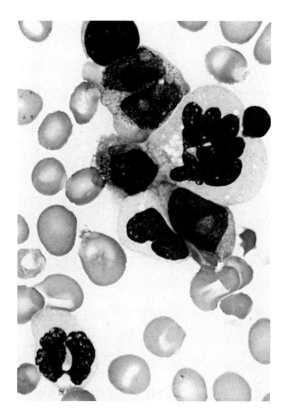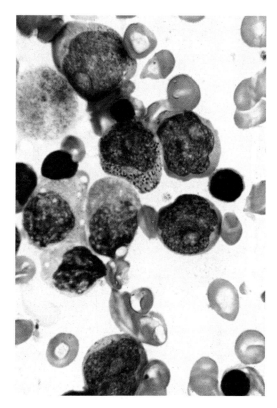

Figure 179
REFRACTORY ANEMIA WITH EXCESS OF BLASTS
Left: Bone marrow smear from an adult man with RAEB. A very large neutrophil with nuclear hyperlobulation and slightly hypogranular cytoplasm is present in the upper right. A single myeloblast with a prominent nucleolus and two neutrophils with markedly hypogranular cytoplasm are also present. (Wright-Giemsa stain)
Right: Bone marrow smear from an adult woman with RAEB showing neutrophil precursors at the promyelocyte and myelocyte stages of maturation and two myeloblasts on the right. (Wright-Giemsa stain)

The bone marrow biopsy in approximately 80 to 90 percent of patients is hypercellular with a panmyeloid hyperplasia; in approximately 10 to 20 percent of patients the marrow is normocellular or hypocellular (figs. 180, 181) (39). The number of blasts in the biopsy sections generally corresponds to the number in the smear or biopsy imprint. In some patients, small foci of immature cells, blasts and promyelocytes, may occur spatially unrelated to their normal paratrabecular or perivascular location. This finding has been referred to as abnormal localization of immature precursors (ALIP) (fig. 182) (60–63). The presence of three or more of these in a bone marrow section has been associated with an increased incidence of leukemic evolution (60). ALIP has been reported in all type of MDS including refractory anemia and RARS. The presence of several foci of myeloblasts and promyelocytes in a bone marrow section in a patient with a diagnosis of refractory anemia or RARS based on aspirate smears warrants careful reevaluation of the smears to determine whether the process should more accurately be classified as RAEB or RAEB-T.

Megakaryocytes may be decreased or numerous (fig. 183). Dysplastic megakaryocytes, particularly micromegakaryocytes, may be more apparent in the marrow sections and can be accentuated with the periodic acid–Schiff (PAS) stain. A slight degree of reticulin fibrosis is present in a minority of patients. Severe fibrosis is uncommon (29,43).

Refractory Anemia with Excess of Blasts in Transformation (RAEB-T). Patients with RAEB-T present with clinical and laboratory features similar to those with RAEB. RAEB-T may occur in an individual with a previously established

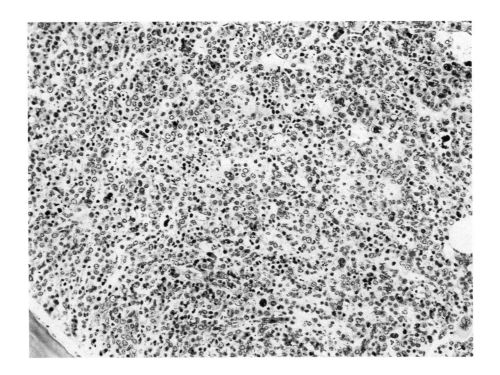

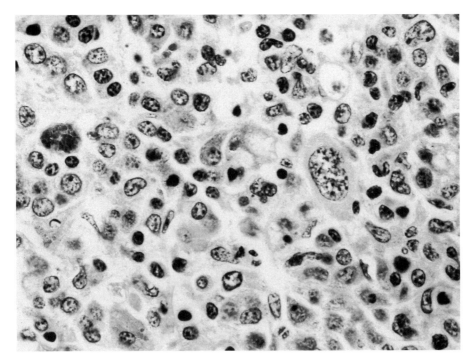

Figure 180
REFRACTORY ANEMIA WITH EXCESS OF BLASTS

Top: Markedly hypercellular bone marrow from an adult woman with pancytopenia and scattered blasts in the blood smear. The marrow smear from this specimen contained 6 percent myeloblasts. (Hematoxylin and eosin stain)

Bottom: High magnification of the specimen on top showing a predominance of immature neutrophils. Scattered red blood cell precursors and a megakaryocyte with a hypolobulated nucleus are present. (Hematoxylin and eosin stain) (Fig. 46.16B from Brunning RD. Myelodysplastic syndromes. In: Knowles DM, ed. Neoplastic hematopathology. Baltimore: Williams & Wilkins, 1992:1367–404.)

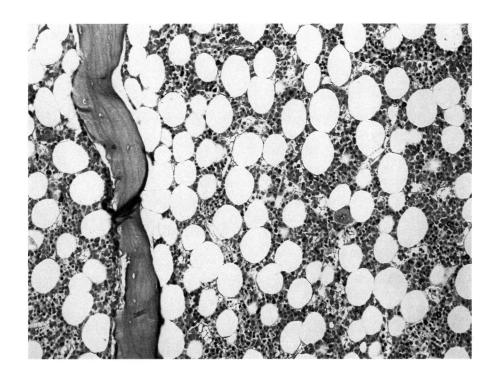

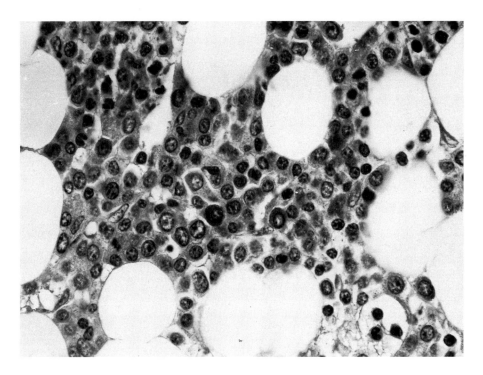

Figure 181
REFRACTORY ANEMIA WITH EXCESS OF BLASTS

Top: Bone marrow biopsy from an adult male with a diagnosis of RAEB. The marrow is moderately hypocellular. (Hematoxylin and eosin stain)

Bottom: High magnification of the specimen on the top. The granulocytes are predominantly promyelocytes and myelocytes. The bone marrow contained 11 percent myeloblasts; the blood showed 2 percent myeloblasts. (Hematoxylin and eosin stain)

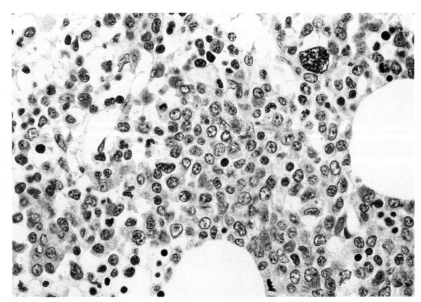

Figure 182
REFRACTORY ANEMIA
WITH EXCESS OF BLASTS:
ABNORMAL LOCALIZATION OF
IMMATURE PRECURSORS
(ALIP)

Bone marrow section from a patient with RAEB showing a loosely structured focus of myeloblasts and promyelocytes. This represents an abnormal localization of immature precursors (ALIP). (Hematoxylin and eosin stain)

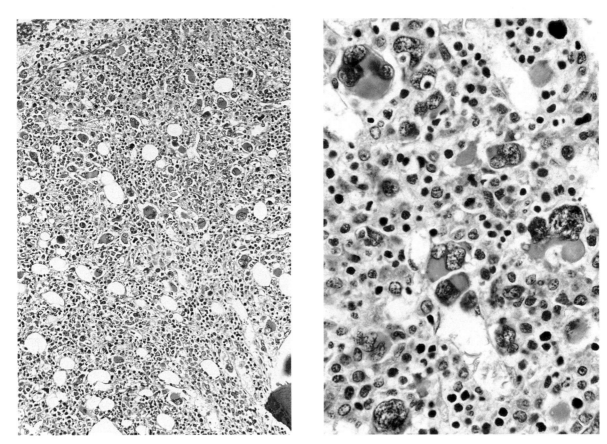

Figure 183
REFRACTORY ANEMIA WITH EXCESS OF BLASTS

Left: Low magnification of a bone marrow biopsy from a patient with RAEB with numerous megakaryocytes that show variation in size. (Hematoxylin and eosin stain)

Right: High magnification of the specimen on the left. The nuclei of some of the megakaryocytes are hypolobulated and have finely dispersed chromatin. (Hematoxylin and eosin stain)

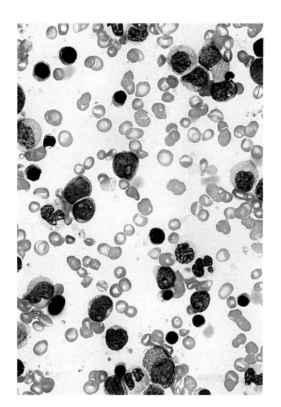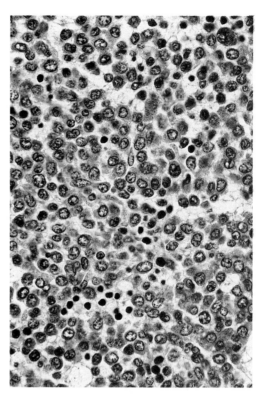

Figure 184
REFRACTORY ANEMIA WITH EXCESS OF BLASTS IN TRANSFORMATION
Left: Bone marrow smear from an adult female with a diagnosis of RAEB-T based on 22 percent myeloblasts in the marrow smear. This field shows several myeloblasts; there are numerous neutrophils at different stages of maturation. (Wright-Giemsa stain)
Right: Portion of a marrow biopsy from the same patient showing a predominance of blasts, promyelocytes, and myelocytes. Erythroid precursors are scattered among the granulocytes. (Hematoxylin and eosin stain)

diagnosis of a lower-grade MDS such as RAEB or in patients with no antecedent hematologic abnormalities. The morphologic changes in the myeloid cells are the same as those found in RAEB. RAEB-T, as defined, may occur in any age group (3). The presence of any one of three findings confirms the diagnosis: 1) 20 to 29 percent type I and II blasts in the bone marrow; 2) 5 to 29 percent type I and II blasts in the blood; 3) the detection of Auer rods in myeloblasts or other cells of the neutrophil cell line in a patient in whom the blasts in the bone marrow or blood is less than 30 percent (figs. 184–188). Auer rods are detected in approximately 70 percent of cases of RAEB-T and is the only criterion present in 50 to 60 percent of cases (37). Occasionally, Auer rods may be detected in blasts or neutrophil precursors when the blast percentage is less than 5; these processes should be classified as RAEB-T (figs. 185, 186). Ringed sideroblasts

may be numerous and, as in RAEB, may exceed 15 percent of the nucleated red blood cells (fig. 188, bottom) (23).

Similar to RAEB, the bone marrow in 80 to 90 percent of patients with RAEB-T is hypercellular; in approximately 10 to 20 percent of patients the marrow is normocellular or hypocellular (fig. 189). The blasts and immature neutrophils may be uniformly distributed or there may be aggregates of blasts and promyelocytes (see fig. 184, right). Megakaryocytes vary from decreased to increased. Abnormal megakaryocytes may be prominent. They may occur in clusters and show dysplastic maturation characterized by marked variation in size and nuclear chromatin pattern. Small megakarocytes may be numerous. Reticulin fibrosis of mild degree is present in approximately 10 percent of cases. Similar to AML, RAEB-T may be complicated by leukemic infiltration at extramedullary sites (fig. 190).

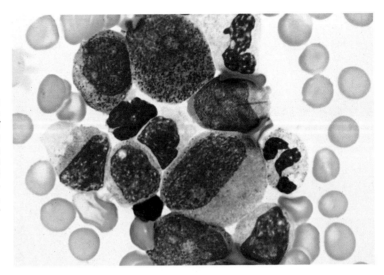

Figure 185
REFRACTORY ANEMIA WITH EXCESS
OF BLASTS IN TRANSFORMATION

Bone marrow smear from an adult man with a diagnosis of RAEB-T. The marrow contained 8 percent myeloblasts. The diagnosis of RAEB-T was based on the detection of Auer rods, one of which is present in a blast at the right of center. The predominant cells are maturing neutrophils. (Wright-Giemsa stain) (Fig. 46.20 from Brunning RD. Myelodysplastic syndromes. In: Knowles DM, ed. Neoplastic hematopathology. Baltimore: Williams & Wilkins, 1992:1367–404.)

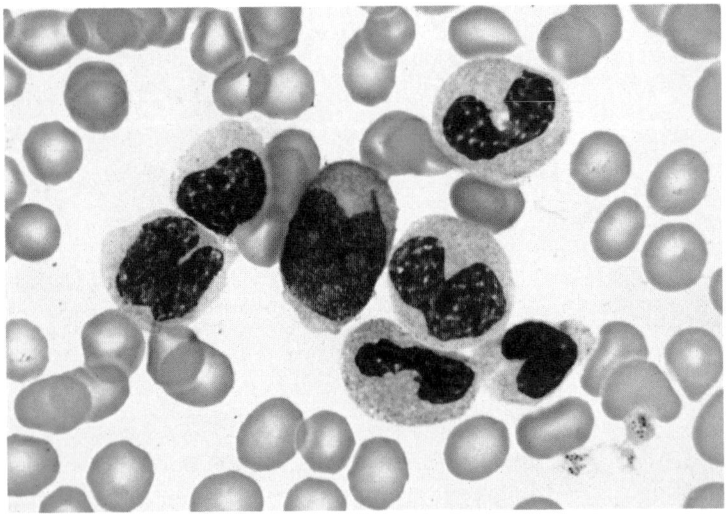

Figure 186
REFRACTORY ANEMIA WITH EXCESS
OF BLASTS IN TRANSFORMATION

Bone marrow smear from a 42-year-old patient with 8 percent myeloblasts. A single myeloblast contains a slender, long Auer rod. The other cells are neutrophils showing nuclear hypolobulation. (Wright-Giemsa stain)

Figure 187
REFRACTORY ANEMIA WITH EXCESS
OF BLASTS IN TRANSFORMATION

Bone marrow smear from a 12-year-old girl with RAEB-T. The marrow contained 6 percent blasts, several of which contained an Auer rod as shown. The maturing and mature neutrophils show marked nuclear hypolobulation. The large cell with abundant cytoplasm is a mature neutrophil with no evidence of nuclear segmentation. Granulation appears normal. (Wright-Giemsa stain)

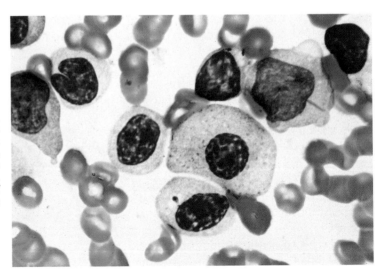

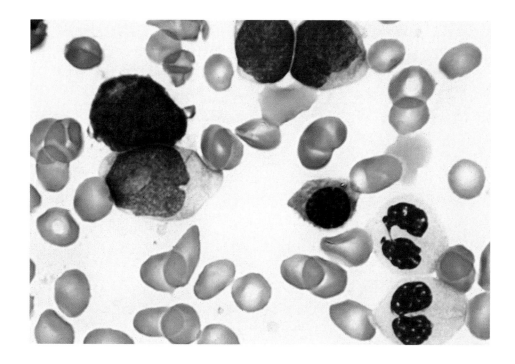

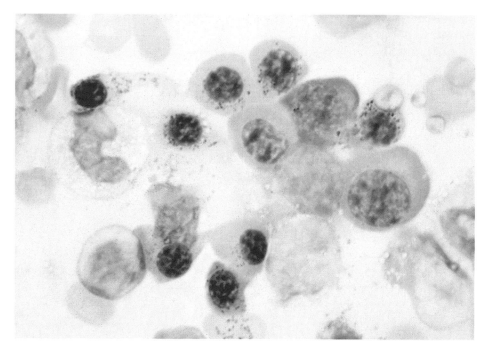

Figure 188
REFRACTORY ANEMIA WITH EXCESS OF BLASTS IN TRANSFORMATION

Top: Bone marrow smear from a 72-year-old male with a 1-year history of macrocytic anemia unresponsive to hematinic therapy. This marrow specimen contained 60 to 65 percent erythroid precursors and 4 percent myeloblasts; one of the myeloblasts in this field shows a delicate Auer rod. Two hypogranular neutrophils with pseudo–Pelger-Huet nuclei are at the lower right. (Wright-Giemsa stain)

Bottom: Iron stain of the specimen on the top showing several ringed sideroblasts. Approximately 40 percent ringed sideroblasts were present. (Prussian blue followed by safranin O stain) (Fig. 46.21B from Brunning RD. Myelodysplastic syndromes. In: Knowles DM, ed. Neoplastic hematopathology. Baltimore: Williams & Wilkins, 1992:1367–404.)

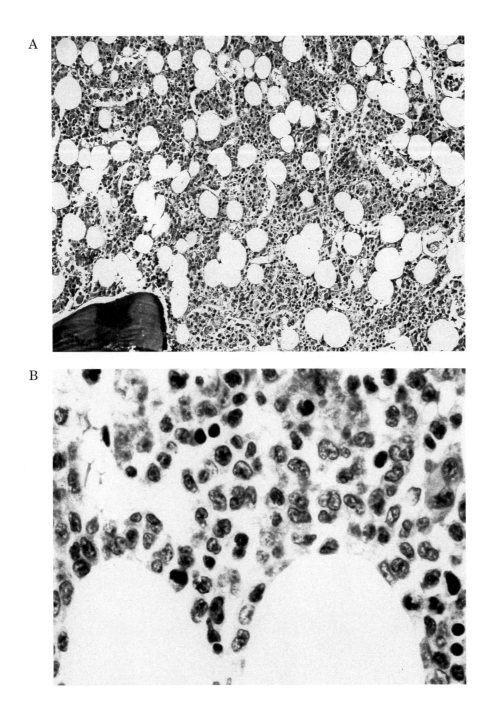

Figure 189

REFRACTORY ANEMIA WITH EXCESS OF BLASTS IN TRANSFORMATION

A. Normocellular bone marrow biopsy obtained August 1, 1987, from a 47-year-old woman with a Hb level of 13.7 g/dL, WBC count of 2.2×10^9/L, and platelet count of 47×10^9/L. The bone marrow smear contained 12 percent myeloblasts; Auer rods were found in occasional blasts and a diagnosis of RAEB-T was made. The patient declined therapy. (Hematoxylin and eosin stain)

B. High magnification of the specimen in A showing a shift to immaturity in the neutrophils. Red blood cell precursors appear normal in number. (Hematoxylin and eosin stain)

C. Bone marrow biopsy from the patient in A and B obtained August 28, 1991. The biopsy is slightly more cellular than the biopsy obtained 4 years before. Hematology values at the time of this biopsy were Hb 10.2 g/dL, WBC 1.1×10^9/L, and platelets 176×10^9/L. The patient had recurrent infections, two requiring hospitalization, but otherwise functioned well. (Hematoxylin and eosin stain)

D. High magnification of the specimen in C showing more immature cells than in B but no significant difference in the number of blasts. (Hematoxylin and eosin stain)

C

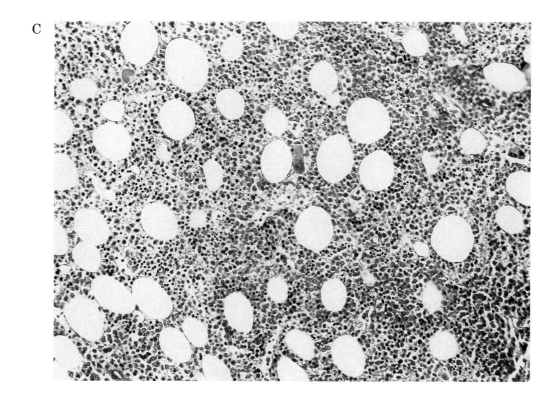

D

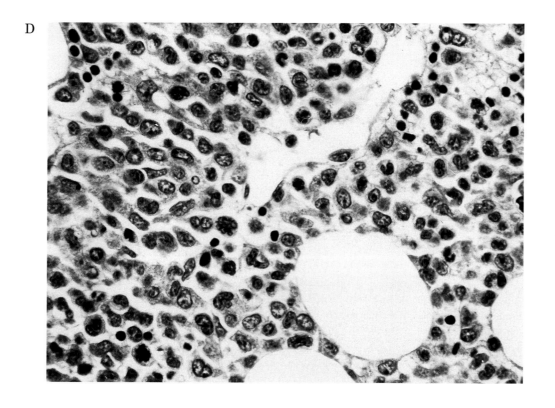

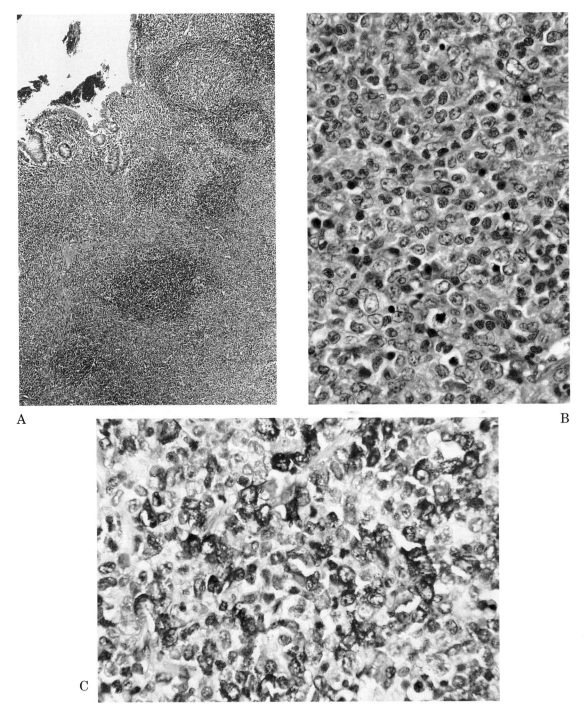

Figure 190
GRANULOCYTIC SARCOMA OF THE APPENDIX IN A PATIENT
WITH BLOOD AND BONE MARROW FINDINGS OF RAEB-T

A. Low magnification of a section of the appendix from a 37-year-old man with the diagnosis of RAEB-T based on 18 percent myeloblasts, some with Auer rods, in the marrow. The patient declined therapy and subsequently developed symptoms of acute appendicitis. The submucosa shows a dense infiltrate of immature cells. (Hematoxylin and eosin stain)

B. High magnification of the specimen in A showing a predominant population of blasts and immature granulocytes. Occasional scattered segmented neutrophils and eosinophils are present. (Hematoxylin and eosin stain)

C. Chloroacetate esterase stain showing a high percentage of reacting cells indicating immature neutrophils.

Chronic Myelomonocytic Leukemia (CMML).
The term CMML may be used in the context of a myelodysplastic syndrome or a myeloproliferative disorder; a qualifying term should be used. The distinction between CMML, myelodysplastic and CMML, myeloproliferative is based primarily on the leukocyte count and the presence of splenomegaly. CMML, myeloproliferative presents with clinical and hematologic features similar to chronic myeloid leukemia. There is an elevated leukocyte count and usually splenomegaly, but studies for the Philadelphia chromosome and the BCR/*abl* rearrangement are negative. The entity is discussed in more detail in the chapter on Chronic Myeloproliferative Diseases.

CMML as a myelodysplastic syndrome presents with hematologic features similar to RAEB. The number of blasts in the bone marrow is less than 20 percent and is less than 5 percent in the blood. The distinguishing finding from RAEB is an absolute blood monocyte count of 1.0×10^9/L or greater (fig. 191). The bone marrow resembles RAEB but there is an increase in monocytes and monocyte precursors (fig. 191, right). In addition to dysplastic changes in the granulocytes, abnormalities in the erythroid precursors and megakaryocytes may be present (fig. 192). The monocytes and precursors are nonspecific esterase (NSE) positive; combination staining with NSE and chloroacetate esterase (CAE) may show individual monocytes reactive for both enzymes, indicating features of both neutrophils and monocytes.

The bone marrow section is hypercellular in most patients. The cell population reflects the proportion of neutrophils and monocytes (fig. 193). The megakaryocytes may be normal or reduced in number. Abnormal localization of immature precursors may be present; these are reported to have the same significance for evolution to acute leukemia as in RAEB (60,63). A relatively high incidence of myelofibrosis has been reported in patients with CMML (33).

CMML, similar to other types of leukemia, may be complicated by leukemic infiltration of extramedullary sites and granulocytic sarcoma (fig. 194).

Approximately 50 percent of patients with CMML have hypergammaglobulinemia, which is usually polyclonal (57).

The criteria for CMML are relatively imprecise in that the monocytic component is recognized by 1.0 or more monocytes in the peripheral blood. The degree of maturation of the monocytes and the magnitude of the monocytosis is not usually addressed. As a result, there is considerable heterogeneity in the disorders reported as CMML; this is reflected in widely differing survivals, ranging from 3 to more than 60 months (57). In considering the possibility of a diagnosis of CMML, both myeloproliferative disorders and acute myelomonocytic leukemia should be excluded. If there is a high percentage of promonocytes, as described in acute myelomonocytic leukemia M4 and acute monocytic leukemia M5B, then these diagnoses should be considered. A careful search for Auer rods is important in all cases.

The morphologic features of the proliferating monocytic cells may be misleading and it is prudent to be cautious in predicting biologic behavior from one observation. It is important to carefully monitor the hematologic status in patients with this disease and to recognize changes that indicate an evolution to acute leukemia. This evolution may be reflected either in an increasing number of blasts and promonocytes or a rapidly increasing leukocytic count due to an increase in monocytes, granulocytes, or both.

Chronic Myelomonocytic Leukemia in Transformation (CMML-T). Patients may present with the hematologic features of CMML and one or more of the three findings associated with RAEB in transformation to acute leukemia. Of these findings, the most frequently noted is the presence of Auer rods (fig. 195). These cases should be designated as CMML in transformation to acute leukemia. The biologic course of this process is similar to RAEB-T with a high incidence of evolution to acute leukemia, most commonly acute myelomonocytic leukemia.

Myelodysplastic Syndrome, Unclassified (MDS-U). Patients may present with the clinical and hematologic features of a MDS that lacks specific categorizing features; the number of blasts in the bone marrow is less than 5 percent and no or only occasional blasts are found in the blood. The feature distinguishing MDS-U from refractory anemia is the degree of dysgranulopoiesis and dysmegakaryocytopoiesis, which may be marked (figs. 196, 197). Ringed sideroblasts may be present. The marrow is usually hypercellular with a panhyperplasia.

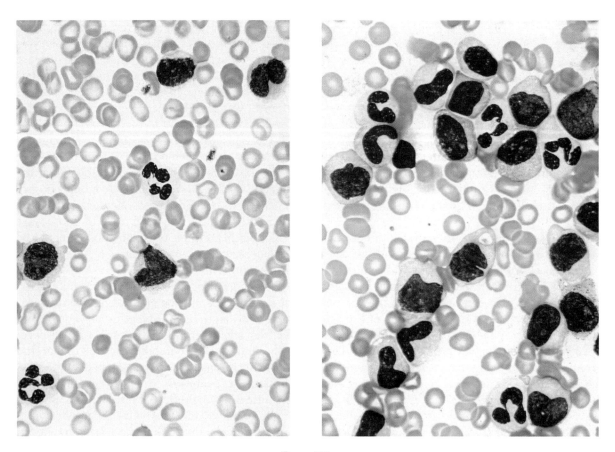

Figure 191
CHRONIC MYELOMONOCYTIC LEUKEMIA
Left: Blood smear from an adult male with CMML. There are three mature monocytes. (Wright-Giemsa stain)
Right: Bone marrow smear from the same patient showing increased monocytes and precursors. (Wright-Giemsa stain)

Figure 192
CHRONIC MYELOMONOCYTIC
LEUKEMIA

Bone marrow smear from a patient with CMML. In addition to the increase in monocyte precursors there are abnormalities in erythroid cell development that manifest primarily as cytoplasmic vacuoles. (Wright-Giemsa stain)

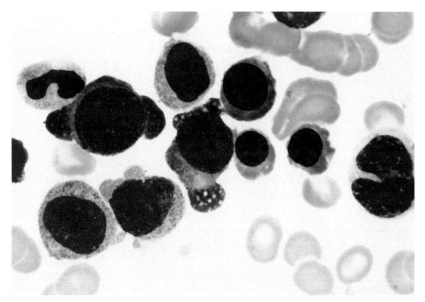

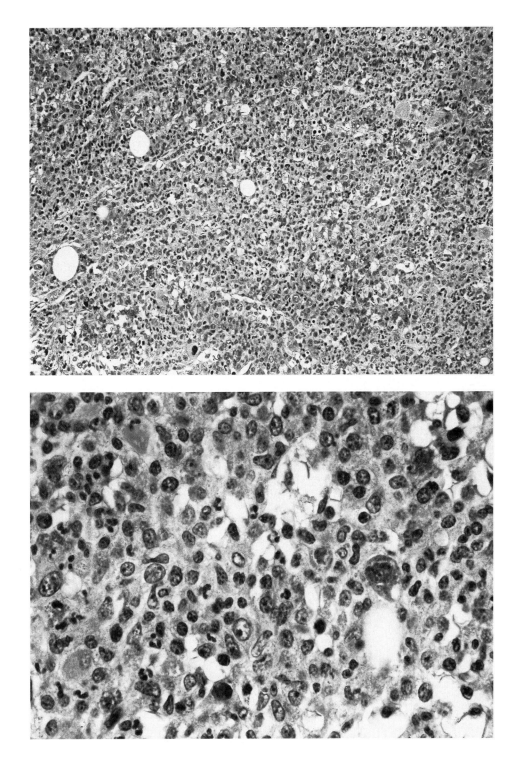

Figure 193
CHRONIC MYELOMONOCYTIC LEUKEMIA

Top: Markedly hypercellular bone marrow biopsy from an adult man with CMML. (Hematoxylin and eosin stain) (Fig. 46.25A from Brunning RD. Myelodysplastic syndromes. In: Knowles DM, ed. Neoplastic hematopathology. Baltimore: Williams & Wilkins, 1992:1367–404.)

Bottom: High magnification of the specimen on the top showing a predominance of monocytes and immature neutrophils. (Hematoxylin and eosin stain)

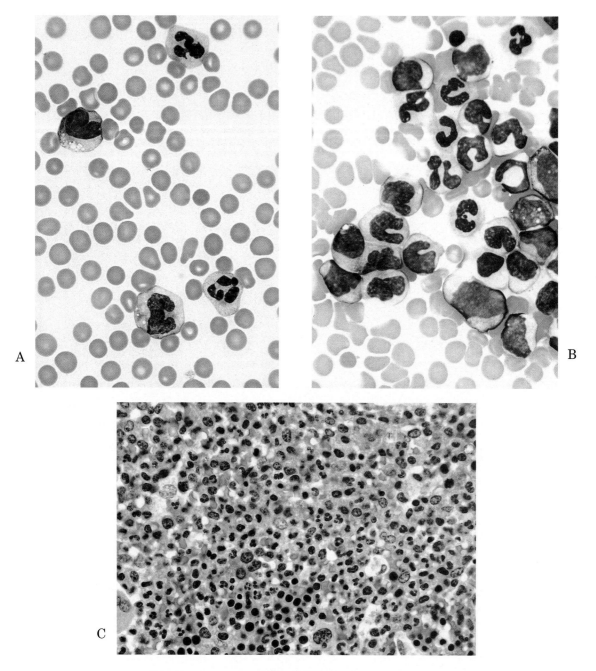

Figure 194
GRANULOCYTIC SARCOMA IN A PATIENT WITH CHRONIC MYELOMONOCYTIC LEUKEMIA

A. Blood smear from an 82-year-old woman with a 10-month history of CMML. There are two neutrophils and two mature monocytes. The blood findings did not change significantly in the 10-month interval. (Wright-Giemsa stain)

B. Bone marrow smear from patient in A with an increased number of monocytes, the majority of which are mature or only slightly immature. An occasional monoblast is present. (Wright-Giemsa stain)

C. Bone marrow section from the patient in A and B. There is evidence of maturation of the myeloid cells; there are no foci of immature cells. (Hematoxylin and eosin stain)

D. Low magnification of one of several subcutaneous lesions from the chest wall biopsied during the same time period as the bone marrow biopsy and blood smear illustrated in A–C. The lesion consists of a predominant population of blast cells with numerous scattered macrophages containing cellular debris. (Hematoxylin and eosin stain)

E. High magnification of the specimen in D. Mitotic figures are present. The blasts reacted with antibody to MPO and lysozyme. (Hematoxylin and eosin stain)

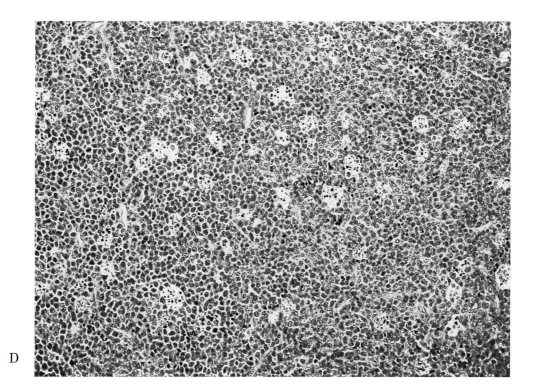

D

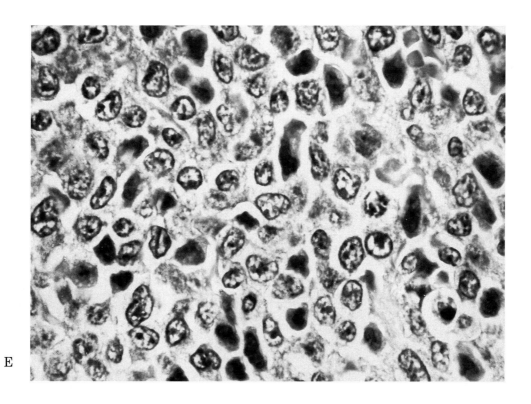

E

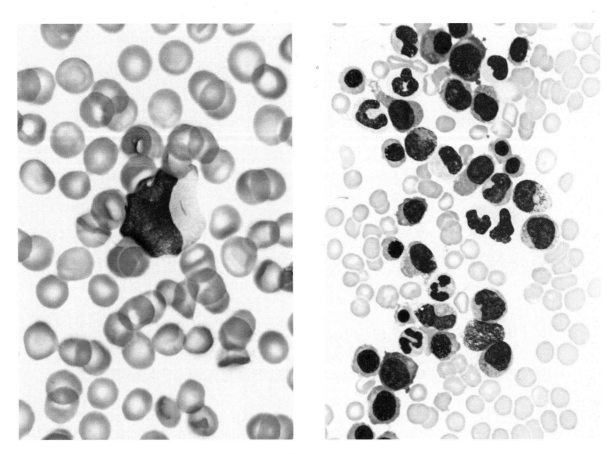

Figure 195
CHRONIC MYELOMONOCYTIC LEUKEMIA IN TRANSFORMATION

Left: Blood smear from a 43-year-old man with CMML-T. The patient had a 6-week history of increasing fatigue. The Hb level was 9.4 g/dL; the leukocyte count was 7×10^9/L. Platelets were normal in number. This field shows a blast with an Auer rod. (Wright-Giemsa stain)

Right: Bone marrow smear from the same patient showing several promonocytes and monocytes in addition to neutrophils and erythrocyte precursors. (Wright-Giemsa stain)

Figure 196
MYELODYSPLASTIC SYNDROME,
UNCLASSIFIED

Bone marrow smear from a 59-year-old woman with pancytopenia. Some of the neutrophils and precursors show abnormally bilobed nuclei. A red blood cell precursor in the upper left shows a lobulated nucleus. There is no increase in blasts, monocytes, or ringed sideroblasts. Because of the lack of specific categorizing findings, no subclassification was designated. (Wright-Giemsa stain)

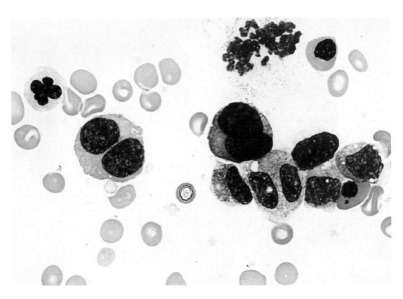

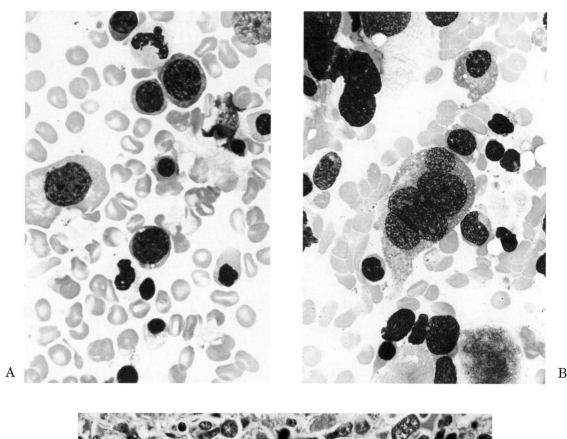

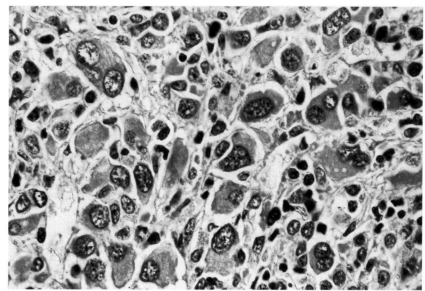

Figure 197
MYELODYSPLASTIC SYNDROME, UNCLASSIFIED

A. Bone marrow smear from a 37-year-old man with pancytopenia. The marrow aspirate smears show erythroid hyperplasia with marked dyserythropoiesis, including megaloblastoid changes. (Wright-Giemsa stain)

B. The marrow aspirate smear shows large erythroid precursors with hyperlobulated nuclei. Numerous ringed sideroblasts were present and occasional dysplastic neutrophils were found. There was no increase in myeloblasts. (Wright-Giemsa stain)

C. Bone marrow section from same patient illustrating a marked increase in megakaryocytes, many with hypolobulated nuclei. There was an increase in reticulin fibers. Cytogenetic studies showed several clonal abnormalities including monosomy 5 and monosomy 7. (Hematoxylin and eosin stain)

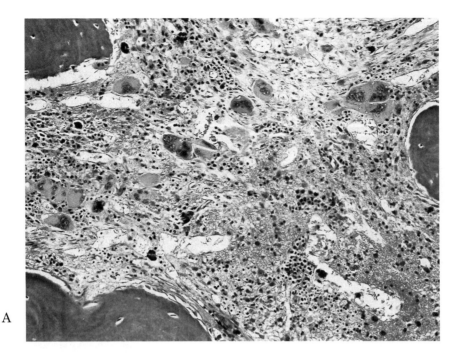

A

Figure 198

MYELODYSPLASTIC SYNDROME WITH MYELOFIBROSIS

A. Bone marrow biopsy from a 6-year-old girl with a 5-month history of severe anemia. The leukocyte and platelet counts were normal. The blood smear contained 1 to 2 percent blasts. Karyotype analysis showed a trisomy for chromosome 8. The marrow is hypercellular with marked fibrosis. Megakaryocytes are increased and occur both singly and in clusters. Islands of red blood cell precursors are scattered throughout the marrow. (Hematoxylin and eosin stain)

B. High magnification of a cluster of megakaryocytes from the specimen shown in A. These megakaryocytes are large and show normal nuclear lobulation. Erythroid precursors are juxtaposed to the megakaryocytes. (Hematoxylin and eosin stain)

C. Bone marrow biopsy 3 months following an allogeneic bone marrow transplant for the patient described in A. There is a marked reduction in connective tissue and cellularity, most notably megakaryocytes. The interstitium is loosely structured. (Hematoxylin and eosin stain)

D. Bone marrow biopsy 1 year following bone marrow transplant for the patient described in A. The marrow cellularity is increased and megakaryocyte proliferation is prominent. Karyotype analysis at this time showed a recurrence of trisomy for chromosome 8. (Hematoxylin and eosin stain)

The designation MDS-U may also be used for patients presenting with thrombocytopenia, neutropenia, or both without a concurrent anemia, or alternatively, the terms refractory thrombocytopenia or refractory neutropenia may be used. The diagnosis of MDS in these instances should only be made if there is convincing evidence of dysplasia of the granulocytes or megakaryocytes.

Myelofibrosis in Myelodysplastic Syndromes. Myelofibrosis may occur in MDS but severe fibrosis is uncommon (29,33,43). The difficulty in establishing the diagnosis of MDS in these instances relates to the inadequacy of aspirate material for determining blast percentage and cell identification in fibrotic bone marrow biopsies. The reported variance in survival of patients with MDS with fibrosis is in part a reflection of the difficulty in precise classification in these cases. The incidence of myelofibrosis in the subclasses of MDS varies (33,43,47). In some cases it may be possible to be specific as to subclassification while in other instances a more general term such as *myelodysplasia with myelofibrosis* should be used (figs. 198, 199). Caution should be exercised when giving an opinion about prognosis in these cases and the process should be carefully monitored clinically and hematologically to ascertain biologic behavior.

Acute myelodysplasia with myelofibrosis is generally an aggressive disorder with a biologic course similar to acute myeloid leukemia and is discussed in that section (55).

Cytochemical Findings. Cytochemical stains are of somewhat limited utility in the diagnosis of the MDSs. A low neutrophil alkaline phosphatase

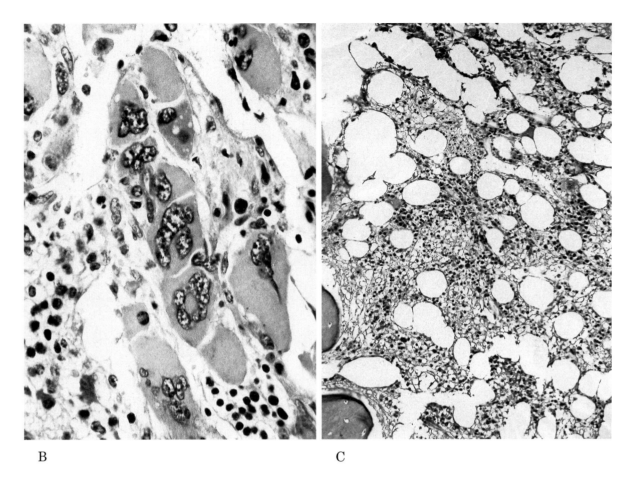

B

C

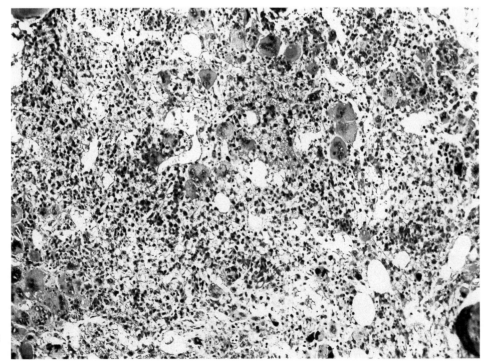

D

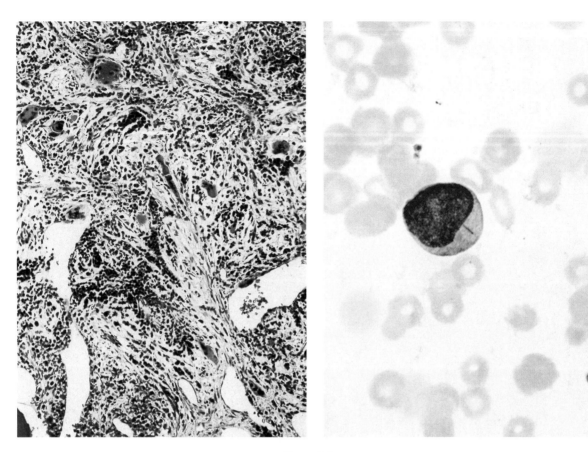

Figure 199
REFRACTORY ANEMIA WITH EXCESS OF BLASTS IN TRANSFORMATION
ASSOCIATED WITH MARKED MYELOFIBROSIS

Left: Bone marrow biopsy from a 62-year-old man with pancytopenia. There is marked fibrosis with a "streaming" effect. Mature megakaryocytes, some in clusters, are scattered throughout the biopsy. There is no apparent marked shift to immaturity in the hematopoietic cells. (Hematoxylin and eosin stain)

Right: Bone marrow aspirate from patient on the left yielded an inadequate specimen with only a few cells. Occasional blasts, rarely with an Auer rod as illustrated, were identified. Based on the rare myeloblasts with an Auer rod the process was classified as RAEB-T. Ten months following this biopsy the blood and bone marrow findings were those of AML-M2. (Wright-Giemsa stain)

level is substantial evidence of abnormal neutrophil development. Myeloperoxidase (MPO), Sudan black B (SBB), and CAE reactivity may be diminished or absent in the neutrophils. These findings should be considered as circumstantial evidence for a MDS; a diagnosis should not be based solely on these observations.

The NSE stain should be used in suspected cases of CMML or CMML-T (fig. 200). Since both the neutrophils and monocytes may have markedly abnormal nuclear and cytoplasmic features, MPO and NSE may be necessary for an accurate quantitation of these two cell lines. A combination of MPO and NSE or CAE and NSE may identify individual cells with cytochemical characteristics of both neutrophils and monocytes. This finding is most frequently noted in CMML and CMML-T.

Immunologic Markers. Morphologic abnormalities in the myeloid cells are the hallmark of the MDSs and there should be no difficulty in distinguishing these disorders from acute lymphoblastic leukemia. The limited role of immunologic markers relates to the recognition of a possible biphenotypic nature of the blasts in those MDSs characterized by increased blast counts. The detection of blasts with biphenotypic characteristics should not alter the primary diagnosis.

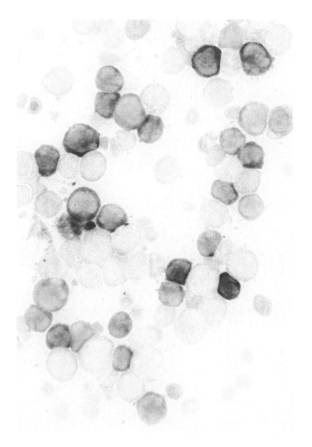

Figure 200
CHRONIC MYELOMONOCYTIC LEUKEMIA:
NONSPECIFIC ESTERASE STAIN
This bone marrow smear from a patient with CMML reacted for NSE. There are numerous positive cells. (Alpha napthyl acetate, methyl green stains)

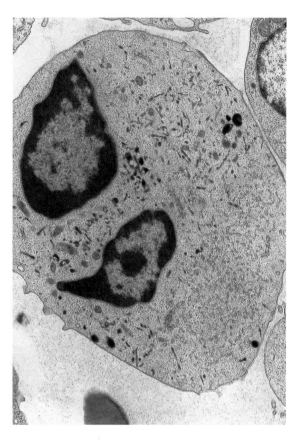

Figure 201
ABNORMAL NEUTROPHIL: ULTRASTRUCTURE
Electron micrograph of a mature neutrophil in a blood specimen from a patient with a myelodysplastic syndrome. The nucleus is hypolobulated; one segment has a nucleolus. The cytoplasm is markedly hypogranular. (Uranyl acetate–lead citrate stains, X14,000) (Fig. 46.3 from Brunning RD. Myelodysplastic syndromes. In: Knowles DM, ed. Neoplastic hematopathology. Baltimore: Williams & Wilkins, 1992:1367–404.)

Ultrastructural Findings. The ultrastructural findings in the myeloid cells of MDS are the same as those in the acute myeloid leukemias (6). The major alterations are due to abnormalities in nuclear and cytoplasmic development. Maturing neutrophils may exhibit decreased primary and secondary granules and granules of abnormal size or shape (fig. 201). Monocyte abnormalities include increased cytoplasmic microfilaments and abnormal granule production (fig. 202). The erythroid abnormalities include large vacuoles, duplications of the nuclear envelope, nuclear blebs, redundant cell membranes, and unusual cell shapes (fig. 203). The type III or ringed sideroblast that is most notable in sideroblastic anemia but that may be present in all types of MDS shows intracristal iron deposits in the mitochondria.

The megakaryocytes may manifest decreased numbers of granules and demarcation membranes; the micromegakaryocytes frequently manifest a decreased number of granules and demarcation membranes (fig. 204). The platelets may be hypogranular or contain very large granules (fig. 205).

Cytogenetic Findings. Cytogenetic studies are an important part of the evaluation of patients with MDS. These may be useful for prognostic purposes and as evidence for the diagnosis in equivocal cases (19,44,49,54,58,70–72). In addition, certain cytogenetic findings appear to identify clinical pathologic entities; a de novo MDS associated with a 5q- chromosome abnormality is characterized by a macrocytic anemia, hypolobulated megakaryocytes, and a prolonged

171

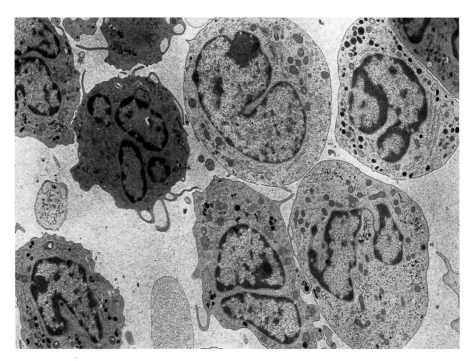

Figure 202
ABNORMAL MONOCYTES: ULTRASTRUCTURE
Electron micrograph of monocytes in a bone marrow specimen from a patient with CMML. Several atypical, very large granules are present. (Uranyl acetate–lead citrate stains, X13,000)

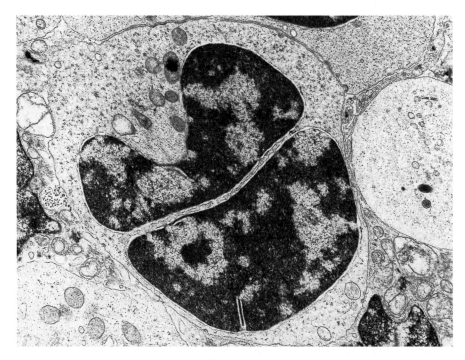

Figure 203
ABNORMAL ERYTHROBLAST: ULTRASTRUCTURE
Electron micrograph of an abnormal erythroblast in a bone marrow specimen from a patient with a myelodysplastic syndrome. The nucleus shows a cleft and splits. (Uranyl acetate-lead citrate stains, X19,000) (Fig. 46.6 from Brunning RD. Myelodysplastic syndromes. In: Knowles DM, ed. Neoplastic hematopathology. Baltimore: Williams & Wilkins, 1992:1367–404.)

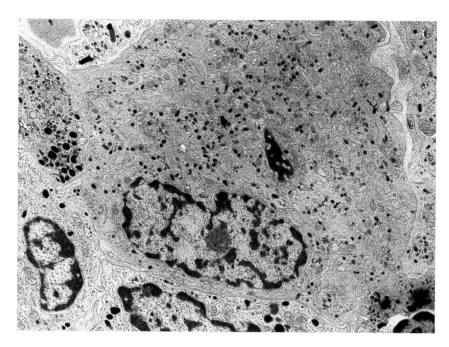

Figure 204
MICROMEGAKARYOCYTE: ULTRASTRUCTURE
Electron micrograph of a micromegakaryocyte in a bone marrow specimen from a patient with a myelodysplastic syndrome. In addition to the small size, the cytoplasm shows deficient granule production. (Uranyl acetate–lead citrate stains, X8,000) (Fig. 46.8 from Brunning RD. Myelodysplastic syndromes. In: Knowles DM, ed. Neoplastic hematopathology. Baltimore: Williams & Wilkins, 1992:1367–404.)

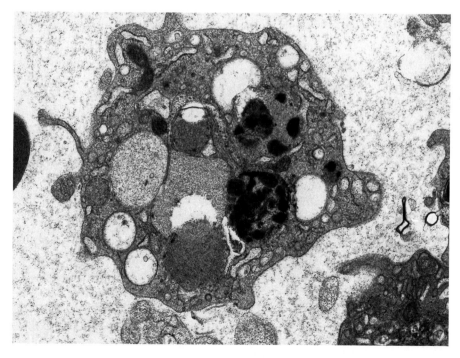

Figure 205
ATYPICAL PLATELET: ULTRASTRUCTURE
Electron micrograph of a platelet in a blood specimen from a patient with a myelodysplastic syndrome. Several atypical, very large granules are present. (Uranyl acetate–lead citrate stains, X32,000)

clinical course (26,34,41,52,56,65). MDSs associated with complex chromosome abnormalities or loss of chromosome 7 or 7q- appear to have an aggressive clinical course (1,11,17).

Chromosome abnormalities have been reported in approximately 70 to 80 percent of cases of primary MDS. The cytogenetic abnormalities have been categorized into eight groups (70–72). The most common cytogenetic abnormality is the presence of complex chromosome defects, i.e., two or more clonal abnormalities, and occurs in approximately 20 to 25 percent of patients. This finding is generally associated with a rapid clinical course irrespective of FAB subtype. The complex abnormalities frequently include monosomy 5 or 5q-, monosomy 7 or 7-, and monosomy 20 or 20q-.

The second most frequent cytogenetic abnormality is monosomy 7 or 7q- as single defects, occurring in approximately 15 percent of patients. These abnormalities may occur in all FAB subtypes and are associated with a high (approximately 70 percent) evolution to acute myeloid leukemia or a higher risk form of MDS.

Other abnormalities occurring with relatively high frequency as single defects are +8, 9q-, and 20q-, each occurring in 5 to 10 percent of patients. All of these defects may be detected in essentially all FAB subtypes.

The relationship of chromosome abnormalities to prognosis in primary or de novo MDS can be summarized by three risk groups (71):

Favorable: normal chromosomes, 5q- (single defect)

Intermediate: +8

Unfavorable: complex defects, monosomy 7 or 7q-

Because of low incidence, the prognostic significance of some chromosome defects is indeterminate. These include 9q-, 20q-, t(1;3), and t(2;11). There is no consistent relationship between FAB subtype of primary MDS and cytogenetic abnormality. However, 80 to 90 percent of patients with RAEB and RAEB-T have abnormal clones (19).

As noted, the cytogenetic abnormalities in the primary MDSs, unlike the acute myeloid leukemias, do not in general relate to FAB subtypes. However, two chromosome abnormalities occurring as isolated cytogenetic findings are associated with relatively well-defined clinical pathologic entities: the 5q- syndrome and isolated monosomy 7 syndrome of childhood.

5q- Syndrome. The de novo 5q- syndrome is a myelodysplastic process associated with an interstitial deletion of the long arm of chromosome 5 involving bands q12 to q32 as the sole chromosome abnormality (26,34,41,52,56,58,65). These patients have no prior history of exposure to chemotherapy or radiotherapy. The 5q syndrome is a rare disorder occurring in adults, with a female predominance (34,65). Splenomegaly has been reported in 16 percent of patients (34). The clinical course is frequently prolonged; evolution to acute leukemia may occur and is usually accompanied by the detection of additional chromosome abnormalities.

The anemia is moderate to severe and usually normochromic macrocytic. The leukocyte count is normal to slightly elevated; the platelet count is normal to elevated.

The 5q syndrome is usually associated with the blood and bone marrow findings of refractory anemia or RAEB (fig. 206A) (34,56,65). The abnormality may also occur with RARS and RAEB-T.

The bone marrow shows decreased erythroid precursors and dysplastic changes in granulocytes. There may be an excess of myeloblasts. One of the most prominent features is the presence of increased megakaryocytes, many of which have round, oval, and nonlobulated nuclei (fig. 206B). Sideroblasts are decreased in some patients.

The bone marrow biopsy shows varying degrees of cellularity. There is usually hypoplasia of the erythroid precursors. Megakaryocytes are increased and frequently cluster. Many of the megakaryocytes have nonlobulated nuclei but relatively abundant cytoplasm in contrast to the usual micromegalokaryocytes observed in the myeloproliferative disorders (fig. 206C). There may be scattered infiltrates of lymphocytes and plasma cells.

Monosomy 7 Syndrome of Childhood. This is a hematologic disorder in young children that is associated with an isolated monosomy 7 (11). It is very rare (1,17,18,51). The age of presentation ranges from 6 months to 8 years; the median age is 10 months. There is a male predominance; the disease has been reported in siblings (51). The major clinical findings are a history of recurrent infections and hepatosplenomegaly; lymphadenopathy is sometimes present. A concurrence of monosomy 7 syndrome and neurofibromatosis has been observed (50).

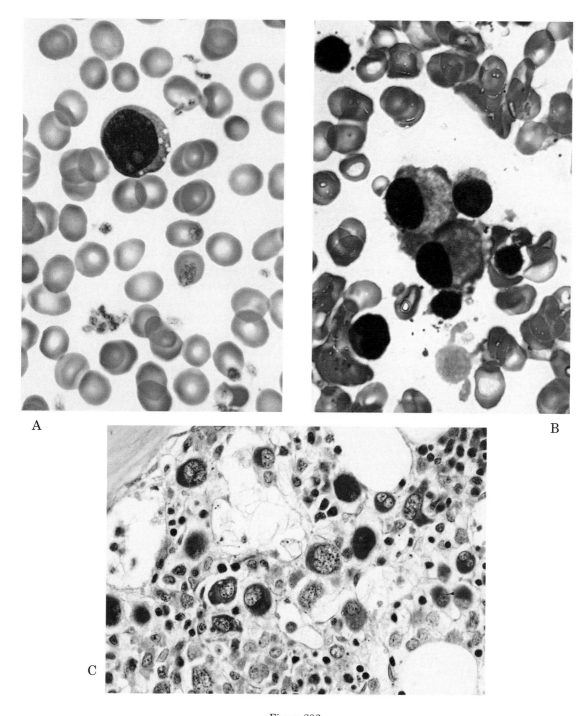

Figure 206

REFRACTORY ANEMIA WITH EXCESS OF BLASTS ASSOCIATED WITH A 5q- CHROMOSOME ABNORMALITY

A. Blood smear from an adult woman with RAEB associated with an isolated 5q- chromosome abnormality. This field shows a blast and numerous platelets. The platelet count was 567×10^9/L. (Wright-Giemsa stain)

B. Bone marrow smear from the patient in A showing three small megakaryocytes with nonlobulated nuclei. There is a relatively abundant amount of cytoplasm. (Wright-Giemsa stain) (Fig. 46.28A from Brunning RD. Myelodysplastic syndromes. In: Knowles DM, ed. Neoplastic hematopathology. Baltimore: Williams & Wilkins, 1992:1367–404.)

C. Bone marrow section from the patient in A and B showing increased megakaryocytes. Many show nuclear hypolobulation. The amount of cytoplasm varies but is relatively abundant in contrast to some micromegakaryocytes which have a sparse amount of cytoplasm. (Periodic acid–Schiff stain)

The patients usually present with anemia and leukocytosis. Fifty percent of patients are thrombocytopenic. The fetal hemoglobin level is usually normal, but may be slightly elevated. Neutrophil function studies show defective chemotaxis (11,51). Chromosome studies show a loss of one chromosome 7 as the only abnormality.

There is usually a monocytosis and leukoerythroblastosis in the blood. Dysplastic changes may be present in the granulocytes and monocytes (fig. 207). The number of blasts is usually less than 2 percent. The bone marrow shows a slight increase in blasts in most patients; a range of 3 to 11 percent, with a mean of 6 percent, was reported in one series (11). Dysplastic changes in the erythroid cells, granulocytes, and monocytes are present in approximately half of the patients. The megakaryocytes are usually morphologically normal, but are reduced in slightly more than 50 percent of patients.

The bone marrow cellularity is usually increased; in some patients it may be hypocellular due to an increase in fat cells and interstitial cell depletion (fig. 208). Slight reticulin fibrosis may be present. The blood and bone marrow abnormalities associated with an isolated monosomy 7 syndrome of childhood may be similar to the findings in juvenile chronic myeloid leukemia, which is discussed in the chapter on Chronic Myeloproliferative Diseases.

Differential Diagnosis. The diagnosis of MDS is based on the demonstration of dysplastic changes in immature and mature cells of the myeloid series, with or without an increase in myeloblasts. The diagnosis should only be established after careful review of the blood and bone marrow findings and clinical history. The designation should not be used for every case with hematologic abnormalities for which there is no apparent etiology; dysplastic changes similar to those found in the MDSs, most notably in red blood cell precursors, may occur as a result of exposure to toxins or drugs.

The possibility of an incorrect diagnosis most commonly occurs in cases in which the diagnosis is based on the interpretation of dysplastic changes without an increase in myeloblasts: refractory anemia, RARS, and MDS-U.

One of the most difficult problems relates to the diagnosis of refractory anemia when the morphologic findings are primarily in the red blood cells without an increase in blasts. It is important that the evaluation of a possible refractory anemia excludes any possibility that the morphologic changes are secondary to nutritional deficiency, drugs or toxins. The most important consideration is megaloblastic anemia due to vitamin B_{12} or folate deficiency. Red blood cell and serum folate, and serum B_{12} levels must be assayed in any patient with suspected refractory anemia. Normal levels are not absolute assurances of normality and it is prudent to treat patients with these vitamins if there is a macrocytic anemia.

Heavy metal intoxication, particularly arsenic, can lead to myelodysplastic changes, primarily in the erythroblasts but also in the neutrophils (28,68). Patients may present with pancytopenia and the morphologic findings may suggest MDS. The red blood cells frequently show coarse basophilic stippling. Exposure to the offending agent may be occupational, accidental, or as a result of homicidal intent (fig. 209).

Congenital dyserythropoietic anemia is most likely to manifest in childhood, but may initially be recognized in the adult years (figs. 210, 211) (31). The erythroid precursors in this group of disorders generally show marked morphologic alterations including nuclear lobulation, megaloblastoid nuclei, nuclear gigantism, and multinucleation. The erythrocytes in the blood smear show varying degrees of anisopoikilocytosis. The granulocytes and megakaryocytes are normal and the platelet and leukocyte counts are in the normal range.

Acute alcohol intoxication may lead to megaloblastic changes in both neutrophils and red blood cell precursors by virtue of interference with folic acid metabolism. Vacuolated erythroblasts and ringed sideroblasts may be transitory findings. Dysplastic changes in myeloid cells may be observed in acquired immune deficiency syndrome (40,59).

In some cases, the major differential diagnosis will be between a myelodysplastic disorder and a myeloproliferative process. This has been noted in the discussion on chronic myelomonocytic leukemia, a term that may be used in the context of a myelodysplastic or myeloproliferative disorder. Occasional cases of sideroblastic anemia present with thrombocytosis (7). The thrombocytosis suggests the possibility of essential thrombocythemia

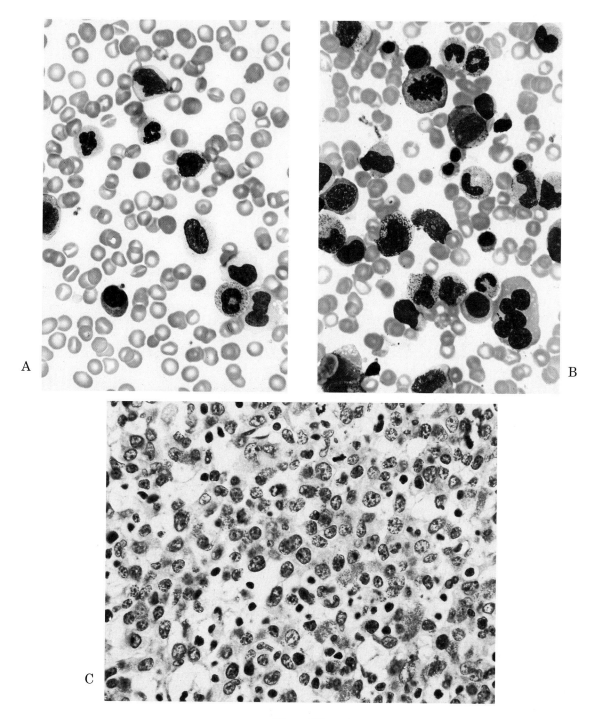

Figure 207

ISOLATED MONOSOMY 7 SYNDROME OF CHILDHOOD

A. Blood smear from a from a 4-year-old child with anemia, thrombocytopenia, and leukocytosis. The leukocytes are predominantly mature monocytes and neutrophils with occasional immature cells. A plasma cell is at the lower left. (Wright-Giemsa stain)

B. Bone marrow smear from the same patient as in A. There is an increased number of monocytes and promonocytes and large multinucleated polychromatic erythroid precursors. (Wright-Giemsa stain)

C. Bone marrow biopsy from the same patient. The marrow is markedly hypercellular with a predominance of immature neutrophils and monocytes. Red blood cell precursors are scattered throughout the marrow; megakaryocytes are reduced. (Hematoxylin and eosin stain)

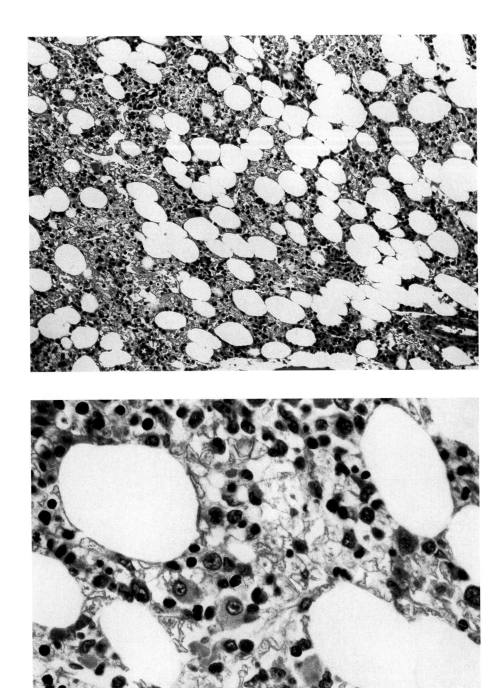

Figure 208

ISOLATED MONOSOMY 7 SYNDROME OF CHILDHOOD WITH A HYPOCELLULAR BONE MARROW

Top: Bone marrow biopsy from a 9-year-old boy with a history of repeated infections. At the time this biopsy was obtained the patient was pancytopenic with mild dysplastic changes in neutrophils and erythroid precursors. An isolated monosomy 7 was found on cytogenetic study. This figure shows a moderately hypocellular marrow with increased adipocytes and hypocellular interstitium. (Hematoxylin and eosin stain)

Bottom: High magnification of the specimen on the top illustrating the hypocellular interstitium. Several small megakaryocytes with hypolobulated nuclei are present. (Hematoxylin and eosin stain)

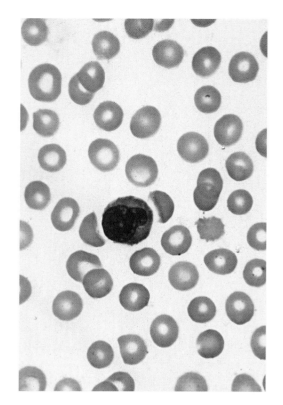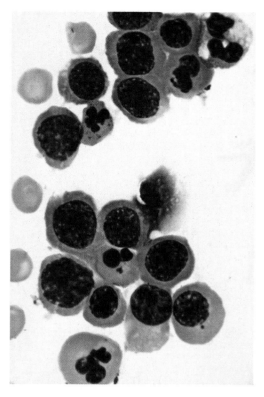

Figure 209
MYELODYSPLASTIC CHANGES RELATED TO ARSENIC INTOXICATION

Left: Blood smear from a 42-year-old male admitted to hospital in an obtunded state. Hematologic studies showed a pancytopenia. An erythroid precursor with a slightly lobulated megaloblastoid nucleus is shown. (Wright-Giemsa stain)

Right: Bone marrow smear from the same patient showing erythroid precursors with marked dysplastic changes including nuclear lobulation and karyorrhexis. Rare giant neutrophil precursors with premature nuclear segmentation were also present. Four days after obtaining this specimen, the patient's wife confessed to adding arsenic to his evening meals. The patient was treated with dimercaprol and completely recovered hematologically and neurologically. (Wright-Giemsa stain)

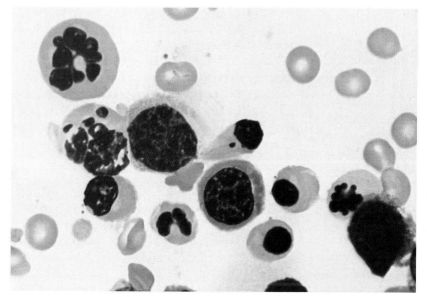

Figure 210
CONGENITAL
DYSERYTHROPOIETIC ANEMIA

Bone marrow specimen from a young child with congenital dyserythropoietic anemia. The red blood cell precursors are marked by nuclear abnormalities including large size, megaloblastoid chromatin, lobulation, and karyorrhexis. (Wright-Giemsa stain) (Fig. 46.33 from Brunning RD. Myelodysplastic syndromes. In: Knowles DM, ed. Neoplastic hematopathology. Baltimore: Williams & Wilkins, 1992:1367–404.)

Figure 211
CONGENITAL
DYSERYTHROPOIETIC
ANEMIA

Bone marrow smear from a 22-year-old male found to have a slightly elevated reticulocyte count and slight hyperbilirubinemia during an insurance medical evaluation. The Hb level was 13.7 g/dL; platelets and leukocytes were normal. Numerous abnormal red blood cell precursors similar to the one illustrated were present. The abnormalities were characterized primarily by gigantism and nuclear hyperlobulation. A diagnosis of congenital dyserythropoiesis was made. The patient is alive and asymptomatic 16 years later. (Wright-Giemsa stain) (Fig. 46.32 from Brunning RD. Myelodysplastic syndromes. In: Knowles DM, ed. Neoplastic hematopathology. Baltimore: Williams & Wilkins, 1992:1367–404.)

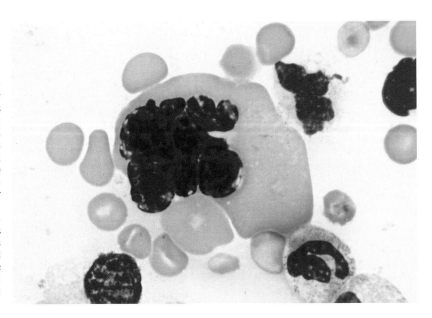

but the dysplastic changes are more compatible with a myelodysplastic process. In general, if there is evidence of bone marrow failure with a decrease in one or more cell lines and prominent dysplastic changes, a myelodysplastic classification is the most appropriate. If a process is characterized by an increase in one or more cell lines, a myeloproliferative classification is appropriate. Dysplastic changes may occur in myeloproliferative disorders but are less marked than in MDSs. If marked dysplastic changes are present in a myeloproliferative disorder, they usually indicate a more aggressive phase.

These guidelines will not resolve all problems and some cases will have to be arbitrarily classified as a myelodysplastic or myeloproliferative disorder. Patients with refractory anemia with ringed sideroblasts and thrombocytosis exemplify this dilemma. Ringed sideroblasts, sometimes in excess of 15 percent of bone marrow nucleated red blood cells, may also be observed in idiopathic myelofibrosis.

Prognosis and Evolution. The biologic course of the MDSs varies substantially with the different types and within types (8,9,12,21,32,42,57,58).

In most patients, RAEB-T and CMML-T are marked by a rapid clinical course similar to acute myeloid leukemia. Those patients who do not develop the definitive criteria of acute myeloid leukemia succumb to the complications of bone marrow failure (37,58). Occasional patients have a prolonged course (see fig. 189).

RAEB has a variable evolution (58). The majority of patients experience rapidly progressive bone marrow failure, with or without the development of overt acute leukemia. A small number of patients have a prolonged clinical course with stable hematologic findings over several years.

Similar to RAEB, CMML has a variable evolution (53,57,58). Some patients have a prolonged clinical course while others transform to acute myelomonocytic leukemia within weeks or months of diagnosis.

Refractory anemia encompasses a heterogeneous group of patients. Although the major finding in this disorder is anemia without an increase in blasts, patients with severe dysplasia of granulocytes and megakaryocytes may be placed in this category because the findings do not satisfy the criteria for one of the other types of MDS, i.e., RAEB or RAEB-T. Those patients with only anemia and mild changes in the erythroid progenitors may have a more stable clinical course than patients with prominent dysplastic changes in the granulocytes, megakaryocytes, and erythroid cells. As noted, MDS-U is a more appropriate designation for the latter group of patients.

Table 21 summarizes the survival periods and the incidence of leukemic evolution in 1081 patients with a diagnosis of MDS. Information was accrued from 11 published studies (8,13,21,

Table 21

**SURVIVAL AND INCIDENCE OF ACUTE LEUKEMIA
IN THE PRIMARY MYELODYSPLASTIC SYNDROMES***

Type	Percent Patients	Survival in Months (Median)	Progression to Leukemia (%)
Refractory anemia	28	18–64 (50)	12
Refractory anemia with ringed sideroblasts	24	14–76+ (51)	8
Refractory anemia with excess of blasts	23	7–16 (11)	44
Refractory anemia with excess of blasts in transformation	16	2.5–11 (5)	60
Chronic myelomonocytic leukemia	9	9–60+ (11)	14

*From reference 58.

22,27,38,53,58,61,64,66,67). This summary includes only those myelodysplastic categories proposed by the FAB group.

As noted in the table, patients with RAEB and RAEB-T have an unfavorable prognosis with a high rate of progression to acute leukemia and a short survival time. The median survival period for patients with CMML is also 'short but the percentage of cases evolving to acute leukemia is relatively low in comparison to RAEB and RAEB-T. The wide survival range of patients with CMML may reflect the application of different criteria for this diagnosis. Patients with refractory anemia and RARS have long median survival times and low rates of evolution to acute leukemia. Similar to CMML, there is a wide survival range in refractory anemia and RARS (58). Although refractory anemia and RARS can generally be viewed as low-risk forms of MDS, caution must be exercised in prognosticating in an individual case.

Scoring Systems. Several scoring systems have been proposed for stratifying patients with MDS, with the exception of RAEB-T, into prognostic groups; RAEB-T is uniformly accepted as a high-risk type of MDS. The Bournemouth system is based on the percent of bone marrow blasts, platelet count, neutrophil count, and hemoglobin level (38). A score of 1 is assigned for each of the following values: marrow blasts of 5 percent or more, platelets 100×10^9/L or less, neutrophils 2.54×10^9/L or less, and a hemoglobin level of less than 10 g/dL. Patients are placed in three prognostic groups based on the score: A (0,1), B (2,3), and C (4); A is the most favorable

group. The differences in survival based on this stratification are statistically significant (38).

Other scoring systems have been based on similar factors and age. Percent of bone marrow blasts, age, and degree of thrombocytopenia are generally found to have prognostic relevance (8,9,12,13,46,48,63,69). Older age, high percent of marrow blasts, and marked thrombocytopenia predict shorter survival periods. The percent of type I blasts in the bone marrow has been reported to have more relevance for prognosis than the combined percent of type I and II blasts (48).

Treatment. In a discussion of the management of patients with primary MDS, it is important to recognize the differences in the biologic course of the different types. Most patients with refractory anemia and RARS have a relatively stable clinical course for a prolonged period, with a low incidence of transformation to acute leukemia (58). The majority of patients with RAEB-T and CMML-T have rapidly progressive bone marrow failure with a high incidence of leukemic evolution. This biologic diversity and the occurrence primarily in middle-aged and older individuals precludes generalizations about therapeutic approaches (42). The lower-grade MDSs, with less potential for transformation to acute leukemia, refractory anemia, and RARS, may be satisfactorily managed with supportive therapy when indicated; the use of biologic response modifiers such as granulocyte stimulating factor, may be efficacious in some patients with neutropenia (32). RAEB-T and CMML-T are similar to acute leukemia and patients with these types of MDS may benefit from aggressive antileukemic therapy. This is particularly true for individuals under the age of 50 with 20 to 30 percent blasts in the bone marrow and Auer rods (37,63). Older individuals are at greater risk for morbidity and mortality with this therapy and caution should be used with this approach.

The management of RAEB and CMML is problematic since the biologic course of these disorders is highly variable. However, patients less than 50 years of age with pronounced bone marrow failure and rapid hematologic deterioration might benefit from antileukemia therapy (63).

THERAPY-RELATED MYELODYSPLASTIC SYNDROMES AND ACUTE MYELOID LEUKEMIA

Definition. Therapy-related MDS and acute myeloid leukemia (AML) occur in individuals previously treated with cytotoxic agents and radiotherapy. Two groups of therapy-related processes are recognized based on the causative agents. The major type occurs in patients treated with alkylating agents and radiotherapy and is usually associated with a panmyelosis and abnormalities of chromosomes 5 and 7 (77–79,81). The other type occurs in patients treated with an epipodophyllotoxin and is frequently associated with abnormalities of 11q23 and AML with a monocytic component (83,86,87).

Incidence and Clinical Findings. The incidence varies with the different causative agents and ranges up to 15 percent in patients with Hodgkin disease treated with nitrogen mustard, vincristine, procarbazine, and prednisone (MOPP) chemotherapy and up to 17 percent in myeloma patients treated with alkylating agents (85). In Hodgkin disease, the peak risk period appears to occur 6 years following initiation of combined modality therapy (73). Risk factors in patients treated with alkylating agents, chemotherapy, and radiotherapy include age, type of agent, duration of treatment, and repetition of exposure to the mutagenic agents (76,78). The time interval from initiation of the causative therapy to manifestation of the MDS or leukemia in this group is 7 to 133 months; medians of 56, 58, and 71 months are reported in different series (78,79,81). The cumulative risk in patients treated with high doses of an epipodophyllotoxin for lung cancer is 15 ±11 percent at 2 years and 44 ±24 percent at 2.5 years (83).

Patients with a therapy-related MDS or acute leukemia most commonly present with fatigue due to anemia; infections resulting from neutropenia and thrombocytopenia may also be presenting manifestations. Because these patients are usually being followed for the disorder for which the causative agents were administered, the detection of laboratory abnormalities may precede the onset of clinical symptoms.

Laboratory Findings. Cytopenias are common. Anemia is virtually always present and thrombocytopenia and neutropenia are seen in the majority of patients (75). Macrocytosis with ovalocytes is common.

The myeloid cells in a high percentage of cases have a clonal chromosome abnormality. The abnormalities in the predominant group of alkylating agent- and radiotherapy-related disorders tend to be multiple and approximately 80 percent involve chromosomes 5 and 7, and include -5, 5q-, -7 and 7q-; when a single abnormality is present it usually involves one of these chromosomes. Extreme karyotypic variability may occur (79). The abnormalities are present in both the MDS and AML phases.

The epipodophyllotoxin-related leukemias have been primarily associated with abnormalities of chromosome 11 at band q23 (83,87).

Blood and Bone Marrow Findings. The blood and bone marrow findings vary depending on the stage at which the problem is initially diagnosed and the therapeutic agents associated with the process. The predominant type, related to alkylating agent therapy and radiotherapy, is separated into MDS and AML based on the percent of blasts; however, these two processes should be viewed as two stages of the same disorder. The majority of cases are characterized by a panmyelosis, which frequently makes precise classification difficult (75,81). The morphologic alterations vary from subtle abnormalities of nuclear development in the erythroblasts, neutrophil precursors, and megakaryocytes to marked abnormalities in size and nuclear and cytoplasmic characteristics (figs. 212–214). Nuclear hypolobulation and cytoplasmic hypogranulation are present in a high percentage of cases. Abnormalities of erythroblast nuclei are present in virtually all cases; marked gigantism and hyperlobulated nuclei are frequent. Ringed sideroblasts occur in approximately 60 percent of cases and range up to 45 percent of the nucleated red blood cells (fig. 215).

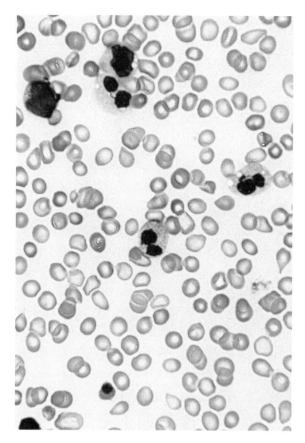

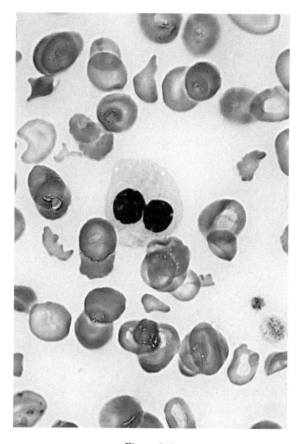

Figure 212
THERAPY-RELATED
MYELODYSPLASTIC SYNDROME

Blood smear from an adult male with a therapy-related MDS. Three neutrophils with pseudo–Pelger-Huet nuclei are present; a normoblast is present in the lower left. (Wright-Giemsa stain) (Fig. 46.34 from Brunning RD. Myelodysplastic syndromes. In: Knowles DM, ed. Neoplastic hematopathology. Baltimore: Williams & Wilkins, 1992:1367–404.)

Figure 213
THERAPY-RELATED
MYELODYSPLASTIC SYNDROME

Blood smear from an adult female with a myelodysplastic syndrome related to radiotherapy and chemotherapy for Hodgkin disease. A hypogranular neutrophil with a pseudo–Pelger-Huet nucleus is shown. The red blood cells show marked poikilocytosis, in part related to postsplenectomy status. (Wright-Giemsa stain)

This finding may be the initial manifestation of a dysplastic process. In some cases, the erythroblasts show marked reactivity with PAS (fig. 216). Increased blood and bone marrow basophils occur in approximately 25 percent of cases and may be one of the earliest manifestations of the disease.

The blood and bone marrow findings in the majority of cases of this type of therapy-related MDS are those of refractory anemia or RAEB. Striking dysplastic changes in all myeloid cell lines may be present in a patient with less than 5 percent marrow blasts. Because of this, subclassification may be difficult and a diagnosis of therapy-related MDS is adequate. The therapy-related acute leukemias are principally of AML-M2, AML-M4, or AML-M6 subtypes (figs. 217, 218). Because of the panmyelosis nature of many of these leukemias, approximately 40 to 50 percent of cases cannot be classified (81).

The epipodophyllotoxin-related leukemias frequently manifest as acute leukemia with a monocytic component, M5 or M4. Presentations with and without an antecedent preleukemic phase have been reported (fig. 219) (83,87).

Histopathologic Findings. The bone marrow is normocellular in approximately 50 percent of cases, hypercellular in 25 percent, and hypocellular in 25 percent (fig. 220) (81). The hypercellular marrows are generally characterized by a panhyperplasia. Megakaryocytes may

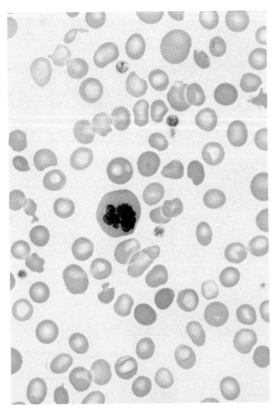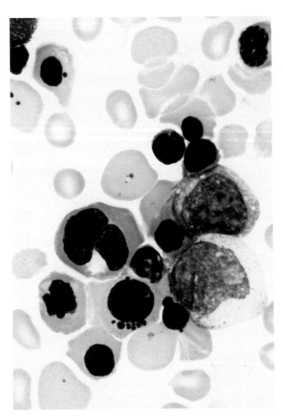

Figure 214
THERAPY-RELATED MYELODYSPLASTIC SYNDROME

Left: Blood smear from an adult woman with a myelodysplastic syndrome related to multiagent chemotherapy for metastatic breast carcinoma. The red blood cells show increased anisopoikilocytosis with numerous macrocytes. A large red blood cell precursor with marked nuclear lobulation is present. (Wright-Giemsa stain)

Right: Bone marrow smear from the same patient showing numerous red blood cell precursors with marked nuclear lobulation. Myeloblasts are not increased. (Wright-Giemsa stain)

Figure 215
THERAPY-RELATED
MYELODYSPLASTIC
SYNDROME

Iron stain of a bone marrow smear from a young woman with a myelodysplastic syndrome following radiotherapy and chemotherapy for Hodgkin disease. One of the early manifestations of myelodysplasia in this patient was the presence of ringed sideroblasts as illustrated. (Prussian blue followed by safranin O stain) (Fig. 46.41 from Brunning RD. Myelodysplastic syndromes. In: Knowles DM, ed. Neoplastic hematopathology. Baltimore: Williams & Wilkins, 1992:1367–404.)

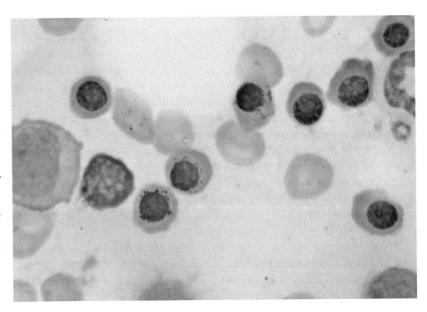

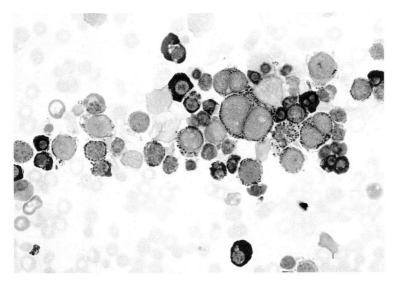

Figure 216
THERAPY-RELATED
MYELODYSPLASTIC
SYNDROME

This bone marrow smear from a patient with therapy-related MDS reacted with PAS. Most of the erythroid precursors are intensely positive. (Periodic acid–Schiff stain)

Figure 217
THERAPY-RELATED ACUTE
MYELOID LEUKEMIA

Blood smear from an adult with acute myeloid leukemia related to chemotherapy for a non-Hodgkin lymphoma. In addition to the high percentage of blasts there was an increase in basophils. (Wright-Giemsa stain)

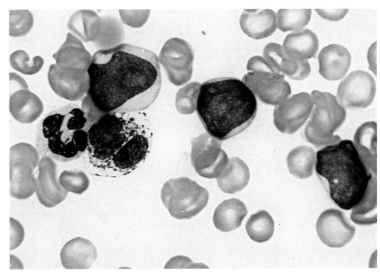

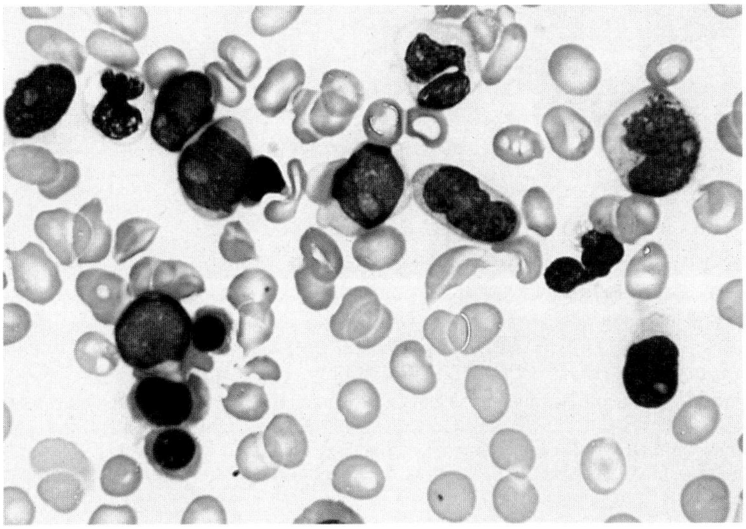

Figure 218
THERAPY-RELATED ACUTE
MYELOID LEUKEMIA

Bone marrow smear from an 18-year-old man with therapy-related AML 4 years following radiotherapy and combination chemotherapy for Hodgkin disease. The smear contained 30 to 35 percent myeloblasts. (Wright-Giemsa stain)

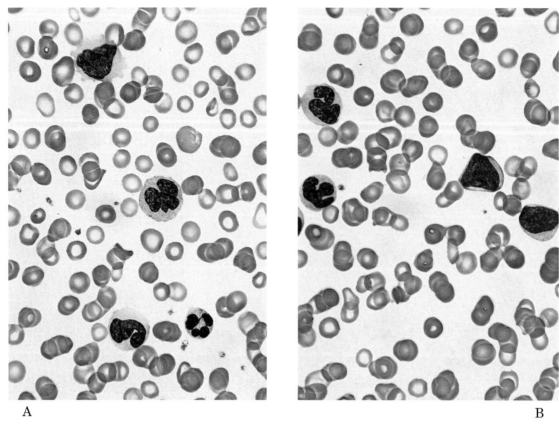

A

B

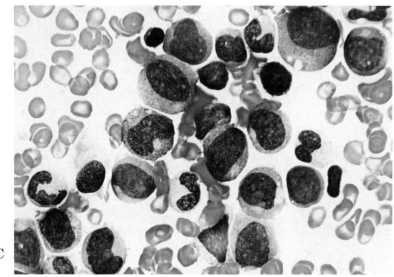

C

Figure 219
ETOPOSIDE-ASSOCIATED MYELODYSPLASTIC SYNDROME
WITH t(9;11)(p21;q23) CYTOGENETIC ABNORMALITY

A. Blood smear from a child treated 2 years previously for acute lymphoblastic leukemia with a regimen that included etoposide. At the time of this smear the hemoglobin level was 10 g/dL, WBC 27×10^9/L, and platelets 116×10^9/L. (Wright-Giemsa stain)

B. There was a marked increase in monocytes, primarily mature, and 3 percent blasts. (Wright-Giemsa stain)

C. Bone marrow smear showing a slight shift to immaturity and 5 percent blasts. Cytogenetic studies from this specimen showed a t(9;11)(p21;q23) chromosome abnormality. (Wright-Giemsa stain)

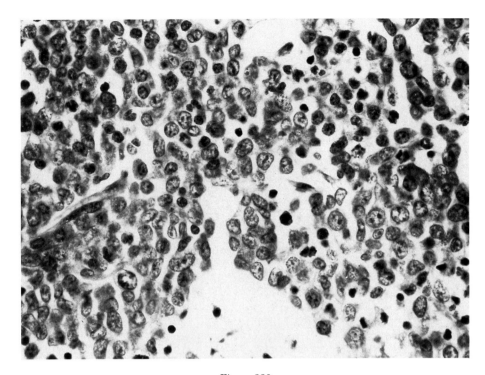

Figure 220
THERAPY-RELATED ACUTE MYELOID LEUKEMIA
Bone marrow biopsy from a patient with therapy-related AML. The marrow is markedly hypercellular due to an increase in blasts and promyelocytes. Segmented neutrophils and megakaryocytes are markedly reduced. (Hematoxylin and eosin stain)

be disproportionately increased and manifest considerable size range with numerous micromegakaryocytes (fig. 221). Clustering of megakaryocytes may be present. Approximately 15 percent of bone marrows show some increase in reticulin fibers (81). A marked increase in reticulin fibers resembling acute myelofibrosis may be present in some patients (84).

The marrow sections may show evidence of the malignant process for which the initial treatment was administered.

Ultrastructural Findings. All myeloid cell lines usually show evidence of abnormal maturation (74,80). Developing neutrophils show decreased primary and secondary granule production and abnormally large and misshapen granules. The monocytes may show increased microfilaments and abnormal granules. The erythroid abnormalities include intracristal mitochondrial iron, vacuoles, duplication of the nuclear envelope, nuclear blebs, a redundant cell membrane, and bizarre cell shape (74,81). Mega-

karyocytes may show decreased granules and demarcation membranes. Micromegakaryocytes and large platelets with decreased or abnormal giant granules may be present.

Prognostic Factors. Therapy-related MDS generally has a more aggressive clinical course than the de novo forms and the marrow findings may evolve rapidly into AML (fig. 222). The overall median survival time is 4 to 8 months. Patients with MDS have only a slightly longer median survival period than patients with AML (81).

Several laboratory findings have been associated with a poor prognosis including cytogenetic abnormalities other than t(15;17), t(8;21), and inv(16); more than 5 percent blasts in the marrow; and a platelet count less than 100×10^9/L (78). Clinical factors associated with an unfavorable prognosis include age over 65 years, Hodgkin disease, myeloma or ovarian cancer as the primary tumor, and therapy with alkylating agents, nitrosoureas, or procarbazine (78).

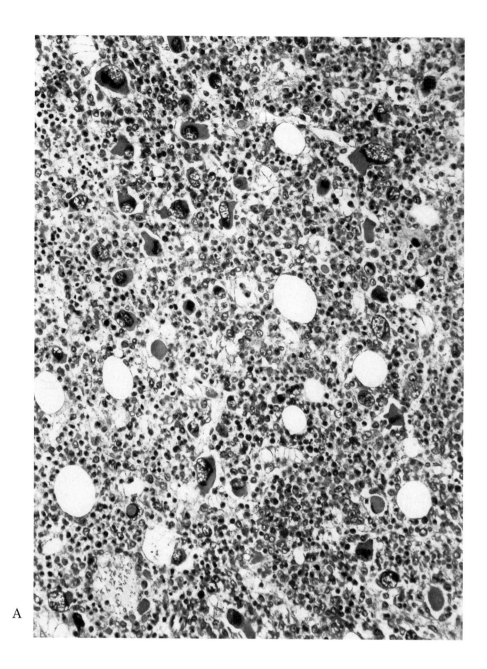

A

Figure 221
THERAPY-RELATED MYELODYSPLASTIC SYNDROME

A. Bone marrow biopsy from an adult male with an 11-year history of non-Hodgkin lymphoma treated with multiple courses of radiotherapy and chemotherapy. The marrow is markedly hypercellular with numerous randomly distributed megakaryocytes. A diagnosis of therapy-related MDS was established from this specimen. There was no evidence of recurrent lymphoma. (Hematoxylin and eosin stain)

B. High magnification of the specimen in A showing numerous varying sized megakaryocytes with nonlobulated and hypolobulated nuclei. The nuclei of most of the megakaryocytes have dispersed chromatin. The neutrophils are predominantly immature forms. (Hematoxylin and eosin stain)

C. A reticulin stain of the specimen in A and B shows a slight increase in reticulin fibers. (Wilder reticulin stain) (Fig. 46.43C from Brunning RD. Myelodysplastic syndromes. In: Knowles DM, ed. Neoplastic hematopathology. Baltimore: Williams & Wilkins, 1992:1367–404.)

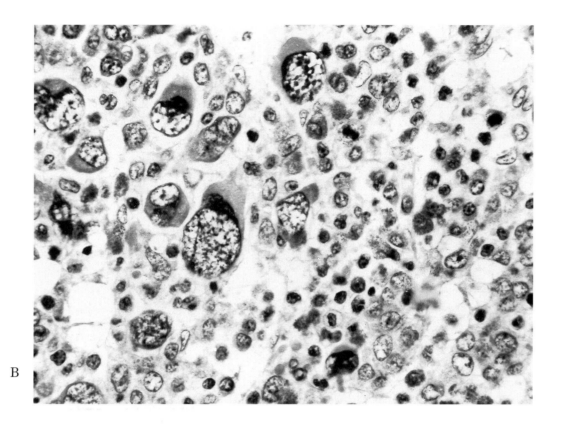

B

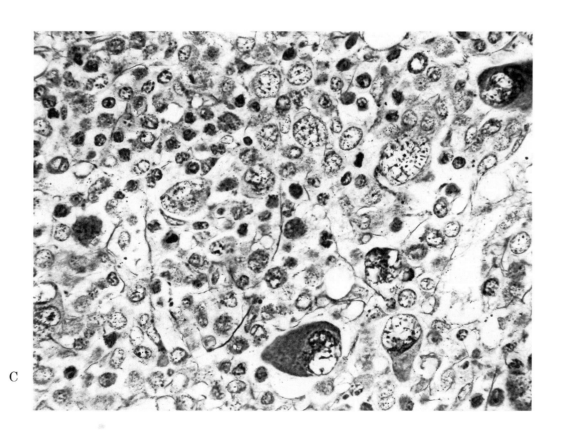

C

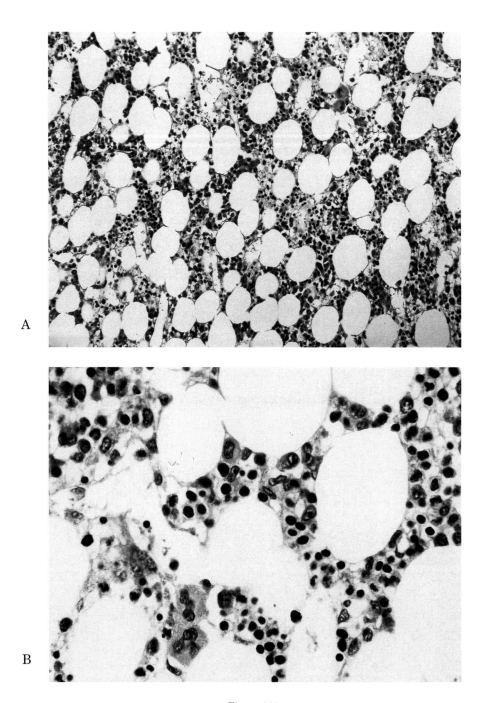

Figure 222

THERAPY-RELATED MYELODYSPLASTIC SYNDROME TRANSFORMING TO ACUTE MYELOID LEUKEMIA

A. Bone marrow biopsy from a patient with a history of radiotherapy and chemotherapy for Hodgkin disease. The patient was pancytopenic at the time of this biopsy June 13, 1982. (Hematoxylin and eosin stain) (Fig. 46.46A from Brunning RD. Myelodysplastic syndromes. In: Knowles DM, ed. Neoplastic hematopathology. Baltimore: Williams & Wilkins, 1992:1367–404.)

B. High magnification of specimen in A showing a slight relative erythroid hyperplasia and megakaryocytes. Neutrophil precursors are slightly reduced. There is no increase in immature cells. (Hematoxylin and eosin stain)

C. Bone marrow biopsy from the same patient obtained 2 months later on August 12, 1982. The marrow is markedly hypercellular. (Hematoxylin and eosin stain)

D. High magnification of the specimen in C showing a predominance of blasts and immature neutrophils. A diagnosis of therapy-related AML was made based on this specimen. (Hematoxylin and eosin stain) (Fig. 46.47B from Brunning RD. Myelodysplastic syndromes. In: Knowles DM, ed. Neoplastic hematopathology. Baltimore: Williams & Wilkins, 1992:1367–404.)

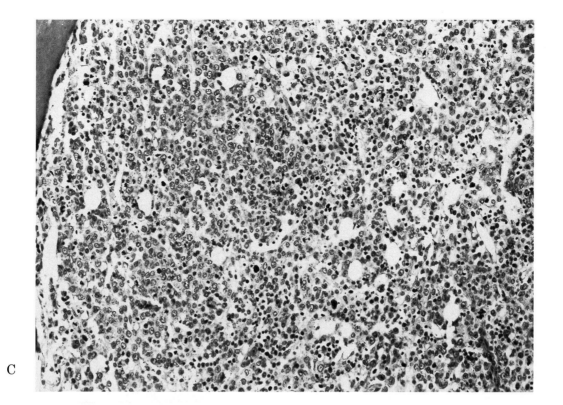

C

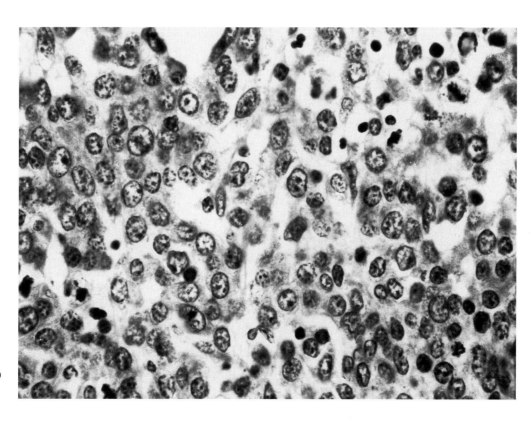

D

REFERENCES

Primary Myelodysplastic Syndromes

1. Baranger L, Baruchel A, Leverger G, Schaison G, Berger R. Monosomy-7 in childhood hemopoietic disorders. Leukemia 1990;4:345–9.
2. Bennett JM, Catovsky D, Daniel MT, et al. Proposals for the classification of the acute leukaemias. Br J Haematol 1976;33:451–8.
3. _____, Catovsky D, Daniel MT, et al. Proposals for the classification of the myelodysplastic syndromes. Br J Haematol 1982;51:189–99.
4. _____, Catovsky D, Daniel MT, et al. Proposed revised criteria for the classification of acute myeloid leukemia. A report of the French-American-British Cooperative Group. Ann Intern Med 1985;103:620–5.
5. Bitter MA, Neilly ME, Le Beau MM, Pearson MG, Rowley JD. Rearrangements of chromosome 3 involving bands 3q21 and 3q26 are associated with normal or elevated platelet counts in acute nonlymphocytic leukemia. Blood 1985;66:1362–70.
6. Brunning RD, Parkin JL, Hanson CA. Hematopoietic and lymphoreticular neoplasms. In: Azar HA, ed. Pathology of human neoplasms. An atlas of diagnostic electron microscopy and immunohistochemistry. New York: Raven Press, 1988:221–303.
7. Case records of the Massachusetts General Hospital (Case 17-1992). N Engl J Med 1992;326:1137–46.
8. Coiffier B, Adeleine P, Gentilhomme O, Felman P, Treille-Ritouet D, Bryon PA. Myelodysplastic syndromes. A multi-parametric study of prognostic factors in 336 patients. Cancer 1987;60:3029–32.
9. _____, Adeleine P, Viala JJ, et al. Dysmyelopoietic syndromes. A search for prognostic factors in 193 patients. Cancer 1983;52:83–90.
10. Dreyfus B. Preleukemic states. I. Definition and classification. II. Refractory anemia with excess of myeloblasts in the bone marrow (smoldering acute leukemia). Nouv Rev Fr Hematol Blood Cells 1976;17:33–45.
11. Evans JP, Czepulkowski B, Gibbons B, Swansbury GJ, Chessells JM. Childhood monosomy 7 revisited. Br J Haematol 1988;69:41–5.
12. Fenaux P, Jouet JP, Zandecki M, et al. Chronic and subacute myelomonocytic leukaemia in the adult: a report of 60 cases with special reference to prognostic factors. Br J Haematol 1987;65:101–6.
13. Foucar K, Langdon RM II, Armitage JO, Olson DB, Carroll TJ Jr. Myelodysplastic syndromes. A clinical and pathologic analysis of 109 cases. Cancer 1985;56:553–61.
14. _____, McKenna RW, Bloomfield CD, Bowers TK, Brunning RD. Therapy-related leukemia: a panmyelosis. Cancer 1979;43:1285–96.
15. Gattermann N, Aul C, Schneider W. Two types of acquired idiopathic sideroblastic anaemia (AISA). Br J Haematol 1990;74:45–52.
16. Groupe Francais de Morphologie Hematologique. French registry of acute leukemia and myelodysplastic syndromes. Age distribution and hemogram analysis of the 4496 cases recorded during 1982–1983 and classified according to FAB criteria. Cancer 1987;60:1385–94.
17. Gyger M, Bonny Y, Forest L. Childhood monosomy 7 syndrome. Am J Hematol 1982;13:329–34.
18. Hutter JJ Jr, Hecht F, Kaiser-McCaw B, et al. Bone marrow monosomy 7: hematologic and clinical manifestations in childhood and adolescence. Hematol Oncol 1984;2:5–12.
19. Jacobs RH, Cornbleet MA, Vardiman JW, Larson RA, Le Beau MM, Rowley JD. Prognostic implications of morphology and karyotype in primary myelodysplastic syndromes. Blood 1986;67:1765–72.
20. Jenkins RB, Tefferi A, Solberg LA Jr, Dewald GW. Acute leukemia with abnormal thrombopoiesis and inversions of chromosome 3. Cancer Genet Cytogenet 1989;39:167–79.
21. Joseph AS, Cinkotai KI, Hunt L, Geary CG. Natural history of smouldering leukaemia. Br J Cancer 1982;46:160–6.
22. Juneja SK, Imbert M, Jouault H, Scoazec JY, Sigaux F, Sultan C. Haematological features of primary myelodysplastic syndromes (PMDS) at initial presentation: a study of 118 cases. J Clin Pathol 1983;36:1129–35.
23. _____, Imbert M, Sigaux F, Jouault H, Sultan C. Prevalence and distribution of ringed sideroblasts in primary myelodysplastic syndromes. J Clin Pathol 1983;36:566–9.
24. Kantarjian HM, Keating MJ. Therapy-related leukemia and myelodysplastic syndrome. Semin Oncol 1987;14:435–43.
25. _____, Keating MJ, Walters RS, et al. Therapy-related leukemia and myelodysplastic syndrome: clinical, cytogenetic, and prognostic features. J Clin Oncol 1986;4:1748–57.
26. Kerkhofs H, Hagemeijer A, Leeksma CH, et al. The 5q-chromosome abnormality in haematological disorders: a collaborative study of 34 cases from the Netherlands. Br J Haematol 1982;52:365–81.
27. _____, Hermans J, Haak HL, Leeksma CH. Utility of the FAB classification for myelodysplastic syndromes: investigation of prognostic factors in 237 cases. Br J Haematol 1987;65:73–81.
28. Kyle RA, Pease GL. Hematologic aspects of arsenic intoxication. N Eng J Med 1965;273:18–23.
29. Lambertenghi-Deliliers G, Orazi A, Luksch R, Annaloro C, Soligo D. Myelodysplastic syndrome with increased marrow fibrosis: a distinct clinico-pathological entity. Br J Haematol 1991;78:161–6.
30. Le Beau MM, Albain KS, Larson RA, et al. Clinical and cytogenetic correlations in 63 patients with therapy-related myelodysplastic syndromes and acute nonlymphocytic leukemia: further evidence for characteristic abnormalities of chromosomes no. 5 and 7. J Clin Oncol 1986;4:325–45.
31. Lewis SM, Verwilghen RL. Dyserythropoiesis and dyserythropoietic anemias. In: Brown EB, Moore CV, eds. Progress in Hematology, Vol. 8. New York: Grune & Stratton, 1973:99–129.
32. List AF, Garewal HS, Sandberg AA. The myelodysplastic syndromes: biology and implications for management. J Clin Oncol 1990;8:1424–41.

33. Maschek H, Georgii A, Kaloutsi V, et al. Myelofibrosis in primary myelodysplastic syndromes: a retrospective study of 352 patients. Eur J Haematol 1992;48:208–14.

34. Mathew P, Tefferi A, Dewald GW, et al. The 5q- syndrome: a single-institution study of 43 consecutive patients. Blood 1993;81:1040–5.

35. Menke DM, Colon-Otero G, Cockerill KJ, Jenkins RB, Noel P, Pierre RV. Refractory thrombocytopenia: a myelodysplastic syndrome that may mimic thrombocytopenia purpura. Am J Clin Pathol 1992;98:502–10.

36. Michels SD, McKenna RW, Arthur DC, Brunning RD. Therapy-related acute myeloid leukemia and myelodysplastic syndrome: a clinical and morphologic study of 65 cases. Blood 1985;65:1364–72.

37. _____, Saumur J, Arthur DC, Robison LL, Brunning RD. Refractory anemia with excess of blasts in transformation: hematologic and clinical study of 52 patients. Cancer 1989;64:2340–6.

38. Mufti GJ, Stevens JR, Oscier DG, Hamblin TJ, Machin D. Myelodysplastic syndromes: a scoring system with prognostic significance. Br J Haematol 1985;59:425–33.

39. Nand S, Godwin JE. Hypoplastic myelodysplastic syndrome. Cancer 1988;62:958–64.

40. Napoli VM, Stein SF, Spira TJ, Raskin D. Myelodysplasia progressing to acute myeloblastic leukemia in an HTLV-III virus-positive homosexual man with AIDS-related complex. Am J Clin Pathol 1986;86:788–91.

41. Nimer SD, Golde DW. The 5q- abnormality. Blood 1987;70:1705–12.

42. Noël P. Management of patients with myelodysplastic syndromes. Mayo Clin Proc 1991;66:485–97.

43. Pagliuca A, Layton DM, Manoharan A, Gordon S, Green PJ, Mufti GJ. Myelofibrosis in primary myelodysplastic syndromes: a clinico-morphological study of 10 cases. Br J Haematol 1989;71:499–504.

44. Pierre RV, Catovsky D, Mufti GJ, et al. Clinical-cytogenetic correlations in myelodysplasia (preleukemia). Cancer Genet Cytogenet 1989;40:149–61.

45. Pintado T, Ferro MT, San Román CC, Mayayo M, Laraña JG. Clinical correlations of the 3q21;q26 cytogenetic anomaly. A leukemic or myelodysplastic syndrome with preserved or increased platelet production and lack of response to cytotoxic drug therapy. Cancer 1985;55:535–41.

46. Ribera JM, Cervantes F, Rozman C. A multivariate analysis of prognostic factors in chronic myelomonocytic leukaemia according to the FAB criteria. Br J Haematol 1987;65:307–11.

47. Ríos A, Cañizo MC, Sanz MA. Bone marrow biopsy in myelodysplastic syndromes: morphologic characteristics and contribution to the study of prognostic factors. Br J Haematol 1990;75:26–33.

48. Sanz GF, Sanz MA, Vallespí T, et al. Two regression models and a scoring system for predicting survival and planning treatment in myelodysplastic syndromes: a multivariate analysis of prognostic factors in 370 patients. Blood 1989;74:395–408.

49. Second International Workshop on chromosomes in leukemia. Chromosomes in preleukemia. Cancer Genet Cytogenet 1980;2:108–13.

50. Shannon KM, Watterson J, Johnson P, et al. Monosomy 7 myeloproliferative disease in children with neurofibromatosis, type 1: epidemiology and molecular analysis. Blood 1992;79:1311–8.

51. Sieff CA, Chessells JM, Harvey BA, Pickthall VJ, Lawler SD. Monosomy 7 in childhood: a myeloproliferative disorder. Br J Haematol 1981;49:235–49.

52. Sokal G, Michaux JL, Van Den Berghe H, et al. A new hematologic syndrome with a distinct karyotype: the 5q- chromosome. Blood 1975;46:519–33.

53. Solal-Celigny P, Desaint B, Herrera A, et al. Chronic myelomonocytic leukemia according to the FAB classification: analysis of 35 cases. Blood 1984;63:634–8.

54. Suciu S, Kuse R, Weh HJ, Hossfeld DK. Results of chromosome studies and their relation to morphology, course, and prognosis in 120 patients with de novo myelodysplastic syndrome. Cancer Genet Cytogenet 1990;44:15–26

55. Sultan C, Sigaux F, Imbert M, Reyes F. Acute myelodysplasia with myelofibrosis: a report of eight cases. Br J Haematol 1981;49:11–6.

56. Swolin B, Weinfeld A, Ridell B, Waldenström J, Westin J. On the 5q- deletion: clinical and cytogenetic observations in ten patients and review of the literature. Blood 1981;58:986–93.

57. Tefferi A, Hoagland HC, Therneau TM, Pierre RV. Chronic myelomonocytic leukemia: natural history and prognostic determinants. Mayo Clin Proc 1989;64:1246–54.

58. Third MIC Cooperative Study Group. Recommendations for a morphologic, immunologic, and cytogenetic (MIC) working classification of the primary and therapy-related myelodysplastic disorders. Report of the workshop held in Scottsdale, Arizona, USA, on February 23–25, 1987. Cancer Genet Cytogenet 1988;32:1–10.

59. Treacy M, Lai L, Costello C, Clark A. Peripheral blood and bone marrow abnormalities in patients with HIV related disease. Br J Haematol 1987;65:289–94.

60. Tricot G, Boogaerts MA, De Wolf-Peeters C, Van den Bergh H, Verwilghen RL. The myelodysplastic syndromes: different evolution patterns based on sequential morphological and cytogenetic investigations. Br J Haematol 1985;59:659–70.

61. _____, De Wolf-Peeters C, Hendrickx B, Verwilghen RL. Bone marrow histology in myelodysplastic syndromes. 1. Histological findings in myelodysplastic syndromes and comparison with bone marrow smears. Br J Haematol 1984;57:423–30.

62. _____, Vlietinck R, Boogaerts MA, et al. Prognostic factors in the myelodysplastic syndromes: importance of initial data on peripheral blood counts, bone marrow cytology, trephine biopsy and chromosomal analysis. Br J Haematol 1985;60:19–32.

63. _____, Vlietinck R, Verwilghen RL. Prognostic factors in the myelodysplastic syndromes: a review. Scand J Haematol 1986;36(Suppl 45):107–13.

64. Vallespi T, Torrabadella M, Julia A, et al. Myelodysplastic syndromes: a study of 101 cases according to the FAB classification. Br J Haematol 1985;61:83–92.

65. Van Den Berghe H, Vermaelen K, Mecucci C, Barbieri D, Tricot G. The 5q- anomaly. Cancer Genet Cytogenet 1985;17:189–255.

66. Varela BL, Chuang C, Woll JE, Bennett JM. Modifications in the classification of primary myelodysplastic syndromes: the addition of a scoring system. Hematol Oncol 1985;3:55–63.

67. Weisdorf DJ, Oken MM, Johnson GJ, Rydell RE. Chronic myelodysplastic syndrome: short survival with or without evolution to acute leukaemia. Br J Haematol 1983;55:691–700.

68. Westhoff DD, Samaha RJ, Barnes A Jr. Arsenic intoxication as a cause of megaloblastic anemia. Blood 1975;45:241–6.

69. Worsley A, Oscier DG, Stevens J, et al. Prognostic features of chronic myelomonocytic leukaemia: a modified Bournemouth score gives the best prediction of survival. Br J Haematol 1988;68:17–21.

70. Yunis JJ, Brunning RD. Prognostic significance of chromosomal abnormalities in acute leukaemias and myelodysplastic syndromes. Clin Haematol 1986;15:597–620.

71. _____, Lobell M, Arnesen MA, et al. Refined chromosome study helps define prognostic subgroups in most patients with primary myelodysplastic syndrome and acute myelogenous leukaemia. Br J Haematol 1988;68:189–94.

72. _____, Rydell RE, Oken MM, Arnesen MA, Mayer MG, Lobell M. Refined chromosome analysis as an independent prognostic indicator in de novo myelodysplastic syndromes. Blood 1986;67:1721–30.

Therapy-Related Myelodysplastic Syndromes and Acute Myeloid Leukemia

73. Blayney DW, Longo DL, Young RC, et al. Decreasing risk of leukemia with prolonged follow-up after chemotherapy and radiotherapy for Hodgkin's disease. N Eng J Med 1987;316:710–4.

74. Brunning RD, Parkin JL, Hanson CA. Hematopoietic and lymphoreticular neoplasms. In: Azar HA, ed. Pathology of human neoplasms. An atlas of diagnostic electron microscopy and immunohistochemistry. New York: Raven Press, 1988:221–303.

75. Foucar K, McKenna RW, Bloomfield CD, Bowers TK, Brunning RD. Therapy-related leukemia: a panmyelosis. Cancer 1979;43:1285–96.

76. Greene MH, Young RC, Merrill JM, DeVita VT. Evidence of a treatment dose response in acute nonlymphocytic leukemias which occur after therapy of non-Hodgkin's lymphoma. Cancer Res 1983;43:1891–8.

77. Kantarjian HM, Keating MJ. Therapy-related leukemia and myelodysplastic syndrome. Semin Oncol 1987;14:435–43.

78. _____, Keating MJ, Walters RS, et al. Therapy-related leukemia and myelodysplastic syndrome: clinical, cytogenetic, and prognostic features. J Clin Oncol 1986;4:1748–57.

79. Le Beau MM, Albain KS, Larson RA, et al. Clinical and cytogenetic correlations in 63 patients with therapy-related myelodysplastic syndromes and acute nonlymphocytic leukemia: further evidence for characteristic abnormalities of chromosomes no. 5 and 7. J Clin Oncol 1986;4:325–45.

80. McKenna RW, Parkin JL, Foucar K, Brunning RD. Ultrastructural characteristics of therapy-related acute nonlymphocytic leukemia: evidence for a panmyelosis. Cancer 1981;48:725–37.

81. Michels SD, McKenna RW, Arthur DC, Brunning RD. Therapy-related acute myeloid leukemia and myelodysplastic syndrome: a clinical and morphologic study of 65 cases. Blood 1985;65:1364–72.

82. _____, Saumur J, Arthur DC, Robison LL, Brunning RD. Refractory anemia with excess of blasts in transformation: hematologic and clinical study of 52 patients. Cancer 1989;64:2340–6.

83. Ratain MJ, Kaminer LS, Bitran JD, et al. Acute nonlymphocytic leukemia following etoposide and cisplatin combination chemotherapy for advanced non-small-cell carcinoma of the lung. Blood 1987;70:1412–7.

84. Sultan C, Sigaux F, Imbert M, Reyes F. Acute myelodysplasia with myelofibrosis: a report of eight cases. Br J Haematol 1981;49:11–6.

85. Tucker MA, Coleman CN, Cox RS, Varghese A, Rosenberg SA. Risk of second cancers after treatment for Hodgkin's disease. N Eng J Med 1988;318:76–81.

86. Whitlock JA, Greer JP, Lukens JN. Epipodophyllotoxin-related leukemia. Identification of a new subset of secondary leukemia. Cancer 1991;68:600–4.

87. Winick NJ, McKenna RW, Shuster JJ, et al. Secondary acute myeloid leukemia in children with acute lymphoblastic leukemia treated with etoposide. J Clin Oncol 1993;11:209–17.

❖❖❖

CHRONIC MYELOPROLIFERATIVE DISEASES

The chronic myeloproliferative diseases are a group of closely related disorders characterized by proliferation of one or more myeloid cell lines. There are four generally recognized entities within this group: chronic myeloid leukemia (CML), polycythemia vera (PV), essential thrombocythemia (ET), and idiopathic myelofibrosis (IM). Idiopathic myelofibrosis is also referred to as agnogenic myeloid metaplasia; this term, however, does not adequately reflect the major pathologic finding in the bone marrow in this disease, which is fibrosis.

Although chronic myelomonocytic leukemia is generally viewed as a myelodysplastic syndrome, there is a somewhat poorly defined proliferative process involving both the granulocytes and monocytes that has features more consistent with a myeloproliferative disease than a myelodysplastic syndrome (49). This entity, described in this chapter as chronic myelomonocytic leukemia, myeloproliferative, has some of the clinical and hematologic features of the reported cases of Philadelphia chromosome–negative chronic myeloid leukemia.

Juvenile chronic myeloid leukemia (JCML), which has morphologic and clinical features similar to the myelodysplastic syndromes or acute myelomonocytic leukemia, was initially proposed as a type of granulocytic leukemia of childhood and for that reason is included in this chapter (17).

The hypereosinophilic syndrome has clinical and morphologic findings that overlap both the acute and chronic myeloproliferative disorders. It could be appropriately classified with either group but because of the more mature cell type involved at initial diagnosis the entity is arbitrarily included in this section.

Classification of the myeloproliferative disorders has been greatly advanced with the advent of cytogenetics and molecular techniques. However, despite the availability of these new technologies, there are some myeloproliferative disorders that cannot be precisely classified. Rather than using a "best fit" classification for these cases, it is appropriate to use the more general term myeloproliferative syndrome, unclassified. In these instances, it is prudent not to predict biologic course and to carefully monitor the hematologic evolution of the process.

CHRONIC MYELOID LEUKEMIA

Definition. A chronic myeloproliferative disorder characterized hematologically by marked leukocytosis, basophilia, and eosinophilia; the leukocytosis is due primarily to an increase in mature and immature neutrophils. Chronic myeloid leukemia (CML) is a clonal disorder associated in virtually all cases with a t(9;22) chromosome translocation, usually manifest as the Philadelphia (Ph) chromosome, and/or molecular evidence of the translocation of the *abl* oncogene from chromosome 9 to the breakpoint cluster region of chromosome 22 (10,24,38).

Incidence and Clinical Findings. CML is primarily a disease of adults, but may occur at any age, including infancy. The median age is 53 years; 36 percent of the patients are older than 60 years (34). There is a slight male predominance (35). The disease is uncommon in children and accounts for less than 5 percent of all cases of childhood leukemia. The most commonly occurring symptoms relate to anemia, splenomegaly, and an increased metabolic rate: fatigue, dyspnea on exertion, sweating, and fever are frequently present (52). Signs of leukostasis are reported in 12 percent of adult patients and 60 percent of individuals less than 20 years of age (44). Spleen size varies: the spleen was palpable more than 10 cm below the left costal margin in greater than 70 percent of patients in one study (34). Hepatomegaly, lymphadenopathy, and signs of spontaneous bleeding may be present. Hyperhistaminemia may occur with unusually high basophil counts (43).

Laboratory Findings. The leukocyte count shows a wide range but is usually in excess of 50×10^9/L. Seventy to 90 percent of patients present with leukocyte counts in excess of 100×10^9/L; the count exceeds 350×10^9/L in approximately 25 percent of cases (34). Marked leukocytosis has been reported to be more frequent in children. In one study, 60 percent of patients less than 20 years of age had a mean leukocyte count of 360×10^9/L in contrast to a mean leukocyte count of 137×10^9/L in individuals over the age of 20 (44). The majority of patients present with anemia: the hemoglobin level in one series ranged from 5.3 to 13.0 g/dL (34). The

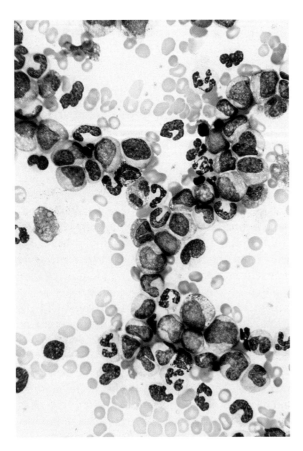

Figure 223
CHRONIC MYELOID LEUKEMIA: CHRONIC PHASE
Blood smear from a 44-year-old woman with newly diagnosed CML and presenting leukocyte count of 425×10^9/L. Neutrophils at all stages of maturation are present with a predominance of segmented forms and myelocytes. (Wright-Giemsa stain)

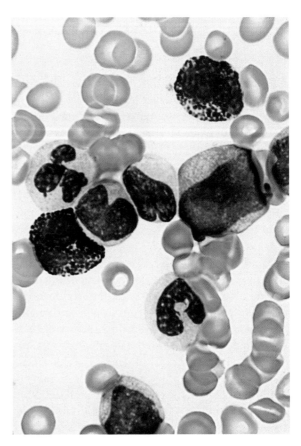

Figure 224
CHRONIC MYELOID LEUKEMIA: CHRONIC PHASE
Blood smear from a patient with untreated CML showing segmented neutrophils, myelocytes, a promyelocyte, and two basophils. (Wright-Giemsa stain)

platelet count ranged from 24 to 1400×10^9/L, with a mean of 484.8×10^9/L; 11 percent of the patients had a platelet count of less than 100×10^9/L.

The neutrophil alkaline phosphatase level is decreased in 90 to 95 percent of untreated patients and is one of the earliest manifestations of the disease (20). The level generally returns to normal following successful treatment. Serum vitamin B_{12} and vitamin B_{12}-binding capacity are increased; the increase in the total and unsaturated B_{12}-binding proteins is due to an increase in transcobalamins I and II (59).

Basophilia, thrombocytosis, and decreased neutrophil alkaline phosphatase levels have been shown to be very early manifestations of CML and may precede the clinical manifestations by several years (20).

Blood and Bone Marrow Findings. The most important hematologic findings are in the peripheral blood, which shows a neutrophilic leukocytosis and basophilia. The basophilia is of critical importance and the diagnosis should not be established in the absence of this finding unless the Ph chromosome or molecular evidence of the BCR/*abl* hybrid gene is present. The neutrophil series is represented by all stages of maturation, from the myeloblast to the segmented neutrophil; myelocytes and segmented stages are the most numerous (figs. 223, 224). Myeloblasts generally do not exceed 2 to 3 percent. As the leukocyte count increases, there is a decrease in the percentage of segmented neutrophils and a corresponding increase in promyelocytes and myelocytes. The neutrophils in the chronic phase of the disease do not usually show

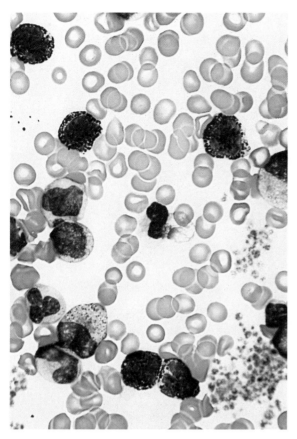

Figure 225
CHRONIC MYELOID LEUKEMIA:
CHRONIC PHASE

Blood smear from a 52-year-old male with newly diagnosed CML. The leukocyte count at presentation was 147×10^9/L; the platelet count was 740×10^9/L. Three basophils and all stages of neutrophil maturation, including two early promyelocytes, are shown. The increased platelets are normal in appearance. (Wright-Giemsa stain)

dysplastic changes. Eosinophilia is usually present but lacks the diagnostic specificity of basophilia. In occasional patients, marked eosinophilia or basophilia may be noted, with numerous immature basophils and eosinophils (fig. 225) (23,43). The majority of patients with CML also manifest an absolute monocytosis. A marked monocytosis occurring in the early phase of CML may suggest chronic myelomonocytic leukemia.

The platelets vary in appearance and atypical platelets characterized by large size and diminished or absent granules may be present. Megakaryocyte nuclei are present in the blood smears in approximately 25 percent of cases. A small

number of nucleated red blood cells and minimal red blood cell anisocytosis and poikilocytosis are present in the majority of patients. Spherocytes may be noted.

Although the vast majority of patients with CML are diagnosed with a marked leukocytosis with some degree of basophilia and neutrophil immaturity, the detection of the Ph chromosome and the BCR/*abl* hybrid gene has made it possible to diagnose CML when there is only minimal expression of hematologic abnormalities, such as thrombocytosis or a slight increase in basophils, in patients with a normal or only slightly increased leukocyte count (fig. 226) (20).

The bone marrow shows a marked increase in neutrophils and precursors. The maturational sequence is essentially normal but the percentage of immature cells, promyelocytes and myelocytes, is usually greater than in the peripheral blood. The megakaryocytes are usually increased. Erythroid precursors are usually reduced. Macrophages containing blue-pigment debris and pseudo–Gaucher cells are found in the marrow in approximately one third of cases (fig. 227). These probably represent two different stages of macrophages that have phagocytosed neutrophils. Similar to Gaucher cells, pseudo–Gaucher cells stain with periodic acid–Schiff (PAS) and Sudan black B (SBB) (22). On ultrastructural examination, the cytoplasmic inclusions in the pseudo–Gaucher cells consist of amorphous material and crystalloid structures.

Histopathologic Findings. The bone marrow is markedly hypercellular with an increase in granulocytes and, frequently, megakaryocytes (fig. 228) (12,28). The neutrophils show normal maturation with an increase in myelocytes. Promyelocytes and myelocytes are usually prominent along the endosteal surface of the bone trabeculae and in perivascular locations (fig. 229). The megakaryocytes may be uniformly distributed or occur in clusters. With progression of disease, megakaryocyte proliferation may be very prominent and numerous micromegakaryocytes may be present. Myelofibrosis is generally associated with advanced disease but may be present in the early stages (fig. 230). Increased reticulin fibers have been reported in bone marrow biopsies specifically stained for reticulin in up to 80 percent of patients evaluated within 3 months of diagnosis (6). The increase in reticulin fibers

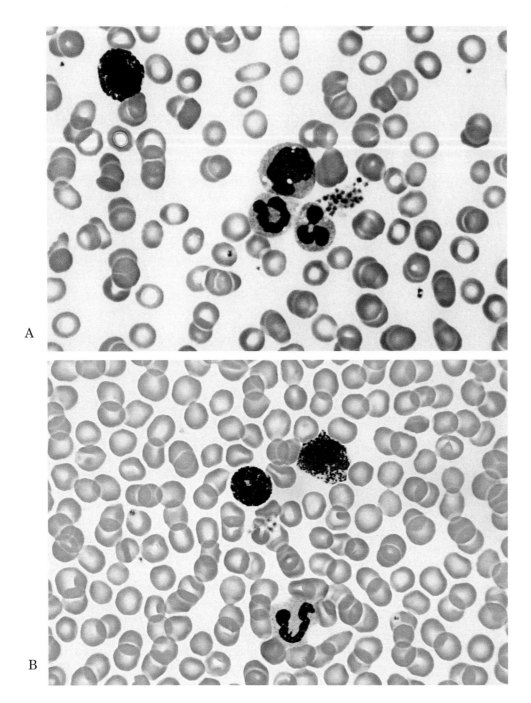

Figure 226

CHRONIC MYELOID LEUKEMIA: EARLY CHRONIC PHASE

A. Blood smear from an 81-year-old woman admitted to hospital for cardiac abnormalities and abdominal pain. Routine hematology studies showed a platelet count of 617×10^9/L and a leukocyte count of 10.6×10^9/L. There was no increase in basophils; immature neutrophils were rare. (Wright-Giemsa stain)

B. Blood smear from the same patient 2 years later. Hematology values at this time showed a platelet count of 736×10^9/L and a leukocyte count of 17.9×10^9/L with 8 percent basophils. There was no splenomegaly; cytogenetic and molecular studies showed a Ph chromosome and a BCR/*abl* hybrid gene. (Wright-Giemsa stain)

C. Bone marrow biopsy obtained at the same time as the smear in B. The marrow is hypercellular for age with a panmyeloid hyperplasia. A moderate amount of adipose tissue is present. (Hematoxylin and eosin stain)

D. High magnification of C showing a group of megakaryocytes. (Hematoxylin and eosin stain)

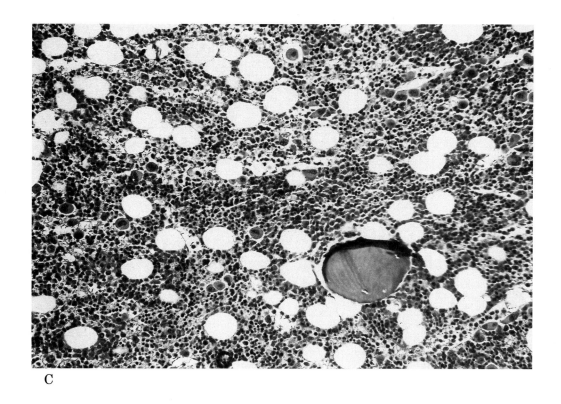

C

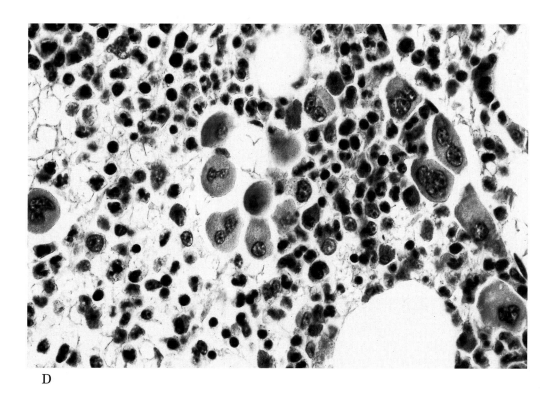

D

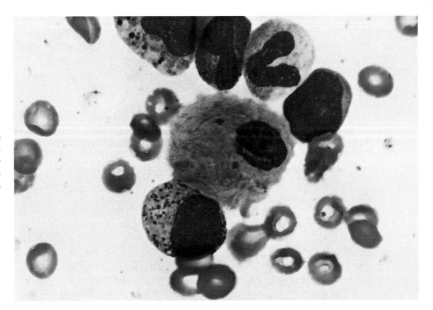

Figure 227
CHRONIC MYELOID
LEUKEMIA:
PSEUDO–GAUCHER CELL
Pseudo–Gaucher cell in a bone marrow smear from a patient with CML. The cytoplasm contains structures resembling the structures in Gaucher cells. (Wright-Giemsa stain)

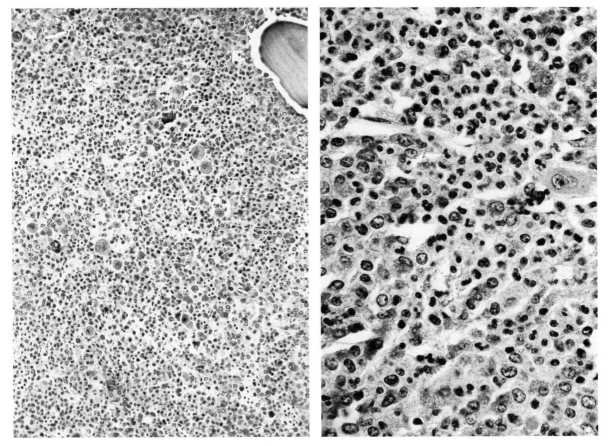

Figure 228
CHRONIC MYELOID LEUKEMIA: CHRONIC PHASE
Left: Bone marrow biopsy from a patient with newly diagnosed CML. The marrow is markedly hypercellular due principally to an increase in granulocytes. Megakaryocytes are also increased. (Hematoxylin and eosin stain)
Right: An area of the specimen on the left showing all stages of granulocyte maturation. In this field there is a predominance of segmented neutrophils. (Hematoxylin and eosin stain)

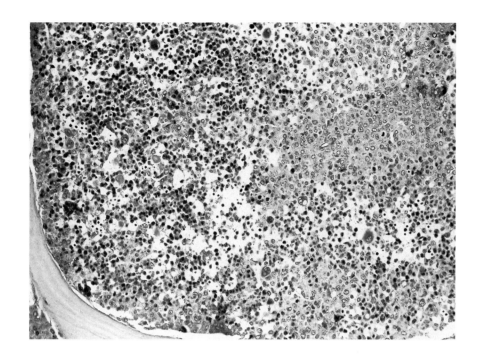

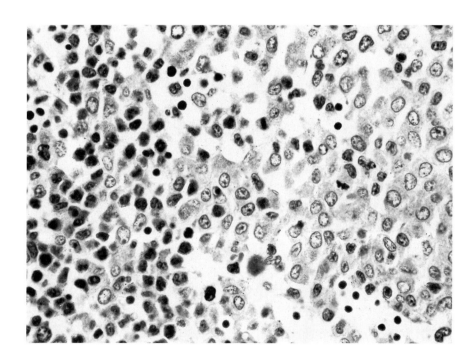

Figure 229
CHRONIC MYELOID LEUKEMIA: CHRONIC PHASE

Top: PAS-stained bone marrow biopsy from a patient with CML, with perivascular and paratrabecular accentuation of promyelocytes and myelocytes. The more lightly-reacting promyelocytes and myelocytes in the perivascular and paratrabecular locations contrast with the more intensely-reacting segmented neutrophils. This pattern of proliferation may be markedly accentuated in CML but should not be interpreted as focal blast transformation. (Periodic acid–Schiff stain)

Bottom: High magnification of the specimen on top showing a focus of promyelocytes and myelocytes adjacent to a vascular structure. (Periodic acid–Schiff stain)

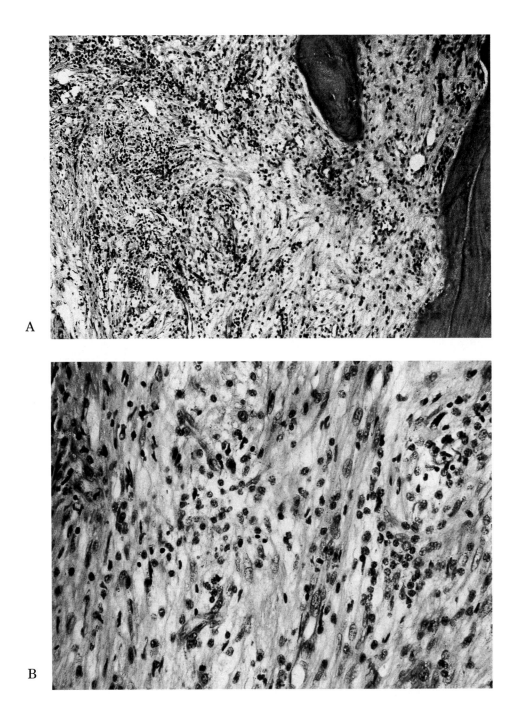

Figure 230
CHRONIC MYELOID LEUKEMIA: BLAST CRISIS AND MYELOFIBROSIS

A. Portion of a bone marrow biopsy from a patient with CML in blast crisis. The marrow shows an increase in stromal and vascular structures. (Hematoxylin and eosin stain)

B. Higher magnification of the specimen in A showing a marked increase in fibroblasts. Hematopoietic cells are scattered throughout the fibrous tissue. (Hematoxylin and eosin stain)

C. An area of the biopsy seen in A and B showing numerous blasts with dispersed chromatin and nucleoli. (Hematoxylin and eosin stain)

D. Reticulin stain of bone marrow biopsy seen in A–C showing a marked increase in coarse reticulin fibers. (Wilder reticulin stain)

E. Bone marrow smear from the same specimen showing four blasts and two basophils. The blasts reacted for MPO. (Wright-Giemsa stain)

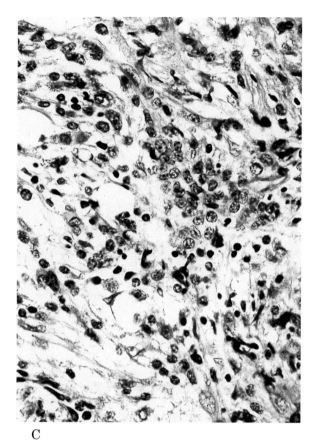

C

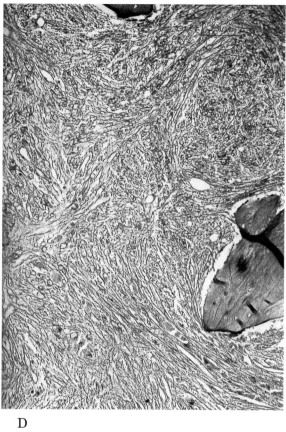

D

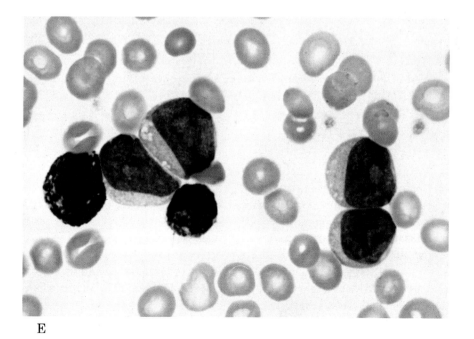

E

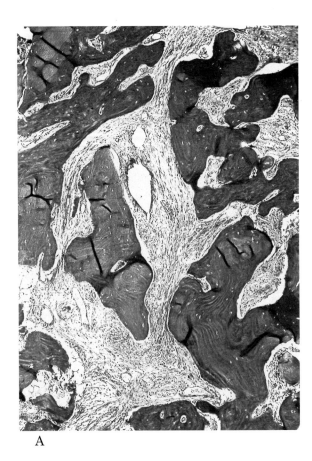 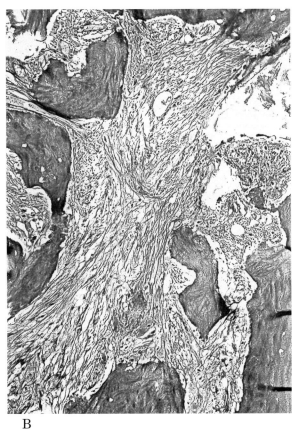

A   B

Figure 231

CHRONIC MYELOID LEUKEMIA WITH OSTEOMYELOSCLEROSIS: BONE MARROW TRANSPLANTATION

A. Bone marrow biopsy from a 26-year-old woman with a 42-month history of CML. The biopsy shows marked osteomyelosclerosis. The bone trabeculae are markedly widened and the medullary space is densely fibrotic. (Hematoxylin and eosin stain)

B. Reticulin stain of the biopsy in A showing a marked increase in coarse reticulin fibers. (Wilder reticulin stain)

C. Bone marrow biopsy from the patient in A 28 days following allogeneic bone marrow transplant. The bone trabeculae are still widened. The fibrotic process has regressed and there is a return of fat cells. (Hematoxylin and eosin stain)

D. Biopsy from the patient in A 5 months following bone marrow transplantation showing a markedly hypocellular marrow with near complete resolution of the fibrotic process. Cytogenetic studies from the specimen showed no chromosome abnormalities. (Hematoxylin and eosin stain)

E. High magnification of the specimen in D showing numerous red blood cell precursors and megakaryocytes. The granulocyte precursors are markedly reduced. The patient died from a graft versus host reaction 230 days following transplant. (Hematoxylin and eosin stain)

may be focal or diffuse. A focal increase is usually more prominent in perivascular locations. With disease progression there is usually evolution of the fibrosis from a focal to a diffuse pattern. The amount of reticulin fibrosis in early stage CML has been associated with degree of splenomegaly, hemoglobin level, marrow and blood blast percentages, and additional karyotypic abnormalities (8). Frank collagen fibrosis is much less frequent than reticulin fibrosis and osteomyelosclerosis is distinctly uncommon (fig. 231). Regression of fibrosis following bone marrow transplantation has been observed (fig. 231) (33).

The onset of fibrosis or the progression from a focal to a diffuse pattern has been viewed as an ominous prognostic factor in some studies. In one group of patients, the mean survival period after the development of myelofibrosis was 4.9 months (14). Although marked fibrosis is generally associated with a shorter survival time, some patients with early stage CML and marked fibrosis have a prolonged course (6).

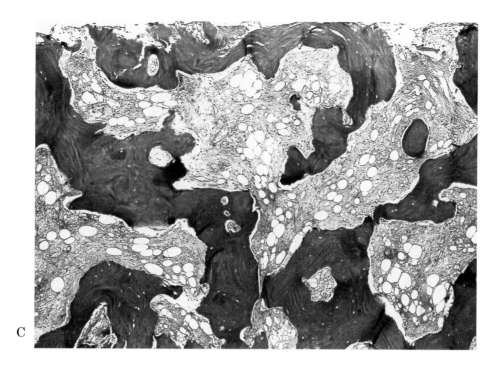

C

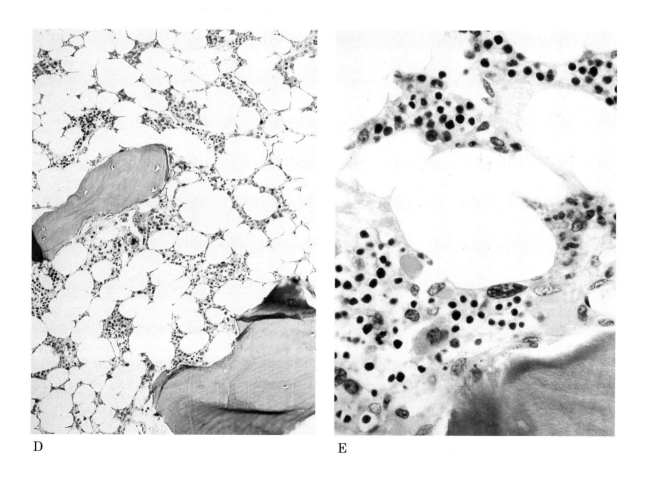

D

E

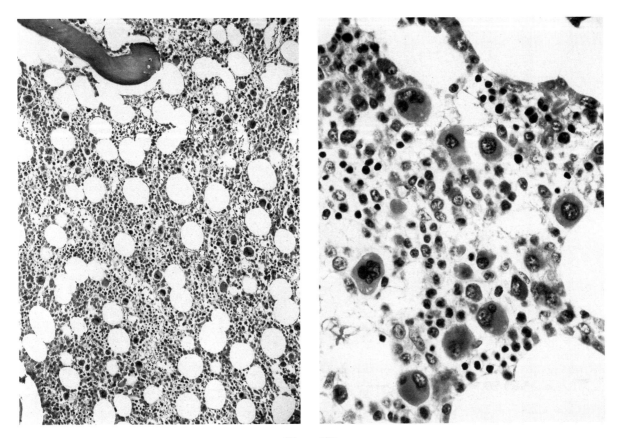

Figure 232
CHRONIC MYELOID LEUKEMIA ON HYDROXYUREA THERAPY
Left: Bone marrow biopsy from a 47-year-old patient with CML following 3 months of hydroxyurea therapy. The marrow is slightly hypercellular with numerous megakaryocytes.
Right: High magnification of the specimen seen on the left. Several of the megakaryocytes are small with hypolobulated nuclei. (Both sides, hematoxylin and eosin stain)

Patients with Ph-positive CML presenting with frank collagen fibrosis in the bone marrow, granulocytic hyperplasia, and a blood picture resembling idiopathic myelofibrosis have been reported (6). The neutrophil alkaline phosphatase level in these patients may be elevated. The survival in this group is variable and it has been suggested that this constellation of findings represents a disease intermediate between CML and idiopathic myelofibrosis.

The histopathology of the bone marrow may change only minimally following therapy or there may be total regression of diagnostic features. Following treatment with hydroxyurea, the marrow ranges from slightly hypocellular to markedly hypercellular (fig. 232). A reduction in the leukocyte and platelet counts is not always paralleled by a substantial reduction in marrow cellularity. Following interferon therapy, the marrow ranges from hypocellular to hypercellular; in some cases there may be no residual morphologic evidence of disease (fig. 233).

Ultrastructural Findings. On ultrastructural examination, the majority of segmented neutrophils from patients with chronic phase CML appear morphologically normal. A small number of neutrophils may have a very low granule count. The neutrophil precursors manifest more abnormalities than segmented neutrophils including bundles of microfilaments in myeloblasts and promyelocytes, deep nuclear folds, and clustering of microfilaments and mitochondria in the hof (55). Other studies have shown mixed granule populations in the granulocytes (47).

Immunologic Findings. Membrane surface markers do not have a significant role in the diagnosis of chronic phase CML. In the blast crisis

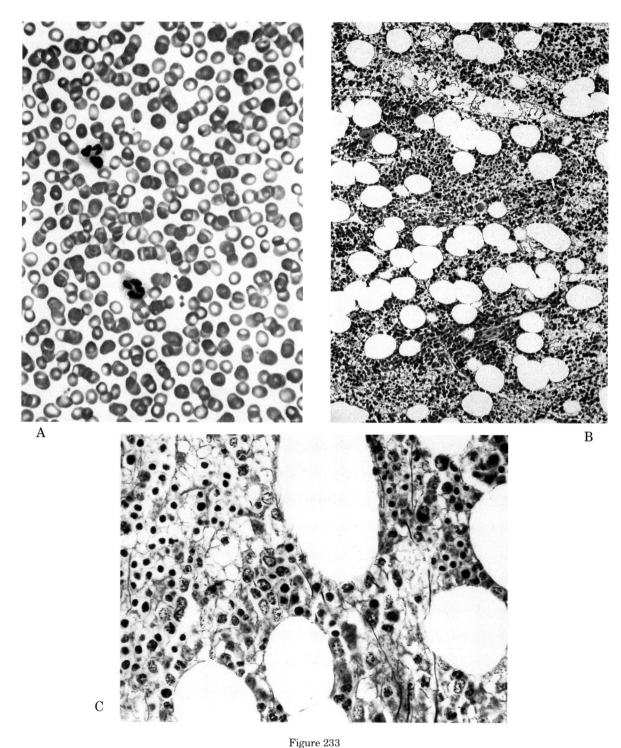

Figure 233
CHRONIC MYELOID LEUKEMIA FOLLOWING INTERFERON THERAPY

A. Blood smear from a 54-year-old man with CML treated with alpha-interferon. The leukocyte count is slightly decreased and there is no morphologic evidence of residual leukemia. (Wright-Giemsa stain)

B. Bone marrow biopsy obtained on the same day as the blood smear in A. The marrow is slightly hypercellular with a normal number of megakaryocytes and slight hyperplasia of the erythroid precursors. (Hematoxylin and eosin stain)

C. High magnification of the specimen in B. The number of neutrophils and precursors is reduced and there is a slight erythroid hyperplasia. The interstitium shows some evidence of cellular depletion with loosely arranged cells. (Hematoxylin and eosin stain)

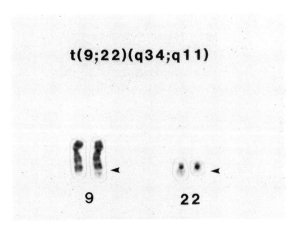

Figure 234
CHRONIC MYELOID LEUKEMIA:
PHILADELPHIA CHROMOSOME
Partial karyotype of a myeloid cell from the bone marrow of a patient with CML showing the typical t(9;22) translocation. (G-banded, Wright-Giemsa stained)

stage, these studies have the same role as in the acute leukemias in distinguishing myeloblastic, megakaryoblastic, and lymphoblastic types.

Spleen. The spleen is infiltrated by granulocytes at all stages of maturation. This occurs primarily in the pulp cords. The cellular infiltrate impinges on the malpighian corpuscles, which gradually diminish in prominence with progression of the disease. Foci of myelopoiesis are present in the sinusoids. These findings have been interpreted as compensatory extramedullary hematopoiesis and are not specific for CML (41).

Cytogenetic Findings. The Ph chromosome, which results from a reciprocal translocation between chromosomes 9 and 22, the t(9;22) (q34;q11), is observed in the myeloid cells in approximately 90 to 95 percent of patients with the typical clinical and hematologic findings of CML. It is found in all of the cells of myeloid lineage including neutrophils, erythroblasts, megakaryocytes, monocytes, eosinophils, and basophils (fig. 234) (5,24,38,45,46,53,54). It is not present in fibroblasts from bone marrow tissue or somatic cells (16,29). In an affected individual, the abnormality is usually present in more than 90 percent of cells; it is also present in myeloid cells in the spleen (26,45,46,53,54).

The Ph chromosome appears to be the first manifestation of CML and may be observed in bone marrow cells when the leukocyte count is less than 10×10^9/L (20). From prospective studies of patients at high risk for developing leukemia, it has been estimated that there is a median period of 6.3 years from the time of occurrence of the first cell with a Ph chromosome in the bone marrow to the accumulation of a leukemic cell mass in the blood of 100×10^9/L.

The molecular changes associated with the t(9;22) abnormality involve the translocation of the *abl* oncogene on chromosome 9 to the major breakpoint cluster region on chromosome 22 (7). This juxtaposition results in the production of an abnormal amount of tyrosine kinase (24). The leukemic cells in approximately 5 percent of cases of CML do not manifest the t(9;22) chromosome abnormality on routine cytogenetic studies but are positive for the BCR/*abl* hybrid gene when studied by molecular techniques. Cases with the characteristic blood and bone marrow findings of CML that are negative for the t(9;22) on routine cytogenetic study should not be viewed as negative for the BCR/*abl* hybrid gene in the absence of molecular studies.

Approximately 5 to 10 percent of cases of CML have variant translocations. Molecular studies in these instances usually confirm the translocation of the *abl* oncogene from chromosome 9 to the major or minor breakpoint cluster regions on chromosome 22 (45).

Blast Transformation. The usual biologic course in most cases of CML is a chronic phase of 3 to 4 years followed by a more aggressive phase of relatively short duration. The aggressive phase occurs in two forms: a blast crisis and an accelerated phase (3,4,21,35,36,42). In some patients, the use of one or the other of these terms is arbitrary.

Blastic transformation of CML is generally defined as 30 percent or more blasts in the blood or bone marrow smears or a focus of blasts in a marrow biopsy or extramedullary site. The transformation may be abrupt in onset, with a rapidly increasing blast percentage in the blood and bone marrow with accompanying bone marrow failure, resulting in worsening anemia and thrombocytopenia similar to de novo acute leukemia. The blasts may show myeloid or lymphoid differentiation morphologically and immunophenotypically (2,36). Approximately 70 percent of cases are myeloid (fig. 235). The morphologic characteristics may resemble acute myeloid leukemia (AML)-M1

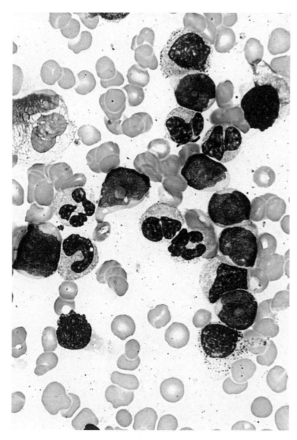

Figure 235
CHRONIC MYELOID LEUKEMIA:
MYELOBLASTIC TRANSFORMATION

Bone marrow smear from a patient with CML in myelo-blastic transformation. Approximately 50 percent of the leukocytes are blasts. (Wright-Giemsa stain)

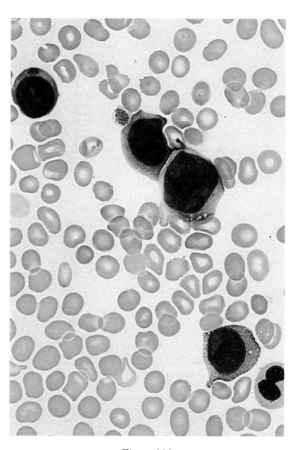

Figure 236
CHRONIC MYELOID LEUKEMIA:
BLAST TRANSFORMATION

Bone marrow smear from a patient with CML showing a poorly differentiated blast and three immature cells interpreted as red blood cell precursors. (Wright-Giemsa stain)

or M2, erythroleukemia, acute monocytic leukemia, acute megakaryoblastic leukemia, myelomonocytic leukemia, or an acute panmyelosis with involvement of more than one myeloid cell line (figs. 236, 237) (1,9,36,42). There frequently is evidence of abnormal neutrophil maturation characterized by nuclear hyposegmentation and diminished specific granules. Megakaryoblastic crisis may be recognized by evidence of maturation of the blasts to micro-megakaryocytes; in some cases there are numerous micromegakaryocytes in the blood accompanied by a marked thrombocytosis (fig. 238). The megakaryoblasts may be undifferentiated or lymphoid in appearance, with minimal or no evidence of maturation to recognizable megakaryocytes (fig. 239). The nature of the blasts in these cases is determined by the demonstration

of platelet peroxidase on ultrastructural examination or reactivity with antiplatelet glycoprotein antibodies utilizing immunocytochemistry or flow cytometry (1,30).

SBB and myeloperoxidase (MPO) reactions may not be as intense in the myeloblasts in myeloid blast crisis as in de novo AML-M1 or M2 and a negative reaction does not exclude the possibility of myeloid differentiation. Rarely, Auer rods may be observed (fig. 240). Ultrastructural and immunologic studies have demonstrated considerable diversity in the blast population in blast transformation and a high percentage of cases involve all the myeloid cell lines with a predominance of one type.

In approximately 25 to 35 percent of cases of blast transformation of CML, the blasts have the morphologic and immunophenotypic features of

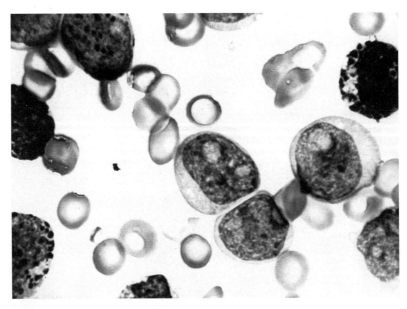

Figure 237
CHRONIC MYELOID LEUKEMIA:
MYELOBLAST TRANSFORMATION
Bone marrow smear from a patient with CML, myeloid blast crisis, showing several myeloblasts and basophils. An immature basophil is at the upper left. (Wright-Giemsa stain)

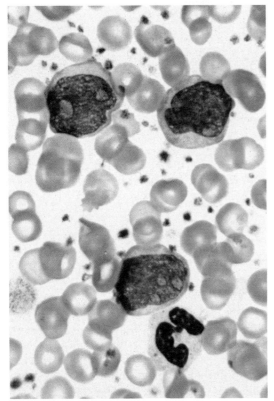

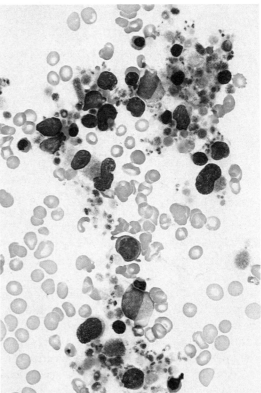

Figure 238
CHRONIC MYELOID LEUKEMIA: MEGAKARYOBLASTIC TRANSFORMATION

Left: Blood smear from a 14-year-old boy with a 27-month history of CML treated with hydroxyurea. He was admitted for bone marrow transplant. The leukocyte count was 47×10^9/L, the platelet count 420×10^9/L, and the hemoglobin level was 11.2 g/dL. This smear contained approximately 60 percent blasts with no differentiating features. Electron microscopic studies showed platelet peroxidase in numerous blasts. (Wright-Giemsa stain)

Right: Blood smear from the same patient obtained 3 weeks following treatment with daunorubicin, cytosine arabinoside, and 6-thioguanine. The leukocyte count was markedly increased with numerous blasts and a high percentage of micromegakaryocytes. (Wright-Giemsa stain)

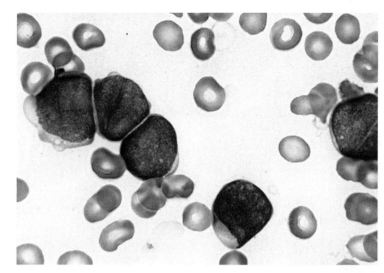

Figure 239
CHRONIC MYELOID
LEUKEMIA: MEGAKARYOBLASTIC
TRANSFORMATION
Poorly differentiated blasts in the blood smear from a patient with a 37-month history of CML. The blasts were TdT, MPO, SBB, and NSE negative. Electron microscopic studies showed evidence of megakaryocyte differentiation. (Wright-Giemsa stain)

Figure 240
CHRONIC MYELOID
LEUKEMIA: MYELOBLASTIC
TRANSFORMATION
Bone marrow smear from a case of CML, blast crisis, showing several myeloblasts, one with a prominent Auer rod. A neutrophil with a bilobed, pseudo–Pelger-Huet nucleus is immediately adjacent to the blast with the Auer rod. (Wright-Giemsa stain)

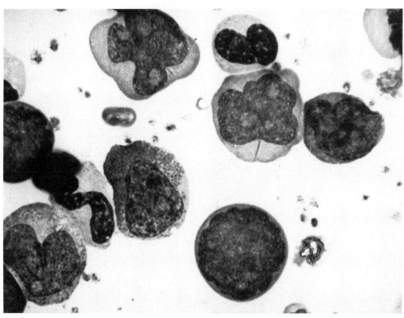

lymphoblasts (fig. 241) (2,15,19,27,32,48). The nuclei have coarse chromatin and may show clefting and folds; nucleoli are inconspicuous. The morphologic features of the blasts in lymphoid blast crisis vary substantially in different cases. In most cases, the blasts resemble the L1 or L2 lymphoblasts of acute lymphoblastic leukemia (ALL) (fig. 241); rarely, they resemble L3 lymphoblasts (fig. 242). In some instances, the blasts have a pseudoerythroblastic appearance but are terminal deoxynucleotidyltransferase (TdT) positive and express lymphoid antigens. In some cases, the blasts have lymphoid characteris-tics; are MPO, chloroacetate esterase (CAE), and SBB negative; express B-cell precursor surface antigens; and contain varying numbers of coarse azurophilic granules. On ultrastructural examination these granules may have the characteristics of basophil, mast cell, or theta granules (fig. 243) (39). In bone marrow sections, lymphoblastic crisis of CML is indistinguishable from de novo ALL (fig. 244).

Similar to the blasts in the majority of cases of de novo ALL, the blasts in lymphoid blast crisis are TdT positive and have the immunophenotypic characteristics of B-cell precursor lymphoblasts.

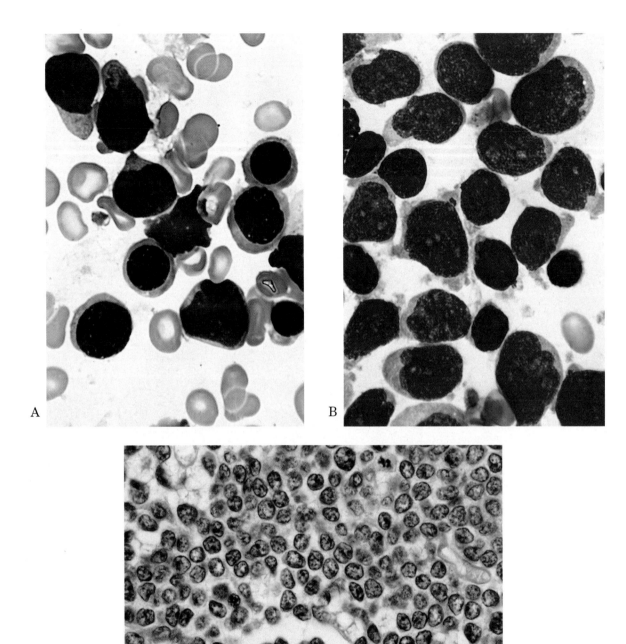

Figure 241
CHRONIC MYELOID LEUKEMIA: LYMPHOBLASTIC TRANSFORMATION
WITH INVOLVEMENT OF LYMPH NODES

A. Bone marrow aspirate from a 34-year-old man with a 23-month history of CML treated with busulfan and hydroxyurea. There was a recent onset of lymphadenopathy. Approximately 40 percent of the cells are blasts as shown. The blasts were MPO negative and TdT positive. (Wright-Giemsa stain)

B. Imprint of a cervical lymph node biopsy from the same patient. There is a uniform population of blasts that was TdT positive. Some of the blasts have coarse azurophilic granules and some of the nuclei are slightly indented. (Wright-Giemsa stain)

C. Section of the lymph node biopsy illustrated in B. There is a uniform population of lymphoblasts, some of which have clefted nuclei. (Hematoxylin and eosin stain)

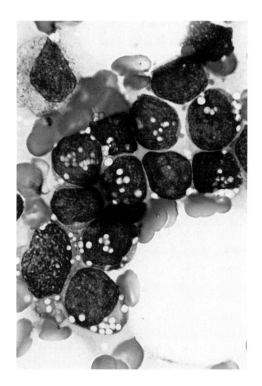

Figure 242
CHRONIC MYELOID LEUKEMIA:
LYMPHOBLASTIC TRANSFORMATION

Bone marrow smear from a patient with lymphoblastic transformation of CML. The lymphoblasts contain numerous, sharply defined vacuoles and resemble the lymphoblasts of ALL-L3. The vacuoles were variably positive with oil red O and were PAS negative. Unlike ALL-L3 lymphoblasts, these cells were TdT positive and lacked surface immunoglobulin. They were CD19+ and CD10+, similar to the lymphoblasts in B-cell precursor ALL. (Wright-Giemsa stain)

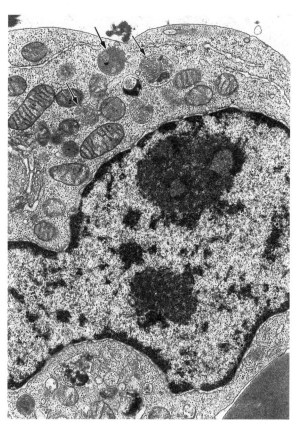

Figure 243
LYMPHOID BLAST CRISIS OF CHRONIC
MYELOID LEUKEMIA: ULTRASTRUCTURE

Electron microscopy of a lymphoblast from a case of CML in blast crisis. The blasts were TdT positive and of B-cell precursor immunophenotype. Several large basophil granules and a theta granule are present. (Uranyl acetate–lead citrate stains, X20,000)

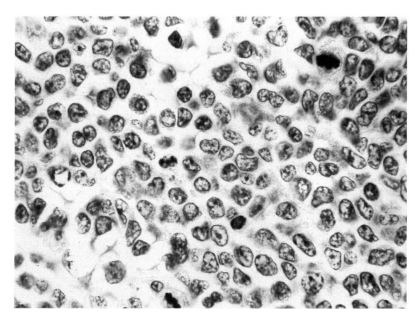

Figure 244
CHRONIC MYELOID
LEUKEMIA: LYMPHOBLASTIC
TRANSFORMATION

Bone marrow biopsy from a patient with CML in lymphoblast crisis showing complete replacement by blast cells, which were of B-cell precursor immunophenotype and TdT positive. Occasional mitotic figures are identified. (Hematoxylin and eosin stain)

213

The majority are common ALL-associated antigen CD10 (CALLA) positive (2). The blasts in some cases have a pre–B-cell phenotype, as demonstrated by the presence of intracytoplasmic µ heavy chains (27,56). Immunoglobulin gene rearrangement studies have confirmed the B-cell lineage of the lymphoblasts (2). Cases of lymphoid blast crisis of CML in which the lymphoblasts were immunophenotyped as T cells have been reported (18). Although the blasts in TdT-positive cases are usually lymphoid in appearance, a number of TdT-positive cases with myeloblastic morphology have been noted (31).

In occasional cases, blastic transformation in CML is characterized by the presence of varying sized foci of blasts in bone marrow sections in which the predominant pattern is chronic phase CML. The foci may consist of myeloblasts, erythroblasts, megakaryoblasts, monoblasts, lymphoblasts, or blasts without differentiating features (figs. 245, 246). These focal areas of blast transformation in the bone marrow must be distinguished from areas of promyelocyte and myelocyte proliferation that occur normally in paratrabecular and perivascular locations and that may be accentuated in the accelerated phase of CML (see fig. 229). In some cases the marrow sections show evidence of both blast transformation and fibrosis (see fig. 230).

Although blastic transformation in the majority of patients is characterized by an increase of blasts in the bone marrow and blood, a number of patients may present with extramedullary manifestations. Sites most commonly involved are the lymph nodes and spleen, but tumors of blasts may occur in virtually any location (11,25, 37,40,58). The extramedullary tumor may resemble a malignant lymphoma (fig. 247). The nature of the myeloid lesions can be clarified with the CAE stain which reacts with cells of the neutrophil series or by reactivity with antibodies to MPO, lysozyme, or other constituents of myeloid cells.

If the extramedullary lesion is composed of undifferentiated cells or lymphoid blasts, the relationship of the lesion to a previously established diagnosis of CML can be determined by cytogenetic or genotypic analysis of the tumor cells and the demonstration of TdT in imprints of the lesion. In some patients, the extramedullary transformation may precede changes in the bone marrow by several months. The blasts in the extramedullary sites may manifest additional chromosome alterations characteristic of the acute phase, similar to blast crisis occurring in the bone marrow.

An increase in basophils, both mature and immature, may accompany the blastic proliferation and it is possible that in some instances the blasts represent basophil precursors. As noted, ultrastructural examination of the blasts may aid in recognizing the basophils. Cells with both basophil and mast cell granules may be present (39).

Infrequently, blast transformation may manifest with cytogenetic and morphologic findings usually noted in de novo AML such as an inv(16)-associated AML-M4 with increased marrow eosinophils. Cytogenetic studies may show cells with both a Ph chromosome and the inv(16) abnormality (fig. 248).

Patients occasionally present in blast transformation without a previously diagnosed chronic phase. This occurs with both the myeloid and lymphoid types. In some of the cases, there may be a substantial number of neutrophils and precursors in the blood and marrow smears and the findings may resemble AML with maturation (M2) (figs. 249, 250). In the lymphoblastic type there is no evidence of maturation of the blasts to promyelocytes and the blasts are usually TdT positive. The distinction of Ph-positive acute lymphoblastic leukemia from CML presenting in lymphoid blast crisis is discussed in the section, Acute Lymphoblastic Leukemias.

Accelerated Phase. In approximately 30 percent of patients with CML, transformation is characterized by one or more findings including myelofibrosis, basophilia in excess of 20 percent, a hemoglobin level of 7.0 g/dL or less, platelets 100×10^9/L or less, karyotypic evolution, and an increase in blasts but less than 30 percent (figs. 251–253) (21,36). Several terms have been applied to this type of transformation but the most frequently used is accelerated phase. There may also be an increase in eosinophils, immature monocytes, megakaryoblasts, and erythroblasts. The mature and maturing myeloid cells may show marked dysplastic changes characterized by nuclear hyposegmentation and hypogranulation in the neutrophils as well as dyserythropoiesis. The bone marrow sections may show a marked increase in hypolobulated megakaryocytes with an accompanying increase in reticulin fibers (fig. 254).

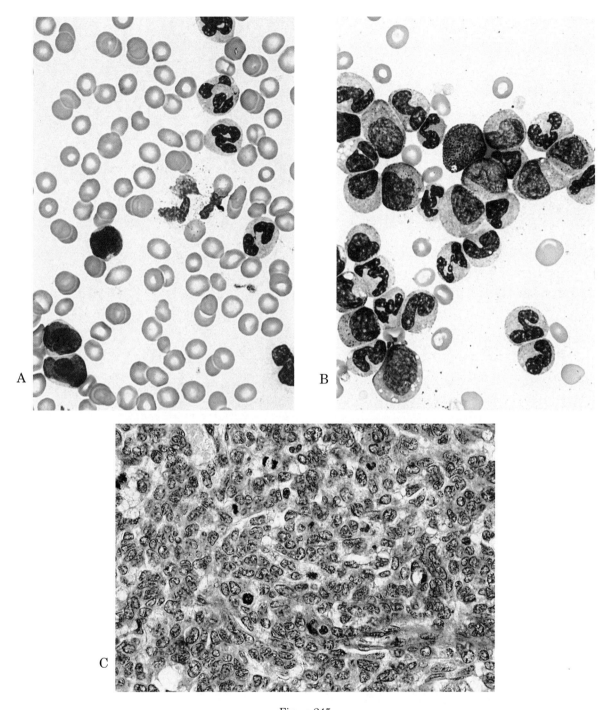

Figure 245
CHRONIC MYELOID LEUKEMIA: FOCAL BLAST TRANSFORMATION

A. Blood smear from a 40-year-old male who presented with massive hepatosplenomegaly and a retroperitoneal mass. This blood specimen contained 22 percent blasts, three examples of which are present at the lower left. The platelets are moderately reduced. (Wright-Giemsa stain)

B. Portion of a bone marrow smear showing neutrophils at all stages of maturation. Although not shown in this area, the smear contained 12 percent blasts, similar to those in the blood. (Wright-Giemsa stain)

C. Portion of the bone marrow biopsy showing one of several foci of blasts. Several mitotic figures are present. Chromosome studies on this marrow specimen showed cells with two Philadelphia chromosomes. Monoclonal antibody studies were not performed. The process was classified as CML presenting in blast transformation. (Hematoxylin and eosin stain)

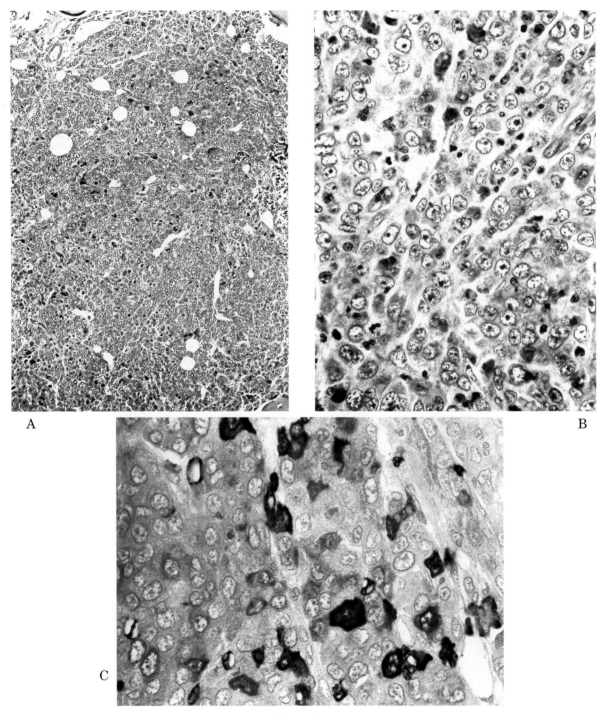

Figure 246
CHRONIC MYELOID LEUKEMIA: FOCAL BLAST TRANSFORMATION

A. A bone marrow biopsy from a patient with CML and less than 5 percent blasts in the marrow smear. Several variably sized well-circumscribed foci of blast cells, similar to the one illustrated, were scattered throughout the marrow. (Hematoxylin and eosin stain)

B. High magnification of the specimen in A showing a predominance of blasts with finely dispersed chromatin, prominent nucleoli, and a variable amount of amphophilic cytoplasm. (Hematoxylin and eosin stain)

C. The specimen in A and B reacted with antibody to hemoglobin A. Several of the blasts are intensely reactive and many show an intermediate degree of reactivity. On the basis of this reaction, the blast foci were interpreted as erythroblasts. (Peroxidase–antiperoxidase stain)

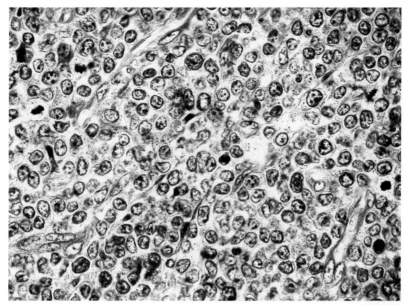

Figure 247
CHRONIC MYELOID LEUKEMIA: LYMPHOBLASTIC TRANSFORMATION PRESENTING IN A LYMPH NODE

Lymph node biopsy from a patient with CML showing diffuse replacement by lymphoblasts of B-cell precursor type and TdT positive. An occasional mitotic figure is identified. (Hematoxylin and eosin stain)

Figure 248
CHRONIC MYELOID LEUKEMIA: TRANSFORMATION TO AML-M4 ASSOCIATED WITH INV(16) CHROMOSOME ABNORMALITY

Bone marrow smear from a patient with a 23-month history of CML who developed a slight monocytosis, increased blasts in the blood and marrow, and an increase in marrow eosinophils with abnormal basophilic-staining granules. Cytogenetic studies showed cells with both a t(9;22) and an inv(16) abnormality. (Wright-Giemsa stain)

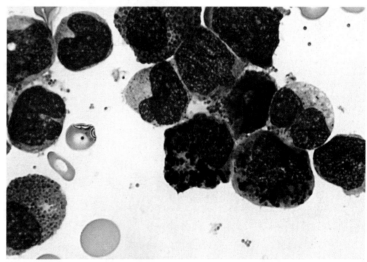

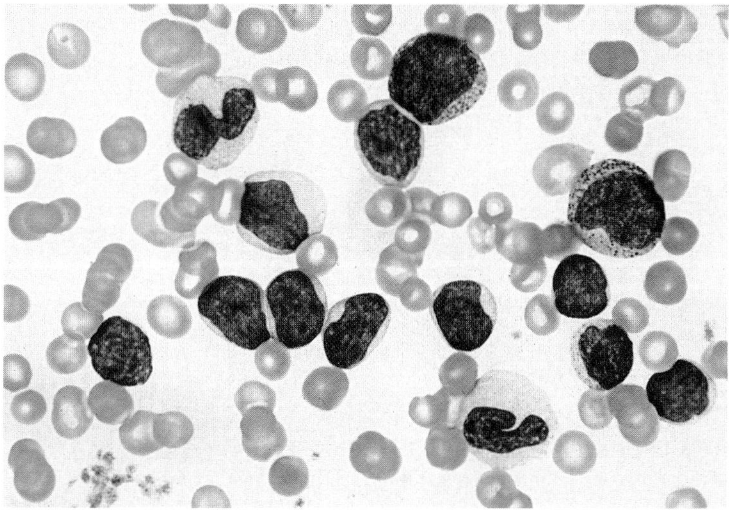

Figure 249
CHRONIC MYELOID LEUKEMIA PRESENTING IN LYMPHOBLAST TRANSFORMATION

Blood smear from a 10-year-old boy who presented with a leukocyte count of 142×10^9/L with 55 percent blasts, 34 percent neutrophils, and 1 percent basophils. There were numerous promyelocytes, myelocytes, and segmented neutrophils. The blasts were TdT positive and had a B-cell precursor immunophenotype; cytogenetic studies showed cells with both single and double Ph chromosomes. Because of the high percentage of neutrophils and precursors this presentation may resemble AML-M2.

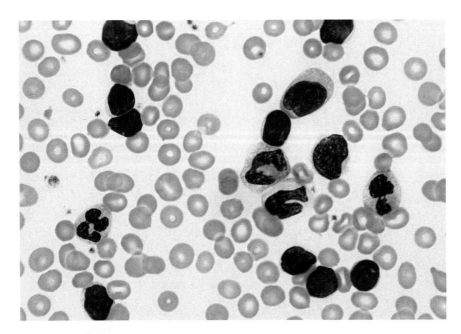

Figure 250
CHRONIC MYELOID LEUKEMIA PRESENTING WITH 41 PERCENT LYMPHOBLASTS
Blood smear from a 56-year-old woman presenting with a leukocyte count of 200×10^9/L, a hemoglobin level of 10 g/dL, and a platelet count of 220×10^9/L. The leukocyte differential consisted of 55 percent neutrophils and precursors, 3 percent monocytes, 1 percent basophils, and 41 percent lymphoblasts. The lymphoblasts are small with a high nuclear-cytoplasmic ratio, condensed nuclear chromatin, and generally indistinct or no evident nucleoli. Virtually all of the lymphocytic cells were TdT positive. Cytogenetic studies showed several metaphases with a single Philadelphia chromosome. The findings are those of both chronic phase CML and lymphoblastic transformation. (Wright-Giemsa stain)

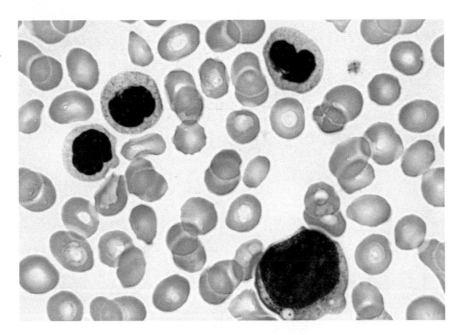

Figure 251
CHRONIC MYELOID LEUKEMIA: ACCELERATED PHASE
Blood smear from a patient with CML in accelerated phase. The mature neutrophils in this field show pronounced nuclear hyposegmentation. (Wright-Giemsa stain)

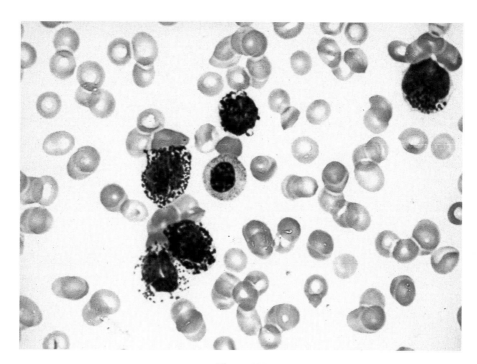

Figure 252
CHRONIC MYELOID LEUKEMIA: ACCELERATED PHASE
Blood smear from a patient in accelerated phase of CML showing five basophils and a mature neutrophil with a nonlobulated, pseudo–Pelger-Huet nucleus. (Wright-Giemsa stain)

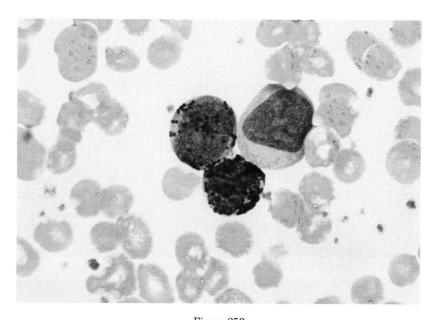

Figure 253
CHRONIC MYELOID LEUKEMIA: ACCELERATED PHASE
Blood smear from a case of CML in accelerated phase showing a blast, an immature basophil, and a mature basophil. The immature basophil has a high nuclear-cytoplasmic ratio, moderately to intensely basophilic cytoplasm, and numerous granules. (Wright-Giemsa stain)

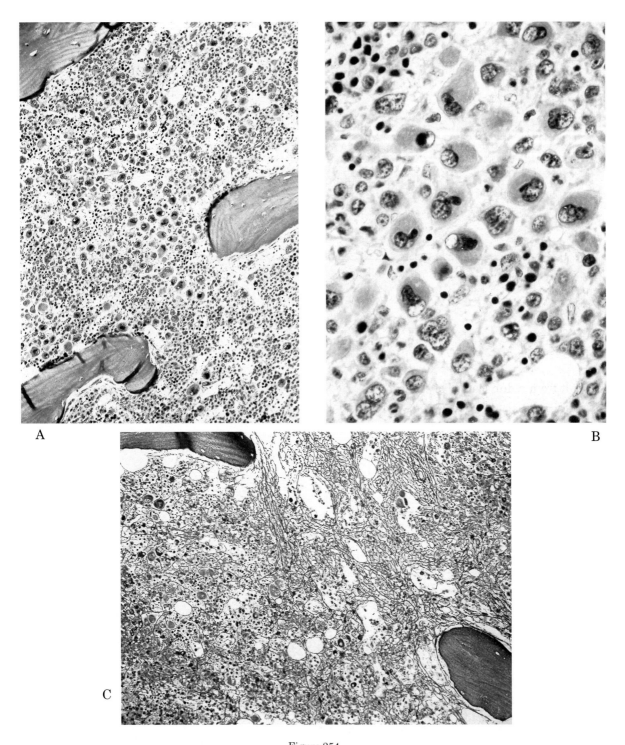

Figure 254
CHRONIC MYELOID LEUKEMIA: ACCELERATED PHASE

A. Markedly hypercellular bone marrow biopsy from a patient with CML in accelerated phase. There are numerous megakaryocytes occurring singly and in clusters. (Hematoxylin and eosin stain)

B. High magnification of the biopsy in A showing a cluster of megakaryocytes which are small to medium sized. Some of the megakaryocytes are micromegakaryocytes with hypolobulated nuclei. (Hematoxylin and eosin stain)

C. Reticulin stain of the specimen in A and B showing a moderate increase in reticulin fibers which are focally accentuated, a common finding in the development of bone marrow fibrosis. (Wilder reticulin stain)

Patients in the accelerated phase usually have evidence of progressive bone marrow failure with increasing anemia and thrombocytopenia, although the clinical course is somewhat more prolonged and unpredictable than in blastic transformation. Progression to a blast phase may occur. Generally, the accelerated phase evolves from a chronic phase. Similar to blast transformation, occasional patients present with hematologic and cytogenetic findings of the accelerated phase without a prior diagnosed chronic phase (fig. 255).

Cytogenetics of Transformation. The clinical and hematologic evolution of CML from the chronic to the accelerated or blastic phase is accompanied by cytogenetic evolution in approximately 70 to 80 percent of patients (26,46). The most commonly observed abnormalities, in addition to the Ph chromosome, are a second Ph chromosome, trisomy 8, isochromosome for the long arm of chromosome 17, +19, and additional aneuploidy. The second Ph chromosome appears to result from a duplication of the original since no additional abnormal chromosome 9 is observed. The additional chromosome abnormalities may precede the hematologic manifestations of transformation by several months.

Differential Diagnosis. The most important entities to be distinguished from CML are leukemoid reactions and the other chronic myeloproliferative syndromes, most notably chronic idiopathic myelofibrosis and polycythemia vera.

Neutrophilic leukocytosis leukemoid reactions that may resemble CML are usually related to bacterial infections or tumors. In both instances there may be a moderate increase in the neutrophils, with an increased number of immature neutrophils. In rare instances, the leukocyte count exceeds 100×10^9/L. When the leukocyte count is markedly elevated there is usually a "shift" to immaturity in the neutrophils but the number of promyelocytes and myelocytes is not as high as in CML. In leukemoid reactions, the neutrophils frequently manifest alterations in the cytoplasm referred to as toxic changes, including increased coarse azurophilic granules and Döhle bodies, findings not present in uncomplicated CML. The absence of basophilia in most leukemoid reactions is a very important distinguishing feature. Basophilia is an uncommon finding exclusive of the myeloproliferative dis-

eases. It occurs in a very limited number of disorders including renal disease, hypothyroidism, hypersensitivity reactions, ulcerative colitis, and systemic mastocytosis. The neutrophil alkaline phosphatase level, which is markedly decreased in CML, is elevated in leukemoid reactions, although occasionally it can be normal. In equivocal cases the presence of the Ph chromosome is definitive. The absence of this chromosome abnormality and the BCR/abl hybrid gene effectively excludes the diagnosis of CML.

The two myeloproliferative disorders that most closely resemble CML hematologically are polycythemia vera and idiopathic myelofibrosis (agnogenic myeloid metaplasia). In both disorders the degree of leukocytosis is generally lower than that found in CML. Other laboratory studies are useful in distinguishing these disorders. When uncomplicated by bleeding, polycythemia vera is characterized by an increased hematocrit and red blood cell mass. The criteria for polycythemia vera proposed by the Polycythemia Vera Study Group exclude cases with the Ph chromosome (57).

Idiopathic myelofibrosis may be somewhat more difficult to distinguish from CML than polycythemia vera. The spleen is usually larger than in CML and the red blood cells show more poikilocytosis with numerous dacryocytes, although in the early stages of idiopathic myelofibrosis the red blood cell changes may be minimal. Normoblastemia, atypical platelets, and micromegakaryocytes are more frequent in the blood than in CML. The total leukocyte count in CML is usually much higher and an increase in basophils is virtually always present, in contrast to idiopathic myelofibrosis in which it is reported in 10 to 20 percent of cases.

Treatment and Prognosis. The major aim of therapy in CML has progressed from lowering the leukocyte count to suppression and eradication of the Ph-positive clone. Busulfan was the first drug found to be effective in CML and was the mainstay of therapy for several decades. Hydroxyurea is equally effective and because of the mutagenic effect of busulfan has largely replaced that drug. The availability of alpha- and gamma-interferon has had a particularly promising impact on CML therapy. These drugs can produce complete hematologic and cytogenetic remission (13,21,50). However, although the interferons suppress the

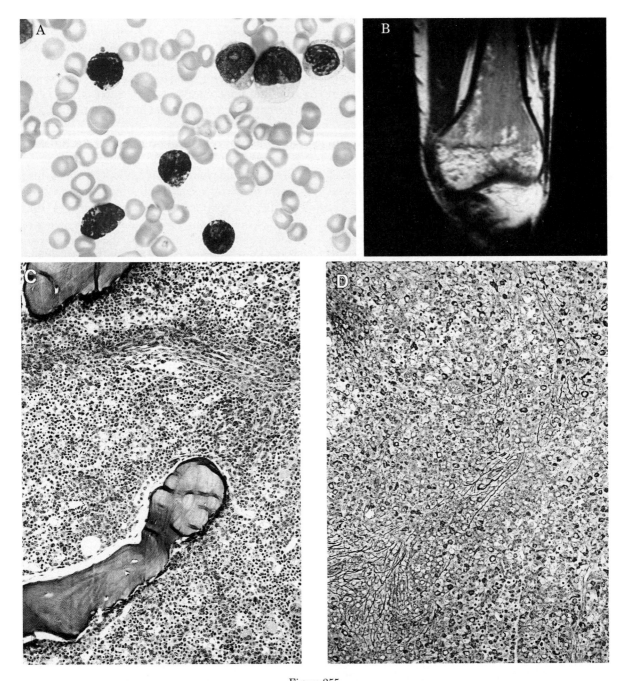

Figure 255
CHRONIC MYELOID LEUKEMIA PRESENTING IN THE ACCELERATED PHASE

A. Blood smear from a 33-year-old man who consulted an orthopedic surgeon for left knee pain. Magnetic resonance imaging of the knee joint and distal femur showed expansion of the red marrow. The radiologist suggested the possibility of a myeloproliferative disease. The leukocyte count was 27×10^9/L with 47 percent basophils and 10 percent blasts. A t(9;22) and i(17q) were found on cytogenetic study. The process was classified as CML presenting in accelerated phase. (Wright-Giemsa stain)

B. Magnetic resonance image of the left knee joint of the same patient. There is marked expansion of the red marrow reflected by the darkened area in the lower portion of the femur. Expansion of the red marrow occurs in patients with CML. (Hematoxylin and eosin stain)

C. Bone marrow biopsy showing marked hypercellularity. A perivascular-associated increase in promyelocytes and myelocytes is present on the right. (Hematoxylin and eosin stain)

D. Reticulin stain of the biopsy in C showing a focal, primarily perivascular-associated increase in reticulin fibers. (Wilder reticulin stain)

Table 22

DIFFERENTIATING FEATURES OF TYPICAL CHRONIC MYELOID LEUKEMIA, ATYPICAL CHRONIC MYELOID LEUKEMIA, AND CHRONIC MYELOMONOCYTIC LEUKEMIA, MYELOPROLIFERATIVE*

	Typical CML	Atypical CML	CMML
Immature granulocytes ≥15 percent in blood	+	+	−
Basophilia >0.14×10^9/L	+	±	−
Monocytes > 3 percent in blood	−**	+	+
Dysgranulopoiesis	−	+	±
Philadelphia chromosome	95%	−	−
BCR/*abl* hybrid gene	100%	−	−

*Modified from Sheperd et al. (62). The term chronic myeloid leukemia is used here instead of chronic granulocytic leukemia, the term used in the cited reference.
**May be present in a few patients in early stages.

proliferation of the Ph-positive clone, they do not totally eradicate Ph-positive stem cells and the long-term effectiveness of these agents is indeterminate.

Bone marrow transplantation is increasingly employed for treatment. It is particularly beneficial for patients less than 40 years of age for whom there is a good HLA-matched donor available (51). Autologous transplantation following effective therapy and the production of large numbers of Ph-negative clones is now being attempted by some transplantation groups.

The median survival period for patients with CML with contemporary approaches to therapy including alpha interferon and bone marrow transplantation is approximately 60 to 65 months (21).

In the majority of patients, CML terminates in the accelerated phase or a blast crisis. The treatment of these events includes drugs employed for acute leukemia. The results are generally unsatisfactory. Complete or partial remission is achieved in approximately 30 percent of patients, with a median survival time of 7 months (52). Nonresponders survive a median of 2 to 3 months. Patients with lymphoblastic crisis of CML have been reported to have a more favorable course than patients with myeloblastic crisis because of the response to regimens that include vincristine and corticosteroids (42).

ATYPICAL CHRONIC MYELOID LEUKEMIA

The term atypical chronic myeloid leukemia has been used to describe a myeloproliferative disorder that has some hematologic features of both Ph-positive CML and chronic myelomonocytic leukemia (Table 22) (60–63). In atypical CML there is no t(9;22) chromosome abnormality or molecular evidence of a BCR/*abl* hybrid gene. In contrast to Ph-positive CML, there are usually dysplastic changes in the neutrophils and the basophils are normal in number or only slightly increased. The leukocyte count ranges from 20 to 180×10^9/L; the median leukocyte count in one study was 54.4×10^9/L (62). The promyelocytes, myelocytes, and metamyelocytes comprise more than 15 percent of the leukocytes in the blood and the monocytes usually exceed 3 percent (fig. 256) (62). A majority of patients have thrombocytopenia; the median platelet count in one series was 79×10^9/L. The hemoglobin level ranges from 3.4 to 14.2 g/dL, with a median of 9.8 g/dL. The bone marrow is hypercellular and may show a higher percentage of erythroid precursors than usually observed in typical Ph-positive CML. The prognosis appears to be less favorable than in typical Ph-positive CML (62).

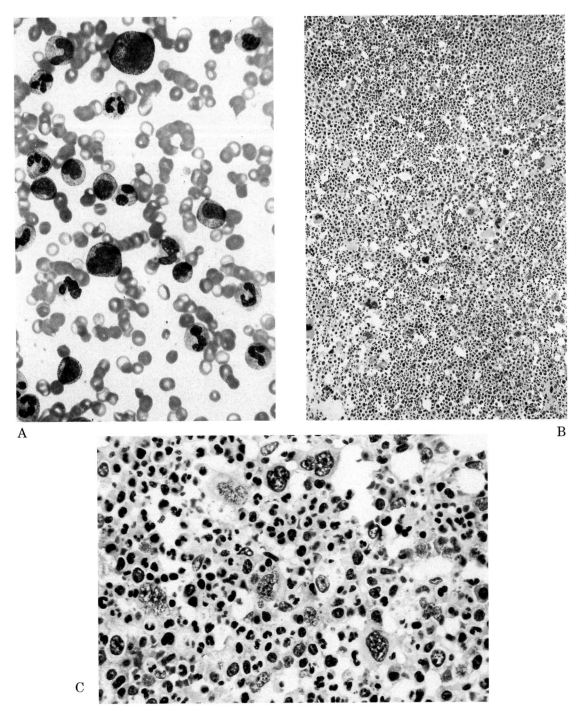

Figure 256
ATYPICAL CHRONIC MYELOID LEUKEMIA

A. Blood smear from a 47-year-old woman with a leukocyte count of 41×10^9/L and a platelet count of 160×10^9/L. The blood smear had numerous (21 percent) promyelocytes and neutrophil myelocytes and 4 percent monocytes. Basophils were not increased. Occasional neutrophils had pseudo–Pelger-Huet nuclei, as in the neutrophil above center. Cytogenetic studies were negative for the Philadelphia chromosome and there was no BCR/*abl* hybrid gene on molecular analysis. (Wright-Giemsa stain)

B. Low magnification of a bone marrow biopsy showing a markedly cellular marrow. (Hematoxylin and eosin stain)

C. High magnification of the biopsy in B showing a marked increase in neutrophils and precursors and several mature-appearing megakaryocytes. (Hematoxylin and eosin stain)

CHRONIC NEUTROPHILIC LEUKEMIA

Chronic neutrophilic leukemia is a rare disorder that is characterized by leukocyte counts in excess of 30×10^9/L and splenomegaly (64,66). The neutrophils are predominantly mature or a mixture of segmented neutrophils and bands. Anemia is a variable manifestation. The neutrophils may contain Döhle bodies and toxic granulation. In contrast to patients with typical CML, the myeloid cells in chronic neutrophilic leukemia do not contain the Ph chromosome and the neutrophil alkaline phosphatase level is frequently increased. Similar to typical CML, the serum vitamin B_{12} level is markedly elevated. This, however, is a nonspecific finding and may also be found in reactive neutrophilia. On histopathologic examination, the spleen shows infiltration of the white and red pulp by mature neutrophils.

This form of leukemia has been reported to occur over a wide age range, 26 to 88 years; the majority of patients are over 60. Survival has ranged from 6 months to 5 years.

The most important differential diagnosis in this disease is a leukemoid reaction. The diagnosis of chronic neutrophilic leukemia should be made with considerable caution and only after all possibilities of a leukemoid reaction have been eliminated.

Other myeloproliferative disorders should be excluded; the diagnosis of chronic neutrophilic leukemia should not be established without cytogenetic and molecular studies for the BCR/*abl* translocation. An association of chronic neutrophilic leukemia with polycythemia vera has been reported and studies to exclude this entity should be performed (65).

CHRONIC MYELOMONOCYTIC LEUKEMIA, MYELOPROLIFERATIVE

Although chronic myelomonocytic leukemia is generally classified as a myelodysplastic syndrome, there is a form of this leukemia which by virtue of the blood, bone marrow, and clinical findings is most appropriately classified as a myeloproliferative disorder. This entity presents with an elevated leukocyte count with increased monocytes and neutrophils, a variable platelet count, anemia, and some degree of splenomegaly (69). Basophils may be slightly increased but this is not a constant finding. Dysplastic changes are minimal or not present. The platelets are usually normal or slightly decreased; an occasional patient has thrombocytosis. Some of these cases closely resemble CML hematologically except for the monocytosis and lack of basophilia. The absence of a Ph chromosome or molecular evidence of the BCR/*abl* hybrid gene effectively excludes the diagnosis of CML. Some of the cases reported as Ph-negative CML are possibly examples of this disorder (67,68,70).

The incidence of chronic myelomonocytic leukemia, myeloproliferative is indeterminate because of differing criteria for the diagnosis. It is primarily a disease of older individuals and is more common in males.

The blood shows varying percentages of neutrophils and monocytes. Immature cells of the neutrophil series, including promyelocytes, are present, but these are usually less than 15 percent. Blasts are occasionally found. The monocytes exceed 3 percent, are primarily mature, and may be indistinguishable from normal monocytes (fig. 257). Occasional promonocytes may be noted. The bone marrow is hypercellular with an increase in both neutrophils and monocytes, although the increase in monocytes may be minimal. The neutrophil hyperplasia includes cells at all stages of maturation. Blasts do not usually exceed 5 percent. The monocytes are primarily mature with a low number of promonocytes. Erythroid precursors and megakaryocytes are generally normal in number. The neutrophil alkaline phosphatase level may be low or normal. The biologic course in chronic myelomonocytic leukemia, myeloproliferative, is usually characterized by increasing immaturity in the monocytes and neutrophils, with progressive bone marrow failure and termination as acute myelomonocytic leukemia. Organ infiltration may be a prominent feature with disease progression.

The differential diagnosis includes CML, atypical CML, a leukemoid reaction, acute myelomonocytic leukemia, and chronic myelomonocytic leukemia, myelodysplastic. CML is excluded by the absence of the Ph chromosome. The distinction from atypical CML is based primarily on the percent of immature granulocytes in the blood (see Table 22). The diagnosis of acute myelomonocytic leukemia is excluded by the less than 30 percent blasts required for a diagnosis of acute leukemia. If there is a high percentage of

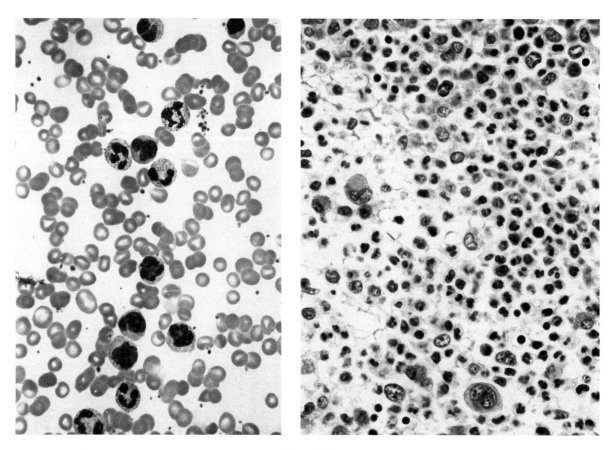

Figure 257
CHRONIC MYELOMONOCYTIC LEUKEMIA, MYELOPROLIFERATIVE
Left: Blood smear from a 58-year-old woman with an elevated leukocyte count, slight thrombocytosis, and splenomegaly. The leukocyte increase was due principally to an increase in mature monocytes and neutrophils. The neutrophil alkaline phosphate level was decreased. Cytogenetic studies showed a trisomy for chromosome 8 but no Ph chromosome. Molecular studies for the BCR/*abl* hybrid gene were negative. (Wright-Giemsa stain)
Right: Bone marrow section from the same patient. The marrow is markedly hypercellular with no shift to immaturity. (Hematoxylin and eosin stain)

promonocytes and the number of myeloblasts, monoblasts, and promonocytes exceeds 30 percent in the blood or bone marrow, the diagnosis of acute myelomonocytic leukemia should be made.

The distinction between chronic myelomonocytic leukemia, myelodysplastic and chronic myelomonocytic leukemia, myeloproliferative may be difficult and arbitrary and there are cases in which a definitive distinction is not possible. In general, a process characterized by leukocytosis with monocytosis and neutrophilia, minimal or no dysplastic changes, a normal platelet count, and splenomegaly is more suggestive of a myeloproliferative process. Essentially, if the clinical and laboratory findings suggest CML but the Ph chromosome and molecular evidence of a BCR/*abl* hybrid gene are absent, the possibility of chronic myelomonocytic leukemia, myeloproliferative should be considered. If bone marrow failure, neutropenia, and dysplastic changes are the predominant findings, chronic myelomonocytic leukemia, myelodysplastic is the more likely diagnosis.

A leukemoid reaction is always an important consideration in patients who present with a monocytosis. These patients must be evaluated for an underlying neoplasm or infectious process. In some instances, the diagnosis can only be established after a period of observation.

The major laboratory findings distinguishing typical CML, atypical CML, and chronic myelomonocytic leukemia, as proposed by Shepherd and colleagues (69), are shown in Table 22.

Treatment of chronic myelomonocytic leukemia, myeloproliferative is similar to that for CML and includes hydroxyurea and interferon. The prognosis for this disorder is reported as poor. However, the reported groups usually include cases of chronic myelomonocytic leukemia, myelodysplastic. In general, the median survival is probably shorter than for patients with Ph-positive CML.

JUVENILE CHRONIC MYELOID LEUKEMIA

Definition. The term *granulocytic leukemia in childhood* was introduced to designate those myeloproliferative disorders in children that have hematologic features identical or similar to CML as it occurs in adults (79). Two major entities were included in this designation: adult type and juvenile type (71,75,78,79,83). The adult type is morphologically, clinically, and cytogenetically identical to CML as it occurs in adults. The juvenile type, referred to as juvenile chronic myeloid leukemia (JCML), is morphologically, cytogenetically, and clinically distinct from Ph-positive CML (79). It is a clinically aggressive disease, more similar in its course to acute myeloid leukemia. Also, in contrast to adult-type CML, which is more common in children 14 to 18 years of age, JCML is more common in very young children.

Incidence and Clinical Findings. JCML is a rare form of leukemia with an acute or subacute course in most patients; the median survival is approximately 10 to 12 months (79,83). Most patients are less than 2 years of age at diagnosis and 95 percent are less than 4 years of age (79). Males outnumber females 2 to 1. Hepatosplenomegaly and lymphadenopathy are common presenting clinical findings. An eczematoid rash, frequently facial, is characteristic. Familial neurofibromatosis has been reported in some cases (72,76,81).

Laboratory Findings. The neutrophil alkaline phosphatase level, as in adult-type CML, is reduced. A very important finding is the level of fetal hemoglobin which is markedly increased, ranging from 40 to 55 percent in most patients (fig. 258) (79). This contrasts to the less than 10 percent in the adult form of CML. The fetal hemoglobin level may increase with disease progression. Additional findings include decreased

levels of hemoglobin A2, reduced erythrocyte carbonic anhydrase, increased glucose 6-phosphate dehydrogenase, reduced I antigen, and a displacement of the oxygen dissociation curve to the left as a result of the increased level of fetal hemoglobin. A polyclonal increase in immunoglobulins is frequent (78). Chromosome studies in JCML have shown no consistent abnormality except for the absence of the Ph chromosome (73,74,81).

Cell culture studies of hematopoietic cells from children with JCML have shown a prominent monocytic component (71,77,78). Two consistent abnormalities have been reported: excessive proliferation of monocyte macrophage colonies in the absence of exogenous colony-stimulating factor and suppression of growth of normal hematopoietic colony formation.

Blood and Bone Marrow Findings. The hemoglobin level is moderately reduced. The leukocyte count is lower than in adult-type CML; a range of 27 to 77×10^9/L was reported in one series (79). Thrombocytopenia is usually present at the outset. The leukocyte differential shows a higher percentage of myeloblasts, monocytes, and lymphocytes than in the adult form and the percentage of segmented neutrophils is lower (fig. 258). Basophilia may be present but is not a constant feature. Nucleated red blood cells are usually present; the number of these cells may increase with progression of the disease. Occasional plasma cells and immunoblasts may be noted.

The bone marrow is hypercellular and contains an increased number of blasts, up to 12 percent, and an increased number of mature and immature monocytes. Megakaryocytes are generally decreased (fig. 258).

Differential Diagnosis. The differential diagnosis may be problematic because of differing concepts of the disease. If a markedly elevated fetal hemoglobin level is included as a diagnostic criterion, in addition to the other clinical and laboratory findings, the disorder is a relatively well-defined entity hematologically.

The hematopoietic disorder in children associated with an isolated monosomy 7 may also present before the age of 2 years with rash, particularly facial, lymphadenopathy, and hepatosplenomegaly. The hematologic findings in isolated monosomy 7 syndrome of childhood, which are described in the section on myelodysplastic syndromes, include moderate anemia, thrombocytopenia,

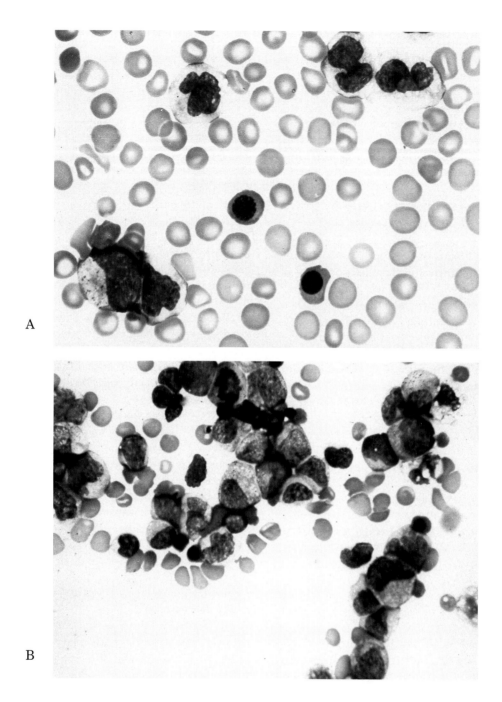

A

B

Figure 258
JUVENILE CHRONIC MYELOID LEUKEMIA

A. Blood smear from a 3 1/2-year-old boy. The increased leukocytes consist predominantly of neutrophils and monocytes, mostly mature. The three leukocytes at the top are monocytes; a neutrophil myelocyte and a monocyte are at the lower left. There are two late polychromatic normoblasts. (Wright-Giemsa stain)

B. Bone marrow smear showing numerous neutrophil myelocytes and a few monocytes. The blasts are only slightly increased. (Wright-Giemsa stain)

C. Bone marrow biopsy showing a markedly cellular marrow. The predominant neutrophils are myelocytes and reflect the cell population in the smear. Red blood cell precursors with round dense nuclei and clear cytoplasm are scattered among the granulocytes. Megakaryocytes are reduced in number. (Hematoxylin and eosin stain)

D. Fetal hemoglobin stain of the same specimen as A. Approximately 50 percent of the cells contain hemoglobin F. (Kleihaur-Betke stain)

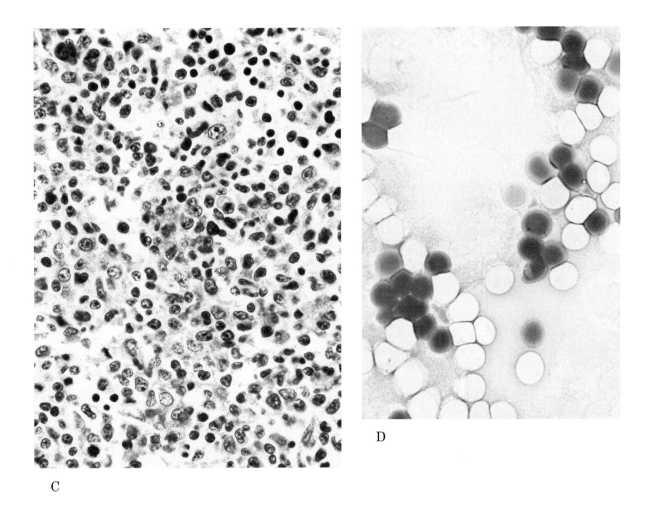

C

D

monocytosis, and erythroid precursors in the blood. Unlike JCML, the fetal hemoglobin level is usually normal or only slightly increased. However, cases of monosomy 7 with a markedly elevated fetal hemoglobin level and cases of JCML with low levels have been observed. The definitive finding is the demonstration of monosomy 7 in the myeloid cells.

Acute myelomonocytic leukemia is distinguished from JCML by a blast count of 30 percent or higher in the blood or bone marrow and a fetal hemoglobin level of less than 10 percent.

The clinical and laboratory findings of JCML have been observed in very young children with persistent Epstein-Barr virus infection (80). These include leukocytosis, thrombocytopenia, hepatosplenomegaly, elevated levels of fetal hemoglobin, and i antigen-positive red blood cells.

Treatment and Prognosis. Patients with JCML have a more acute clinical course than those with the adult type, with a median survival period of 10 to 12 months. Progressive bone marrow failure with increasing evidence of myelodysplasia and an increasing blast percentage are part of the evolution in most cases. Unlike adult-type CML, abrupt transformation to a blast phase does not usually occur (83). Patients with JCML do not typically respond to busulfan or hydroxyurea and acute myeloid leukemia regimens have limited success (78). Allogeneic bone marrow transplantation has been beneficial in some patients (82).

POLYCYTHEMIA VERA

Definition. A clonal myeloproliferative disease characterized by excessive production of all myeloid cells: red blood cells, granulocytes, and megakaryocytes (84). This disease usually evolves through three successive stages: the proliferative phase, in which the cardinal manifestation is an increased red blood cell mass, a stable phase, and the spent or myeloid metaplasia phase (90,97,98). A low number of patients develop acute myeloid leukemia (90,93).

Definitive criteria for the diagnosis of polycythemia vera were established by the Polycythemia Vera Study Group (PVSG) in 1971 (87). The diagnostic criteria are categorized into two groups: A, major criteria, and B, minor criteria (Table 23).

The diagnosis of polycythemia vera is established if the following combinations are present: A1 (increased red blood cell mass) plus A2 (normal arterial oxygen saturation) plus A3 (splenomegally) or A1 plus A2 and any two criteria from category B.

Incidence and Clinical Findings. Polycythemia vera is a rare disorder; the annual incidence is 5 to 10 cases per million individuals (95). The male to female ratio is 1.2 to 1 and the median age of onset is 60 years. There is an increased incidence in individuals of Jewish descent and a decreased incidence in American blacks (95).

The presenting symptoms relate primarily to the increased red blood cell mass and include headache, weakness, pruritus, and dizziness. Splenomegaly is the most common physical finding and is one of the major criteria.

The onset of the disease in patients under 40 years of age appears to be marked by greater clinical severity and a higher frequency of life-threatening complications related to thrombosis or hemorrhagic events (95).

Laboratory Findings. An increased red blood cell mass is the sine qua non for diagnosis. The hemoglobin level, red blood cell count, and hematocrit are elevated. The leukocyte count is increased in more than 80 percent of patients, usually in the range of 10 to 20×10^9/L (87). There is a neutrophilic leukocytosis with a slight left shift. Modest basophilia is present in approximately 60 to 70 percent of patients and eosinophilia is frequent. The platelet count is increased in 50 to 80 percent of patients and platelet aggregation is abnormal in approximately 50 percent (85,96).

Table 23

PVSG CRITERIA FOR THE DIAGNOSIS OF POLYCYTHEMIA VERA*

A criteria:
- A1 Increased red blood cell mass
  - males: ≥36 mL/kg
  - females: ≥32 mL/kg
- A2 Normal arterial oxygen saturation ≥92 percent
- A3 Splenomegaly

B criteria:
- B1 Thrombocytosis: $>400 \times 10^9$/L
- B2 Leukocytes: $>12 \times 10^9$/L in the absence of fever or infection
- B3 Increased neutrophil alkaline phosphatase level in the absence of fever or infection
- B4 Increased serum vitamin B_{12} level or unsaturated B_{12}-binding protein

* From reference 87.

Blood and Bone Marrow Findings. In the initial phases of the disease the red blood cells are generally normal in appearance or there may be slight poikilocytosis (fig. 259). In patients who have undergone repeated phlebotomy, the red blood cells may be microcytic and hypochromic. Large, hypogranular platelets and fragmented naked megakaryocyte nuclei may be present.

The bone marrow is marked by a panhyperplasia with an increase in all myeloid cells, the most marked increase occurring in the red blood cell precursors. There is no significant shift to immature cells. Stains for iron usually show decreased to absent iron stores (90).

Histopathologic Findings. The bone marrow biopsy is the most important part of the pathologic examination in polycythemia vera. The marrow is markedly hypercellular in the majority of patients; a mean cellularity of 82 percent with a range of 37 to 100 percent was reported by the PVSG (90). In approximately 15 percent of patients, the cellularity is less than 60 percent. There is a panhyperplasia, with the most marked increase occurring in the megakaryocytes and erythroid precursors. The increase in megakaryocytes may be particularly pronounced (fig. 260). The megakaryocytes usually show considerable variation in size from small to unusually large with

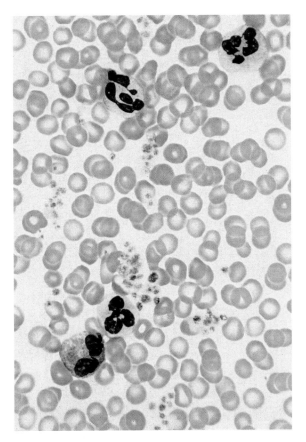

Figure 259
POLYCYTHEMIA VERA

Blood smear from a 38-year-old woman with polycythemia vera who presented with a Hb of 19 g/dL, WBC count of 12.8×10⁹/L, platelet count of 555×10⁹/L, and splenomegaly. Radioisotope studies showed an increased red blood cell mass. (Wright-Giemsa stain)

hyperlobulated nuclei (100). Clustering of megakaryocytes may occur. An increase in reticulin fibers is present in 25 percent of cases at the time of initial diagnosis (90). Approximately 10 percent of pretreatment cases show a marked increase in reticulin fibers. The increased reticulin generally corresponds to increased cellularity.

Evolution. *Post-Polycythemia Myeloid Metaplasia.* The initial and stable phases of polycythemia vera are 5 to 20 years in duration. In approximately 10 to 20 percent of patients, the stable phase is succeeded by a myeloid metaplasia or "spent" phase, marked by a decreasing red blood cell mass, increasing splenomegaly, leukoerythroblastosis, tear drop poikilocytosis, extramedullary hematopoiesis, and bone marrow fibrosis (figs. 261–263) (90,93,97,98). The marrow

biopsies from patients in the post-polycythemia myeloid metaplasia phase show a moderate to marked increase in reticulin fibers; collagenous fibrosis may be present.

Acute Leukemia in Patients with Polycythemia Vera. Patients with polycythemia vera are at increased risk for the development of acute myeloid leukemia (93,101). The results of the PVSG randomized study demonstrated that the incidence of this complication is higher in patients treated with ³²P or chlorambucil than in patients treated with phlebotomy only (93). The time interval from the initial diagnosis of polycythemia vera to the onset of leukemia varied from 2.6 to 5.2 years in the group treated with phlebotomy only, from 2.1 to more than 11 years in chlorambucil-treated patients, and 3.2 to 12.5 years in the ³²P-treated patients. The incidence of this complication was higher in the patients who developed a myeloid metaplasia phase, 23 percent, as compared to those not evolving to myeloid metaplasia, 7 percent.

Cytogenetic Findings. The incidence of chromosome abnormalities in patients with polycythemia vera varies widely in different series but overall appears to be in the range of 40 to 50 percent (89). The incidence appears to increase with progression of the disease. The most common abnormalities include +8, +9, and 20q-. Patients with abnormal clones at diagnosis appear to have a shorter survival than patients without an abnormal clone (89).

Differential Diagnosis. The major difficulty in the differential diagnosis of polycythemia vera occurs in the proliferative phase of the disease and relates to the elevated hematocrit. Polycythemia vera must be distinguished from other causes of an increased hematocrit. Adherence to the diagnostic criteria proposed by the PVSG, especially measurement of the red blood cell mass, is critical to the diagnosis (87).

The first step in the differential diagnosis of an elevated hematocrit is determining whether the erythrocytosis is absolute or relative (86,87). When there is a relative erythrocytosis, the red blood cell mass is not increased; the erythrocytosis may be stress related or spurious (102).

If the red blood cell mass is increased, the arterial oxygen saturation must be determined. An arterial oxygen saturation of less than 92 percent suggests hypoxemia as a factor in the polycythemia. If the arterial oxygen saturation is normal,

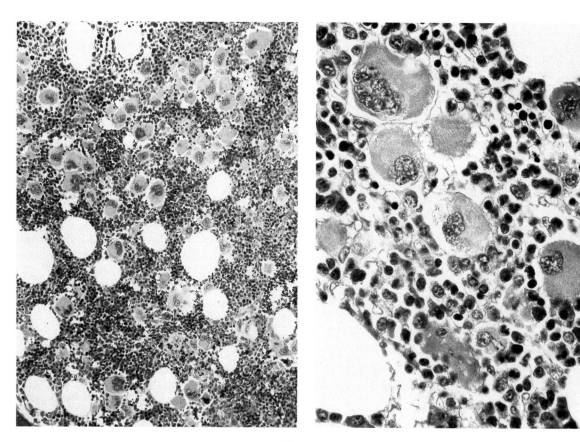

Figure 260
POLYCYTHEMIA VERA

Left: Bone marrow biopsy from a 64-year-old man with polycythemia vera. The marrow is markedly hypercellular with a marked increase in megakaryocytes. (Hematoxylin and eosin stain)

Right: High magnification of the biopsy specimen on the left showing a predominance of erythroid precursors and megakaryocytes. (Hematoxylin and eosin stain)

Figure 261
POLYCYTHEMIA VERA:
MYELOID METAPLASIA PHASE

Blood smear from a 68-year-old woman with a 13-year history of polycythemia vera treated with phlebotomy, ^{32}P, and hydroxyurea. There was a 6- to 7-month history of decreasing hemoglobin level and platelet count. There are three red blood cell precursors present and slight to moderate anisopoikilocytosis. (Wright-Giemsa stain)

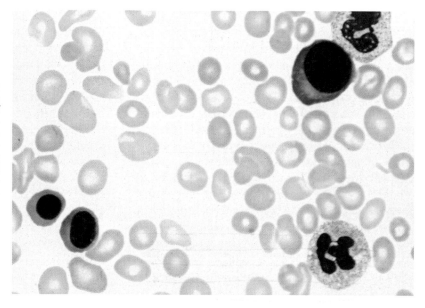

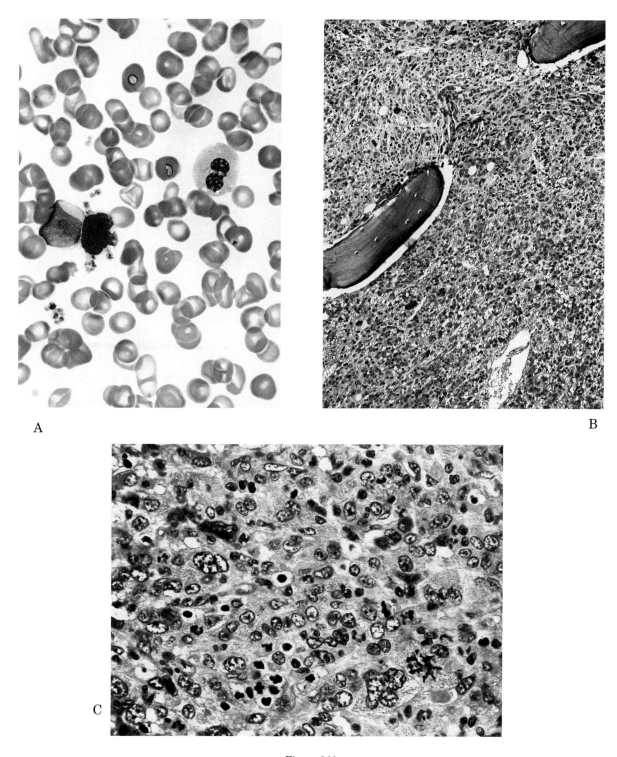

Figure 262
POLYCYTHEMIA VERA: MYELOID METAPLASIA PHASE

A. Blood smear from a 47-year-old woman with an 8-year history of polycythemia vera treated with phlebotomy, splenectomy, and hydroxyurea. A blast, micromegakaryocyte, and hypolobulated neutrophil are shown. (Wright-Giemsa stain)

B. Bone marrow biopsy from the same patient. The marrow is markedly hypercellular. (Hematoxylin and eosin stain)

C. High magnification of the specimen in B showing a predominance of immature cells. Some of the nucleated red blood cells show dysplastic features. (Hematoxylin and eosin stain)

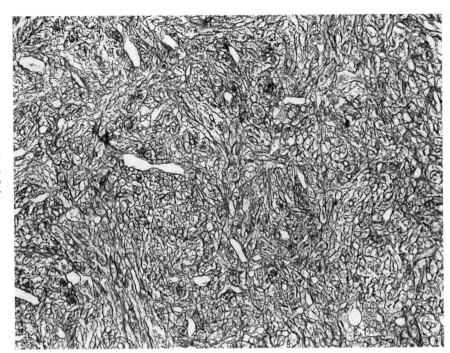

Figure 263
POLYCYTHEMIA VERA:
MYELOID
METAPLASIA PHASE
Reticulin stain of the specimen in figure 262 showing a marked increase in coarse reticulin fibers. (Wilder reticulin stain)

there are several considerations including smokers' polycythemia which is diagnosed by elevated levels of carboxyhemoglobin, and erythropoietin-producing tumors such as renal cell carcinoma. High oxygen affinity hemoglobins may lead to polycythemia and can be excluded by oxygen dissociation curves or P_{50}; the P_{50} is usually less than 20 (88). Patients with a familial history of polycythemia should be investigated for this possibility. Elevated erythropoietin levels indicate a secondary erythrocytosis; normal levels are indeterminate (88). In these various disorders, the bone marrow lacks the typical histopathologic pattern of the panmyeloid hyperplasia characteristic of polycythemia vera. The megakaryocytes are usually normal in number, size, and pattern of distribution.

The myeloid metaplasia and acute leukemia phases do not usually present a diagnostic problem because of the prior history. However, the detection of fibrosis in the bone marrow of a patient with polycythemia vera should always be viewed with the same differential diagnosis as bone marrow fibrosis in other patients (fig. 264) (94).

Treatment and Prognosis. Treatment is principally directed at lowering the hematocrit and platelets. Because of the demonstrated leukemogenic effect of alkylating agents, these drugs are no longer generally used. In patients less than 50 years of age, phlebotomy only is preferred (91). If thrombotic or hemorrhagic complications occur or if there is a high frequency of phlebotomy, myelosuppressive therapy, principally hydroxyurea, is used (92). Anagrelide is an effective drug for lowering the platelet count (99). In patients between the ages of 50 and 70 years, phlebotomy, with or without hydroxyurea, is used (91). In patients over the age of 70, ^{32}P or hydroxyurea plus phlebotomy are used. The general principal of therapy in polycythemia vera is to avoid leukemogenic agents in patients of all ages and to avoid myelosuppressive therapy in individuals less than 50.

Patients in the myeloid metaplasia phase are managed with supportive therapy. The acute leukemia that occurs in 9 to 10 percent of patients is frequently refractory to therapy; multiagent chemotherapy is employed in younger individuals.

Untreated patients survive 1.5 to 3 years. The major causes of death are thrombotic and hemorrhagic complications. Patients treated with either phlebotomy, chlorambucil, or ^{32}P as single therapeutic modalities have median survival periods of 8.9 to 13.9 years: 13.9 years for phlebotomy only, 8.9 years for chlorambucil only, and 11.8 years for ^{32}P only (86). Thromboembolic complications are the most frequent cause of death.

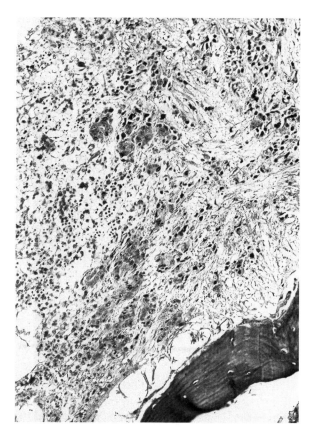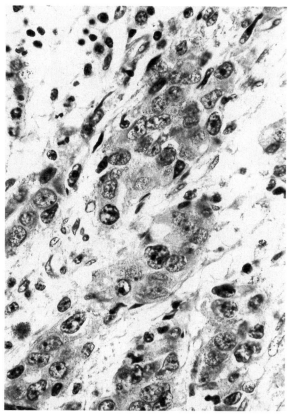

Figure 264

POLYCYTHEMIA VERA WITH MYELOFIBROSIS SECONDARY TO METASTATIC CARCINOMA

Left: Bone marrow biopsy from a 64-year-old man with a 3-year history of polycythemia vera treated with ^{32}P and phlebotomy. The marrow biopsy was preceded by a short history of seizures, memory loss, and hypercalcemia. This marrow biopsy shows extensive fibrosis with several clusters of metastatic tumor. (Hematoxylin and eosin stain)

Right: High magnification of the specimen on the left showing clusters of tumor cells. The myelofibrosis was interpreted as secondary to the metastatic tumor. Subsequent autopsy showed widespread prostatic carcinoma. (Hematoxylin and eosin stain)

ESSENTIAL THROMBOCYTHEMIA

Definition. A myeloproliferative disorder in which the principal manifestation is a marked increase in the platelet count. Evidence indicates that essential or primary thrombocythemia (ET) is a clonal disorder with origin in a multipotential stem cell (108). The criteria for diagnosis proposed by the PVSG are shown in Table 24 (112).

Incidence and Clinical Findings. Essential thrombocythemia is an uncommon disorder. The annual reported incidence for Olmstead County, Minnesota is 7 per million people (110). The age range of the 37 patients studied by the PVSG was 21 to 84 years, with a median of 61 (112). The male to female ratio is 1 to 1.

Prominent presenting clinical manifestations are abnormal bleeding and symptoms related to

Table 24

PVSG CRITERIA FOR THE DIAGNOSIS OF ESSENTIAL THROMBOCYTHEMIA*

1. Platelet count $\geq 600 \times 10^9$/L

2. Hemoglobin level ≤ 13 g/dL or normal red blood cell mass

3. Stainable iron in marrow or no response to iron therapy

4. No Ph chromosome or molecular evidence of the BCR/*abl* hybrid gene

5. Collagen fibrosis of marrow

    a. absent

    b. less than 1/3 of biopsy without both splenomegaly and a leukoerythroblastic reaction

6. No demonstrable cause for thrombocytosis

* From reference 112.

central nervous system and peripheral vascular ischemia. A mild degree of splenomegaly is reported in 38 percent of patients (112).

Although essential thrombocythemia usually occurs in an older age group, the disease may present in younger individuals. In this age group the incidence of thrombohemorrhagic complications is lower and there is a more favorable long-term prognosis (110).

Laboratory Findings. The principal laboratory finding is thrombocytosis. Although a minimum platelet count of 600×10^9/L has been proposed for diagnosis by the PVSG, the majority of patients have platelet counts of 1000×10^9/L or higher (112). The hemoglobin range reported by the PVSG was 10.0 to 18.8 g/dL, with a median of 13.8 g/dL; the leukocyte count ranged from 6 to 41×10^9/L, with a median of 11.5×10^9/L. The neutrophil alkaline phosphatase level is usually normal but may be decreased or increased (109,112). Platelet aggregation studies show hypoaggregation in the majority of patients; a small number show spontaneous aggregation (105,106,111).

Blood and Bone Marrow Findings. The platelets in the blood smear may be normal in appearance or show marked variation in size. Numerous large, atypical, hypogranular forms may be present (fig. 265).

Histopathologic Findings. Bone marrow cellularity is reported as increased in 90 percent of patients and moderately to markedly hypercellular in 70 percent (fig. 265) (112). The marrow may be normocellular or only slightly hypercellular (fig. 266). The megakaryocytes are disproportionately increased and may show considerable variation in size, similar to the findings in polycythemia vera. Erythroid and granulocytic hyperplasia may also be present. Reticulin fibers are increased in approximately 20 to 50 percent of cases (104,112). In younger patients, reticulin fibers are increased in the bone marrow in only about 6 percent of cases (110).

Differential Diagnosis. The differential diagnosis of essential thrombocythemia includes causes of secondary thrombocytosis and closely related myeloproliferative disorders, most notably polycythemia vera, idiopathic myelofibrosis, and CML (103).

Reactive thrombocytosis may be associated with several conditions including iron deficiency anemia, neoplasms, and inflammatory processes and is an almost universal finding following splenectomy. The platelet counts in the secondary thrombocytoses are not usually in the range found in essential thrombocythemia and are less than 1000×10^9/L; the magnitude of the count, however, is not in itself a distinguishing feature. A scoring system for distinguishing essential thrombocythemia from reactive thrombocytosis based on splenomegaly on radiologic scan, unstimulated BRU-E–derived colonies, elevated platelet ATP-ADP, elevated platelet distribution width, and evidence of clinical ischemia has been used. The scoring system had a predictive value of 89 percent in distinguishing the two disorders (106).

Distinguishing essential thrombocythemia from polycythemia vera may be difficult, if not impossible, on histologic grounds in some cases; the megakaryocytes may be morphologically similar in both number and appearance in both disorders. The criteria proposed by the PVSG for the diagnosis of these disorders should be used for distinction (105). CML may present with a marked thrombocytosis but the leukocyte count is usually much higher. The presence of basophilia is supportive evidence for CML and the presence of the Ph chromosome is definitive. Idiopathic myelofibrosis is accompanied by distinct bone marrow fibrosis in contrast to essential thrombocythemia in which myelofibrosis is not present or is minimal.

Patients with a myelodysplastic syndrome or acute myeloid leukemia associated with the de novo 5q- chromosome abnormality or inv(3) may present with thrombocytosis. The megakaryocytes in the 5q- syndrome are usually smaller than in essential thrombocythemia and, characteristically, the nuclei are hypolobulated or nonlobulated. The process associated with abnormalities of chromosome 3 has features more of an acute process, either acute myeloid leukemia or a myelodysplastic syndrome, with dysplastic changes in the erythroid and granulocytic cells; the megakaryocytes are small with nonlobulated nuclei.

Treatment and Prognosis. The principal aim of therapeutic intervention in essential thrombocythemia is to decrease the platelet count and platelet aggregation so as to diminish the risk of thromboembolic and hemorrhagic phenomena; large vessel thrombosis is the primary clinical complication. Myelosuppressive options include treatment with hydroxyurea, busulfan, and ^{32}P. Because of the possible long-term complications of

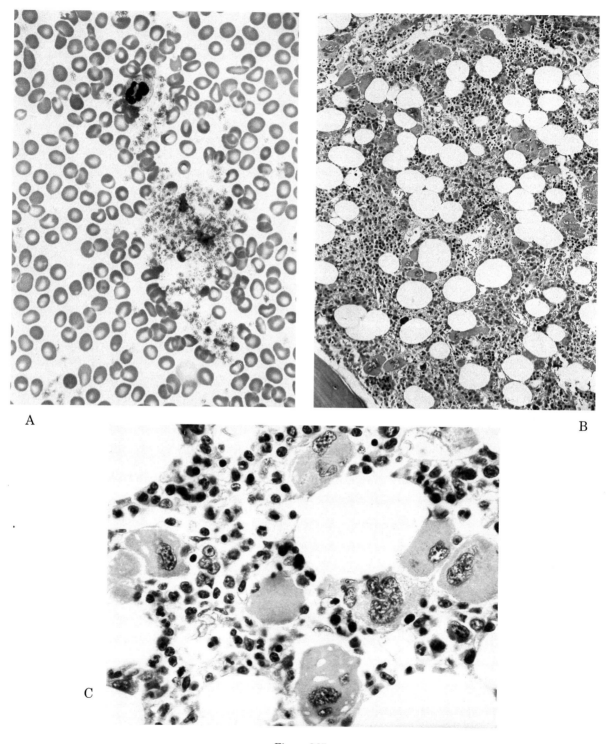

Figure 265
ESSENTIAL THROMBOCYTHEMIA

A. Blood smear from a 57-year-old male with a platelet count of 1700×10⁹/L. There is a cluster of large platelets. (Wright-Giemsa stain)

B. Bone marrow biopsy obtained at the same time as the specimen in A. There is a marked increase in megakaryocytes which occur both singly and in aggregates. Many of the megakaryocytes are unusually large. (Hematoxylin and eosin stain)

C. High magnification of the specimen in B. (Hematoxylin and eosin stain)

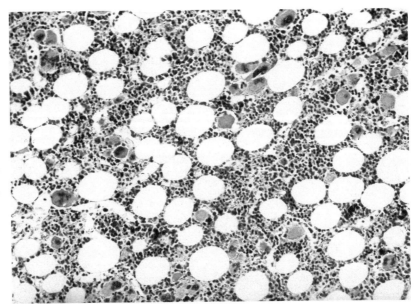

Figure 266
ESSENTIAL
THROMBOCYTHEMIA
Bone marrow biopsy from a 66-year-old woman with a platelet count of 1200×10⁹/L and a normal hemoglobin level and leukocyte count. The marrow is slightly hypercellular for the age of the patient. Megakaryocytes are increased. (Hematoxylin and eosin stain)

busulfan and ³²P therapy, hydroxyurea is the preferred approach. Antiplatelet aggregating agents that may be used include aspirin and dipyridamole (111). Anagrelide, a drug with a potent antiaggregating effect on platelets, has been successful in decreasing the platelet count in essential thrombocythemia, polycythemia vera, and CML with minimal side effects (113).

Essential thrombocythemia in patients less than 40 years of age appears to be accompanied by a more benign clinical course than in older individuals (110). It is frequently detected incidentally in this age group and the incidence of serious thrombotic hemorrhagic complications is low. Because of this, it has been suggested that these patients may be managed more conservatively than older patients.

Eighty percent of patients with essential thrombocythemia survive 5 to 8 years. A 2 to 5 percent incidence of evolution to acute leukemia has been reported (104,107,109).

CHRONIC IDIOPATHIC MYELOFIBROSIS (AGNOGENIC MYELOID METAPLASIA)

Definition. A chronic myeloproliferative disorder characterized by a panmyelosis, bone marrow fibrosis, and extramedullary hematopoiesis. Idiopathic myelofibrosis (IM) appears to be a clonal disorder of hematopoietic cells; the fibrosis is an epiphenomenon (120,128).

Incidence and Clinical Findings. Idiopathic myelofibrosis occurs primarily in adults, with a median age of approximately 60 to 67 years; rare cases have been reported in children (124,128). There is a male predominance in most reported series (125,126).

The patients usually present with fatigue, weight loss, fever, and hepatosplenomegaly. Lymphadenopathy is uncommon at the onset of the disease.

Laboratory Findings. The hematologic parameters may show considerable variability at the time of diagnosis (119,123). In one reported series, the hemoglobin level was less than 10 g/dL in 50 percent of patients and less than 8 g/dL in 20 percent (123). The leukocyte count also varies substantially and may be low, normal, or increased (123,126). Forty percent of patients in one study had counts between 10×10⁹/L and 25×10⁹/L. The platelet count was less than 150×10⁹/L in 37 percent of patients and exceeded 500×10⁹/L in 13 percent (126). Reticulocytosis may be present. The neutrophil alkaline phosphatase level is usually elevated but may be normal or decreased (128). Positive acid and sucrose hemolysis tests, similar to the findings in paroxysmal nocturnal hemoglobinuria, have been reported (121).

Radiologic evidence of sclerosis may be present (128). The proximal portions of the long bones and the axial skeleton are most frequently involved.

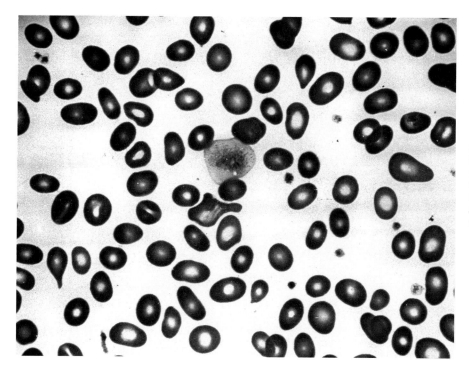

Figure 267
CHRONIC IDIOPATHIC
MYELOFIBROSIS
Blood smear from a patient with newly diagnosed idiopathic myelofibrosis. The red blood cells show moderate anisopoikilocytosis with dacryocytes and elliptocytes. An atypical platelet is present. (Wright-Giemsa stain)

Blood and Bone Marrow Findings. The most consistent findings in the blood are leukoerythroblastosis and increased red blood cell poikilocytosis with dacryocytes (fig. 267). These findings, however, may not be present at the time of initial diagnosis in a substantial number of patients (123). Atypical, large and hypogranular platelets and abnormal megakaryocytes including micromegakaryocytes, promegakaryocytes, and megakaryocyte nuclei are frequently present (figs. 267, 268). There may be a slight increase in basophils. The abnormalities in the blood may be particularly marked following splenectomy (fig. 269). Blasts are present in the blood in approximately 40 percent of patients but do not usually exceed 10 percent. An increased percentage of blasts in the blood is not always associated with rapidly progressive disease and patients may have blasts of 12 to 14 percent for many months with a relatively stable hematologic status. With progression of disease there is a tendency for increasing leukocytosis with an increased number of immature cells: megakaryoblasts, promegakaryocytes, and micromegakaryocytes are frequently observed (fig. 270). Leukopenia may occur in some patients. Ringed sideroblasts may be observed and may be 15 percent or more of the nucleated red blood cells in the bone marrow.

Histopathologic Findings. The bone marrow is hypercellular in virtually all cases; the hypercellularity is usually diffuse but may be patchy. There are varying proportions of hematopoietic cells and connective tissue elements. All three major myeloid cell lines are present in the cellular areas although one cell type may predominate (fig. 271). Megakaryocytes are increased in approximately 90 percent of cases and frequently occur in clusters. Dysplastic megakaryocytes with markedly condensed and distorted nuclei are characteristic and may be particularly prominent in biopsies with collagenous fibrosis. The marrow sinusoids are usually distended and contain hematopoietic cells; intrasinusoidal megakaryocytes may be particularly prominent (fig. 272) (118,129). The proportion of hematopoietic cells and fibrosis may vary in biopsies obtained from different sites and in different areas of the same biopsy (117,118,126,129).

The degree of fibrosis varies considerably. In the majority of patients the early changes manifest as an increase in reticulin fibers; dense collagenous fibrosis is uncommon. At this stage the bone marrow cells may show a streaming pattern due to the reticulin framework (fig. 271C). Megakaryocytes may be markedly distorted (fig. 271B)

239

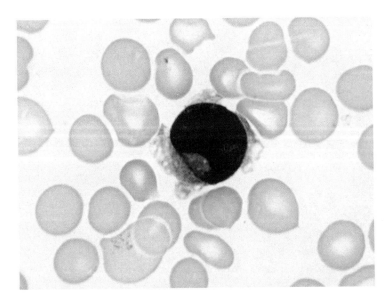

Figure 268
CHRONIC IDIOPATHIC MYELOFIBROSIS
Promegakaryocyte in a blood smear from a 67-year-old woman with a 6-year history of idiopathic myelofibrosis with 15 percent blasts in the blood. The cell illustrated is intermediate in development to a megakaryoblast and a micromegakaryocyte. One of the cytoplasmic buds has a dense area of granulation. (Wright-Giemsa stain)

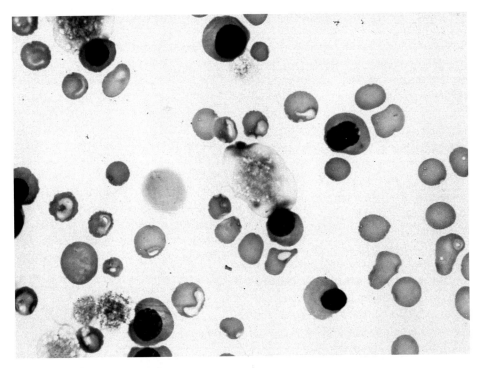

Figure 269
CHRONIC IDIOPATHIC MYELOFIBROSIS: POST-SPLENECTOMY
Blood smear from a 52-year-old man with a 4-year history of idiopathic myelofibrosis treated with hydroxyurea and splenectomy. Following splenectomy the patient developed marked normoblastemia, 600 nucleated red blood cells per 100 leukocytes, and thrombocytosis. In addition to several normoblasts there are very large and atypical platelets; one of the platelets in the center is large and partially agranular. (Wright-Giemsa stain)

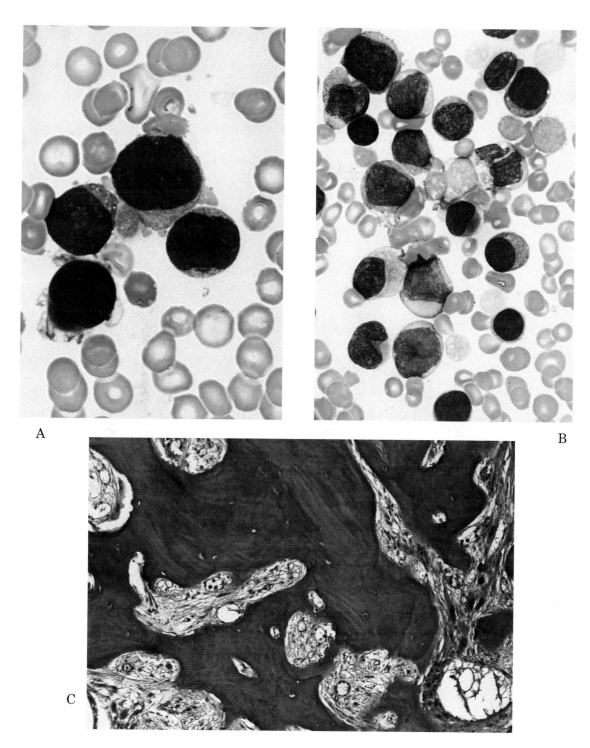

Figure 270
CHRONIC IDIOPATHIC MYELOFIBROSIS: BLAST TRANSFORMATION

A. Four immature cells in the blood smear of a patient with a 9-year history of idiopathic myelofibrosis and splenectomy. Three of the cells have a blast nucleus. The cell in the lower left is an abnormally small, late stage promegakaryocyte. (Wright-Giemsa stain)

B. Bone marrow aspirate smear obtained at the same time as the specimen in A. There are numerous blasts. Several of the immature cells are small with basophilic cytoplasm and slightly clumped nuclear chromatin. Fine azurophilic granules are present in the cytoplasm of some of the smaller cells which were interpreted as promegakaryocytes.

C. Bone marrow biopsy showing marked osteomyelosclerosis. (Hematoxylin and eosin stain)

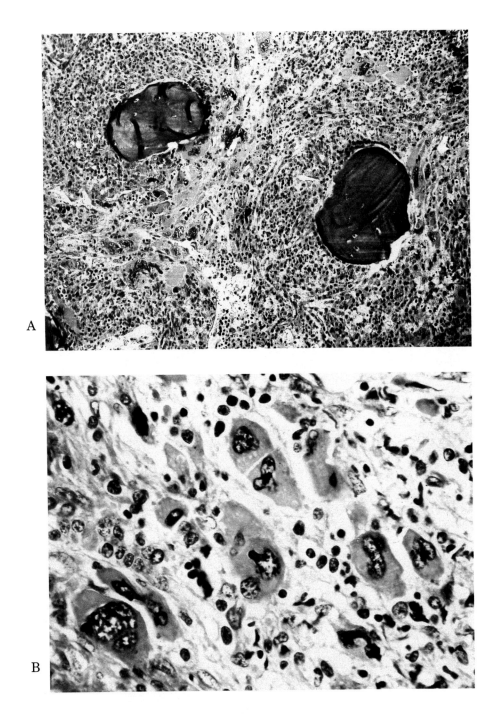

Figure 271
CHRONIC IDIOPATHIC MYELOFIBROSIS: HISTOPATHOLOGY OF BONE MARROW
A. Bone marrow biopsy from a 56-year-old woman with marked splenomegaly. The marrow is markedly hypercellular with a predominance of granulocytes and megakaryocytes. The megakaryocytes are present in band-like clusters. (Hematoxylin and eosin stain)
B. High magnification of the specimen in A showing numerous megakaryocytes, many of which are markedly distorted. (Hematoxylin and eosin stain)
C. An area of the specimen in A and B showing a predominance of granulocytes at all stages of maturation. There is a streaming effect due to reticulin fibrosis. (Hematoxylin and eosin stain)
D. Reticulin stain showing a marked increase in coarse reticulin fibers. (Wilder reticulin stain)

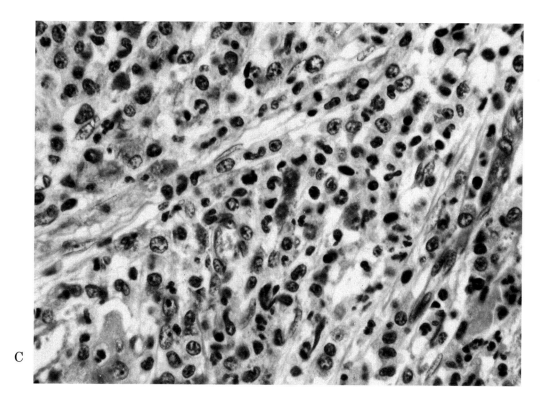

C

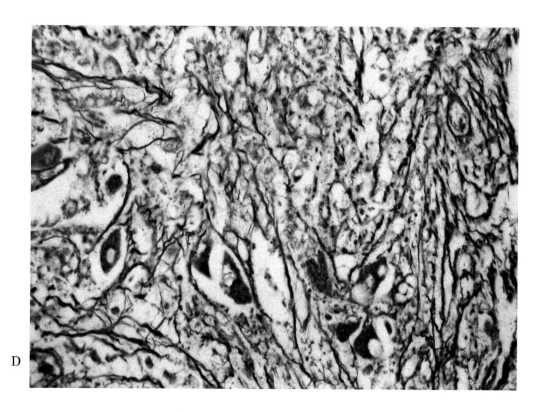

D

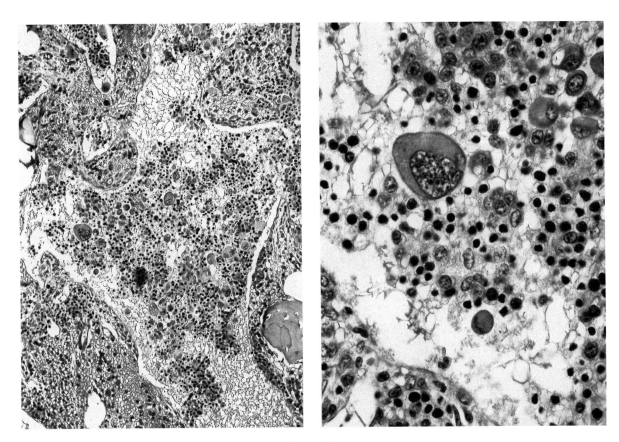

Figure 272
CHRONIC IDIOPATHIC MYELOFIBROSIS: INTRASINUSOIDAL HEMATOPOIESIS
Left: Bone marrow biopsy from a patient with long-standing idiopathic myelofibrosis. The widely dilated sinusoid contains a large number of hematopoietic cells. (Hematoxylin and eosin stain)
Right: High magnification of the specimen on the left illustrating intrasinusoidal erythroid precursors, granulocytes, and megakaryocytes. (Hematoxylin and eosin stain)

(118,128). The degree of osteosclerosis varies widely in different cases and the incidence, as reported in two series, was 54 and 36 percent (125,127). In cases with osteosclerosis, the bone trabeculae are irregularly shaped and thickened (see fig. 270C). Osteoblasts and osteoclasts are sparse (122,127).

Ward and Block (127) described three principal histologic patterns in a series of 39 biopsies obtained from patients diagnosed with idiopathic myelofibrosis: panhyperplasia, myeloid atrophy and fibrosis, and myelofibrosis and osteosclerosis. The panhyperplasia group was characterized by hyperplasia of the three myeloid cell lines: erythroblasts, granulocytes, and megakaryocytes. These cells occupied 70 percent or more of the bone marrow space. Some increase in reticulin fibers was present but there was no

collagenous fibrosis. Occasional aggregates of lymphocytes were present in a minority of patients with this pattern. The findings in these cases were similar to the findings in polycythemia vera. The myeloid atrophy with fibrosis pattern showed small areas of hematopoiesis separated by reticulin and collagen fibers, plasma cells, and stromal cells. All myeloid cell lines were usually present in the hematopoietic foci but megakaryocytes predominated. Osteosclerosis was not prominent although some biopsies showed a mild increase in the size of bone trabeculae. An absence of granulocytes was noted in some cases. The third pattern was marked by myelofibrosis and osteosclerosis. In these biopsies the bone trabeculae occupied 30 percent or more of the marrow space and were thickened and twisted. Osteoblasts and osteoclasts were not present. The amount of fibrotic tissue correlated with the amount of bone. The hematopoietic cells present were primarily megakaryocytes.

On the basis of bone marrow histopathology, Thiele et al. (123) divided idiopathic myelofibrosis at initial diagnosis into two groups. The biopsies in the first group were hypercellular with atypical megakaryocytes and left-shifted granulocytes and erythroid precursors. There was no, or only a slight, increase in reticulin fibers, primarily around vascular structures, but no evidence of collagen. The biopsies in the second group showed a moderate to marked decrease in marrow hematopoietic cells with conspicuous fibro-osteosclerotic changes. In addition to dense reticulin fibrosis, there were coarse bundles of collagen and dispersed areas of adipose tissue. These changes were accompanied by pronounced and atypical megakaryocyte proliferation. Patients in the second group had lower platelet counts and hemoglobin levels, more normoblasts in the blood, and more marked splenomegaly than the patients in the first group. The overall survival time was not significantly different in the two groups.

Other observers have reported a patchy distribution of the fibrotic process as well as a lack of correlation between amount of bone marrow fibrosis and degree of splenomegaly, duration of disease, and amount of splenic myeloid metaplasia (129).

Spleen, Liver, and Lymph Nodes. The spleen shows widely separated trabeculae and malpighian corpuscles that are small and atrophic (122). Varying proportions of the three major myeloid cell lines, erythroblasts, granulocytes, and megakaryocytes, are present in the sinusoids. The megakaryocytes, because of their size, are usually the most conspicuous. The hematopoietic cells in the liver are sinusoidal in distribution. In involved lymph nodes, the distribution of the myeloid cells is usually sinusoidal but may show a pronounced perifollicular infiltration. As in the spleen, the megakaryocytes are the most conspicuous (fig. 273). Infiltrates of other organs may occur. Fibrous hematopoietic tumors arising in extramedullary sites including the retroperitoneum, pelvis, mesentery, and pleura have been reported (116). Amyloidosis has also been observed (114).

Differential Diagnosis. Bone marrow fibrosis can occur with several disorders, both hematologic and nonhematologic. The hematologic disorders include both myeloproliferative and lymphoproliferative processes. The myeloproliferative disorders in the differential diagnosis of idiopathic myelofibrosis include CML, polycythemia vera, and essential thrombocythemia. All of these disorders have the potential to manifest bone marrow fibrosis, which usually occurs in the advanced stage of the disease. The most distinctive feature of CML is the Ph chromosome; this finding excludes the diagnosis of idiopathic myelofibrosis. The criteria for polycythemia vera and essential thrombocythemia are described in the sections on these disorders. In some patients, distinguishing between "spent" phase polycythemia vera and idiopathic myelofibrosis may be very difficult. The distinction should be based on clinical and hematologic history.

Acute myelofibrosis is marked by an aggressive clinical course. The red blood cells in the blood show minimal or no poikilocytosis and there is no or minimal splenomegaly. In addition to the fibrosis in the bone marrow, there is evidence of panmyeloid involvement and an increase in immature cells and blasts (115).

Bone marrow involvement in the non-Hodgkin lymphomas may be accompanied by varying degrees of fibrosis. The monomorphous cell population in these lesions contrasts with the polycellular population in idiopathic myelofibrosis. Marrow lesions of Hodgkin disease, particularly those with diffuse involvement, may mimic idiopathic myelofibrosis. Characteristic Reed-Sternberg cells with prominent nucleoli contrast with the megakaryocytes, which frequently have contorted hyperchromatic nuclei and inconspicuous nucleoli. A panel of antibodies should aid in distinguishing Hodgkin disease and non-Hodgkin lymphoma from idiopathic myelofibrosis.

Metastatic tumor in the bone marrow should always be considered in patients with bone marrow fibrosis, even in the context of a myeloproliferative disorder (see fig. 264). The clinical and laboratory findings in idiopathic myelofibrosis are usually sufficiently characteristic for this distinction, although immunohistochemical evaluations with panels of monoclonal antibodies may be necessary in some cases.

Treatment and Prognosis. Treatment in the early phase of idiopathic myelofibrosis is primarily supportive, with red blood cell transfusions

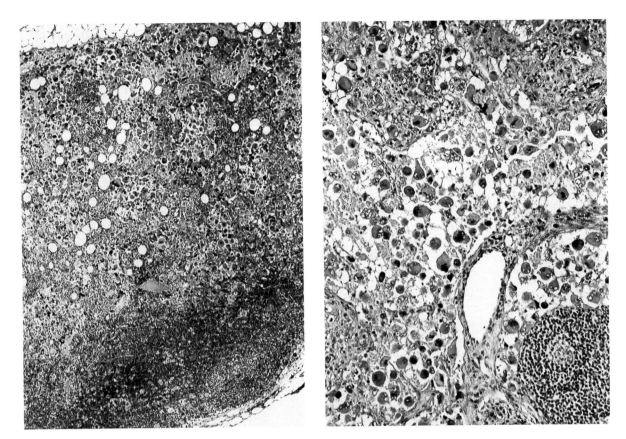

Figure 273
CHRONIC IDIOPATHIC MYELOFIBROSIS: LYMPH NODE

Left: Lymph node biopsy from a patient with idiopathic myelofibrosis and lymphadenopathy showing marked sinusoidal infiltration by myeloid cells, predominantly megakaryocytes. (Hematoxylin and eosin stain)

Right: High magnification of the specimen on the left showing numerous megakaryocytes predominantly in the sinusoid but also infiltrating the lymphoid tissue. Many of the megakaryocytes are large with hyperlobulated nuclei. (Hematoxylin and eosin stain)

as necessary to correct the anemia. Hydroxyurea may be used to control very high leukocyte and platelet counts. Splenic irradiation and splenectomy have a role in those patients with serious complications related to hypersplenism.

The biologic course in the majority of patients is prolonged; approximately 60 percent of patients live 5 years and a significant number live 10 years. The median survival period in one large series was 5.1 years, with a range of 6 months to more than 9 years (125). Favorable prognostic factors at diagnosis include hemoglobin levels of more than 10 g/dL and platelet counts of more than 100×10^9/L. The total leukocyte count, percentage of blasts and immature granulocytes in the blood, and degree of splenomegaly do not appear to be significant in predicting survival (126).

HYPEREOSINOPHILIC SYNDROME

Definition. Persistent unexplained eosinophilia of 1.5×10^9/L or greater for 6 months or longer or death before 6 months associated with signs and symptoms of the hypereosinophilic syndrome. All known causes of eosinophilia must be excluded and there should be presumptive evidence of unexplained organ involvement or dysfunction including hepatosplenomegaly, heart murmur, congestive heart failure, diffuse or focal central nervous system abnormalities, pulmonary fibrosis, fever, weight loss, or anemia (130,131,133,135–137).

Incidence and Clinical Findings. The incidence of hypereosinophilic syndrome is undetermined but the entity is very rare. The disease may manifest at any age; 70 percent of patients are between 20 and 50 years of age. There is a marked male predominance, with a male to female ratio of 9 to 1 (136,137).

Hypereosinophilic syndrome is a multisystem disease that can involve virtually any organ. Presenting signs and symptoms include weakness, fatigue, cough, dyspnea, myalgias, angioedema, and rash (130,135,136). The major manifestations are in the heart, central nervous system, skin, and lungs. Changes in these organs appear to be related to the release of injurious products from the eosinophil granules, particularly major basic protein and eosinophil cationic protein (138).

Laboratory Findings. The defining hematologic feature of this disease is an increase in eosinophils (132,137). Absolute eosinophil counts of 3.3 to 132×10^9/L have been reported (137). Mild anemia is frequent but severe anemia is unusual. The platelet count varies considerably and thrombocytosis may be present; approximately 25 to 30 percent of patients have slight thrombocytopenia. Severe thrombocytopenia is uncommon. Blood neutrophil counts are usually in the normal range but may increase concurrent with increasing eosinophils.

The vitamin B_{12} level is elevated in 60 percent of patients (130). The neutrophil alkaline phosphatase level may be normal, elevated, or decreased. Patients with more advanced disease have a higher incidence of elevated serum B_{12} levels and decreased neutrophil alkaline phosphatase scores.

Both normal and abnormal karyotypes have been reported. The reported cytogenetic abnormalities have shown no consistent pattern and include hyperdiploidy and aneuploidy, isochromosome 17, short Y, trisomy X, and trisomy 8 (130,137). The presence of a Ph chromosome, t(9;22), has been reported (130). These cases, however, should be interpreted as CML with eosinophilia.

Blood and Bone Marrow Findings. The eosinophils may manifest a wide spectrum of morphologic changes including large size, degranulation, cytoplasmic vacuolization, and nuclear hypersegmentation and hyposegmentation (fig. 274). Neutrophil promyelocytes and myelocytes, and occasionally myeloblasts may be present in the blood. In some patients the neutrophils are characterized by dysplastic changes including hypogranularity and hyposegmentation. Basophilia is present in approximately 20 to 25 percent of patients. Normoblasts may be seen.

The bone marrow is hypercellular with a marked increase in eosinophils at all stages of development (fig. 274). Macrophages with Charcot-Leyden crystals are usually present. Increased myeloblasts and promyelocytes, and dysplastic changes in developing granulocytes may be present. Megakaryocytes are usually normal in number but may be decreased. With progression of the disorder there may be an increasing percentage of blasts, immature neutrophils, myelodysplasia, and fibrosis (fig. 275).

Ultrastructural Findings. The eosinophil granules may be reduced in number. They may be homogeneous in appearance, in contrast to normal eosinophil granules which have a dense core surrounded by a less dense capsule (fig. 276).

Clinical Course. Hypereosinophilic syndrome can follow a benign or aggressive clinical course. A grading system based on the laboratory and clinical findings has evolved to predict prognosis (135). Patients with evidence of cardiac or neurologic complications or splenomegaly have a more aggressive course. The presence of myeloblasts in the blood has also been associated with a poor prognosis (136).

Differential Diagnosis. The most important point in establishing the diagnosis of hypereosinophilic syndrome is the exclusion of all possible etiologies of secondary eosinophilia. This includes parasitic infections, hypersensitivity states, allergic conditions, skin diseases, tumors, angioimmunoblastic lymphadenopathy, peripheral T-cell lymphoma, and connective tissue disorders (fig. 277).

Marked eosinophilia may occur in CML or other myeloproliferative disorders. Studies for the Ph chromosome or the BCR/*abl* hybrid gene should be performed before establishing a diagnosis; the presence of either is evidence for CML with eosinophilia.

Distinguishing between hypereosinophilic syndrome and eosinophilic leukemia is difficult, if not impossible, in some patients (134). Because of the damaging effect of the proteins produced by the eosinophil granules on various organ systems, patients may die even though the process may not be neoplastic. The characterization of a hypereosinophilic process as leukemic has been based on the presence of immature cells in the blood or blast transformation. Although blast transformation should be considered as evidence for leukemia, the

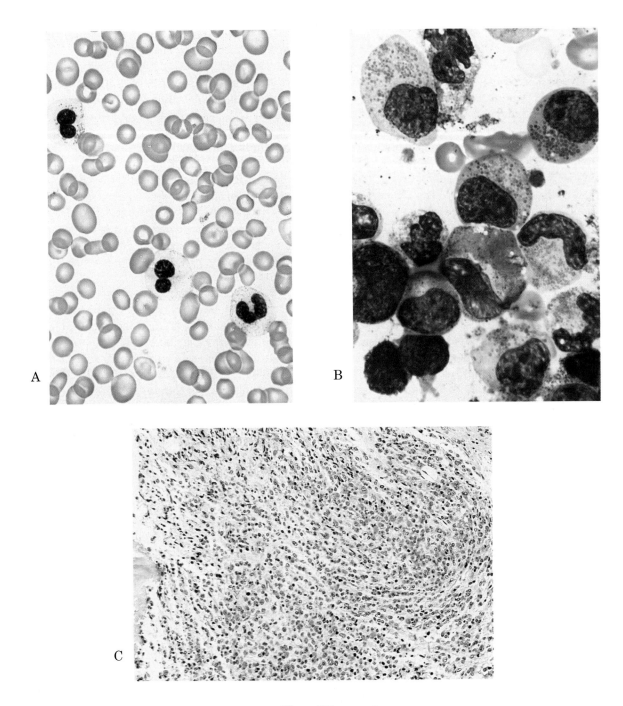

Figure 274
HYPEREOSINOPHILIC SYNDROME

A. Blood smear from a 50-year-old male with a 3-year history of hypereosinophilic syndrome with progressive bone marrow failure and multiple organ involvement. The three eosinophils show marked hypogranulation. (Wright-Giemsa stain)

B. Bone marrow smear from the patient in A showing a marked increase in eosinophils at all stages of maturation. Some of the granules in immature eosinophils have a basophilic color and two of the eosinophil myelocytes have a diminished number of granules. (Wright-Giemsa stain)

C. Bone marrow biopsy showing marked hypercellularity due primarily to an increase in eosinophils and precursors. Megakaryocytes are markedly reduced. Increased reticulin fibers are present. Despite intensive chemotherapy there was a progressive increase in marrow fibrosis and number of blasts (see fig. 275). The patient died of central nervous system failure 17 months after this specimen was obtained. (Hematoxylin and eosin stain)

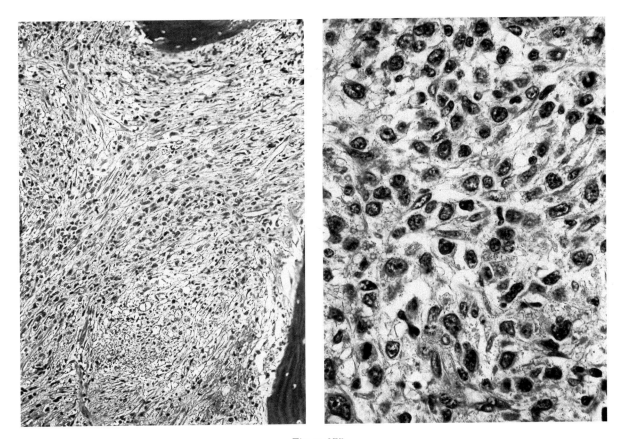

Figure 275
HYPEREOSINOPHILIC SYNDROME WITH MYELOFIBROSIS
Left: Bone marrow biopsy done 7 months after the biopsy shown in figure 274. The marrow is markedly fibrotic. (Hematoxylin and eosin stain)
Right: High magnification of the specimen on the left. Blasts and immature cells are scattered throughout the fibrotic tissue. (Hematoxylin and eosin stain)

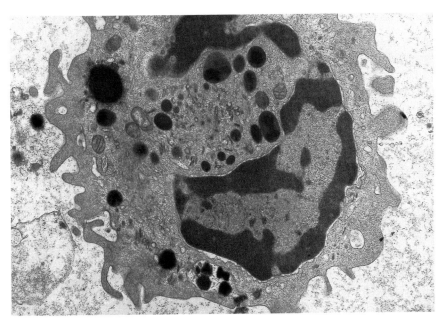

Figure 276
HYPEREOSINOPHILIC
SYNDROME:
ULTRASTRUCTURE
Electron micrograph of an abnormal eosinophil from the specimen in figure 274B. There is a decreased number of granules. The majority of the granules present are homogeneous in contrast to normal eosinophil granules which have a dense core surrounded by a less dense capsule. (Uranyl acetate–lead citrate stains, X20,000)

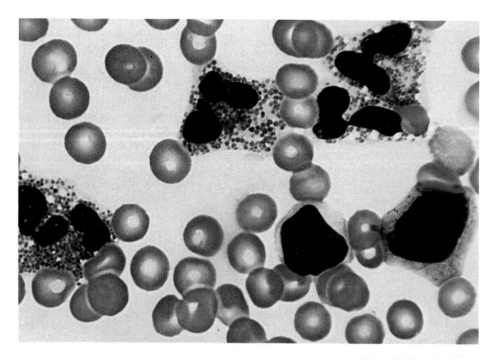

Figure 277
REACTIVE EOSINOPHILIA

Blood smear from a 5-month-old boy with 83 percent eosinophils. The number and size of the eosinophil granules are normal. A few vacuoles are present and the nuclei are slightly hyperlobulated. The eosinophilia gradually regressed with no evidence of organ dysfunction. No etiologic basis for the eosinophilia was identified. (Wright-Giemsa stain)

presence of immature cells of the granulocyte series in the blood is not in itself sufficient for a diagnosis of leukemia. In the absence of a clonal chromosome abnormality it is probably most appropriate to use the term hypereosinophilic syndrome for processes presenting with a sustained eosinophilia for which there is no demonstrated etiologic basis and in which the number of blasts is low. The treatment of these patients will be dictated in most instances by the organ damage resulting from the release of proteins from the eosinophil granule. Although the biologic evolution of individual cases may be more compatible with leukemia, the evidence for this may not be unequivocal at the onset of the process. When clearer evidence of leukemia is present, the diagnostic terminology should reflect the evolution.

Treatment and Prognosis. Therapy is principally focused on reducing the eosinophil count in order to obviate the toxic effects of the products of the eosinophil granules on various organs. Patients who are asymptomatic may be managed conservatively.

Corticosteroid therapy is generally the first used. Hydroxyurea and vincristine have also been beneficial in lowering the eosinophil count; more aggressive regimens employing multiagent therapy are used in cases resistant to less toxic drugs.

Scoring systems based on hematologic and clinical findings have been proposed to predict prognosis (135). Evidence of bone marrow failure and other features associated with acute myeloid leukemia or a myelodysplastic syndrome are adverse factors. Evidence of advanced organ dysfunction, particularly cardiac, central nervous system, and pulmonary is predictive of aggressive disease. Survival of 80 percent at 5 years has been achieved with aggressive therapeutic approaches (131).

REFERENCES

Chronic Myeloid Leukemia

1. Bain B, Catovsky D, O'Brien M, Spiers AS, Richards GH. Megakaryoblastic transformation of chronic granulocytic leukaemia. An electron microscopy and cytochemical study. J Clin Pathol 1977;30:235–42.

2. Bakhshi A, Minowada J, Arnold A, et al. Lymphoid blast crises of chronic myelogenous leukemia represent stages in the development of B-cell precursors. N Eng J Med 1983;309:826–31.

3. Barton JC, Conrad ME. Current status of blastic transformation in chronic myelogenous leukemia. Am J Hematol 1978;4:281–91.

4. Canellos GP. Clinical characteristics of the blast phase of chronic granulocytic leukemia. Hematol Oncol Clin North Am 1990;4:359–67.

5. Champlin RE, Golde DW. Chronic myelogenous leukemia: recent advances. Blood 1985;65:1039–47.

6. Clough V, Geary CG, Hashmi K, Davson J, Knowlson T. Myelofibrosis in chronic granulocytic leukaemia. Br J Haematol 1979;42:515–26.

7. de Klein A, van Kessel AG, Grosveld G, et al. A cellular oncogene is translocated to the Philadelphia chromosome in chronic myelocytic leukemia. Nature 1982;300:765–7.

8. Dekmezian R, Kantarjian HM, Keating MJ, Talpaz M, McCredie KB, Freireich EJ. The relevance of reticulin stain-measured fibrosis at diagnosis in chronic myelogenous leukemia. Cancer 1987;59:1739–43.

9. Ekblom M, Borgström G, von Willebrand E, Gahmberg CG, Vuopio P, Andersson LC. Erythroid blast crisis in chronic myelogenous leukemia. Blood 1983;62:591–6.

10. Fialkow PJ, Jacobson RJ, Papayannopoulou T. Chronic myelocytic leukemia: clonal origin in a stem cell common to the granulocyte, erythrocyte, platelet and monocyte/macrophage. Am J Med 1977;63:125–30.

11. Garfinkel LS, Bennett DE. Extramedullary myeloblastic transformation in chronic myelocytic leukemia simulating a coexistent malignant lymphoma. Am J Clin Pathol 1969;51:638–45.

12. Georgii A, Vykoupil KF, Thiele J. Classification of myeloproliferative diseases by bone marrow biopsies. Hematological and cytogenetic findings and clinical course. Bibl Haematol 1984;50:41–56.

13. Goldman JM, Lu DP. New approaches in chronic granulocytic leukemia—origin, prognosis, and treatment. Semin Hematol 1982;19:241–56.

14. Gralnick HR, Harbor J, Vogel C. Myelofibrosis in chronic granulocytic leukemia. Blood 1971;37:152–62.

15. Greaves MF, Verbi W, Reeves BR, et al. "Pre-B" phenotypes in blast crisis of Ph[1]-positive CML: evidence for a pluripotent stem cell "target." Leuk Res 1979;3:181–91.

16. Greenberg BR, Wilson FD, Woo L, Jenks HM. Cytogenetics of fibroblastic colonies in Ph[1]-positive chronic myelogenous leukemia. Blood 1978;51:1039–44.

17. Hardisty RM, Speed DE, Till M. Granulocytic leukemia in childhood. Br J Haematol 1964;10:551–66.

18. Hernandez P, Carnot J, Cruz C. Chronic myeloid leukaemia blast crisis with T-cell features [Letter]. Br J Haematol 1982;51:175–7.

19. Janossy G, Greaves MF, Revesz T, et al. Blast crisis of chronic myeloid leukaemia (CML). II. Cell surface marker analysis of "lymphoid" and myeloid cases. Br J Haematol 1976;34:179–92.

20. Kamada N, Uchino H. Chronologic sequence in appearance of clinical and laboratory findings characteristic of chronic myelocytic leukemia. Blood 1978;51:843–50.

21. Kantarjian HM, Deisseroth A, Kurzrock R, Estrov Z, Talpaz M. Chronic myelogenous leukemia: a concise update. Blood 1993;82:691–703.

22. Kattlove HE, Williams JC, Gaynor E, Spivack M, Bradley RM, Brady RO. Gaucher cells in chronic myelocytic leukemia: an acquired abnormality. Blood 1969;33:379–90.

23. Kauer GL Jr, Engle RL Jr. Eosinophilic leukaemia with Ph[1]-positive cells. Lancet 1964;2:1340.

24. Kurzrock R, Gutterman JU, Talpaz M. The molecular genetics of Philadelphia chromosome-positive leukemias. N Engl J Med 1988;319:990–8.

25. Kwaan HC, Pierre RV, Long DL. Meningeal involvement as first manifestation of acute myeloblastic transformation in chronic granulocytic leukemia. Blood 1969;33:348–52.

26. Lawler SD. The cytogenetics of chronic granulocytic leukaemia. Clin Haematol 1977;6:55–75.

27. LeBien TW, Hozier J, Minowada J, Kersey JH. Origin of chronic myelocytic leukemia in a precursor of pre-B lymphocytes N Engl J Med 1979;301:144–7.

28. Lorand-Metze I, Vassalo J, Souza CA. Histological and cytological heterogeneity of bone marrow in Philadelphia-positive chronic myelogenous leukaemia at diagnosis. Br J Haematol 1987;67:45–9.

29. Maniatis AK, Amsel S, Mitus WJ, Coleman N. Chromosome pattern of bone marrow fibroblasts in patients with chronic granulocytic leukaemia. Nature 1969;222:1278–9.

30. Marie JP, Vernant JP, Dreyfus B, Breton-Gorius J. Ultrastructural localization of peroxidases in "undifferentiated" blasts during the blast crisis of chronic granulocytic leukaemia. Br J Haematol 1979;43:549–58.

31. Marks SM, Baltimore D, McCaffrey R. Terminal transferase as a predictor of initial responsiveness to vincristine and prednisone in blastic chronic myelogenous leukemia: a cooperative study. N Engl J Med 1978;298:812–4.

32. McCaffrey R, Greaves M, Harrison TA, Revezs T, Beard M, Baltimore D. Biochemical and immunological evidence for lymphoblastic conversion in chronic myelogenous leukemia [Abstract]. Blood 1975;46:1043.

33. McGlave PB, Brunning RD, Hurd DD, Kim TH. Reversal of severe bone marrow fibrosis and osteosclerosis following allogeneic bone marrow transplantation for chronic granulocytic leukaemia. Br J Haematol 1982;52:189–94.

34. Medical Research Council's Working Party for Therapeutic Trials in Leukaemia. Chronic granulocytic leukaemia: comparison of radiotherapy and busulfan therapy. BMJ 1968;1:201–8.

35. Moloney WC. Natural history of chronic granulocytic leukaemia. Clin Haematol 1977;6:41–53.

36. Muehleck SD, McKenna RW, Arthur DC, Parkin JL, Brunning RD. Transformation of chronic myelogenous leukemia: clinical, morphologic, and cytogenetic features. Am J Clin Pathol 1984;82:1–14.

37. Neiman RS, Barcos M, Berard C, et al. Granulocytic sarcoma: a clinicopathologic study of 61 biopsied cases. Cancer 1981;48:1426–37.

38. Nowell PC, Hungerford DA. Chromosome studies in human leukemia. II. Chronic granulocytic leukemia. JNCI 1961;27:1013–21.

39. Parkin JL, McKenna RW, Brunning RD. Philadelphia chromosome-positive blastic leukaemia: ultrastructural and ultracytochemical evidence of basophil and mast cell differentiation. Br J Haematol 1982;52:663–77.

40. Pascoe HR. Tumors composed of immature granulocytes occurring in the breast in chronic granulocytic leukemia. Cancer 1970;25:697–704.

41. Rappaport H. Tumors of the hematopoietic system. Atlas of Tumor Pathology, 1st Series, Fascicle 8. Washington, DC: Armed Forces Institute of Pathology, 1966;263–7.

42. Rosenthal S, Canellos GP, Whang-Peng J, Gralnick HR. Blast crisis of chronic granulocytic leukemia. Morphologic variants and therapeutic implications. Am J Med 1977;63:542–7.

43. _____, Schwartz JH, Canellos GP. Basophilic chronic granulocytic leukaemia with hyperhistaminaemia. Br J Haematol 1977;36:367–72.

44. Rowe JM, Lichtman MA. Hyperleukocytosis and leukostasis: common features of childhood chronic myelogenous leukemia. Blood 1984;63:1230–4.

45. Rowley JD. Biological implications of consistent chromosome rearrangements in leukemia and lymphoma. Cancer Res 1984;44:3159–68.

46. _____. Chromosomes in leukemia and lymphoma. Semin Hematol 1978;15:301–19.

47. Schmidt U, Mlynek ML, Leder LD. Electron-microscopic characterization of mixed granulated (hybridoid) leucocytes of chronic myeloid leukaemia. Br J Haematol 1988;68:175–80.

48. Secker-Walker LM, Summersgill BM, Swansbury GJ, Lawler SD, Chessells JM, Hardisty RM. Philadelphia-positive blast crisis masquerading as acute lymphoblastic leukaemia in children. Lancet 1976;2:1405.

49. Shepherd PC, Ganesan TS, Galton DA. Haematological classification of the chronic myeloid leukaemias. Baillieres Clin Haematol 1987;1:887–906.

50. Silver RT. Chronic myeloid leukemia. A perspective of the clinical and biologic issues of the chronic phase. Hematol Oncol Clin North Am 1990;4:319–35.

51. Sokal JE, Baccarini M, Tura S, et al. Prognostic discrimination among younger patients with granulocytic leukemia: relevance to bone marrow transplantation. Blood 1985;66:1352–7.

52. Spiers AS. The clinical features of chronic granulocytic leukaemia. Clin Haematol 1977;6:77–95.

53. Tjio JH, Carbone PP, Whang J, Frei E III. The Philadelphia chromosome and chronic myelogenous leukemia. JNCI 1966;36:567–84.

54. Tough IM, Jacobs PA, Court Brown WM, Baikie AG, Williamson ER. Cytogenetic studies on bone-marrow in chronic myeloid leukæmia. Lancet 1963;1:844–6.

55. Ullyot JL, Bainton DF. Azurophil and specific granules of blood neutrophils in chronic myelogenous leukemia: an ultrastructural and cytochemical analysis. Blood 1974;44:469–82.

56. Vogler LB, Crist WM, Vinson PC, Sarrif A, Brattain MG, Coleman MS. Philadelphia-chromosome-positive pre-B cell leukemia presenting as blast crisis of chronic myelogenous leukemia. Blood 1979;54:1164–70.

57. Wasserman LR. The management of polycythaemia vera. Br J Haematol 1971;21:371–6.

58. Woodson DL, Bennett DE, Sears DA. Extramedullary myeloblastic transformation of chronic myelocytic leukemia. Lymph node infiltration one year before marrow blastic change. Arch Intern Med 1974;134:523–6.

59. Zittoun J, Zittoun R, Marquet J, Sultan C. The three transcobalamins in myeloproliferative disorders and acute leukaemia. Br J Haematol 1975;31:287–98.

Atypical Chronic Myeloid Leukemia

60. Kantarjian HM, Kurzrock R, Talpaz M. Philadelphia chromosome-negative chronic myelogenous leukemia and chronic myelomonocytic leukemia. Hematol Oncol Clin North Am 1990;4:389–404.

61. Krsnik I, Srivastava PC, Galton DA. Chronic myelomonocytic leukaemia and atypical chronic myeloid leukaemia. In: Schmalzl F, Mufti GJ, eds. Myelodysplastic syndromes. New York: Springer Verlag, 1992:131–9.

62. Shepherd PC, Ganesan TS, Galton DA. Haematological classification of the chronic myeloid leukaemias. Baillieres Clin Haematol 1987;1:887–906.

63. Wiedemann LM, Kahri KK, Shivjil MK, et al. The correlation of breakpoint cluster rearrangement and p210 ph1/ab1 expression with morphological analysis of Ph-negative chronic myeloid leukemia and other myeloproliferative diseases. Blood 1988;71:349–55.

Chronic Neutrophilic Leukemia

64. Bareford D, Jacobs P. Chronic neutrophilic leukemia [Letter]. Am J Clin Pathol 1983;73:837.

65. Foa P, Iurlo A, Saglio G, Guerrasio A, Capsoni F, Maiolo AT. Chronic neutrophilic leukaemia associated with polycythaemia vera: pathogenetic implications and therapeutic approach. Br J Haematol 1991;78:286–8.

66. You W, Weisbrot IM. Chronic neutrophilic leukemia. Report of two cases and review of the literature. Am J Clin Pathol 1979;72:233–45.

Chronic Myelomonocytic Leukemia, Myeloproliferative

67. Kantarjian HM, Kurzrock R, Talpaz M. Philadelphia chromosome-negative chronic myelogenous leukemia and chronic myelomonocytic leukemia. Hematol Oncol Clin North Am 1990;4:389–404.

68. Pugh WC, Pearson M, Vardiman JW, Rowley JD. Philadelphia chromosome-negative chronic myelogenous leukaemia: a morphologic reassessment. Br J Haematol 1985;60:457–67.

69. Shepherd PC, Ganesan TS, Galton DA. Haematological classification of the chronic myeloid leukaemias. Baillieres Clin Haematol 1987;1:887–906.

70. Travis LB, Pierre RV, Dewald GW. Ph[1]-negative chronic granulocytic leukemia: a nonentity. Am J Clin Pathol 1986;85:186–93.

Juvenile Chronic Myeloid Leukemia

71. Altman AJ, Palmer CG, Baehner RL. Juvenile "chronic granulocytic" leukemia: a panmyelopathy with prominent monocytic involvement and circulating monocyte colony-forming cells. Blood 1974;43:341–50.

72. Bader JL, Miller RW. Neurofibromatosis and childhood leukemia. J Pediatr 1978;92:925–9.

73. Berg SL, Phebus CK, Wenger SL. Juvenile chronic myelogenous leukemia with abnormalities of chromosomes 4 and 5. Cancer Genet Cytogenet 1990;44:55–9.

74. Brodeur GM, Dow LW, Williams DL. Cytogenetic features of juvenile chronic myelogenous leukemia. Blood 1979;53:812–9.

75. Castro-Malaspina H, Schaison G, Passe S, et al. Subacute and chronic myelomonocytic leukemia in children (juvenile chronic myelogenous leukemia). Clinical and hematologic observations, and identification of prognostic factors. Cancer 1984;54:675–86.

76. Clark RD, Hutter JJ Jr. Familial neurofibromatosis and juvenile chronic myelogenous leukemia. Hum Genet 1982;60:230–2.

77. Estrov Z, Grunberger T, Chan HS, Freedman MH. Juvenile chronic myelogenous leukemia: characterization of the disease using cell cultures. Blood 1986;67:1382–7.

78. Freedman MH, Estrov Z, Chan HS. Juvenile chronic myelogenous leukemia. Am J Pediatr Hematol Oncol 1988;10:261–7.

79. Hardisty RM, Speed DE, Till M. Granulocytic leukaemia in childhood. Br J Haematol 1964;10:551–6.

80. Herrod HG, Dow LW, Sullivan JL. Persistent Epstein-Barr virus infection mimicking juvenile chronic myelogenous leukemia: immunologic and hematologic studies. Blood 1983;61:1098–104.

81. Kaneko Y, Maseki N, Sakurai M, et al. Chromosome pattern in juvenile chronic myelogenous leukemia, myelodysplastic syndrome, and acute leukemia associated with neurofibromatosis. Leukemia 1989;3:36–41.

82. Sanders JE, Buckner CD, Thomas ED, et al. Allogeneic marrow transplantation for children with juvenile chronic myelogenous leukemia. Blood 1988;71:1144–6.

83. Smith KL, Johnson W. Classification of chronic myelocytic leukemia in children. Cancer 1974;34:670–9.

Polycythemia Vera

84. Adamson JW, Fialkow PJ, Murphy S, Prchal JF, Steinmann L. Polycythemia vera: stem-cell and probable clonal origin of the disease. N Engl J Med 1976;295:913–6.

85. Anger B, Haug U, Seidler R, Heimpel H. Polycythemia vera. A clinical study of 141 patients. Blut 1989;59:493–500.

86. Berk PD, Goldberg JD, Donovan PB, Fruchtman SM, Berlin NI, Wasserman LR. Therapeutic recommendations in polycythemia vera based on Polycythemia Vera Study Group protocols. Semin Hematol 1986;23:132–43.

87. Berlin NI. Diagnosis and classification of the polycythemias. Semin Hematol 1975;12:339–51.

88. Charache S, Weatherall DJ, Clegg JB. Polycythemia associated with a hemoglobinopathy. J Clin Invest 1966; 45:813–22.

89. Diez-Martin JL, Graham DL, Petitt RM, Dewald GW. Chromosome studies in 104 patients with polycythemia vera. Mayo Clin Proc 1991;66:287–99.

90. Ellis JT, Peterson P, Geller SA, Rappaport H. Studies of the bone marrow in polycythemia vera and the evolution of myelofibrosis and secondary hematologic malignancies. Semin Hematol 1986;23:144–55.

91. Hocking WG, Golde DW. Polycythemia: evaluation and management. Blood Rev 1989;3:59–65.

92. Kaplan ME, Mack K, Goldberg JD, Donovan PB, Berk PD, Wasserman LR. Long-term management of polycythemia vera with hydroxyurea: a progress report. Semin Hematol 1986;23:167–71.

93. Landaw SA. Acute leukemia in polycythemia vera. Semin Hematol 1986;23:156–65.

94. Laszlo J. Myeloproliferative disorders (MPD): myelofibrosis, myelosclerosis, extramedullary hematopoiesis, undifferentiated MPD and hemorrhagic thrombocythemia. Semin Hematol 1975;12:409–32.

95. Najean Y, Mugnier P, Dresch C, Rain JD. Polycythaemia vera in young people: an analysis of 58 cases diagnosed before 40 years. Br J Haematol 1987;67:285–91.

96. Schafer AI. Bleeding and thrombosis in the myeloproliferative disorders. Blood 1984;64:1–12.

97. Silverstein MN. The evolution into and the treatment of late stage polycythemia vera. Semin Hematol 1976; 13:79–84.

98. _____. Postpolycythemia myeloid metaplasia. Arch Intern Med 1974;134:113–7.

99. _____, Petitt RM, Solberg LA Jr, Fleming JS, Knight RC, Schacter LP. Anagrelide: a new drug for treating thrombocytosis. N Engl J Med 1988;318:1292–4.

100. Vykoupil KF, Thiele J, Stangel W, Krmpotic E, Georgii A. Polycythemia vera. I. Histopathology, ultrastructure and cytogenetics of the bone marrow in comparison with secondary polycythemia. Virchows Arch [A] 1980;389:307–24.

101. _____, Thiele J, Stangel W, Krmpotic E, Georgii A. Polycythemia vera. II. Transgression towards leukemia with special emphasis on histological differential diagnosis, cytogenetics and survival. Virchows Arch [A] 1980;389:325–41.

102. Weinreb NJ, Shih CF. Spurious polycythemia. Semin Hematol 1975;12:397–407.

Essential Thrombocythemia

103. Adams JA, Barrett AJ, Beard J, McCarthy DM. Primary polycythaemia, essential thrombocythaemia and myelofibrosis—three facets of a single disease process? Acta Haematol 1988;79:33–7.

104. Bellucci S, Janvier M, Tobelem G, et al. Essential thrombocythemias. Clinical evolutionary and biological data. Cancer 1986;58:2440–7.

105. Berlin NI. Diagnosis and classification of the polycythemias. Semin Hematol 1975;12:339–51.

106. Dudley JM, Messinezy M, Eridani S, et al. Primary thrombocythaemia: diagnostic criteria and a simple scoring system for positive diagnosis. Br J Haematol 1989;71:331–5.

107. Fenaux P, Simon M, Caulier MT, Lai JL, Goudemand J, Bauters F. Clinical course of essential thrombocythemia in 147 cases. Cancer 1990;66:549–56.

108. Fialkow PJ, Faguet GB, Jacobson RJ, Vaidya K, Murphy S. Evidence that essential thrombocythemia is a clonal disorder with origin in a multipotent stem cell. Blood 1981;58:916–9.

109. Hehlmann R, Jahn M, Baumann B, Köpcke W. Essential thrombocythemia. Clinical characteristics and course of 61 cases. Cancer 1988;61:2487–96.

110. McIntyre KJ, Hoagland HC, Silverstein MN, Petitt RM. Essential thrombocythemia in young adults. Mayo Clin Proc 1991;66:149–54.

111. Mitus AJ, Schafer AI. Thrombocytosis and thrombocythemia. Hematol Oncol Clin North Am 1990;4:157–78.

112. Murphy S, Iland H, Rosenthal D, Laszlo J. Essential thrombocythemia: an interim report from the Polycythemia Vera Study Group. Semin Hematol 1986; 23:177–82.

113. Silverstein MN, Petitt RM, Solberg LA Jr, Fleming JS, Knight RC, Schacter LP. Anagrelide: a new drug for treating thrombocytosis. N Engl J Med 1988;318:1292–4.

Chronic Idiopathic Myelofibrosis (Agnogenic Myeloid Metaplasia)

114. Akikusa B, Komatsu T, Kondo Y, Yokota T, Uchino F, Yonemitsu H. Amyloidosis complicating idiopathic myelofibrosis. Arch Pathol Lab Med 1987;111:525–9.

115. Bearman RM, Pangalis GA, Rappaport H. Acute ("malignant") myelosclerosis. Cancer 1979;43:279–93.

116. Beckman EN, Oehrle JS. Fibrous hematopoietic tumors arising in agnogenic myeloid metaplasia. Hum Pathol 1982;13:804–10.

117. Block M, Burkhardt R, Chelloul N, et al. Myelofibrosis-osteosclerosis syndrome. Pathology and morphology. Adv Biosci 1975;16:219–40.

118. Burkhardt R, Bartl R, Beil E, et al. Myelofibrosis-osteosclerosis syndrome—review of literature and histomorphology. Adv Biosci 1975;16:9–56.

119. Geary CG. Clinical and hematological aspects of chronic myelofibrosis. In: Lewis SM, ed. Myelofibrosis: pathophysiology and clinical management. New York: Marcell Dekker, 1985:15–50.

120. Jacobson RJ, Salo A, Fialkow PJ. Agnogenic myeloid metaplasia: a clonal proliferation of hematopoietic stem cells with secondary myelofibrosis. Blood 1978;51:189–94.

121. Kuo CY, Van Voolen GA, Morrison AN. Primary and secondary myelofibrosis: its relationship to "PNH- like defect." Blood 1972;40:875–80.

122. Rappaport H. Tumors of the hematopoietic system. Atlas of Tumor Pathology, 1st Series, Fascicle 8. Washington, DC: Armed Forces Institute of Pathology 1966;308–17.

123. Thiele J, Zankovich R, Steinberg T, Fischer R, Diehl V. Agnogenic myeloid metaplasia (AMM)—correlation of bone marrow lesions with laboratory data: a longitudinal clinicopathological study on 114 patients. Hematol Oncol 1989;7:327–43.

124. Tobin MS, Tan C, Argano SA. Myelofibrosis in pediatric age group. NY State J Med 1969;69:1080–3.

125. Varki A, Lottenberg R, Griffith R, Reinhard E. The syndrome of idiopathic myelofibrosis. A clinicopathologic review with emphasis on the prognostic variables predicting survival. Medicine (Baltimore) 1983;62:353–71.

126. Visani G, Finelli C, Castelli U, et al. Myelofibrosis with myeloid metaplasia: clinical and haematological parameters predicting survival in a series of 133 patients. Br J Haematol 1990;75:4–9.

127. Ward HP, Block MH. The natural history of agnogenic myeloid metaplasia (AMM) and a critical evaluation of its relationship with the myeloproliferative syndrome. Medicine (Baltimore) 1971;50:357–420.

128. Weinstein IM. Idiopathic myelofibrosis: historical review, diagnosis and management. Blood Rev 1991; 5:98–104.

129. Wolf BC, Neiman RS. Myelofibrosis with myeloid metaplasia: pathophysiologic implications of the correlation between bone marrow changes and progression of splenomegaly. Blood 1985;65:803–9.

Hypereosinophilic Syndrome

130. Chusid MJ, Dale DC, West BC, Wolff SM. The hypereosinophilic syndrome: analysis of fourteen cases with review of the literature. Medicine (Baltimore) 1975; 54:1–27.

131. Fauci AS, Harley JB, Roberts WC, Ferrans VJ, Gralnick HR, Bjornson BH. NIH Conference. The idiopathic hypereosinophilic syndrome. Clinical, pathophysiologic, and therapeutic considerations. Ann Intern Med 1982; 97:78–92.

132. Flaum MA, Schooley RT, Fauci AS, Gralnick HR. A clinicopathologic correlation of the idiopathic hypereosinophilic syndrome. I. Hematologic manifestations. Blood 1981;58:1012–20.

133. Hardy WR, Anderson RE. The hypereosinophilic syndromes. Ann Intern Med 1968;68:1220–9.

134. Kueck BD, Smith RE, Parkin J, Peterson LC, Hanson CA. Eosinophilic leukemia: a myeloproliferative disorder distinct from the hypereosinophilic syndrome. Hematol Pathol 1991;5:195–205.

135. Schooley RT, Flaum MA, Gralnick HR, Fauci AS. A clinicopathologic correlation of the idiopathic hypereosinophilic syndrome. II. Clinical manifestations. Blood 1981;58:1021–6.

136. Schwartz LB. Hypereosinophilic syndrome: a review. Va Med 1984;111:350–5.

137. Spry CJ. The hypereosinophilic syndrome: clinical features, laboratory findings and treatment. Allergy 1982;37:539–51.

138. Weller PF. The immunobiology of eosinophils. N Engl J Med 1991;324:1110–8.

❖❖❖

SMALL LYMPHOCYTIC LEUKEMIAS AND RELATED DISORDERS

The diseases that are collectively included in the category of small lymphocytic leukemias are morphologically, immunologically, and clinically heterogeneous; there is no term that adequately reflects the morphologic and immunologic diversity that may be present in these leukemias. Although the term small is generally used to describe the lymphocytes in these leukemias, the term may be misleading for some disorders in which the lymphocytes are of medium to large size, most notably prolymphocytic leukemia. The term chronic is equally problematic; although the majority of cases have an indolent course, a small number are similar to acute leukemia in their biologic behavior. As a result, although the term small lymphocytic leukemia is used for the diseases included in this chapter, the limitations of the term must be recognized.

The majority of small lymphocyte proliferations in the western hemisphere and Europe are of B-cell origin; these are uncommon in Japan and China. Small T-lymphocyte proliferations are uncommon in Europe and the western hemisphere. Because of the epidemiology of human T-cell leukemia-lymphoma virus infection, areas of Japan have a relatively high number of cases of adult T-cell leukemia-lymphoma. However, the incidence of other small T-lymphocyte proliferations in these areas may not be significantly higher than in other areas of the world.

As a reflection of the important interrelationship of morphology and immunologic markers in the classification of the small lymphocyte proliferations, these leukemias will be presented as two major immunologic groups: small B-lymphocyte leukemias and small T-lymphocyte leukemias.

The leukemias presented in this chapter are generally recognized entities. It is important to recognize that the classification and discussion do not include all the possible proliferative processes involving small lymphocytes. There are leukemias or leukemias/lymphomas of small lymphocytes involving the blood and bone marrow that present with such unusual morphologic or immunologic features that they preclude classification. It is prudent to admit the limits of classification in these processes and to use a more general diagnostic term, such as small lymphocyte proliferation, type unspecified. It is equally important in these instances to be cautious in predicting biologic behavior. This is particularly relevant to some of the small T-lymphocyte proliferations.

The monoclonal antibodies have been an important adjunct to the classification of the small lymphocyte proliferations. However, the results of antibody studies must be interpreted in the context of the morphologic findings. Both immunology and morphology have a major role in the classification.

B-CELL SMALL LYMPHOCYTIC LEUKEMIAS

Table 25 lists the B-cell small lymphocytic leukemias and related disorders included in this chapter. A discussion of the leukemic phase of mantle cell (intermediate differentiated lymphocytic) lymphoma and small cleaved cell lymphoma is included in the differential diagnosis of B-cell chronic lymphocytic leukemia because of the sometimes overlapping clinical and morphologic features of these disorders. The bone marrow manifestations of these lymphomas are discussed in more detail in the chapter, Bone Marrow Lymphomas.

Table 25

B-CELL SMALL LYMPHOCYTIC LEUKEMIAS

Chronic lymphocytic leukemia
    Typical
    Mixed cell type

B-prolymphocytic leukemia

Chronic lymphocytic leukemia/prolymphocytic
    leukemia

Hairy cell leukemia

Hairy cell leukemia variant

Splenic lymphoma with villous lymphocytes

Table 26

RAI CLASSIFICATION

Stage	Clinical and Laboratory Features	Median Survival (months)
0	Lymphocytosis in blood and bone marrow only	>120
I	Lymphocytosis and lymphadenopathy	95
II	Lymphocytosis and hepatomegaly or splenomegaly, or both; enlarged lymph nodes may or may not be present	72
III	Lymphocytosis and anemia (Hb <10 g/dL); lymph nodes, spleen, and liver may or may not be enlarged	30
IV	Lymphocytosis and thrombocytopenia (platelets <100×10^9/L); anemia and organomegaly may or may not be present	30

Table 27

BINET CLASSIFICATION

Stage	Clinical and Laboratory Features	Median Survival (months)
A	Hemoglobin ≥10 g/dL; platelets ≥100×10^9/L; < three anatomic sites involved*	>120
B	Hemoglobin ≥10 g/dL; platelets ≥100×10^9/L; ≥ three anatomic sites involved*	61
C	Hemoglobin <10 g/dL; platelets <100×10^9/L; or both regardless of the anatomic sites involved*	32

* Anatomic sites include cervical, axillary, and inguinal lymph nodes (unilateral or bilateral), spleen, and liver.

B-Cell Chronic Lymphocytic Leukemia

Definition. A sustained proliferation of light chain restricted, well-differentiated lymphocytes in the blood and bone marrow (5,30,32). The absolute lymphocyte count is usually in excess of 5×10^9/L.

Incidence and Clinical Findings. The annual incidence of B-cell chronic lymphocytic leukemia (B CLL) in the United States is three cases per 100,000 people (30). The disease is uncommon in Japan where it constitutes 2.5 percent of adult leukemias. The disease is uncommon in individuals under 40; rare cases in children have been reported (63). The incidence increases with advancing age; the annual incidence of newly diagnosed cases in individuals 65 to 69 years of age in 1984 to 1988 in the United States averaged 12.3 per 100,000 (56). The male to female ratio is approximately 2 to 1 (30).

The initial clinical findings relate to organ infiltration and include lymphadenopathy, splenomegaly, and hepatomegaly. Staging systems for B CLL based on laboratory and clinical findings have been developed. The two most widely used are the Rai (Table 26) and Binet (Table 27) systems (6,54). These staging systems are intended to reflect tumor burden and prognosis as noted in the median survival periods (32).

Laboratory Findings. The absolute lymphocyte count is usually in the range of 10 to 150×10^9/L; counts in excess of 400×10^9/L may occur. The hemoglobin level, platelet count, and absolute number of neutrophils may be normal or decreased. Anemia may be the result of a shortened red blood cell survival or bone marrow failure.

Fifty to 75 percent of patients with B CLL are hypogammaglobulinemic (20). This may be marked in some patients; a decrease in IgG is the

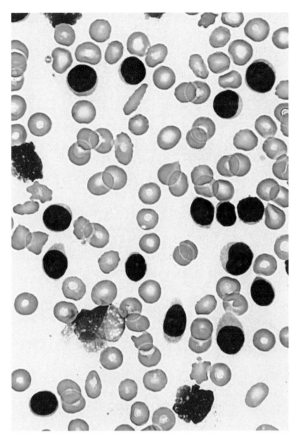

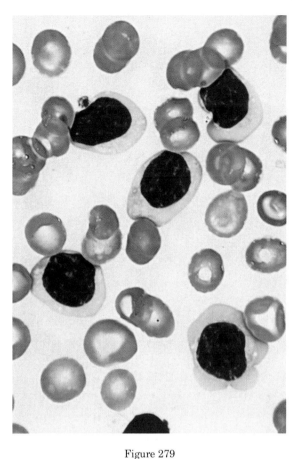

Figure 278
B-CELL CHRONIC LYMPHOCYTIC LEUKEMIA
Blood smear from an adult male with a marked lymphocytosis. The predominant lymphocytes have very sparse pale cytoplasm, round to slightly oval nuclei, and no evident nucleoli. Three damaged cells are present. This morphology is characteristic of the majority of cases of B CLL. (Wright-Giemsa stain)

Figure 279
B-CELL CHRONIC LYMPHOCYTIC LEUKEMIA
Blood smear from a woman with B CLL with a predominant population of large lymphocytes with abundant pale agranular cytoplasm; the nuclear chromatin is clumped. Nucleoli are not evident or are inconspicuous. This morphologic pattern occurs in approximately 20 to 30 percent of cases of B CLL. (Wright-Giemsa stain)

most frequent abnormality. IgM gammopathy has been reported in a low number of patients (20).

Fifteen to 35 percent of patients with B CLL develop IgG-related autoimmune hemolytic anemia, thrombocytopenia, or neutropenia. Primary red blood cell aplasia may also occur.

Blood and Bone Marrow Findings. In the majority of cases of B CLL, the lymphocytes in the blood are small, slightly larger than a red blood cell, with a high nuclear-cytoplasmic ratio. The nuclear chromatin is clumped and may show a compartmentalization phenomenon. Nucleoli are inconspicuous or not visible (fig. 278). The cytoplasm is sparse and clear to lightly basophilic. In approximately 20 to 30 percent of cases, the predominant lymphocytes are medium to

large size with a moderate amount of clear to slightly basophilic cytoplasm which usually lacks azurophilic granules (fig. 279). The nucleus is round and the chromatin is clumped; inconspicuous nucleoli and, occasionally, distinct nucleoli may be present.

The term *mixed cell type* is used for cases of B CLL in which there is a heteromorphous population of lymphocytes. Two morphologic subtypes have been included in this group (5). In one, referred to in this chapter as *mixed cell type chronic lymphocytic leukemia*, there are both large and small lymphocytes (fig. 280). The larger lymphocytes have moderately abundant, pale to lightly basophilic cytoplasm. The nuclear chromatin is clumped and nucleoli are variably prominent.

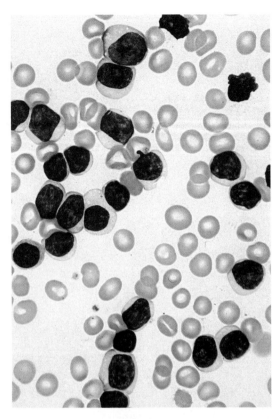 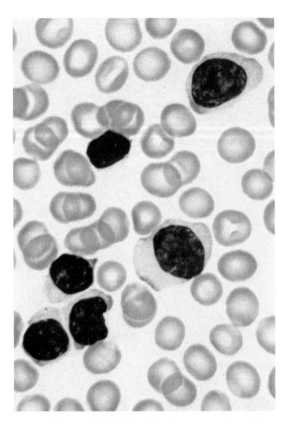

Figure 280

B-CELL CHRONIC LYMPHOCYTIC LEUKEMIA, MIXED CELL TYPE

Left: Blood smear from a man with recently diagnosed B CLL and a leukocyte count of 175×10^9/L. There is variability in the size of the lymphocytes. The larger cells have abundant pale cytoplasm. Some cells have nucleoli that are not prominent. One cell has features of a prolymphocyte. (Wright-Giemsa stain)

Right: Blood smear from a woman with B CLL with a heteromorphous population of lymphocytes; small and medium to large size lymphocytes are present. The larger lymphocytes have clumped nuclear chromatin; one has a distinct but not prominent nucleolus. (Wright-Giemsa stain)

The number of prolymphocytes is 10 percent or less. The other mixed cell type, *chronic lymphocytic leukemia/prolymphocytic leukemia (CLL/PL)*, is discussed later in this section.

In a small number of cases of B CLL, the lymphocyte cytoplasm contains clear rod-like structures which on electron microscopy contain crystalline structures (fig. 281). With immunofluorescent studies, the crystals are shown to contain immunoglobulin.

The lymphocytes in the bone marrow smears from cases of B CLL have the same cytologic features as those in the blood, although many appear to have less cytoplasm. There is no increase in lymphoblasts but prolymphocytes may be present.

Histopathologic Findings. The pattern of bone marrow involvement is generally catego-

rized into three types: diffuse, focal, and interstitial (36,57). Combinations of these types, such as focal and interstitial, occur. In the diffuse type there is extensive replacement of fat in large areas of the bone marrow (fig. 282); the entire expanded interstitium between bone trabeculae is replaced by small lymphocytes. In some cases, there is a substantial number of residual normal hematopoietic cells scattered throughout the lymphocytic infiltrate and islands of erythroid and granulocytic precursors may be present; megakaryocytes may be scattered among the lymphocytes. The focal pattern is characterized by distinct, randomly distributed aggregates of lymphocytes (fig. 283). There are usually abundant residual normal hematopoietic cells. In the interstitial pattern, there is preservation of the

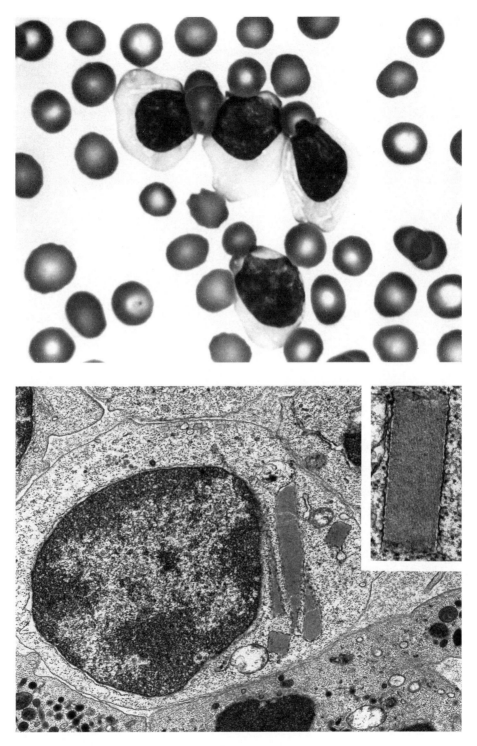

Figure 281
B-CELL CHRONIC LYMPHOCYTIC LEUKEMIA: CYTOPLASMIC INCLUSIONS

Top: Blood smear from a patient with B CLL showing three lymphocytes with rectangular, lucent cytoplasmic inclusions. The inclusions were IgM-kappa positive on fluorescent study. (Wright-Giemsa stain)

Bottom: Electron micrograph of a lymphocyte from the specimen on top. Several membrane-bound crystalline structures are present. Inset: high magnification of one of the inclusions showing a periodicity in the crystalline structure. (Uranyl acetate–lead citrate stains, X18,000; inset X54,000)

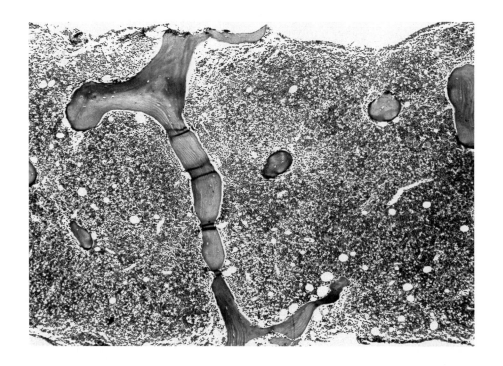

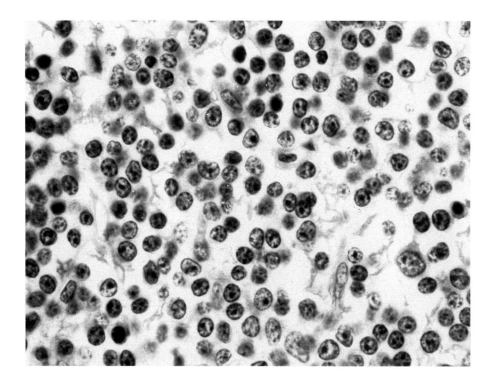

Figure 282
B-CELL CHRONIC LYMPHOCYTIC LEUKEMIA: DIFFUSE BONE MARROW INVOLVEMENT
Top: Bone marrow biopsy from a patient with B CLL showing a diffuse pattern of involvement. Virtually the entire marrow is replaced by small lymphocytes, with a marked reduction in fat cells and normal hematopoietic cells. (Hematoxylin and eosin stain)
Bottom: High magnification of the specimen on top showing a predominant population of small lymphocytes with condensed nuclear chromatin and small but distinct nucleoli. A small number of lymphocytes with more prominent nucleoli are present. There are no mitotic figures. (Hematoxylin and eosin stain)

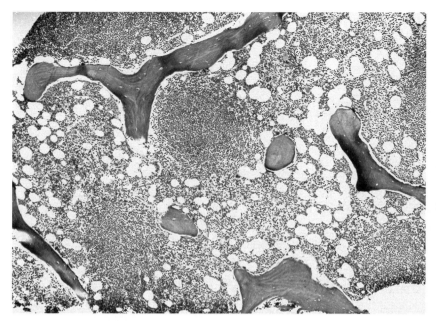

Figure 283
B-CELL CHRONIC
LYMPHOCYTIC
LEUKEMIA: FOCAL BONE
MARROW INVOLVEMENT
Bone marrow biopsy from a case of B CLL showing relatively well-demarcated focal collections of well-differentiated lymphocytes. The surrounding marrow is normal. (Hematoxylin and eosin stain)

overall marrow architecture (fig. 284). The lymphocytes infiltrate the interstitium to a greater or lesser degree. This type is usually accompanied by substantial residual normal hematopoiesis (fig. 284). In some instances the interstitium shows almost complete replacement of normal hematopoietic cells by small lymphocytes despite the preservation of fat tissue.

There can be substantial variability in the pattern of involvement in different areas of a biopsy. If any area fulfills the criteria for diffuse involvement, the process should be classified as diffuse.

The lymphocytes in bone marrow sections reflect the cytology in the smear; they generally have a high nuclear-cytoplasmic ratio, condensed nuclear chromatin, and inconspicuous nucleoli. Mitotic figures are sparse or not found. It is important to distinguish mitotic figures in normoblasts from lymphocytes.

In some cases of B CLL, the bone marrow sections show prolymphocytes with less condensed chromatin and distinct nucleoli. The number of prolymphocytes may be greater than anticipated from the smears. They may be randomly scattered or in foci of transformation similar to those that occur in the lymph nodes in B CLL and well-differentiated lymphocytic lymphoma. The foci of transformation may also contain cells larger than prolymphocytes, with finely dispersed nuclear chromatin and prominent, eosinophilic nucleoli

(fig. 285). Foci of transformation do not necessarily herald a more aggressive stage of the disease.

Reticulin stains show an increase in reticulin fibers in approximately 25 percent of cases.

Cytochemical Findings. Cytochemistry has no major role in the diagnosis of B CLL. The cells in some cases are periodic acid–Schiff (PAS) positive but this is a nonspecific finding.

Ultrastructural Findings. The small lymphocyte in B CLL typically has a moderate amount of cytoplasm with single ribosomes and polyribosomes, a small Golgi region, rare profiles of rough endoplasmic reticulum, and a small number of electron-dense granules (9). The nuclei are round to slightly indented with condensed chromatin and small nucleoli; cytoplasmic inclusions are present in some lymphocytes in 10 to 20 percent of cases and include ribosome-lamella complexes, globular immunoglobulin inclusions, and crystalline immunoglobulin inclusions (see fig. 281). Ribosome-lamella complexes, which have been most frequently associated with hairy cell leukemia and which are composed of a cylindrical arrangement of ribosome-like particles and filamentous lamellae, may be observed occasionally in B CLL.

Immunologic Findings. The proliferating lymphocytes in B CLL express light chain restricted surface immunoglobulin (SIg); intracytoplasmic immunoglobulin (CIg) has been

261

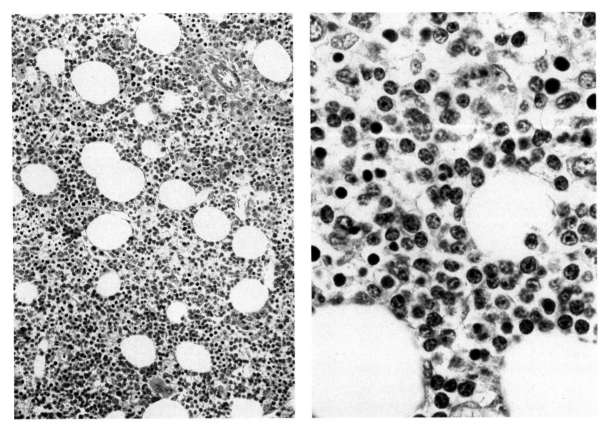

Figure 284

B-CELL CHRONIC LYMPHOCYTIC LEUKEMIA: INTERSTITIAL PATTERN OF BONE MARROW INVOLVEMENT

Left: Bone marrow biopsy from a case of B CLL showing preservation of the normal architecture. The mature lymphocytes infiltrate the interstitium with substantial sparing of normal hematopoietic cells. There is an increase in red blood cell precursors. (Hematoxylin and eosin stain)

Right: High magnification of the specimen on the left showing an area of interstitium with a predominant population of small, well-differentiated lymphocytes. Scattered normoblasts and granulocytes are present. (Hematoxylin and eosin stain)

Figure 285
B-CELL CHRONIC
LYMPHOCYTIC
LEUKEMIA: FOCUS
OF TRANSFORMATION

Bone marrow biopsy from a patient with B CLL showing one of several small foci of transformed lymphocytes. The transformed lymphocytes are larger than the mature lymphocytes at the periphery of the field, have more dispersed chromatin, and distinct, variably prominent nucleoli. (Hematoxylin and eosin stain)

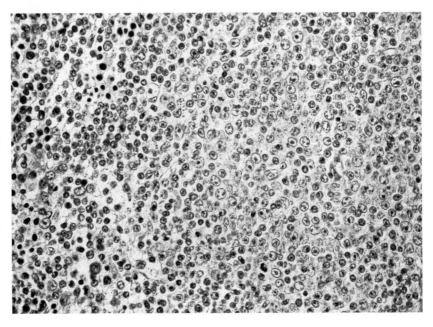

Table 28

IMMUNOPHENOTYPE OF SMALL B-LYMPHOCYTE PROLIFERATIONS*

	SIg**	SIg Intensity	CD5	CD10	CD11c	CD22	CD23	CD24	CD25	B-ly-7	MR+	FMC7
CLL	μ, μ+δ, δ	+	+	−	−/+	−/+	+	+	+/−	−	+	−/+
PL	μ, μ+δ	++	+/−	−/+	−	+/−	−/+	+	−	−	−	+
HCL	γ, γ+, other	++	−	−	+	+	−	−/+	+	+	−/+	+
SLVL	μ, μ+δ, γ	++	−/+	−/+	+/−	+	−/+	+	−	−/+	−	+
MCL	μ, μ+δ, μ+γ	++	+	−/+	−	+	−/+	+	−	−	−/+	+
SCCL	μ, μ+δ, γ+	++	−	+	−	+	−/+	+	−	−	−/+	+

*The lymphocytes in all disorders express pan–B-cell antigens (CD19, CD20) and are negative for terminal deoxynucleotidyltransferase (TdT)
**Heavy chain type; μ=IgM, δ=IgD, γ=IgG
+Mouse red blood cell rosettes

CLL: Chronic lymphocytic leukemia
PL: Prolymphocytic leukemia
HCL: Hairy cell leukemia
SLVL: Splenic lymphoma with villous lymphocytes
MCL: Mantle cell (intermediate differentiated lymphocytic) lymphoma
SCCL: Small cleaved cell lymphoma

reported by some observers (25,27,51). The intensity of the surface immunoglobulin varies but is usually faint, less than on normal small B lymphocytes. In approximately 20 to 30 percent of cases of B CLL the lymphocytes manifest no or very weak surface immunoglobulin (23,27). IgM is the prevalent heavy chain type followed by IgM and IgD, or IgD alone (23,25,27). A high percentage of the lymphocytes form spontaneous rosettes with mouse erythrocytes; this finding is highly correlated with B CLL (5).

Lymphocytes from cases of B CLL react with monoclonal antibody directed against the human leukocyte antigen, D-related (HLA-DR) locus and cells from the majority of cases express CD5 and CD23. The lymphocytes also express CD19, CD20, and CD24. Approximately 25 percent of cases express CD22 (3,20,23), about 15 to 20 percent faintly express CD11c, and 50 percent faintly express CD25 (23,28,68). In some studies, the lymphocytes in a higher percent of cases of B CLL express CD11c and CD25, but less intensely than in hairy cell leukemia (56a). The lymphocytes in 20 to 30 percent of cases express myelomonocytic antigens (51a). B CLL lymphocytes show immunoglobulin gene rearrangement. The immunophenotypic characteristics of B

CLL and other major small B-lymphocyte proliferations are presented in Table 28.

Cytogenetic Findings. Clonal cytogenetic abnormalities can be demonstrated in 50 to 60 percent of patients with B CLL when B-cell mitogenic stimulation is used. The most frequently occurring abnormalities are trisomy for chromosome 12 and abnormalities of 13q, 14q, 6q, and 11 (figs. 286, 287) (33).

Differential Diagnosis. The differential diagnosis of B CLL includes several disorders that are discussed elsewhere in this chapter. Additional considerations include lymphomas of small lymphocytes with blood involvement and persistent polyclonal B lymphocytosis.

The primary discussion of the non-Hodgkin lymphomas is presented in the chapter, Bone Marrow Lymphomas. However, because blood involvement in mantle cell and small cleaved cell lymphomas may be confused with B CLL, a brief discussion of the blood manifestations of these two lymphomas is presented here (18,62). The magnitude of the lymphocytosis is not a reliable distinguishing feature since both small cleaved cell lymphoma and mantle cell lymphoma may present with a marked lymphocytosis.

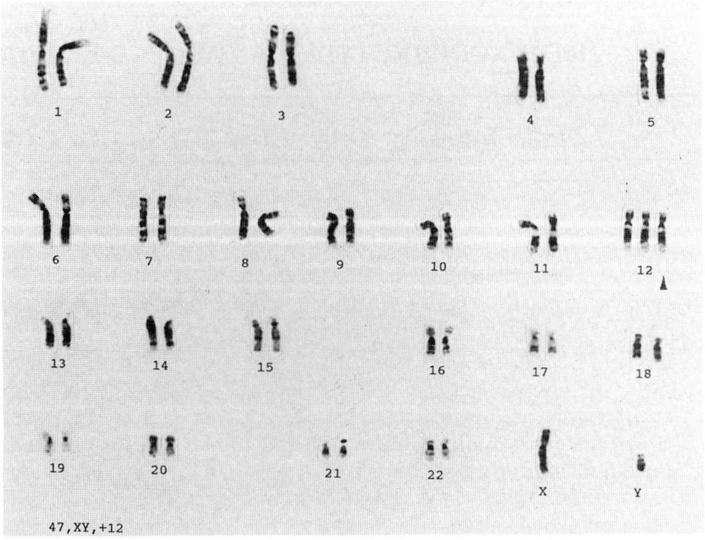

Figure 286
B-CELL CHRONIC
LYMPHOCYTIC LEUKEMIA:
TRISOMY FOR CHROMOSOME 12
Karyotype of a lymphocyte from a patient with
B CLL showing an extra copy of chromosome 12.
(G-banded, Wright-Giemsa stained)

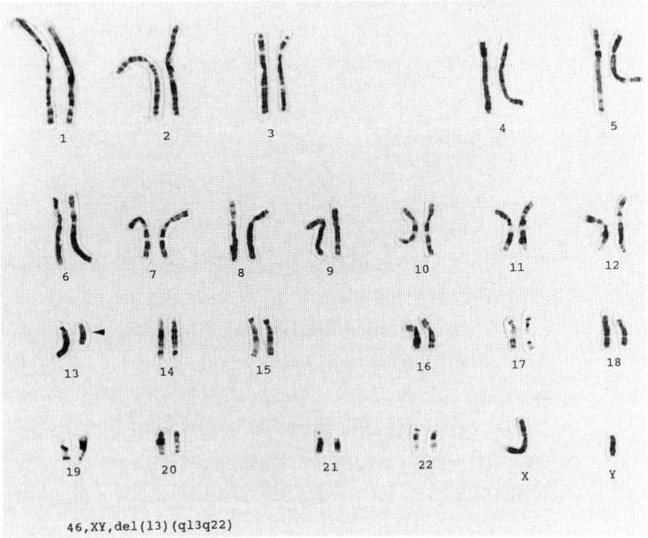

Figure 287
CHRONIC LYMPHOCYTIC LEUKEMIA:
13q- CHROMOSOME ABNORMALITY
Karyotype of a lymphocyte from a patient with
newly diagnosed B CLL. There is a clonal abnormality involving partial deletion of the long arm of chromosome 13 at bands q13q22. (G-banded, Wright-
Giemsa stained)

The lymphocytes in the blood in small cleaved cell lymphoma are usually relatively uniform in size and have a very high nuclear-cytoplasmic ratio. The chromatin is clumped and nucleoli are not usually present. The nuclei of a varying proportion of the lymphocytes are deeply cleft, frequently appearing bisected (fig. 288). If more than an occasional lymphocyte with a deeply cleft nucleus is present in what appears to be B CLL, membrane surface markers should be performed. The small cleaved cell lymphoma cells express CD10, are CD5 and CD23 negative, and have intense surface immunoglobulin, all of which contrast to the immunologic characteristics of the small lymphocytes of B CLL (Table 28) (70). The bone marrow biopsy in

small cleaved cell lymphoma usually is characterized by a paratrabecular distribution of the lymphocytic infiltrate, whereas in CLL focal marrow involvement is random.

The leukocyte count in the leukemic phase of mantle cell lymphoma may be markedly increased; in one series the counts ranged from 26 to 269×10^9/L (18). The lymphocytes in blood and marrow smears show more variability in size and nuclear-cytoplasmic characteristics than the lymphocytes of typical B CLL and range from small lymphocytes with condensed nuclear chromatin to larger cells with more open chromatin and distinct nucleoli (fig. 289). The majority of the lymphocytes are of medium size. The nuclear contour varies from round to markedly

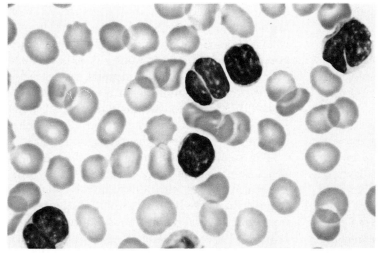

Figure 288
SMALL CLEAVED CELL LYMPHOMA:
BLOOD INVOLVEMENT

Blood smear from a man presenting with a leukocyte count of 40×10^9/L. The majority of lymphocytes were as illustrated, with a high nuclear-cytoplasmic ratio, clumped nuclear chromatin, and cleft or irregularly shaped nuclei. A lymph node biopsy showed a follicular, small cleaved cell lymphoma. (Wright-Giemsa stain)

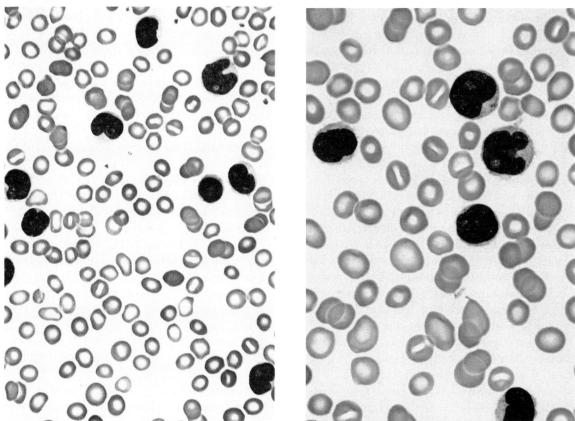

Figure 289
MANTLE CELL LYMPHOMA: BLOOD INVOLVEMENT

Left: Blood smear from a 47-year old-man with a leukocyte count of 47×10^9/L and the lymph node findings of intermediate lymphocytic lymphoma. There is considerable variability in the appearance of the lymphocytes, which expressed CD19, CD5, and intense surface immunoglobulin, and were CD10 negative. The lymphocytes range from small to large; lymphocytes with distorted nuclei and relatively prominent nucleoli are present. (Wright-Giemsa stain)

Right: High magnification of a blood smear from a man with a leukocyte count of 34×10^9/L. The lymphocytes show variability in size, nuclear shape, appearance of nucleoli, and amount of cytoplasm. The smaller lymphocytes have sparse cytoplasm, irregularly shaped nuclei, and indistinct nucleoli. The large cells have relatively prominent nucleoli and a moderate amount of basophilic cytoplasm. One of the cells contains coarse azurophilic granules. These lymphocytes expressed CD5 and CD19, were negative for CD10, and had strong expression of surface immunoglobulin similar to the case illustrated on the left. (Wright-Giemsa stain)

irregular; lymphocytes with cleft or lobulated nuclei are usually present. The cytoplasm may be abundant, is usually pale to slightly basophilic, and may contain coarse azurophilic granules.

The bone marrow biopsy in mantle cell lymphoma shows diffuse or focal involvement; the focal involvement may be random or, preferentially, paratrabecular. Uncommonly, the infiltrate contains naked germinal centers similar to those in the lymph nodes. The lymphocytes vary in size and degree of nuclear irregularity. Distinct nucleoli are present in some cells. The number of mitotic figures varies.

The lymphocytes of mantle cell lymphoma show kappa or lambda light chain restriction and the amount of surface immunoglobulin is usually moderate to intense, in contrast to the lymphocytes of B CLL which have weak surface immunoglobulin. The cells express pan–B-cell antigens including CD19 and CD20. In a minority of cases, a significant percentage of the lymphocytes express CD10 (18). Similar to B CLL, the lymphocytes in mantle cell lymphoma express CD5, a T-cell–associated antigen, but in contrast to B CLL, the lymphocytes in mantle cell lymphoma are usually CD23 negative (see Table 28) (70).

Persistent polyclonal B lymphocytosis is a rare disorder. There is an absolute lymphocytosis with a reported range of 3780 to 13,000/mm^3 (26,38,58). There is a female predominance. The disorder has been associated with cigarette smoking in some cases. An association with Epstein-Barr virus infection has also been reported (16). Some patients have a polyclonal increase in serum IgM and decreased IgG and IgA. The lymphocytes are small to medium sized with round to irregular nuclei. Immunophenotypic analysis shows increased polyclonal B lymphocytes. There is an accompanying decrease in natural killer (NK) lymphocytes in some instances. On molecular analysis, the lymphocytes usually show multiple B-cell clones or no clonal rearrangements. One patient in a series of five cases developed B CLL (58).

Treatment and Prognosis. The prognosis in B CLL is remarkably variable. Some patients may live for several years with few untoward consequences of the leukemic process while others have a rapidly progressive clinical course complicated by repeated infections and immune-related cytopenias. The clinical staging systems of Rai and Binet, which are a measure of tumor burden, have been shown to have prognostic relevance (see Tables 26 and 27). The median survival periods for Rai stages 0, I, and II are over 120, and 95 and 72 months, respectively (32,54), and is 30 months for stages III and IV. In the Binet system, the median survival times for stages A, B, and C are more than 120 months, 61 months, and 32 months, respectively (32).

The relevance of bone marrow histology to prognosis has been shown in several studies. In general, patients with diffuse involvement are usually Rai stage III or IV (36,57). Patients with a nondiffuse pattern, either focal, interstitial, or both, are Rai stage 0, I, or II. In addition to these staging systems, risk categories based on clinical and biochemical findings have proven relevant to prognosis (20,30).

Cytogenetic studies have shown a correlation between karyotypic abnormalities and survival in B CLL (33). Patients with a normal karyotype or only a single clonal abnormality have a longer survival time than patients with complex clonal abnormalities.

Membrane surface marker studies have shown that high intensity surface IgM, high expression of FMC7, and low expression of CD23 are associated with short survival (25). CD13 and CD33 expressions have been associated with diffuse marrow involvement and advanced clinical stage (51a).

Not all patients with B CLL need treatment when initially diagnosed and some patients may do satisfactorily for several years without therapeutic intervention. Treatment, when necessary, has generally included corticosteroids and alkylating agents such as chlorambucil or cyclophosphamide (15,30). Nucleoside analogs such as fludarabine are increasingly used with beneficial results (15).

Prolymphocytoid Transformation of B-Cell Chronic Lymphocytic Leukemia. In some cases of B CLL there is a morphologic and clinical evolution referred to as prolymphocytoid transformation. This is characterized by increasing splenomegaly and lymphadenopathy, and an increasing number of prolymphocytes in the blood (fig. 290) (21,35,40). The bone marrow sections may show large foci of prolymphocytes in transformation centers or prolymphocytes evenly dispersed in the small lymphocyte infiltration. There may be a relatively sharp demarcation

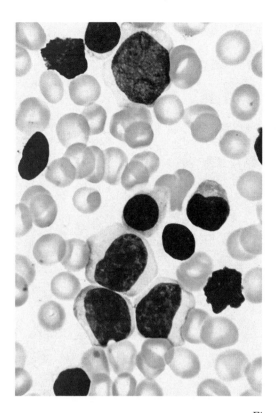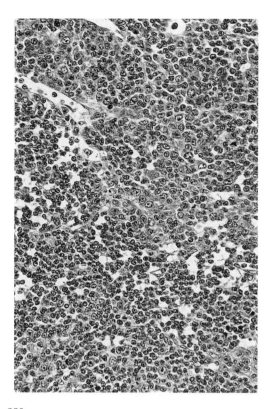

Figure 290
B-CELL CHRONIC LYMPHOCYTIC LEUKEMIA: PROLYMPHOCYTOID TRANSFORMATION

Left: Blood smear from a 57-year-old woman with a 2-year history of untreated CLL. The leukocyte count at diagnosis was 11×10^9/L with 73 percent small lymphocytes. The leukocyte count at the time of this smear was 187×10^9/L. There are small lymphocytes and prolymphocytoid lymphocytes with abundant, lightly basophilic cytoplasm, fine chromatin, and variably prominent nucleoli. Approximately 50 percent of the lymphocytes are prolymphocytoid forms. At the time of this smear the patient had splenomegaly and generalized lymphadenopathy. (Wright-Giemsa stain)

Right: Bone marrow biopsy from the same case showing a focus of prolymphocytoid lymphocytes partially surrounded by small lymphocytes. (Hematoxylin and eosin stain)

between the prolymphocytes and the smaller lymphocytes (fig. 290). Prolymphocytoid transformation occurs following a variable period of chronic phase CLL; in the original report of the entity, the time interval for the preexisting chronic phase varied from 1.3 to 5 years (21). The "prolymphocytoid" cells in prolymphocytoid transformation have the same surface immunoglobulin as the previously predominant small lymphocytes. In the initial report, the prolymphocytoid cells had sparse amounts of surface immunoglobulin similar to the small lymphocytes in chronic phase CLL. Subsequent studies have demonstrated that the prolymphocytoid lymphocytes in some cases have moderate to intense surface immunoglobulin (35). The prolymphocytes may retain expression of CD5 and form spontaneous rosettes with mouse erythrocytes; in some instances, however, they lose reactivity for antibody to CD5 and rosetting capacity for mouse erythrocytes and gain expression of FMC7 and FRA4 (41).

The blood and bone marrow findings in prolymphocytoid transformation may be indistinguishable from chronic lymphocytic leukemia/prolymphocytic leukemia. The prolymphocytoid cells are frequently more heteromorphous than the prolymphocytes in de novo B PL. The term prolymphocytoid transformation should be reserved for those cases for which there is evidence of a previously existent CLL.

Richter Transformation. Richter transformation is a rare complication of B CLL marked by weight loss, fever, localized lymphadenopathy, dysgammaglobulinemia, and histopathologic evidence of a pleomorphic malignant lymphoma that frequently contains multinucleated cells that

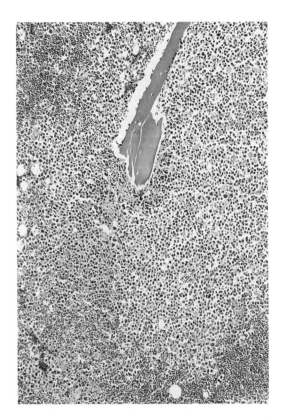 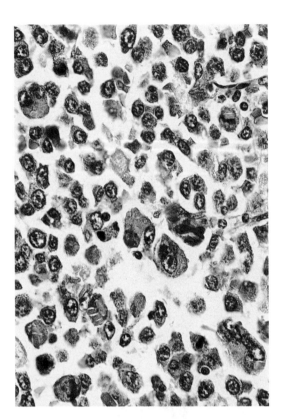

Figure 291
CHRONIC LYMPHOCYTIC LEUKEMIA: RICHTER TRANSFORMATION
Left: A marrow biopsy from a patient with a history of B CLL with a recent onset of weight loss and fatigue. The marrow biopsy shows a large focus of pleomorphic cells which reacted with B-cell antibodies. The large cells are partially encircled by small lymphocytes. (Hematoxylin and eosin stain)
Right: Some of the large cells have abundant cytoplasm containing large crystalline-like structures. The findings were interpreted as a B-cell immunoblastic lymphoma. (Hematoxylin and eosin stain)

may resemble Reed-Sternberg cells (55). The incidence is reported as 3 to 10 percent of cases of B CLL (66). Similar transformations are reported in well-differentiated lymphocytic lymphoma and plasmacytoid lymphoma. The pleomorphic lymphoma may be present in the lymph nodes, spleen, or bone marrow, or in non-hematopoietic organs. A high incidence of associated lytic bone lesions has been reported (66). Lymphocytopenia may be present; the lymphoma cells are not usually present in the blood. The bone marrow may show juxtaposition of the pleomorphic lymphoma and small lymphocyte infiltration (fig. 291). The clinical course is usually rapidly progressive and refractory to chemotherapy.

The biologic events eventuating in Richter transformation are not completely understood but dedifferentiation of the small lymphocytes has been proposed. This hypothesis is supported by studies that have shown similarities in membrane surface markers on the lymphocytes of the CLL phase and the cells of the pleomorphic lymphoma. Differences in immunophenotypic profile have also been reported and the issue is not completely resolved (20).

Another process related to the transformation of the small lymphocytes is the paraimmunoblast variant of large cell lymphoma, which has morphologic features intermediate to prolymphocytoid transformation and Richter transformation (figs. 292, 293) (53). A rare instance of evolution to a small noncleaved cell lymphoma has been noted (fig. 294) (37). These processes should be viewed as part of the morphologic spectrum of lymphocyte transformation that may occur in small lymphocyte proliferations.

The occurrence of a true histiocytic lymphoma in a patient with B CLL has been reported (67).

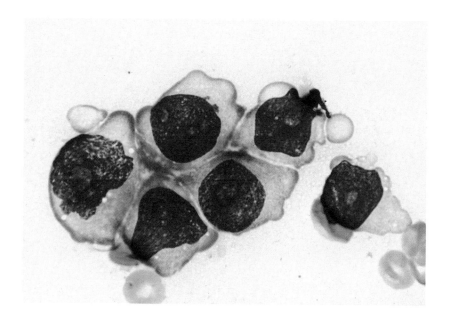

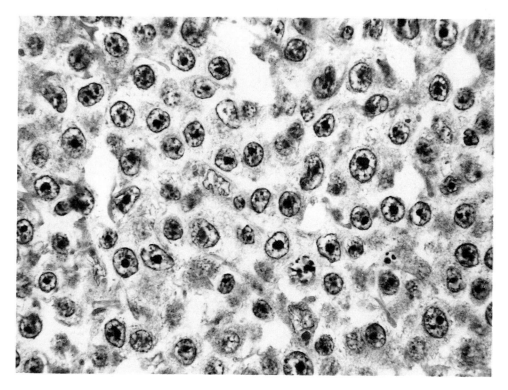

Figure 292
CHRONIC LYMPHOCYTIC LEUKEMIA: PROLYMPHOCYTOID PARAIMMUNOBLASTIC TRANSFORMATION

Top: Bone marrow smear from a 72-year-old male with an 11-year history of CLL. This marrow biopsy was preceded by a 3- to 4-month history of decreasing lymphocytes in the blood and progressive marrow failure. This bone marrow smear shows coalescent aggregates of very large cells with abundant slightly to moderately basophilic cytoplasm, slightly coarse chromatin, and prominent, usually single nucleoli. Rare cells of this type were present in the blood smear. (Wright-Giemsa stain)

Bottom: A portion of the bone marrow biopsy from the same patient showing extensive infiltration by prolymphocytes and large cells with abundant cytoplasm, dispersed chromatin, and prominent single nucleoli. The larger cells were interpreted as paraimmunoblasts, which are larger and have a more prominent nucleolus than a prolymphocyte. (Hematoxylin and eosin stain)

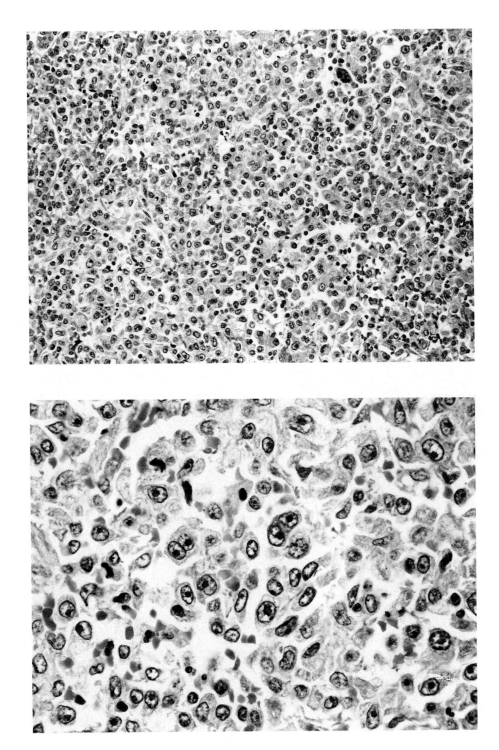

Figure 293
CHRONIC LYMPHOCYTIC LEUKEMIA:
PROLYMPHOCYTOID PARAIMMUNOBLASTIC TRANSFORMATION IN SPLEEN

Top: Portion of a spleen from a patient with a 9-year history of CLL. The red and white pulp is densely infiltrated by large cells with abundant amphophilic to slightly basophilic cytoplasm and nuclei with dispersed chromatin and prominent nucleoli. (Hematoxylin and eosin stain)

Bottom: High magnification of the same specimen showing numerous large lymphocytes with dispersed nuclear chromatin and prominent nucleoli. The abnormal cells are present both in the sinusoids and cords. (Hematoxylin and eosin stain)

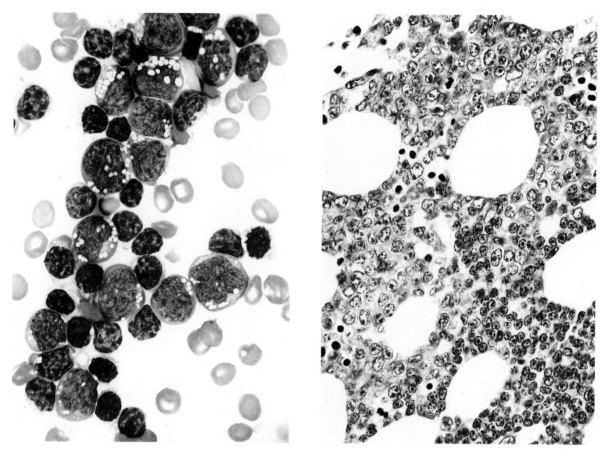

Figure 294
SMALL NONCLEAVED CELL LYMPHOMA ARISING IN A PATIENT
WITH CHRONIC LYMPHOCYTIC LEUKEMIA

Left: Bone marrow smear from a 50-year-old male with a 10-year history of B CLL treated with chlorambucil and prednisone, with a recent onset of night sweats, fever, myalgia, and prominent axillary, cervical, and inguinal lymphadenopathy. The bone marrow, as illustrated, contained two populations of lymphocytes, small well-differentiated lymphocytes and small noncleaved lymphoma cells. Cytogenetic studies of the marrow specimen showed a t(8;22)(q24;q11) chromosome abnormality in 18 of 20 metaphases. Both the small lymphocytes and small noncleaved lymphoma cells expressed IgM kappa and both cell types had the same kappa light chain restriction fragment on molecular analysis. (Wright-Giemsa stain)

Right: Bone marrow biopsy showing a predominant population of small noncleaved lymphoma cells. In the lower right is a focus of well-differentiated lymphocytes. (Hematoxylin and eosin stain)

B-Prolymphocytic Leukemia

Clinical and Laboratory Findings. Prolymphocytic leukemia was initially described in 1974 as a rare variant of CLL in which the predominant lymphocytes are prolymphocytes, large cells with coarse nuclear chromatin, prominent vesicular nucleoli, and a moderate rim of lightly to moderately basophilic cytoplasm (24,65). Two forms of prolymphocytic leukemia are recognized: B and T. Approximately 70 percent of cases are B type. The description in this section applies to B-prolymphocytic leukemia (B PL); T-prolymphocytic leukemia is discussed in the section on post-thymic T-cell proliferations.

B PL occurs primarily in older individuals; the mean age of the patients in the initial series was 64 with a range of 46 to 77 years (24). The male to female ratio is 2 to 1. Patients usually have marked splenomegaly and minimal or no palpable peripheral lymphadenopathy. Retroperitoneal lymphadenopathy may be found on radiologic examination and atypical cases with marked peripheral lymphadenopathy have been reported (49).

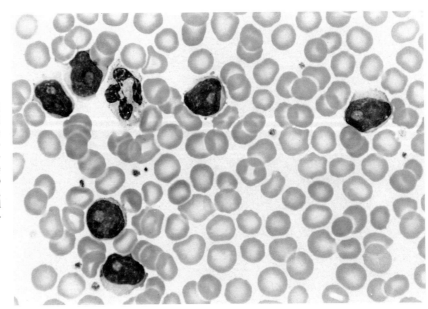

Figure 295
B-PROLYMPHOCYTIC
LEUKEMIA
Blood smear from a 71-year-old man who presented with marked splenomegaly and a leukocyte count of 50×10^9/L with a predominance of prolymphocytes. The prolymphocytes in this smear are large cells with abundant, clear to lightly basophilic cytoplasm, coarse nuclear chromatin, and prominent single nucleoli. (Wright-Giemsa stain)

The leukocyte count is usually markedly elevated and may exceed 1000×10^9/L. Anemia and thrombocytopenia are frequent manifestations (24,65). The prolymphocytes comprise 55 percent or more of the lymphocytes. The nuclear chromatin of the prolymphocyte is variably described as coarse or clumped; the chromatin density is intermediate to that of a blast and a mature lymphocyte (fig. 295). The nucleus is usually round or oval but may show some degree of indentation. There is perinucleolar chromatin condensation. The cytoplasm is slightly to moderately basophilic; some variation is usually present in different cells in the same case. Vacuoles or coarse azurophilic granules may be present. The smaller more mature lymphocytes with more condensed nuclear chromatin may also have distinct, and sometimes prominent, nucleoli. There is a monocytosis in some patients.

Histopathologic Findings. The bone marrow biopsy usually shows a diffuse or a mixed focal and interstitial pattern of involvement (fig. 296A). The prolymphocytes are medium to large with a distinct rim of cytoplasm and a round to oval nucleus. The nuclear chromatin is dispersed and a single, variably prominent nucleolus is usually present; occasional prolymphocytes have multiple nucleoli (fig. 296B). The prolymphocyte proliferation is accompanied by a population of small lymphocytes which may also have relatively prominent nucleoli. Cells larger than pro-

lymphocytes, with very prominent nucleoli and abundant cytoplasm, may be present. The term *paraimmunoblast* has been used for this cell. Focal accumulations of prolymphocytes may resemble pseudofollicles or foci of transformation. Scattered mitotic figures may be noted but are substantially fewer than found in the high-grade, large cell lymphomas with which the process may be confused.

The lymph nodes from patients with B PL show complete obliteration of the architecture in some areas and partial preservation of the sinuses in other areas (4). Most cells are prolymphocytes with prominent nucleoli; pseudofollicular growth patterns may be prominent (fig. 296C).

The spleen shows extensive infiltration of both the red and white pulp with a pseudofollicular pattern (4). The periarteriolar white pulp infiltrate may show an inverse pseudofollicular pattern, with the inner portion consisting of mature lymphocytes encircled by a rim of prolymphocytes with dispersed nuclear chromatin and prominent nucleoli. Mitotic figures are more frequent in the prolymphocytes in the white pulp area than in the smaller lymphocytes (fig. 297) (35a). The leukemic cells also diffusely infiltrate the cords and sinuses. The morphology of the prolymphocytes in the spleen is similar to that in the lymph nodes and marrow sections. Despite the immature appearance of the prolymphocytes, the mitotic rate is usually low; the combination

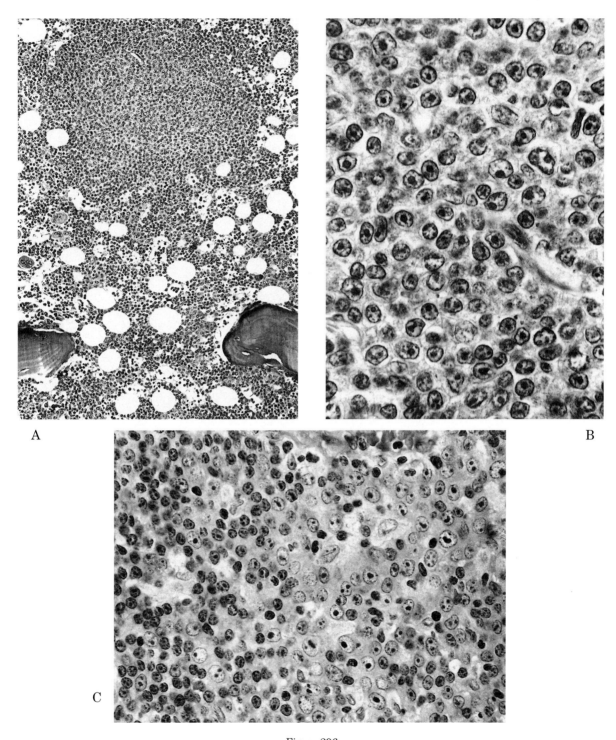

Figure 296
B-PROLYMPHOCYTIC LEUKEMIA: BONE MARROW AND LYMPH NODE

A. Bone marrow biopsy from a case of B-prolymphocytic leukemia. There is a distinct focus of lymphocytes, with spreading into the adjacent interstitium. (Hematoxylin and eosin stain)

B. High magnification of the lesion in A showing numerous prolymphocytes with dispersed chromatin and single, prominent nucleoli. (Hematoxylin and eosin stain)

C. Lymph node biopsy from the same patient. The lymph node showed a diffuse pattern of involvement with pseudo-proliferation centers containing numerous prolymphocytes and paraimmunoblasts. (Hematoxylin and eosin stain)

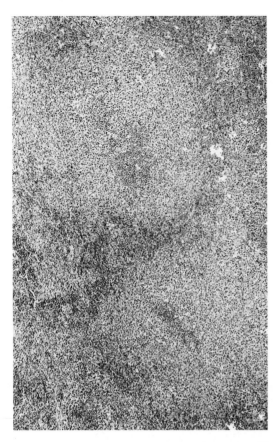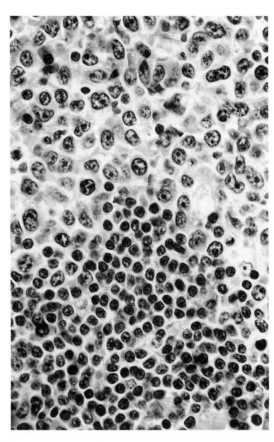

Figure 297
B-PROLYMPHOCYTIC LEUKEMIA

Left: Low magnification of a portion of a spleen removed from a patient with B-prolymphocytic leukemia. The periarteriolar white pulp shows a small central focus of small well-differentiated lymphocytes encircled by a wide margin of prolymphocytes. (Hematoxylin and eosin stain)

Right: High magnification of the specimen on the left showing the large prolymphocytes juxtaposed to the small well-differentiated lymphocytes. Mitotic figures were frequent in the prolymphocyte population. (Hematoxlyin and eosin stain)

of immature appearance and low mitotic activity has been cited as a histopathologic feature of pro-lymphocytic leukemia (4). Atypical cases with high mitotic activity have been reported (49).

Ultrastructural Findings. The pro-lymphocyte has a moderate amount of cytoplasm which contains single ribosomes and polyribo-somes, rare profiles of rough endoplasmic retic-ulum, and occasional clusters of electron-dense granules (fig. 298). Ribosome-lamella complexes and immunoglobulin crystals have been infre-quently observed. The nuclear chromatin varies from fine to moderately condensed; the single large nucleolus is centrally located.

Immunologic Findings. In contrast to the lymphocytes in typical CLL which have weak expression of surface immunoglobulin, the pro-

lymphocytes express dense surface immuno-globulin of either IgM or IgM and IgD type (39). The cells express the pan–B-cell markers CD19, CD20, and CD24. They are usually negative for CD11c and CD23 and variably positive for CD5 and CD22; they may show weak expression of CD10 (3). The prolymphocytes strongly express FMC7, in contrast to the small lymphocytes in typical B CLL (24). Unlike the small lymphocytes in typical B CLL, only a few prolymphocytes form rosettes with mouse red blood cells.

Differential Diagnosis. The differential di-agnosis of B PL includes mixed cell type CLL, large cell lymphomas, T-prolymphocytic leuke-mia, and acute monoblastic leukemia.

CLL of mixed cell type has a heterogeneous population of lymphocytes. The larger cells are

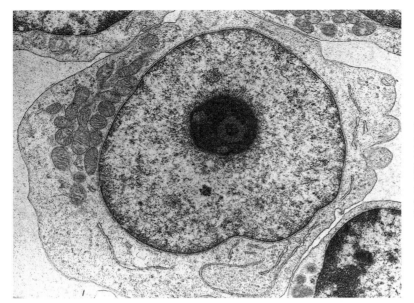

Figure 298
B-PROLYMPHOCYTIC
LEUKEMIA:
ULTRASTRUCTURE
Electron micrograph of a prolymphocyte in a blood specimen from a
patient with B-prolymphocytic leukemia. The nuclear chromatin is finely dispersed and there is a prominent nucleolus. The cytoplasm contains numerous
mitochondria and a few strands of rough
endoplasmic reticulum. (Uranyl acetate–lead citrate stains, X14,000)

approximately the size of prolymphocytes (see fig.
280). The nuclear chromatin, in contrast to that in
the prolymphocyte, is more uniformly clumped;
nucleoli may be present but are not as prominent as
in a prolymphocyte. The usually abundant cytoplasm is pale to slightly basophilic. Occasional prolymphocytes may be present in this type of CLL but
number 10 percent or less.

It may not be possible to distinguish B-prolymphocytic leukemia and T-prolymphocyte leukemia morphologically; membrane surface
markers are definitive.

Large cell lymphomas and transformations of
small cell lymphomas may uncommonly manifest
in the blood (1). The lymphoma cells in these
processes generally show more morphologic variability; the largest cells are usually larger than
prolymphocytes. The cytoplasm is variably and
sometimes deeply basophilic in many of the lymphoma cells; sharply defined clear vacuoles are
frequently, but not invariably, present.

Acute monoblastic leukemia (M5A) may present with a uniform population of cells that closely
resemble prolymphocytes. Because of Fc receptors
(CD16), the monoblasts may possess surface immunoglobulin that can be misinterpreted as indicating
B-cell lineage. This problem is resolved by blocking
the Fc receptors. The nonspecific esterase (NSE)
reaction is moderately to intensely positive in the
monoblasts in the majority of cases of acute monoblastic leukemia and negative in B PL.

Treatment and Prognosis. B PL is usually
an aggressive disease for which there is no treatment of choice. Multiagent chemotherapy, splenic
radiation, splenectomy, and the nucleoside analogs have been used with limited success (41).

Chronic Lymphocytic Leukemia/
Prolymphocytic Leukemia

In typical B CLL the number of prolymphocytes
in the blood is 10 percent or less; in B PL it is 55
percent or more. The cases with 11 to 54 percent
prolymphocytes in the blood are designated chronic
lymphocytic leukemia/prolymphocytic leukemia
(CLL/PL) (fig. 299) (39–41). The bone marrow sections may contain foci of transformation or an admixture of small lymphocytes and prolymphocytes
(fig. 300). Patients with CLL/PL have clinical findings intermediate to CLL and B PL (39). Both
lymphadenopathy and splenomegaly are present;
the degree of splenomegaly is frequently disproportionate to the degree of lymphadenopathy. Patients
with CLL/PL have a variable clinical course; some
cases may be marked by rapid progression. CLL/PL
and prolymphocytoid transformation of CLL may
have similar blood findings in that prolymphocytes
are present in both disorders. The distinction between these two processes should be based on clinical history. If there is a prior history of typical B
CLL, prolymphocytoid transformation is the appropriate diagnostic term. If there is no prior evidence
of B CLL, CLL/PL is the preferred diagnostic term.

Figure 299
B-CELL CHRONIC LYMPHOCYTIC LEUKEMIA/ PROLYMPHOCYTIC LEUKEMIA

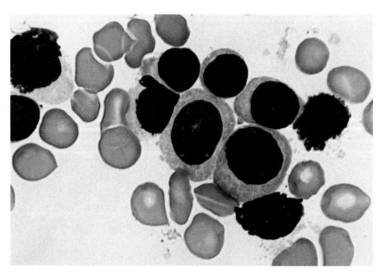

Blood smear from a patient with a marked lymphocytosis. There is a spectrum of lymphocytes from small cells with clumped nuclear chromatin and no nucleoli to large prolymphocytes with abundant basophilic cytoplasm and prominent nucleoli. The chromatin in the prolymphocytes has a density intermediate to a blast and mature lymphocyte. This pattern is characteristic of chronic lymphocytic leukemia/prolymphocytic leukemia in which the prolymphocytes are in the range of 11 to 54 percent. The prolymphocytes in this entity are distinct from the large lymphocytes observed in mixed type CLL as shown in figure 280. (Wright-Giemsa stain)

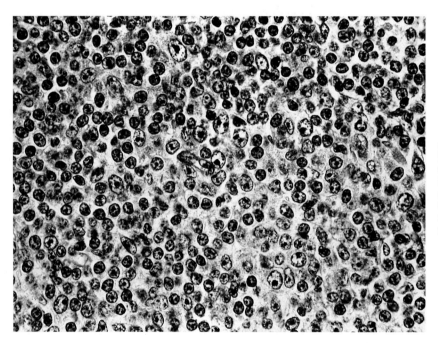

Figure 300
B-CELL CHRONIC LYMPHOCYTIC LEUKEMIA/ PROLYMPHOCYTIC LEUKEMIA

Bone marrow biopsy from the patient whose blood smear is shown in figure 299. This area shows a focus of prolymphocytes with prominent nucleoli surrounded by well-differentiated lymphocytes. Despite the immature-appearing nuclei, mitotic figures are uncommon. (Hematoxylin and eosin stain)

Hairy Cell Leukemia

Definition. A low-grade lymphoproliferative process of B-cell origin with primary manifestations in the blood, bone marrow, and spleen.

Incidence and Clinical Findings. Hairy cell leukemia (HCL) is an uncommon disorder of adults, with a peak incidence in the fifth and sixth decades (7,8,11,22). There is a marked male predominance, with a male to female ratio of 4–5 to 1.

The majority of patients present with splenomegaly and pancytopenia. Peripheral lympha-denopathy at the time of initial diagnosis is uncommon. Massive abdominal lymphadenopathy has been reported in a series of 12 patients primarily with relapse disease following therapy (43). This finding appears to be associated with a blastic type of transformation.

Unusual clinical manifestations including spinal cord compression and gastric mucosal infiltration have been reported (8).

Laboratory Findings. Most patients present with a normocytic normochromic anemia. Thrombocytopenia is present in more than 50 percent of

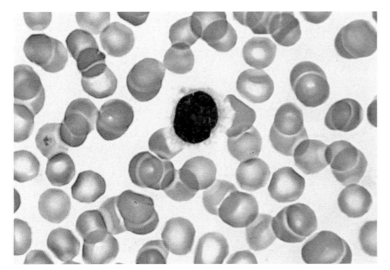

Figure 301
HAIRY CELL LEUKEMIA
A hairy cell in a blood smear from a man presenting with pancytopenia including monocytopenia and splenomegaly. Only rare cells of the type illustrated were identified. (Wright-Giemsa stain)

Figure 302
HAIRY CELL LEUKEMIA
Two hairy cells and a plasmacytoid lymphocyte in a blood smear from a patient with HCL. The cytoplasm of the hairy cells is abundant and somewhat "fluffy" when compared to the cytoplasm of the plasmacytoid lymphocyte which has a sharply demarcated cytoplasmic outline. The hairy cell cytoplasm is clear to slightly basophilic and contains several small, poorly defined vacuoles. (Wright-Giemsa stain)

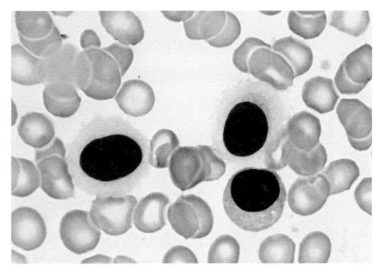

cases (7,11,22,50). The leukocyte count varies but leukopenia is present in the majority of patients, neutropenia is present in more than 75 percent of patients, and monocytopenia is an almost constant feature (7,11,22,50).

Blood and Bone Marrow Findings. The number of leukemic cells in the blood varies but is usually low. In occasional patients rare or no hairy cells are found (fig. 301). In 10 to 20 percent of patients, the number of leukemic cells is 5×10^9/L or more (50). The hairy cells are small to medium in size, with a generally round to oval to slightly lobulated or monocytoid nucleus. The nuclear chromatin is coarse but not as clumped as in the predominant lymphocytes in B CLL. Nucleoli are usually inconspicuous.

The cytoplasmic characteristics serve as the primary basis for the recognition of HCL. The descriptive term "hairy" was suggested because of the appearance of the cells in phase microscopy preparations (61). On air-dried films, the cytoplasm retains some of these characteristics. The cytoplasm, which is clear to lightly basophilic, varies in amount in different cases and in different cells in the same case; it has an irregular outline as a result of varying sized projections (figs. 301–303). The term "shaggy" has been used to describe this characteristic (50). Small vacuoles may be present. In a small number of cases, parallel basophilic bands may be present in the cytoplasm; these correspond to the ribosome-lamella complexes that may be observed on electron microscopy (fig. 304). A blastic variant has been

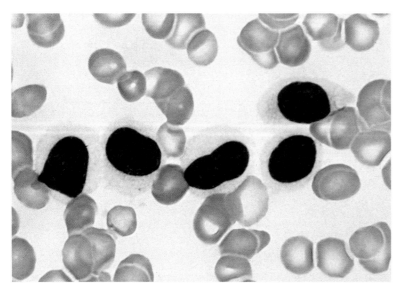

Figure 303
HAIRY CELL LEUKEMIA
Five hairy cells in a blood smear from a 43-year-old man with a high count HCL; severe neutropenia, anemia, and thrombocytopenia were present. The hairy cells in this specimen have abundant, irregularly distributed cytoplasm. The nuclei vary from round to oval to slightly lobulated. Following splenectomy the leukocyte count decreased for a short period and then rose to 70×10^9/L. The rise in the leukocyte count was accompanied by progressive bone marrow failure. The patient did not respond to interferon. He was then treated with deoxycoformycin and achieved complete remission which has lasted 8 years. (Wright-Giemsa stain)

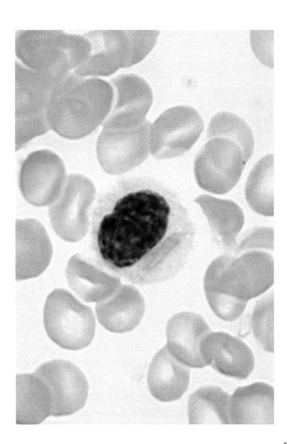

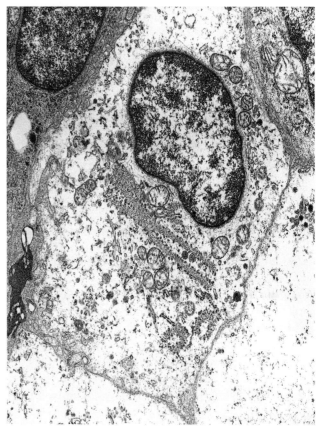

Figure 304
HAIRY CELL LEUKEMIA: RIBOSOME-LAMELLA COMPLEX
Left: Typical hairy cell in the blood smear of a patient with HCL. The cytoplasm contains parallel basophilic structures which represent the light microscopy manifestation of the ribosome-lamella complex seen in on the right. (Wright-Giemsa stain)
Right: Electron micrograph of a hairy cell showing a ribosome-lamella complex which is composed of fibrous lamella with attached ribosomes. (Uranyl acetate–lead citrate stains, X8,000)

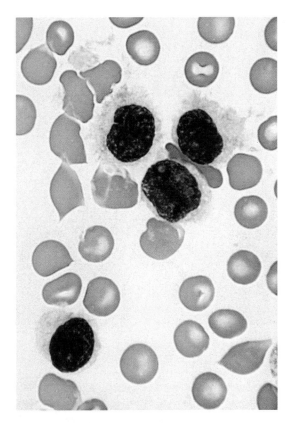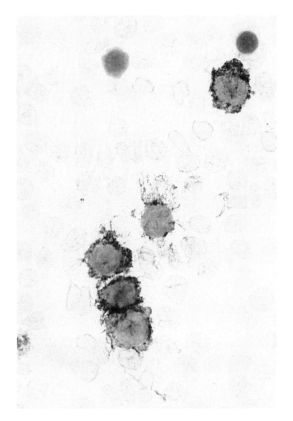

Figure 305
HAIRY CELL LEUKEMIA: BONE MARROW SMEAR

Left: Four hairy cells in a bone marrow smear from a 62-year-old man presenting with severe pancytopenia and splenomegaly. The hairy cells are approximately twice the size of red blood cells; the abundant cytoplasm is irregularly distributed around the nucleus. The nuclei vary from round to oval to slightly indented. Nucleoli are visible but not prominent. (Wright-Giemsa stain)

Right: Bone marrow smear from the same specimen reacted with antibody to CD11c. The hairy cells are uniformly and intensely reactive. (Alkaline phosphatase–antialkaline phosphatase stain)

reported (19). Bone marrow aspiration is frequently difficult but diagnostic specimens can usually be obtained (fig. 305). The hairy cells in marrow aspirate smears and biopsy imprints are similar to those in the blood.

Histopathologic Findings. The bone marrow trephine biopsy is very important for diagnosis because of the relatively unique histopathologic features of this disorder in most cases (2,10,12). The marrow is generally hypercellular. Involvement may be diffuse or focal; the terms partial or patchy have been used to describe focal lesions (10). The diffuse pattern is most common; large areas of marrow are replaced (fig. 306). Residual foci of normal hematopoietic cells may be observed; these foci are usually indistinctly demarcated from the leukemic infiltrate. The extent of involvement is accentuated in sections reacted with antibodies to

B lymphocytes (fig. 307). In partial involvement, there are randomly distributed, irregularly shaped foci of leukemic cells that have a tendency to almost imperceptibly infiltrate the surrounding normal bone marrow; the noninvolved marrow may be hypercellular (fig. 308). Antibodies to B lymphocytes reactive in paraffin-embedded sections can aid considerably in demonstrating partial involvement (fig. 309). In approximately 10 to 20 percent of patients with HCL, the bone marrow is uniformly or focally hypocellular (fig. 310).

The hairy cell infiltrate is very characteristic in the majority of cases fixed in Zenker, B5, or formalin and embedded in paraffin; it is loosely structured with poorly defined clear areas separating the leukemic cells. The hairy cell nuclei are round, oval, or slightly lobulated (figs. 307, 310B) (2,10,12).

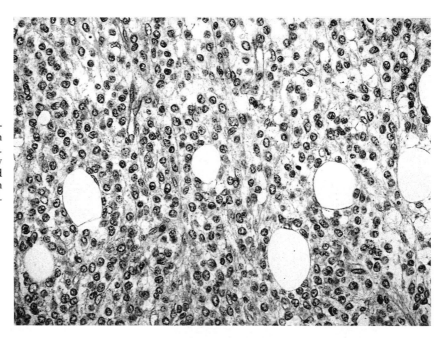

Figure 306
HAIRY CELL LEUKEMIA:
DIFFUSE BONE MARROW
INVOLVEMENT

Bone marrow biopsy from a patient with hairy cell leukemia with a diffuse pattern of involvement. The leukemic infiltrate is loosely spaced in contrast to CLL and small lymphocytic lymphoma in which the cells are closely apposed. (Hematoxylin and eosin stain)

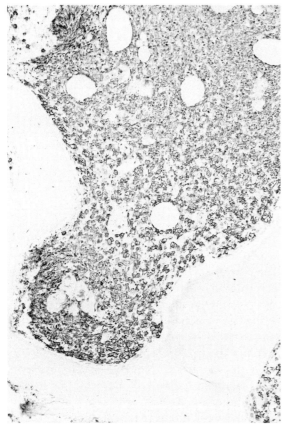

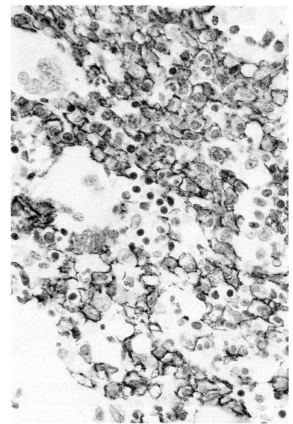

Figure 307
HAIRY CELL LEUKEMIA: IMMUNOHISTOLOGY

Left: Bone marrow biopsy from a patient with HCL reacted with antibody to CD20 (L26). The positive-reacting hairy cells form a loosely structured infiltrate; nonreacting erythroid precursors are scattered among the leukemic cells.

Right: High magnification of the same specimen. (Peroxidase-antiperoxidase stain)

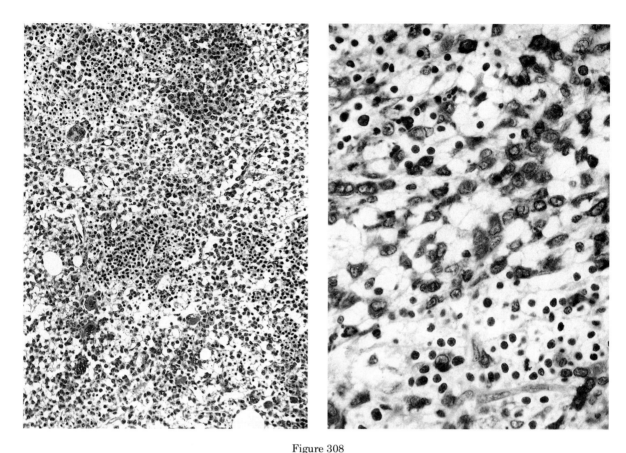

Figure 308
HAIRY CELL LEUKEMIA: PARTIAL BONE MARROW INVOLVEMENT
Left: Bone marrow biopsy from a patient with HCL showing partial involvement. The leukemic infiltrate is irregularly distributed and poorly delimited from the adjacent normal marrow. The loose structure of the leukemic infiltrate contrasts with the more closely aligned normal marrow cells including foci of erythroid precursors. (Hematoxylin and eosin stain)
Right: High magnification of the same specimen showing a poorly demarcated infiltration of hairy cells with adjacent erythroid precursors at the upper and lower margins. (Hematoxylin and eosin stain)

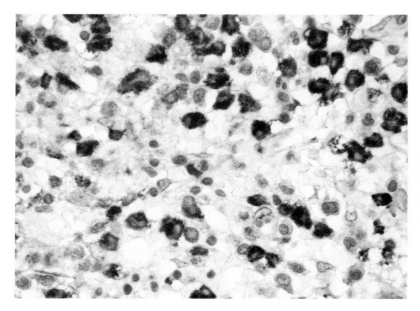

Figure 309
HAIRY CELL LEUKEMIA:
IMMUNOHISTOLOGY IN
PARTIAL BONE MARROW
INVOLVEMENT

An area of a bone marrow biopsy from a patient with HCL with partial involvement reacted with antibody to CD20. There are several positive-reacting hairy cells intermixed with nonreacting normal marrow cells. (Peroxidase-antiperoxidase stain)

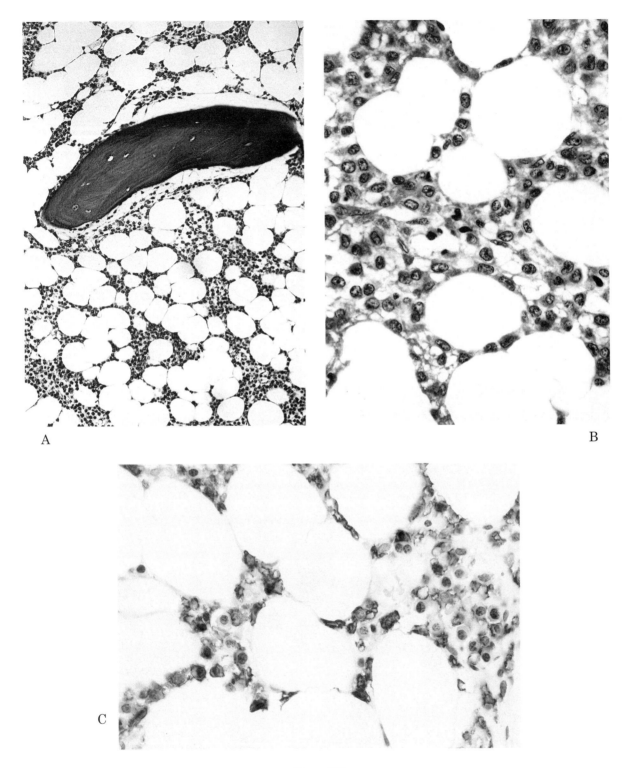

Figure 310
HAIRY CELL LEUKEMIA: HYPOCELLULAR BONE MARROW

A. Hypocellular bone marrow biopsy from a patient with untreated HCL. (Hematoxylin and eosin stain)

B. High magnification of the same specimen showing infiltration of the interstitium by a population of loosely spaced hairy cells. (Hematoxylin and eosin stain)

C. The same specimen reacted with antibody L26 (CD20). The hairy cells are intensely reactive. (Peroxidase-antiperoxidase stain)

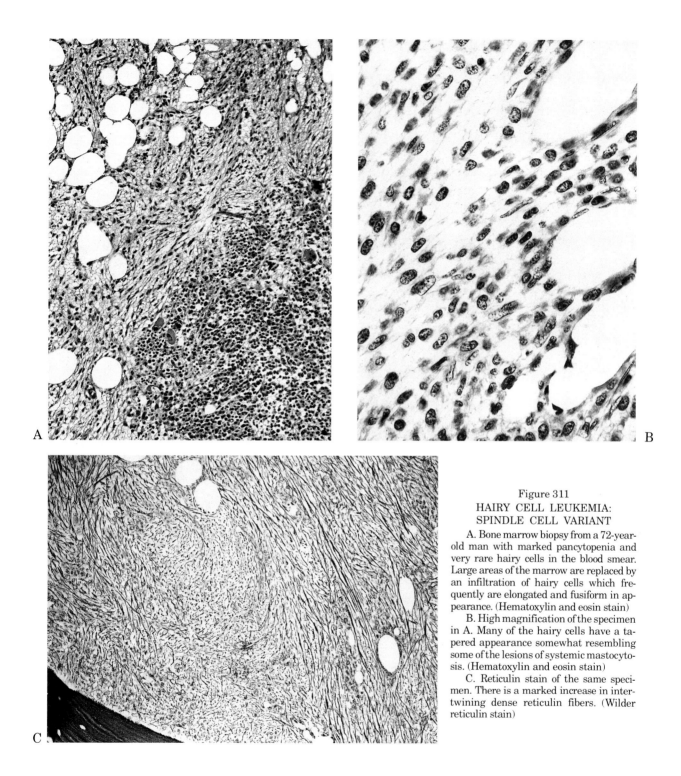

Figure 311
HAIRY CELL LEUKEMIA:
SPINDLE CELL VARIANT

A. Bone marrow biopsy from a 72-year-old man with marked pancytopenia and very rare hairy cells in the blood smear. Large areas of the marrow are replaced by an infiltration of hairy cells which frequently are elongated and fusiform in appearance. (Hematoxylin and eosin stain)

B. High magnification of the specimen in A. Many of the hairy cells have a tapered appearance somewhat resembling some of the lesions of systemic mastocytosis. (Hematoxylin and eosin stain)

C. Reticulin stain of the same specimen. There is a marked increase in intertwining dense reticulin fibers. (Wilder reticulin stain)

Small distinct nucleoli are present. Mitotic figures are not usually identified. In a small number of cases, the hairy cells are elongated and spindly in appearance (fig. 311). The lesions in some of these cases may resemble systemic mastocytosis. A multilobulated variant in which the nuclei have a very irregular, lobulated appearance has been reported (fig. 312) (2,29).

Reticulin stains of the bone marrow biopsy show a moderate to marked increase in reticulin fibers

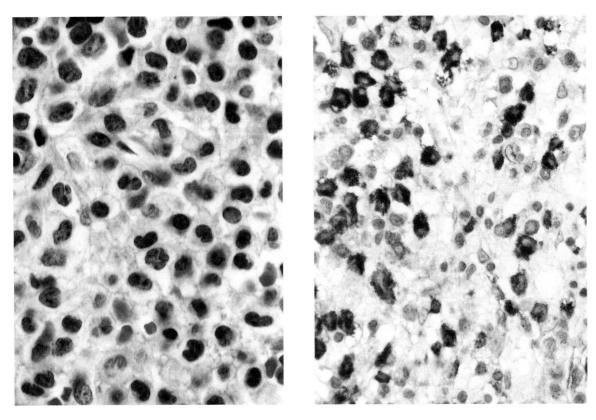

Figure 312
HAIRY CELL LEUKEMIA: MULTILOBULAR VARIANT

Left: Bone marrow biopsy from a patient with splenomegaly and marked pancytopenia. Rare hairy cells were present in the blood and were TRAP positive. The biopsy shows marked infiltration of the marrow by cells that have moderately abundant cytoplasm and nuclei with clumped chromatin. Cells with markedly lobulated nuclei are numerous. Mitotic figures are sparse. The cells expressed CD19, CD11c, and CD25 and were interpreted as hairy cells with multilobulated nuclei. The patient was treated with alpha-interferon which resulted in normalization of the hematology values. (Hematoxylin and eosin stain)

Right: Specimen from the same biopsy reacted with antibody to CD20 (L26). The darkly staining hairy cells form a loose infiltrate with scattered small foci of nonreacting normal marrow cells. (Peroxidase-antiperoxidase stain)

(fig. 311C). The reticulin fibers in some instances appear to individually circumscribe the hairy cells. In cases with partial bone marrow involvement, the reticulin network usually extends into the adjacent normal-appearing marrow.

Some patients with HCL have an increased predisposition to infectious processes including tuberculosis; granulomatous lesions may be identified in the marrow biopsy. Appropriate stains and cultures should be done in these instances.

Examination of bone marrow biopsies for residual leukemia following treatment with the interferons or the nucleoside analogs is facilitated with immunohistology, using antibodies to B lymphocytes reactive with paraffin-embedded tissue. A panel including MB2, L26 (CD20), and DBA.44 is usually adequate for this purpose.

Cytochemical Findings. An important study in the diagnosis of HCL is the demonstration of tartrate-resistant acid phosphatase (TRAP) (50,69). The number and intensity of reacting hairy cells varies; in some cases only a minority of cells are TRAP positive. Slides not treated with tartrate show reactivity in neutrophils, monocytes, platelets, and lymphocytes in addition to the hairy cells. Following incubation with tartaric acid, the activity is present only in the hairy cells. The ablation of the enzyme activity in the nonleukemic cells usually highlights the reactivity in the leukemic cells. When performed according to the method of Yam et al. (69), the TRAP reactivity is a brilliant red granular precipitate (fig. 313). Occasional nonleukemic small lymphocytes may contain coarse amber

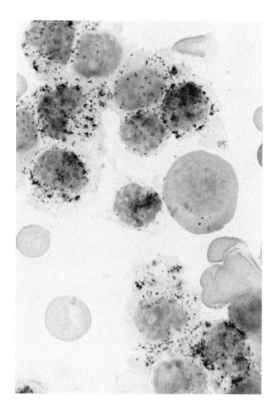

Figure 313
HAIRY CELL LEUKEMIA: TARTRATE-
RESISTANT ACID PHOSPHATASE (TRAP)

Tartrate-resistant acid phosphatase (TRAP) reaction on a bone marrow smear from a patient with HCL. The red reaction product is intense in the hairy cells. (Acid phosphatase stain, following tartrate incubation)

colored crystalline material. This finding should be interpreted as negative. These deposits occur more commonly when aged reagents are used. If the TRAP reaction is negative, other evidence for establishing the diagnosis, including bone marrow histopathology, clinical findings, and membrane surface markers, must be unequivocal.

The specificity of TRAP for HCL in the small lymphocyte proliferations is not absolute; it may be present in a small number of cases of small lymphocytic lymphoma of intermediate differentiation and T-prolymphocytic leukemia (47). The enzyme may also be found in a small number of cases of small B-lymphocyte proliferations which have some features in common with HCL. These will be discussed in the differential diagnosis.

Hairy cells may show positivity with NSE (50). A focal, crescent shaped reaction resistant to sodium fluoride incubation has been shown

with alpha-naphthyl butyrate as the substrate. Hairy cells may be PAS positive but this finding lacks specificity.

Immunologic Findings. Immunologic markers and molecular studies are evidence of the B-cell origin of HCL (17,50). The cells are positive for light chain restricted surface and cytoplasmic immunoglobulins. The heavy chain type is usually IgG alone or in combination with other heavy chain types. Hairy cells express the B-cell–associated antigens C19, CD20, CD24, and HLA-DR and CD22 (3,5,50). The cells are negative for CD21, a marker of early B-cell differentiation. The cells in most cases express CD25, which is also present on monocytes and activated T cells, and CD11c, which is also present on monocytes, neutrophils, activated T cells, and NK cells. In most studies, the hairy cells are negative for CD5, a pan–T-cell antigen that is also present on the lymphocytes in the majority of cases of B CLL. In contrast to the lymphocytes in CLL, hairy cells express B ly-7, an activation/differentiation-associated antigen (13,56a). Antibodies with varying degrees of specificity to hairy cells, such as HC2, have also been developed (5).

Immunohistochemical reactions on bone marrow biopsy specimens can be very useful for identifying the extent of marrow infiltration in HCL, both at the time of initial diagnosis and following therapy. Hairy cells react with most of the pan–B-cell monoclonal antibodies including L26 (CD20), LN2 (CD74), MB2, and DBA.44 (see figs. 307, 309) (31). These antibodies do not react with the same degree of intensity in every case, and the reactivity may be affected by the type of fixative. The reactions with pan–B-cell antibodies are not specific for HCL and their major utility in this disorder is in the estimation of extent of marrow involvement.

Ultrastructural Findings. On transmission electron microscopy, hairy cells are characterized by cytoplasmic projections or microvilli and pseudopods (fig. 314). The nuclear configuration varies considerably, ranging from oval to notched to bilobed; frequently the nucleus shows a deep indentation. The cytoplasm contains pinocytotic vesicles, multivesicular bodies, azurophilic granules, and lysozomal inclusions. Ribosome-lamella complexes may be observed in varying numbers in approximately 40 percent of the cases of HCL (see fig. 304). These structures are not specific for this entity and have been reported in other lymphoproliferative disorders (9).

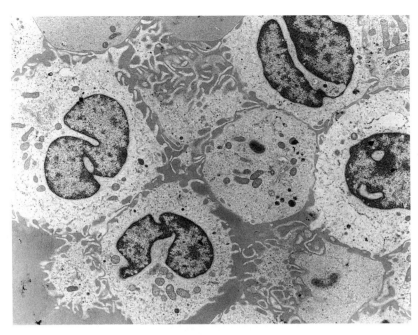

Figure 314
HAIRY CELL
LEUKEMIA:
ULTRASTRUCTURE
Electron micrograph of several hairy cells in a blood specimen. The hairy cells have numerous villous projections. The nuclei are round to very irregular with moderately dispersed chromatin and inconspicuous nucleoli. (Uranyl acetate–lead citrate stains, X6000)

Cytogenetic Findings. Cytogenetic studies have shown clonal chromosome abnormalities in approximately 10 percent of patients with HCL. The abnormalities include 14q+, 14q-, 6q-, -22, +2, 3q+, and +12 (59). These findings lack specificity.

Spleen, Liver, and Lymph Nodes. The spleen shows a diffuse, dense infiltration of the red pulp cords and engorgement of the sinuses by the malignant cells (11). The massive cellular infiltration encroaches on the white pulp and may result in reduction in the size of the malpighian corpuscles. Distended spaces filled with erythrocytes resembling dilated sinuses may be prominent (45). These spaces are lined by hairy cells and have been referred to as pseudosinuses.

The liver shows a diffuse infiltration of the sinuses by the hairy cells. Involved lymph nodes show a diffuse infiltration of the subcapsular sinuses, cortex, and medullary cords (11). Lymphoid follicles and islands of residual lymphocytes surrounded and separated by leukemic cells are present.

Differential Diagnosis. The differential diagnosis of HCL is one of the more difficult problems in bone marrow pathology and includes other small lymphocyte proliferations that are usually associated with splenomegaly. Although the cytologic features of the hairy cells are described as being characteristic of this process, in practice the diagnosis may be difficult because of

similar clinical, cytologic, and cytochemical findings in other small lymphocyte proliferations including splenic lymphoma with villous lymphocytes, hairy cell leukemia variant, and monocytoid B-cell lymphoma (5,13,14,42,46,47). Prolymphocytic leukemia may be considered in the differential diagnosis of HCL because of the associated splenomegaly and lack of lymphadenopathy but should be readily distinguished on the basis of the cytology of the prolymphocytes and the magnitude of the white blood cell count.

There are other small B-lymphocyte proliferations that are uncommon and that resemble HCL (46,47). Monocytoid B-cell lymphoma involves the marrow in approximately 30 percent of cases (46). Unlike HCL, the marrow pattern is usually focally paratrabecular and sharply demarcated.

The variant of HCL in which the cells have an elongated or spindly appearance may resemble systemic mastocytosis. Patients with mastocytosis may have splenomegaly but do not generally have the pancytopenia and monocytopenia found in most cases of HCL. Immunohistochemical reactions readily distinguish these two disorders. The hairy cells are positive with B-cell antibodies and mast cells are negative. The mast cells are positive with toluidine blue, Giemsa, and chloroacetate esterase stains and react with antibodies to mast cells; hairy cells are negative with these reactions.

Treatment and Prognosis. For many years the therapeutic approach to HCL was primarily observation or splenectomy in patients with severe pancytopenia. HCL does not generally respond to the chemotherapeutic agents effective in the non-Hodgkin lymphomas and chronic lymphocytic leukemia. The introduction of the interferons improved the outlook for patients with HCL; partial and complete responses have been obtained. The most important therapeutic advances occurred with the introduction of two nucleoside analogs, deoxycoformycin and 2-chlorodeoxyadenosine (52,64). The initial therapeutic trials with these agents have shown significant treatment response. Prognostic data for HCL preceding the use of the interferons and nucleoside analogs are no longer relevant. There are insufficient data at the writing of this Fascicle to ascertain the full impact of the new agents on survival but initial results are very promising.

Rarely, patients with hairy cell leukemia develop a second B cell malignancy.

Hairy Cell Leukemia Variant

Hairy cell leukemia variant is a rare lymphoproliferative disorder that has cytologic features intermediate to B-prolymphocytic leukemia and HCL. The disorder has been reported under a variety of names (5,14,60). The male to female ratio is 4 to 1; the median age at onset is 61 years. In contrast to most cases of HCL, there is a marked elevation of the leukocyte count, usually in excess of 40×10^9/L. Also, unlike HCL, there usually is no associated neutropenia and monocytopenia.

The leukemic cells in the hairy cell variant are larger than hairy cells, have a higher nuclear-cytoplasmic ratio, and a round to oval nucleus that has coarse chromatin and a relatively prominent nucleolus (fig. 315). The cytoplasm is moderately basophilic and shows delicate to coarse projections. The nuclear features and the cytoplasmic basophilia resemble those of a B prolymphocyte; the cytoplasmic projections are similar to the hairy cell. Although the TRAP reaction is reported as negative, it may be positive in some cases (14,60).

The leukemic cells in the hairy cell variant express CD19, CD20, and CD22 (5). They have light chain restricted surface immunoglobulins and usually IgG heavy chains. The cells are usually CD5 and CD25 negative. In some cases the cells express CD11c.

The bone marrow is infiltrated by the leukemic process but unlike HCL there is not a marked increase in reticulin and the marrow is readily aspirated in most cases (fig. 315). The spleen is reported to show a red pulp infiltration similar to HCL (60).

The disease follows a chronic course. In contrast to typical HCL, the HCL variant does not usually respond to interferons (60).

A variant of HCL occurring in Japan is characterized by higher leukocyte counts than in the typical HCL in western countries; the hairy cells in a minority of cases with this variant are TRAP negative (34). The histopathology in the bone marrow and spleen is reported as similar to typical HCL. Unlike the majority of cases reported in western countries, the hairy cells in the Japanese variant usually express CD10 and in approximately 50 percent of the cases express CD5.

Splenic Lymphoma with Villous Lymphocytes

Splenic lymphoma with villous lymphocytes (SLVL) is a small B-lymphocyte proliferation that may have clinical, laboratory, and cytologic features similar to HCL (5,42,44,47). Similar to HCL, the disease is more common in men than women. The reported mean age at diagnosis is 72 years. Marked splenomegaly is usually but not invariably present; a reported 18 percent of patients do not have a palpable spleen. Anemia and thrombocytopenia are present in approximately 50 percent of cases. The leukocyte count is usually moderately increased; uncommonly, it exceeds 25×10^9/L. Approximately 50 to 60 percent of patients have a modest monoclonal gammopathy, usually of the IgM type; in occasional patients it is IgG (42,44).

The lymphocytes in the blood smear are of medium size, are larger than normal small lymphocytes, and have round to oval nuclei with clumped nuclear chromatin. There may be a single distinct, slightly prominent nucleolus but this is not a consistent finding. The cytoplasm is moderately basophilic and usually marked by the presence of short villi (fig. 316). The villous projections may have a polar distribution. Villous lymphocytes have less cytoplasm than hairy cells. Plasmacytoid cells may be present. Unlike HCL there is no monocytopenia.

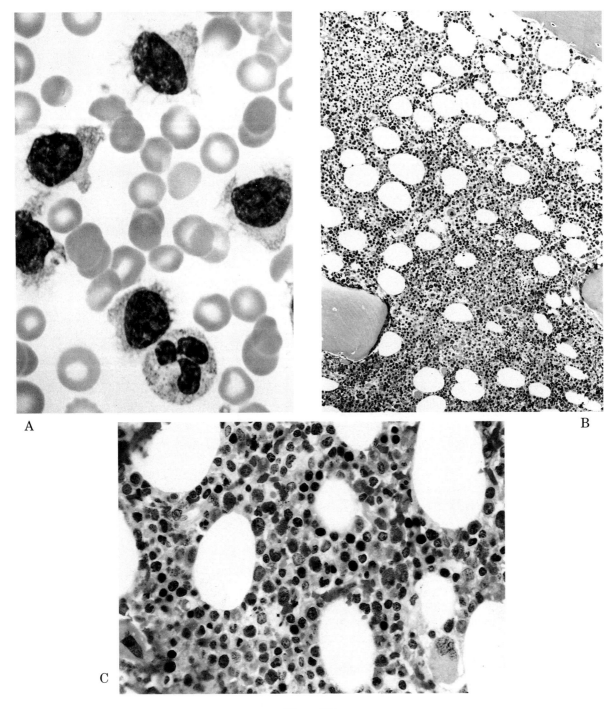

Figure 315
HAIRY CELL LEUKEMIA VARIANT

A. Blood smear from an adult male with a 2-year history of marked lymphocytosis. The lymphocytes are medium to large cells with prominent, irregular cytoplasmic projections. A single distinct, sometimes prominent, nucleolus is present. (Wright-Giemsa stain)

B. Bone marrow biopsy showing an essentially normal architectural pattern with abundant fat. There is an erythroid hyperplasia and megakaryocytes appear adequate. (Hematoxylin and eosin stain)

C. High magnification of the same specimen showing an interstitial infiltration by lymphocytes. There is substantial sparing of normal marrow cells. Numerous red blood cell precursors with round nuclei and condensed nuclear chromatin are intermixed with the lymphocytes. The lymphocytes are larger than the red blood cell precursors and have a finer nuclear chromatin; occasional cells have nucleoli. (Hematoxylin and eosin stain)

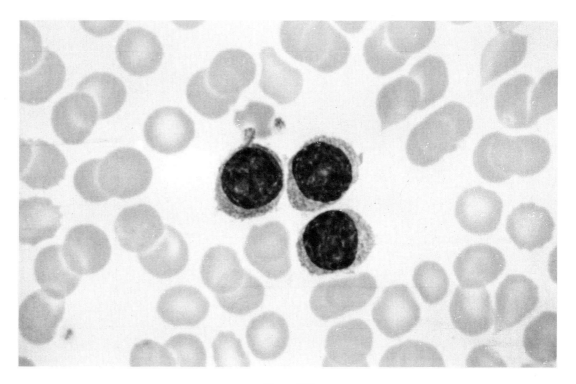

Figure 316
SPLENIC LYMPHOMA WITH VILLOUS LYMPHOCYTES
Three lymphocytes in the blood of a patient with splenomegaly and a small IgM monoclonal gammopathy. The cells have sparse cytoplasm with small villous projections. One of the cells has a distinct nucleolus. (Wright-Giemsa stain)

The extent of bone marrow involvement varies from numerous, small, irregularly shaped aggregates to coalescent infiltrations that replace large areas of marrow (47). The distribution may be random or paratrabecular (fig. 317).

The spleen shows expansion of the white pulp, with spreading into the red pulp in some cases (fig. 318). A relatively high association with sarcoid-like granulomas was reported in one series (47).

In the initial studies proposing SLVL as a specific entity, the villous lymphocytes were reported as TRAP negative. However, in an earlier study of similar cases, the TRAP reaction was positive in some instances (47).

The villous lymphocytes express B-lymphocyte–associated antigens including CD19, CD20, and CD24 (5,42,44). The abnormal cells in approximately 50 percent of cases are CD11c positive. The cells are usually CD5 and CD25 negative.

Cytogenetic analysis has shown a t(11;14) or variant t(11;22) translocation in 22 percent of cases (48). This finding has also been associated with malignant lymphoma of intermediate differentiation.

Patients with SLVL may not need therapy for several years. If the pancytopenia is severe, splenectomy is recommended as the initial therapeutic approach. The disease has a favorable prognosis with a median survival period exceeding 10 years (44).

SLVL may represent several closely related small lymphocyte proliferations. The findings of monoclonal gammopathy and plasmacytoid lymphocytes suggest a close relationship to plasmacytoid lymphoma in some cases. The t(11;14) chromosome abnormality in some patients suggests a relationship to intermediate differentiated lymphoma.

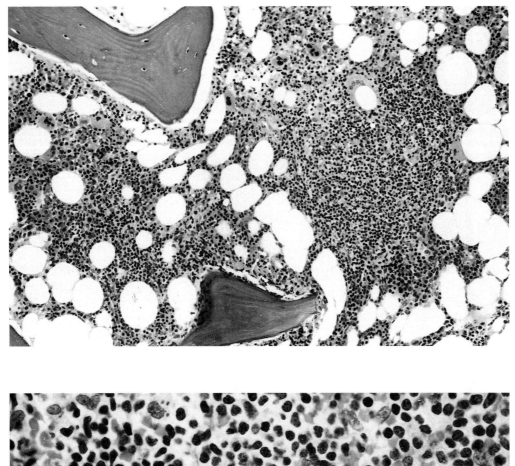

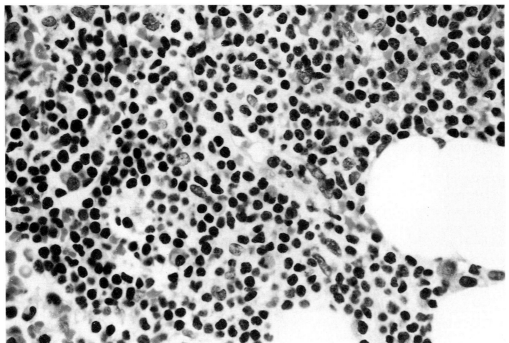

Figure 317
SPLENIC LYMPHOMA WITH VILLOUS LYMPHOCYTES: BONE MARROW

Top: Low magnification of a bone marrow biopsy from an adult male with splenic lymphoma with villous lymphocytes. There are two large focal aggregates of lymphocytes. (Hematoxylin and eosin stain)

Bottom: High magnification of the lesion illustrated on the top showing a predominant population of small lymphocytes with scattered plasma cells. No mitotic figures were observed. (Hematoxylin and eosin stain)

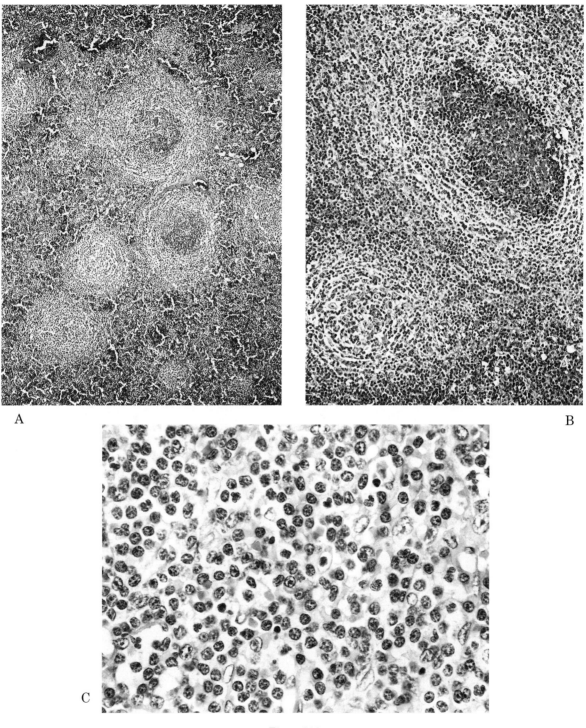

Figure 318
SPLENIC LYMPHOMA WITH VILLOUS LYMPHOCYTES: SPLEEN

A. Sections of spleen from the patient whose blood smear is illustrated in figure 315. Both the white pulp and red pulp are involved by the lymphoproliferative process. Some malpighian corpuscles show a deposition of proteinaceous material.

B. High magnification of the same specimen showing a malpighian corpuscle with a central deposition of eosinophilic proteinaceous substance.

C. Lymphocytes in the red pulp are predominantly mature with moderately clumped chromatin. A small number of cells have nucleoli. Cells with plasmacytoid features are present. (Figures A–C: Hematoxylin and eosin stain)

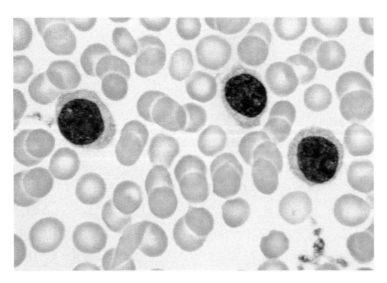

Figure 319
SMALL B-LYMPHOCYTE PROLIFERATION: AMBIGUOUS MORPHOLOGY AND IMMUNOPHENOTYPE
Three lymphocytes in the blood of a 76-year-old asymptomatic woman with a leukocyte count of 14.6×10^9/L, hemoglobin level of 14.2 g/dL, and platelet count of 246×10^9/L. There was no lymphadenopathy or splenomegaly. The lymphocytes, which comprised 72 percent of the blood leukocytes, were small with a slight rim of lightly basophilic cytoplasm. An inconspicuous nucleolus was present in many. The lymphocytes expressed strong IgM kappa, CD19, CD20, CD24, CD5, CD11c, and weakly expressed CD25; the cells reacted negatively for tartrate-resistance acid phosphatase. The bone marrow sections showed a subtle interstitial infiltration of small lymphocytes.
The morphologic and immunophenotypic characteristics of these lymphocytes are not typical for any of the recognized small lymphocyte proliferations. The lymphocytes share some morphologic features of both CLL and splenic lymphoma with villous lymphocytes and immunologic features of CLL, hairy cell leukemia, and mantle cell lymphoma. The case was tentatively classified as a small B-lymphocyte proliferation. An acceptable alternative diagnosis is CLL, CD11c, CD25 positive. The clinical and hematologic status was unchanged after 22 months of observation only. (Wright-Giemsa stain)

Small B-Cell Lymphoproliferative Disorder, Unclassified

Sometimes a patient presents with a proliferation of small lymphocytes in the blood and bone marrow that have morphologic and immunologic features that preclude a precise classification (fig. 319). In these instances, it is important that all clinical and laboratory findings be reviewed. The extent of lymphadenopathy should be determined; a lymph node biopsy should be performed if adenopathy is present. If, after all relevant studies have been reviewed, a recognized entity cannot be diagnosed, it is acceptable to use the term small B-cell lymphoproliferative disorder, unclassified. In these instances, as stated earlier, it is prudent to be cautious about predicting clinical course. The biology of the process will usually be evident in the first few months of observation. The presence of any degree of mitotic activity should always be viewed with concern and careful observation of clinical and hematologic status should be advised.

T-CELL SMALL LYMPHOCYTIC PROLIFERATIONS

The T-lymphocyte–derived leukemias are immunologically distinguished as thymic and post-thymic in origin. The thymic based T-cell leukemias are the TdT-positive lymphoblastic leukemias and are described in the section, Acute Lymphoblastic Leukemias. The T-cell small lymphocytic leukemias that are post-thymic are TdT negative and include a morphologically diverse group of proliferations with considerable clinical, immunologic, and biologic heterogeneity. The recognition of these disorders is based on a combination of morphologic and immunologic characteristics.

There are four major post-thymic T-cell lymphoproliferative processes that manifest primarily in the blood and bone marrow: T-prolymphocytic leukemia, adult T-cell leukemia, large granulated lymphocyte leukemia, and Sézary syndrome. In addition, there are probably several other post-thymic lymphoproliferative processes that are distinct from the above group and which, because of their rarity, are presently not well characterized. Peripheral T-cell lymphoma, a lymph node or spleen based disease, may involve the blood and bone marrow and is discussed in the section on lymphomas in bone marrow and in the differential diagnosis of T-prolymphocytic leukemia in this section. The major post-thymic T-cell lymphoproliferative disorders that manifest in blood and bone marrow and their immunophenotypic characteristics are summarized in Tables 29 and 30.

T-Prolymphocytic Leukemia

Definition. A proliferation of post-thymic T lymphocytes with the cytologic features of prolymphocytes (72,81,89,99,124).

Incidence and Clinical Findings. T-prolymphocytic leukemia (T PL) is a rare disorder. The median age in the largest reported series is 69 years, with a range of 33 to 91 years (99). There is a slight male predominance.

The principal clinical findings are splenomegaly, hepatomegaly, lymphadenopathy, serous effusions, and skin lesions (99). The cutaneous lesions include a generalized or focal maculopapular rash or nodules. There is a possible increased incidence of T PL in patients with ataxia telangiectasia.

Laboratory Findings. There is usually a marked leukocytosis. The reported median white blood cell count is 200×10^9/L, with a range of 16 to 1000×10^9/L (99). Seventy five percent of patients have leukocyte counts in excess of 100×10^9/L, although some patients present with only a slight lymphocytosis. Approximately 50 percent of patients are anemic and thrombocytopenic. The hemoglobin level is less than 10 g/dL in 36 percent of patients and the platelet count is less than 100×10^9/L in 50 percent (99).

The serum calcium level is normal. Serologic studies for the human T-cell leukemia-lymphoma virus, HTLV-1, are negative.

Blood and Bone Marrow Findings. The blood smear serves as the primary diagnostic specimen in T PL. Although the unifying characteristic of the disorder is the morphologic features of the predominant cell, the prolymphocyte, there is considerable variation in what is accepted as T PL and the term may be somewhat misleading (77). The prolymphocytes in the majority of cases of T PL are medium sized, with coarse nuclear chromatin and a single prominent nucleolus (fig. 320). The nuclei are round to oval in 50 percent of cases and irregular with convolutions and folds in the remainder. The two nuclear morphologies may

Table 29

T-CELL SMALL LYMPHOCYTIC PROLIFERATIONS

T-Prolymphocytic leukemia

Large granulated lymphocyte leukemia

Adult T-cell leukemia

Sézary syndrome

Table 30

LABORATORY CHARACTERISTICS OF SMALL T-LYMPHOCYTE PROLIFERATIONS*

	CD4	CD8	CD25	HTLV-1	Cytogenetics
T-Prolymphocytic leukemia	+	–/+	+/–	–	inv(14)(q11q32)**
Large granulated lymphocyte leukemia[+]	–	+		–	
Adult T-cell leukemia	+	–	+	+	
Sézary syndrome	+	–	–	–	

* All disorders variably express pan–T-cell antigens (CD2, CD3, CD5) and are terminal deoxynucleotidyl-transferase (TdT) negative.
**In 76 percent of cases, a translocation involving breakpoints at these two chromosomal bands is present (99).
[+]A natural killer cell type of LGL is CD3 and CD8 negative and CD56 positive.

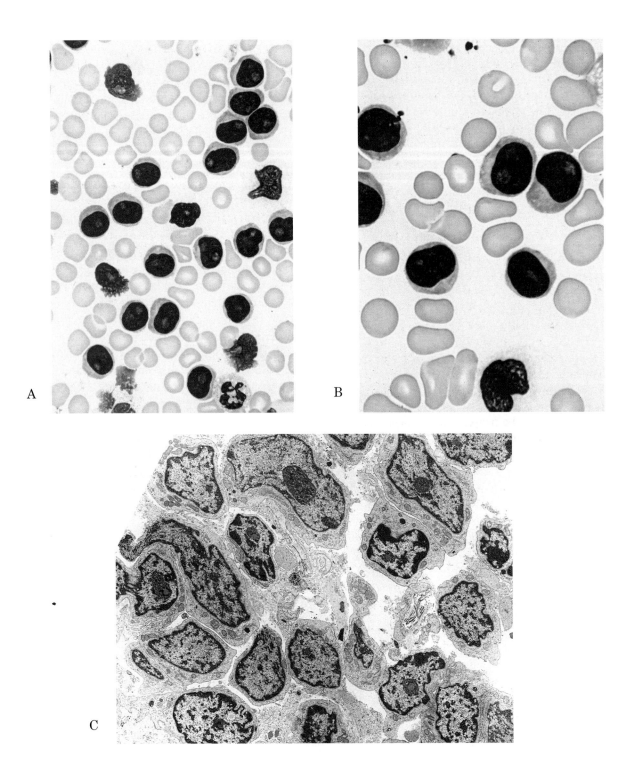

Figure 320
T-PROLYMPHOCYTIC LEUKEMIA

A and B. Blood smear from a 78-year-old man who had a leukocyte count of 110×10^9/L with a predominant population of prolymphocytes that have abundant basophilic cytoplasm, round nuclei with coarse chromatin, and prominent nucleoli. These cells formed spontaneous rosettes with sheep erythrocytes and were surface immunoglobulin negative. The specimen predated monoclonal antibody studies. (Wright-Giemsa stain)

C. Electron micrograph of a portion of a lymph node from the same patient. The nuclear chromatin in the prolymphocytes is marginated along the nuclear membrane. Several of the cells have prominent nucleoli. (Uranyl acetate–lead citrate stains, X5200)

be observed in the same case although one pattern predominates (99). The degree of nuclear irregularity is usually substantially less than that observed in Sézary syndrome or adult T-cell leukemia. However, cases with lymphocytes with polylobulated nuclei or nuclei resembling those in Sézary cells have been observed in the spectrum of T PL (99,100). The cytoplasm is moderately to intensely basophilic and some of the cells may have cytoplasmic projections.

In approximately 20 percent of cases, the lymphocytes lack the distinctive features of a prolymphocyte; the nucleolus is not prominent in specimens examined by light microscopy but is identified by electron microscopy (figs. 321, 322). These cases have been designated as the *small cell variant* of T PL. The prolymphocytes in the small cell variant may have a high nuclear-cytoplasmic ratio with a sparse rim of basophilic cytoplasm. In some cases there is evolution from a predominant population of small lymphocytes to a population of lymphocytes more characteristic of prolymphocytes (figs. 323, 324). Azurophilic granules may be present in a minority of cells.

Histopathologic Findings. The degree of bone marrow involvement varies considerably and is reported to range from 30 to 50 percent. There may be discordance between the magnitude of the leukocyte count and the degree of bone marrow involvement in that patients with marked leukocytosis may have a modest degree of marrow infiltration with substantial sparing of normal hematopoietic cells (fig. 321B). The pattern of infiltration may be diffuse, interstitial, diffuse plus interstitial, or focal plus interstitial. A focal pattern only was not found in the largest series of cases reported (99). A moderate increase in reticulin fibers is usually present.

Ultrastructural Findings. On electron microscopic examination, the nuclei of the T prolymphocytes vary from round to irregular with varying degrees of nuclear enfolding; some lymphocytes may show a polylobulated or cerebriform nuclear outline (figs. 320C, 322A, 325). The heterochromatin is marginated along the nuclear membrane. The cytoplasm frequently contains long or circular strands of smooth or rough endoplasmic reticulum, usually associated with clusters of ribosomes and polyribosomes. Large to medium sized dense granules are present in the prolymphocytes in a majority of patients (100).

Cytochemical Findings. The prolymphocytes usually manifest some acid phosphatase activity which may be tartrate resistant (99,100, 124). The cells may also show NSE reactivity. NSE activity utilizing alpha-naphthyl acetate as a substrate is focal or dot-like (99,100,124).

Immunologic Findings. T prolymphocytes have immunologic characteristics of post-thymic lymphocytes. The cells are TdT negative and express the pan–T-cell markers CD2, CD3, and CD5; CD7 is expressed in over 90 percent of cases and CD25 in about 20 percent. In approximately 70 percent of cases the prolymphocytes express a helper cell phenotype, CD4+, CD8- (Table 30) (99). CD4+, CD8+ is expressed in approximately 20 percent of cases, and CD4-, CD8+ in 10 percent.

Cytogenetic Findings. The most consistent chromosome abnormality in T PL, present in 76 percent of cases, occurs on chromosome 14 with a translocation involving breakpoints at 14q11 and 14q32; the affected 14q11 band is the locus for the T-cell alpha- and delta-receptor genes (fig. 321D). In the majority of cases, the abnormality is an inv(14)(q11q32). Approximately 50 percent of patients also have a trisomy for chromosome 8 in addition to the abnormalities involving chromosome 14 (74,99).

Differential Diagnosis. The differential diagnosis of T PL has to be viewed from two perspectives: distinction from B-prolymphocytic leukemia and distinction from other post-thymic T-cell proliferations.

Although both B- and T-prolymphocytic leukemias were initially reported as a single morphologic entity, it is apparent that the generalizations about clinical findings in the original report do not always apply to T PL (81,89). B-prolymphocytic leukemia usually presents with marked splenomegaly and no peripheral lymphadenopathy. In contrast, approximately half of the patients with T PL have lymphadenopathy and one fourth have skin lesions. There is also much more heterogeneity in the morphology of the leukemic cells in T PL. The prolymphocyte is a large cell with a relatively low nuclear-cytoplasmic ratio, round to oval nucleus, moderately stippled chromatin, and a single prominent nucleolus. The abundant cytoplasm is lightly to moderately basophilic. The T prolymphocyte may have a higher nuclear-cytoplasmic ratio, more intensely basophilic cytoplasm, and coarser nuclear chromatin.

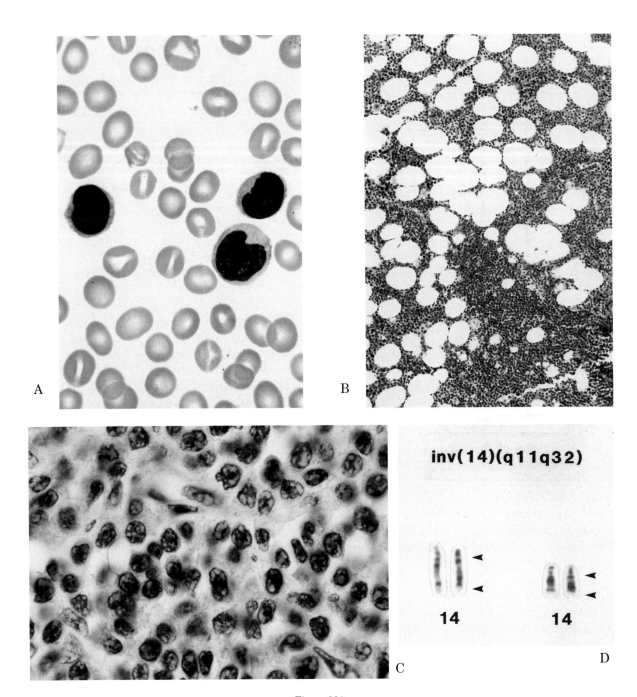

Figure 321
T-PROLYMPHOCYTIC LEUKEMIA

A. Blood smear from a 38-year-old woman who had a leukocyte count of 40×10^9/L with a CD4+, CD8- T-cell lymphocytosis; there was minimal lymphadenopathy on physical examination. The lymphocytes varied in size but were generally small with a slight amount of moderately basophilic cytoplasm and clumped chromatin. Indistinct nucleoli are noted in two of the cells. The lymphocytes from this specimen showed an inv(14) (q11q32) chromosome abnormality. (Wright-Giemsa stain)

B. Bone marrow biopsy obtained at the same time as the specimen in A. The photograph shows one of several aggregates of lymphocytes. A substantial portion of the marrow is uninvolved. (Hematoxylin and eosin stain)

C. High magnification of the lymphocytic aggregate in B showing lymphocytes with markedly irregular nuclei. Many of the lymphocytes have distinct but not prominent nucleoli. The diagnosis of prolymphocytic leukemia is not suggested by this specimen. (Hematoxylin and eosin stain)

D. Portion of a karyotype of a lymphocyte from the specimen shown in B showing an inv(14)(q11q32) abnormality. (G banded, Wright-Giemsa stained)

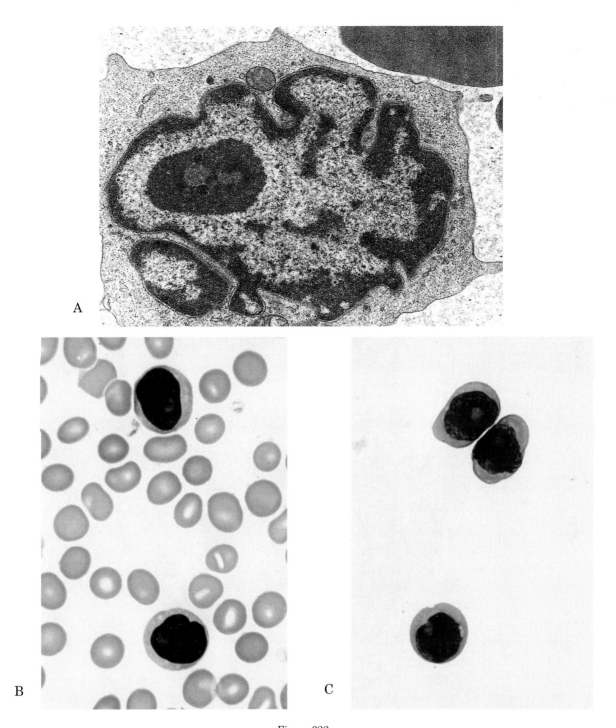

Figure 322
T-PROLYMPHOCYTIC LEUKEMIA

A. Electron micrograph of a prolymphocyte from a blood specimen obtained at the same time as the specimen in 321A. The nuclear outline is irregular; there is a single prominent nucleolus. (Uranyl acetate–lead citrate stains, X21,000)

B. Blood smear from the same patient as in figure 321A 22 months following bone marrow transplantation and 27 months following diagnosis. At this time the patient presented with occipital cortex and sinus masses. The blood contained numerous lymphocytes of the type illustrated. The cells are large, with moderately abundant basophilic cytoplasm and relatively prominent nucleoli. (Wright-Giemsa stain)

C. Prolymphocytes in a cytospin of a spinal fluid specimen obtained at the same time as the specimen in B. The cells are identical to those in the blood. (Wright-Giemsa stain)

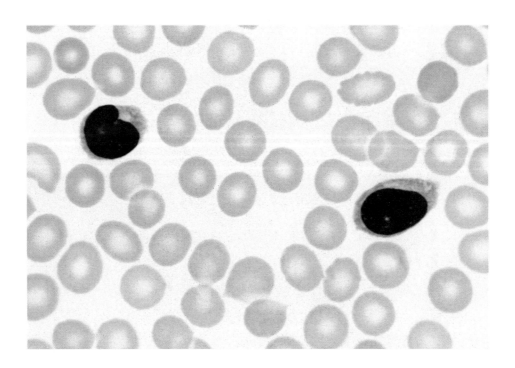

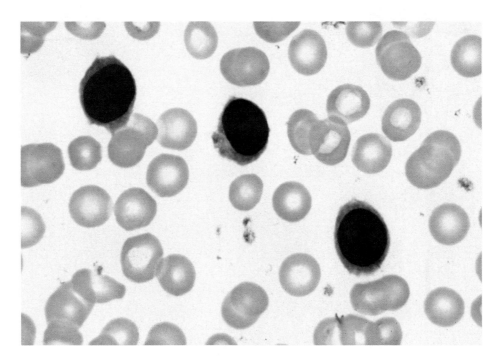

Figure 323
T-PROLYMPHOCYTIC LEUKEMIA: SMALL CELL VARIANT SHOWING EVOLUTION TO LARGE CELLS

Top: Blood smear from a 58-year-old woman with splenomegaly and a leukocyte count of 11.2×10^9/L with 70 percent lymphocytes. As illustrated, the lymphocytes had a rim of moderately basophilic cytoplasm. The nuclear chromatin is clumped. Small nucleoli are present. (Wright-Giemsa stain)

Bottom: Blood smear from the same patient 2 months later. The leukocyte count at this time was 33×10^9/L with 84 percent lymphocytes. The lymphocytes are similar to those in A but nucleoli are slightly more prominent. (Wright-Giemsa stain)

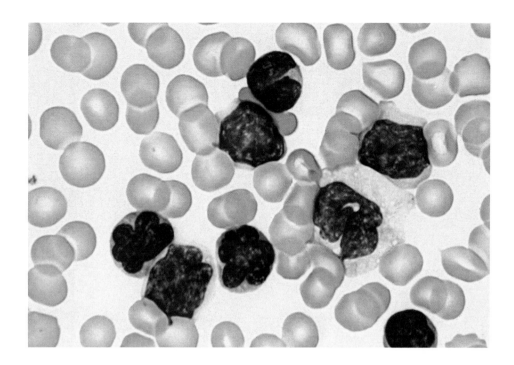

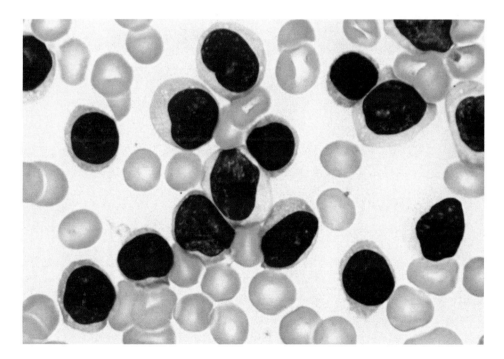

Figure 324

T-PROLYMPHOCYTIC LEUKEMIA: SMALL CELL VARIANT SHOWING EVOLUTION TO LARGE CELLS

Top: Blood smear from the patient in figure 323 14 months later. The leukocyte count at this time was 212×10^9/L. The lymphocytes show marked variation in nuclear shape; some nuclei are markedly lobulated. A monocyte with abundant cytoplasm and lobulated nucleus is also present. The electron micrographs in figure 325 are from this specimen. (Wright-Giemsa stain)

Bottom: Blood smear 21 months after the specimen in 323A. The leukocyte count was 477×10^9/L, Hb 11.7 g/dL, and platelets 42×10^9/L. Both large and small lymphocytes are present. Some of the lymphocytes have distinct but not unusually prominent nucleoli. The lymphocytes from all specimens were CD5+, CD7+, CD4+, CD8-, and TdT negative. The patient died 2 days after this smear was obtained. (Wright-Giemsa stain)

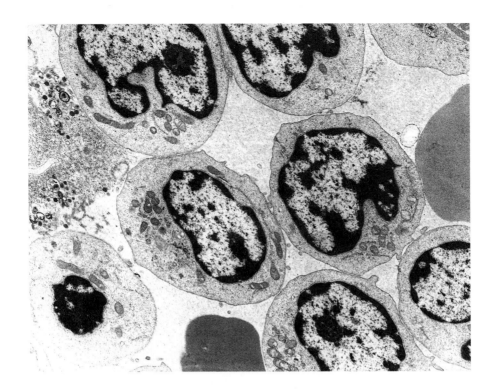

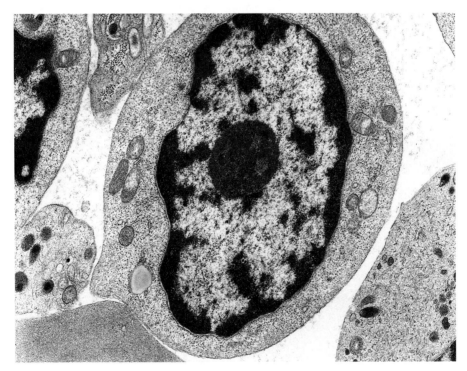

Figure 325
T-PROLYMPHOCYTIC LEUKEMIA: ULTRASTRUCTURE

Top: Electron micrograph of the specimen in figure 324, top. The lymphocytes show variability in nuclear contour. (Uranyl acetate–lead citrate stains, X75,000)

Bottom: A prolymphocyte from the specimen on top with a prominent nucleolus. The cytoplasm is abundant with numerous free ribosomes. (Uranyl acetate–lead citrate stains, X18,000)

The nuclear outline may be round, oval, or irregular with folds and convolutions. The definitive method for distinguishing these two disorders is by immunophenotyping. The B prolymphocyte has light chain restricted surface immunoglobulin and reacts with B-cell–associated antibodies; the T prolymphocyte reacts with T-cell–associated monoclonal antibodies.

The two major entities to be considered in the context of the post-thymic T-cell lymphoproliferative disorders are adult T-cell leukemia and T-cell chronic lymphocytic leukemia. Adult T-cell leukemia is distinguished by positive serology for HTLV-1. In addition, the leukemic cells in adult T-cell leukemia have marked nuclear lobulation; the nuclear contour has been characterized as "flower" shaped. This type of polylobulation may occur in T PL but is uncommon.

The distinction of T PL from T-cell chronic lymphocytic leukemia is partly conceptual (87, 99,104). It has been suggested that T-cell chronic lymphocytic leukemia is not a distinct entity and that all post-thymic T-cell proliferations can be categorized as either large granulated lymphocyte leukemia, prolymphocytic leukemia, or HTLV-1 related adult T-cell leukemia (87). It is important that all high white blood cell count lymphocytic leukemias be immunophenotyped. If a process is of T-cell origin, cytogenetic studies and serologic studies for HTLV-1 should be performed. If abnormalities involving translocations of band q11 and q32 on chromosome 14 are present, the diagnosis of T-prolymphocytic leukemia should be strongly considered if the membrane surface markers and morphology are consistent.

There are some post-thymic T-lymphocyte proliferations involving the blood and bone marrow that do not satisfy the morphologic criteria of T PL, large granulated T-lymphocyte leukemia, or Sézary syndrome, and have negative serology for HTLV-1. Some of these cases have the clinical and lymph node or other organ manifestations of peripheral T-cell lymphoma (figs. 326, 327). In other instances, the findings are less clear (figs. 328, 329). These cases may be categorized as post-thymic T-lymphocyte proliferations; in the majority of cases these probably represent cases of peripheral T-cell lymphoma. Because of the frequent lack of correspondence between morphology and clinical behavior in some of these diseases, the qualifying term "chronic" should be avoided, even in those cases in which the lymphocytes appear well differentiated. The biology of these processes may become clear only after a period of careful clinical and hematologic observation.

Treatment and Prognosis. T PL is a rapidly progressive disease with a median survival time of 7.5 months. The therapy used in B-cell lymphomas generally has little effect. The use of a nucleoside analog, 2' deoxycoformycin, has resulted in some responses of relatively brief duration (99).

Adult T-Cell Leukemia-Lymphoma

Definition. A post-thymic lymphoproliferative process of helper T lymphocytes with an onset in adult life. The characteristic lymphocytes have markedly lobulated nuclei (122). Adult T-cell leukemia-lymphoma (ATCL) usually has an acute course but smoldering and chronic forms have been reported (93,120,129). The disease may present primarily as a lymphoma with no or minimal involvement of the blood and bone marrow or with leukocyte counts of 500×10^9/L. The disease is associated with the human T-cell leukemia-lymphoma virus, type 1 (HTLV-1) infection in most cases (75,88).

A clinical pathologic classification of ATCL based on the number of leukemic cells in the blood and the presence of lymphadenopathy at the time of diagnosis has been proposed (115). Patients with 10 percent or more leukemic cells in the blood and no detectable lymphadenopathy are classified as having leukemia. Patients with one or more enlarged lymph nodes and few or no leukemic cells in the blood are classified as having lymphoma. Patients with both lymphadenopathy and 10 percent or more leukemic cells in the blood are classified in an intermediate or mixed type group (113,115). Thirty-one percent of patients in one series presented with leukemia, 50 percent with lymphoma, and 19 percent with the mixed type. Patients initially presenting with a lymphoma usually develop blood involvement at some time during the course of the illness (115).

Incidence and Clinical Findings. The highest number of cases of ATCL is reported from southwestern Japan, the Caribbean basin, and west Africa (82,102,118,122). ATCL is rare in other parts of the western hemisphere and in Europe. It is essentially a disease of adults; a rare pediatric case has been reported. A mean

A

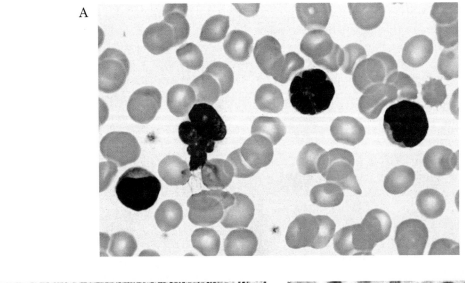

B

C

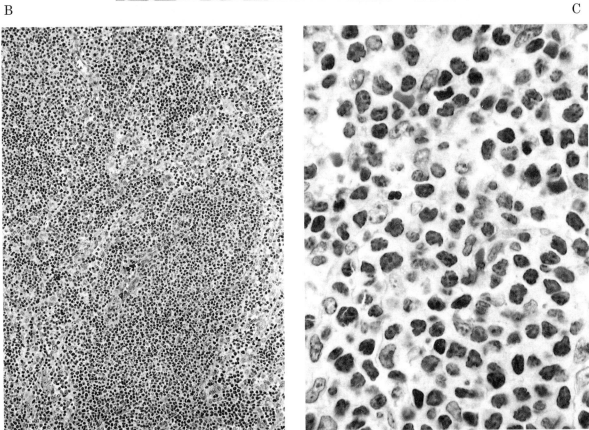

Figure 326
PERIPHERAL T-CELL LYMPHOMA WITH BLOOD INVOLVEMENT

A. Blood smear from a 53-year-old male who presented with lymphocytosis, slight thrombocytopenia, and marked spleno-megaly. The majority of lymphocytes had sparse cytoplasm, clumped chromatin, and markedly lobulated nuclei as shown. The lymphocytes expressed CD2, CD3, CD5, CD7, and CD8. The cells were CD4 and TdT negative. HTLV-1 serology was negative. (Wright-Giemsa stain)

B. Lymph node biopsy from the patient whose blood smear is illustrated in A. There is complete effacement of the lymph node architecture; vascular structures are prominent. (Hematoxylin and eosin stain)

C. High magnification of the specimen in A showing numerous lymphocytes with convoluted nuclei. Some of the lymphocytes have distinct nucleoli. (Hematoxylin and eosin stain)

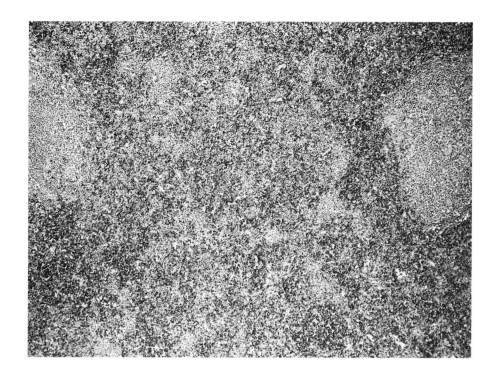

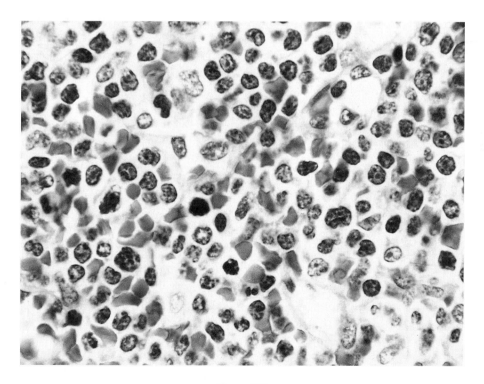

Figure 327
PERIPHERAL T-CELL LYMPHOMA WITH BLOOD INVOLVEMENT

Top: Area of the spleen from the patient in figure 326 showing involvement of both the white and red pulp. (Hematoxylin and eosin stain)

Bottom: High magnification of the same specimen showing red pulp infiltration. Several mitotic figures are present in this field. (Hematoxylin and eosin stain)

Figure 328
POST-THYMIC T-CELL
LEUKEMIA-LYMPHOMA

Blood smear from a 47-year-old male who presented with lymphocytosis and lymphadenopathy. The event initiating hospitalization was the sudden onset of seizures. The majority of lymphocytes in the blood were medium sized with markedly lobulated nuclei and clumped nuclear chromatin. The lymphocytes expressed CD3, CD4, and CD5; they were CD8 and TdT negative. Serologic studies for HTLV-1 were negative. The serum calcium level was normal. Despite intensive chemotherapy the patient had a rapidly progressive clinical course and died 7 months following diagnosis. Autopsy findings showed extensive organ involvement, including the skin and central nervous system. Note the similarity of this lymphocyte to the lymphocyte in figure 330. (Wright-Giemsa stain)

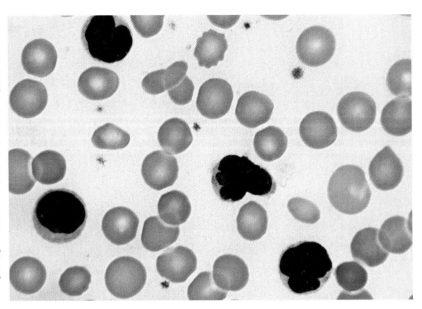

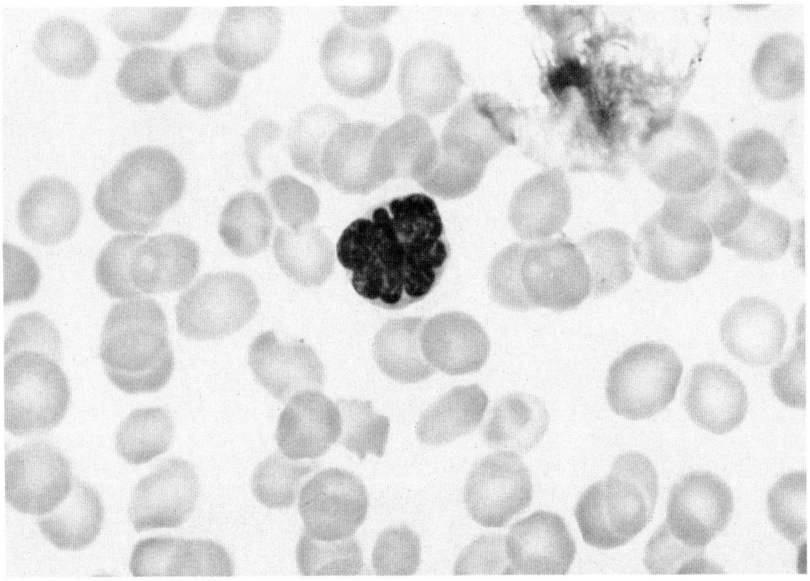

Figure 329
POST-THYMIC T-CELL
LEUKEMIA-LYMPHOMA

Lymphocyte in the blood of a 77-year-old male with marked splenomegaly and lymphadenopathy. The patient was a life-long resident of Minnesota and had never received a blood transfusion. The leukocyte count at the time of this specimen was 19×10^9/L with 74 percent lymphocytes. Many of the lymphocytes had markedly polylobulated nuclei similar to the one shown. The leukocyte count rapidly increased and 6 days later was 70×10^9/L with 94 percent lymphocytes. The lymphocytes expressed CD3, CD4, and CD5. Serology for HTLV-1 was negative. The serum calcium level was normal. The patient died 21 days after the initial specimen was obtained. (Wright-Giemsa stain)

age of 57 years has been reported (102). The male to female ration is 1–1.7 to 1 (94,102,118,122).

Lymphadenopathy is the major clinical finding and is present in approximately 70 to 85 percent of cases (94,102,117,118); splenomegaly is present in 38 to 51 percent of cases and hepatomegaly in 33 to 77 percent. Skin lesions are found in 45 to 50 percent and are characteristically a maculopapular rash or nodules, frequently preceding leukemic manifestations. Generalized erythroderma is rare. Central nervous system involvement occurs in approximately 10 percent of patients (121).

HTLV-1 infection is also associated with tropical spastic paraparesis and the rare concurrence of ATCL- and HTLV-1–associated myelopathy has been reported (79,80).

Laboratory Findings. The major laboratory finding, in addition to the hematologic abnormalities, is a positive serology for HTLV-1 (88). A small number of patients with seronegative ATCL have been reported from Japan (116).

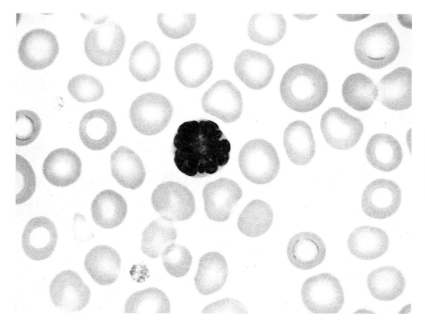

Figure 330
ADULT T-CELL LEUKEMIA
Blood smear from a patient from the Kyushu region of Japan with HTLV-1–positive adult T-cell leukemia. The lymphocyte has a markedly lobulated, "flower" shaped nucleus. (Wright-Giemsa stain)

Anemia is relatively mild: the hemoglobin is less than 10 g/dL in 14 percent of patients (102, 115). Platelet counts of less than 100×10^9/L occur in 17 percent of patients. The leukocyte count may range up to 500×10^9/L. Serum immunoglobulin levels are usually normal. The calcium level is increased in up to 75 percent of patients at some time during the course of the disease; 20 to 50 percent of cases have increased levels at diagnosis (94,95,117,120). Associated osteolytic lesions may be present. The mechanism of the hypercalcemia is increased osteoclast activity, possibly related to the elaboration of a parathyroid related hormone by the leukemic cells (125).

Blood and Bone Marrow Findings. The morphology of the leukemic cells in ATCL is one of the most striking of all leukemic proliferations. The characteristic feature is marked lobulation of the nucleus, which has led to the designation "flower-like" (fig. 330). This degree of hyperlobulation may not be present in all cases. The cells can be predominantly of one size or show marked variation in an individual case (figs. 331, 332). The amount of cytoplasm varies and is slightly to moderately basophilic.

Japanese investigators have categorized ATCL into three clinical morphologic groups: acute, chronic, and smoldering (93,120). In the acute type, there are numerous abnormal lymphocytes in the blood. The lymphocytes show marked variation in size and degree of nuclear irregularity; the

cytoplasm is variably basophilic. In the chronic type, the leukemic cells are relatively uniform in size; the nuclei show relatively uniform bilobulation or enfolding. In the smoldering type, there is 0.5 to 3 percent abnormal lymphocytes in the blood. The cells are described as relatively large with indented, clefted, or bilobed nuclei.

Histopathologic Findings. The bone marrow may have only minimal involvement in the form of a sparse diffuse infiltration or poorly demarcated focal lesions. The marrow biopsies from patients with hypercalcemia usually show bone resorption with prominent osteoclastic activity (fig. 333). These findings are unrelated to the degree of marrow involvement by the lymphoma and may be present in specimens without marrow evidence of lymphoma.

Cytochemical Findings. The leukemic cells may show focal positivity with acid phosphatase, beta-glucuronidase, and NSE. The reactions are nonspecific and may be similar to reactions in other lymphocytic leukemias of the post-thymic T-cell type.

Ultrastructural Findings. The lymphocytes show nuclear pleomorphism with varying degrees of nuclear lobulation. Condensed heterochromatin is distributed along the nuclear border. Nuclear pockets containing tubuloreticular filamentous structures are characteristic. Clustered dense bodies may be observed in the cytoplasm (85).

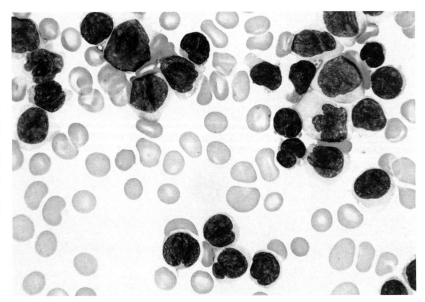

Figure 331
ADULT T-CELL LEUKEMIA
Blood smear from a woman from Louisiana presenting with a leukocyte count of 280×10^9/L, skin lesions, and positive serology for HTLV-1; the serum calcium level was normal. There is marked variation in the size of the lymphocytes. The nuclei vary from round to lobulated; some have Sézary cell–type nuclear convolutions. The lymphocytes expressed CD2, CD3, CD4, CD5, and CD25 and were negative for CD8 and TdT. (Wright-Giemsa stain)

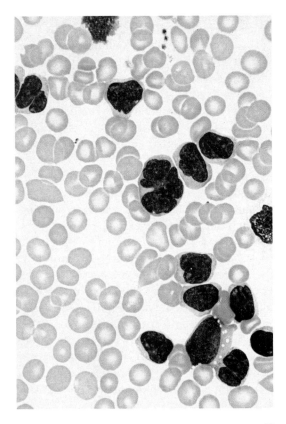

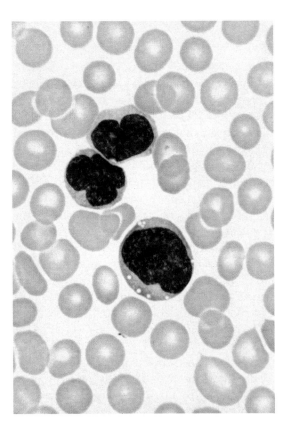

Figure 332
ADULT T-CELL LEUKEMIA
Left: Blood smear from a 34-year-old woman residing in the upper midwest of the United States after emigrating from Liberia 2 years previously. The presenting leukocyte count was 180×10^9/L; serology was positive for HTLV-1 and the serum calcium level was 14.6 mg/dL. The lymphocytes vary in size and degree of nuclear lobulation. Some of the cells have round or only slightly lobulated nuclei. The lymphocytes expressed CD3, CD4, CD5, and CD25 and were CD8 and TdT negative. (Wright-Giemsa stain)
Right: High magnification of the same smear. (Wright-Giemsa stain)

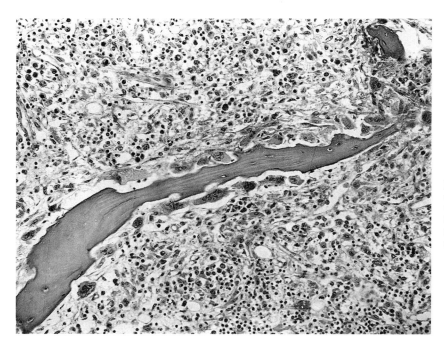

Figure 333
ADULT T-CELL LEUKEMIA:
BONE MARROW BIOPSY
WITH INCREASED
OSTEOCLASTIC ACTIVITY

Bone marrow biopsy from a patient from the Kyushu region of Japan with HTLV-1–positive adult T-cell leukemia. There is marked osteoclastic activity with erosion of bone trabeculae. (Hematoxylin and eosin stain)

Immunologic Findings. The proliferating lymphocytes in ATCL are post-thymic cells and express the pan–T-cell antibodies CD2, CD3, and CD5. They are TdT negative (75,117,118,128). The lymphocytes from most cases express a helper cell phenotype, CD4+, CD8-; rare cases are CD8+. The cells frequently express CD25 and are negative for CD7 in contrast to the lymphocytes in T-prolymphocytic leukemia which express CD7.

Cytogenetic Findings. The cytogenetic abnormalities reported in ATCL are nonspecific and include trisomies for chromosomes 3, 7, and 21, monosomy for chromosome X in females, and loss of a Y in males. The most frequent structural abnormalities include translocations involving 14q32 or 14q11 and deletion of 6q; other structural abnormalities include deletion of 10p, 3q, 5q, 9q, 13q, 1p, and 7p. The combination of rearrangement in 14q32 and monosomy X, or deletion of 10p and trisomy 3 and deletion in 6q21 has been reported as occurring only in the acute type (92,98,107,116,119).

A correlation between the clinical stage and the cytogenetic findings has been reported (109). The chromosome number ranges from diploid to pseudodiploid to hyperdiploid in acute ATCL, from hypodiploid to hyperdiploid in the chronic type, and is diploid in the smoldering type. Patients with the acute form have a high incidence of trisomy for

3, trisomy for 7, or both. These findings are not present in the chronic or smoldering types.

Differential Diagnosis. ATCL has two important features, positive HTLV-1 serology and the markedly lobulated nuclei of the leukemic cells, which aid in distinguishing it from diseases with which it may possibly be confused.

The lymphocytes in T-prolymphocytic leukemia and Sézary syndrome may occasionally suggest the possibility of ATCL but the negative HTLV-1 serology excludes these disorders; hypercalcemia is absent in both.

Although most cases of ATCL are positive for HTLV-1, a small number of HTLV-1–negative ATCL cases have been reported from Japan and elsewhere. These are described as clinically and hematologically indistinguishable from HTLV-1–positive ATCL but are serologically negative and show no evidence of integration of the HTLV-1 proviral genome into chromosomal DNA. Sera from relatives of these patients are also negative for HTLV-1 (116). These patients have chromosome findings and an incidence of hypercalcemia similar to patients with HTLV-1–positive ATCL. These features should aid in distinguishing these patients from those with T-prolymphocytic leukemia.

Treatment and Prognosis. The acute form of ATCL is an aggressive disease; 50 percent of patients are dead within 4.4 months of diagnosis.

The chronic and smoldering forms have a somewhat indolent course until the acute or crisis phase supervenes, at which time there is rapid progression (93,120). Some cases of smoldering leukemia remain in that stage for several years.

For ATCL patients presenting primarily with leukemia, i.e., leukemic cells comprising more than 10 percent of the blood leukocytes, the median survival time is 13.5 months; for those with a lymphomatous presentation the median survival is 10.5 months (115). Patients with a mixed type presentation have the shortest survival, 3 months. The magnitude of the leukocyte count and the absolute number of leukemic cells in the blood appear to correlate with prognosis; higher counts are associated with a more aggressive clinical course (113). Other unfavorable prognostic factors include high corrected calcium level, advanced performance status, elevated lactic acid dehydrogenase level, and age over 40 years (98,113).

Treatment primarily consists of multiagent chemotherapy and radiotherapy. Only a small number of patients achieve a durable remission (114).

Large Granulated Lymphocyte Leukemia

Definition. A proliferation of medium to large granulated lymphocytes. The lymphocytes in the majority of cases are CD3+, CD8+, and CD4-. In a minority of cases the granulated lymphocytes express natural killer cell markers and are CD3 and CD8 negative.

Incidence and Clinical Findings. Large granulated lymphocyte leukemia (LGL) is a rare disorder occurring primarily in adults. There is a slight male predominance; the median age at diagnosis ranges from 55 to 65 years. The disorder may occur in young adults and rare cases have been reported in children (73,96,103,106).

Because of the severe neutropenia associated with this process in the majority of patients with CD3+ and CD8+ lymphocytes, many of the patients present with a history of recurrent bacterial infection; a minority of patients have the clinical features of rheumatoid arthritis (73,96, 103,106). Patients with CD3- and CD8- granulated lymphocytoses do not usually have severe neutropenia or the findings of rheumatoid arthritis (83).

Splenomegaly is observed in more than half of the cases. Hepatomegaly occurs in a small number. Lymphadenopathy related to the proliferative process is uncommon (73,96,103,106); however, lymphadenopathy related to regional bacterial infection may be present and may be prominent.

Laboratory Findings. The major hematologic finding is a lymphocytosis. The increase in lymphocytes may be modest and is less than 20×10^9/L in 95 percent of cases (73,96). There is usually an associated neutropenia that may be marked: 40 to 60 percent of patients have neutrophil counts of less than 0.5×10^9/L (73,96,103). Cases of cyclic neutropenia have been reported (96). A normocytic normochromic or macrocytic normochromic anemia is present in approximately one third of patients. Thrombocytopenia is reported in 22 to 36 percent (73,96,103).

Polyclonal hypergammaglobulinemia, a positive rheumatoid factor, and antinuclear antibodies are found in slightly more than half of the patients and circulating immune complexes in 75 to 100 percent (73,96,103). Antineutrophil antibodies are present in 50 to 65 percent of patients and antiplatelet antibodies in 90 percent.

Blood and Bone Marrow Findings. The major finding in the blood is an increase in medium to large lymphocytes that have abundant clear to very slightly basophilic cytoplasm containing coarse azurophilic granules. The granules vary in number and size (83,101). The nucleus is round to slightly ovoid (fig. 334). The nuclear chromatin is condensed and nucleoli are indistinct or absent. These lymphocytes are similar to the reactive or Downy II lymphocytes that may be observed in infectious mononucleosis and other viral infections. The hypergammaglobulinemia is reflected by increased rouleaux formation.

The bone marrow smear shows a modest increase in granulated lymphocytes in most cases (fig. 334) (83,101). Neutrophils and erythroid precursors are usually normal to slightly decreased in number, with a full maturation spectrum. Cases with a shift to immaturity or "maturation arrest" at the promyelocyte and myelocyte stage have been reported (103).

Histopathologic Findings. The bone marrow is usually hypercellular. The pattern of infiltration of the granulated lymphocytes is usually interstitial; there may be focal aggregates in some cases (fig. 334C). In some patients the amount of infiltration may be minimal and essentially imperceptible in routine preparations (101). Mild to moderate reticulin fibrosis is noted in some patients.

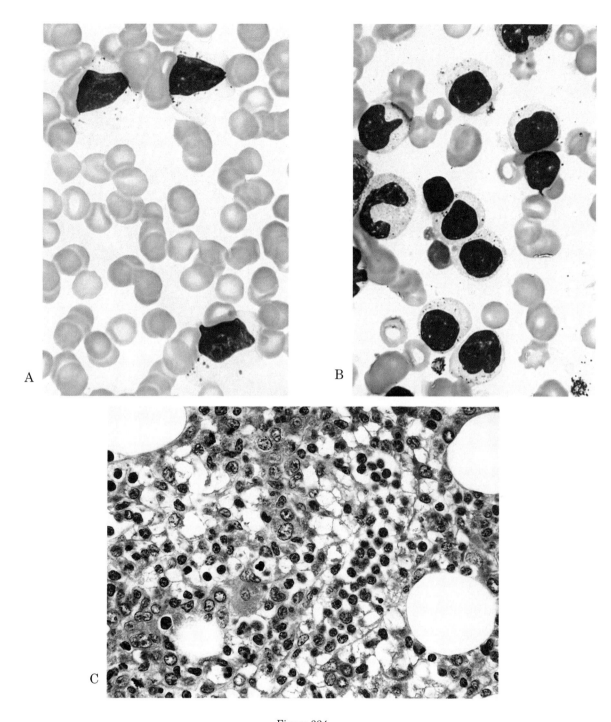

Figure 334
LARGE GRANULATED T-LYMPHOCYTE LEUKEMIA

A. Blood smear from a 23-year-old man with a leukocyte count of 18×10^9/L with 98 percent lymphocytes and 2 percent neutrophils. The majority of lymphocytes were large with abundant pale cytoplasm containing several coarse azurophilic granules. The lymphocytes expressed CD3, CD5, and CD8. (Wright-Giemsa stain)

B. Bone marrow obtained at the same time as the specimen in A showing six lymphocytes with several azurophilic granules. (Wright-Giemsa stain)

C. Bone marrow biopsy from the same patient. There is an accumulation of small lymphocytes to the right of center. Other lymphocytes, fewer in number, are scattered throughout the interstitium. Approximately half of the field consists of neutrophil precursors with abundant granular cytoplasm and round to slightly indented nuclei. (Hematoxylin and eosin stain)

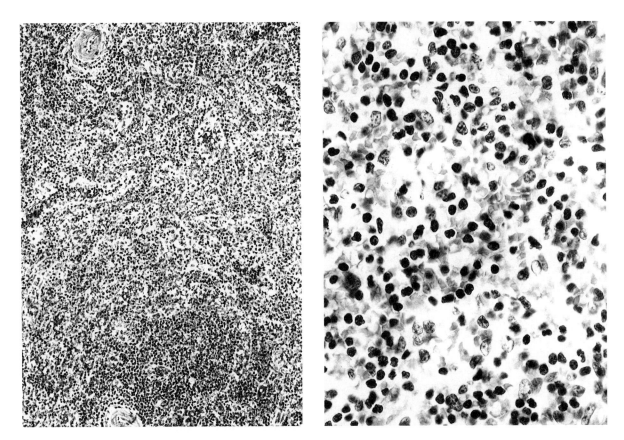

Figure 335
LARGE GRANULATED LYMPHOCYTE LEUKEMIA: SPLEEN
Left: Area of an enlarged spleen from a patient with LGL leukemia. There is diffuse involvement of the red pulp. The malpighian corpuscles are infiltrated by the leukemic cells and the demarcation between the white and red pulp is obscured. Both the cords and sinuses of the red pulp are involved by the leukemic process. (Hematoxylin and eosin stain)
Right: High magnification of the same specimen. (Hematoxylin and eosin stain)

The splenic architecture remains basically intact. The red pulp is expanded and infiltrated by the leukemic cells (fig. 335) (71). The infiltrate is predominantly sinusoidal but may involve the splenic cords. The follicles appear normal in number; germinal centers have been described as both prominent and absent. The liver shows a sinusoidal pattern of involvement; portal infiltration may be present in cases with extensive involvement (71). Lymphocyte infiltration has been reported in other sites including skeletal muscle, myocardium, kidney, lung, gastrointestinal tract, and adrenals (71).

Cytochemical Findings. The large granulated lymphocytes show reactivity for beta-glucuronidase and tartrate-sensitive acid phosphatase (101).

Ultrastructural Findings. The principal and only significant ultrastructural finding in the majority of patients with LGL leukemia is the presence of bundles of parallel tubular arrays in the granular structures (fig. 336) (101). In the subset of patients with CD3- lymphocytes, the granules contain amorphous substance and no evidence of parallel tubular arrays (83).

Immunologic Findings. Although some immunologic heterogeneity has been reported for LGL leukemia, there are two major immunophenotypic groups. The most common of these is the CD3+, CD4-, CD8+ group (73,83,96, 101,103,106). The lymphocytes in this type are variable for expression of CD16, CD57, and HLA-DR; the cells lack natural killer cell function but show a variable degree of antibody dependent

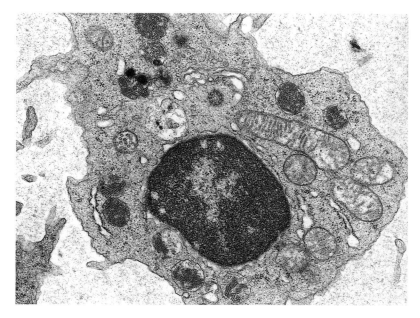

Figure 336
GRANULATED
T-LYMPHOCYTE LEUKEMIA:
ULTRASTRUCTURE
Electron micrograph of a lymphocyte from the same patient as in figure 334 showing several membrane-bound bundles of parallel tubular arrays. (Uranyl acetate–lead citrate stains, X27,000)

cell-mediated cytotoxicity (83). In the second major type, the lymphocytes are CD3-, CD8-, CD56+ and have natural killer and cell-mediated antibody activity (83). The lymphocytes in the CD3+, CD4-, CD8+ type may show T-cell receptor rearrangement while cells of the second type have been reported as negative for this rearrangement (83).

Cytogenetic Findings. Cytogenetic studies have not shown consistent clonal abnormalities.

Differential Diagnosis. The differential diagnosis of LGL leukemia relates principally to two processes: B-cell chronic lymphocytic leukemia and a reactive lymphocytosis.

The distinction of LGL leukemia from B-cell chronic lymphocytic leukemia is based primarily on the morphology of the lymphocytes and immunologic studies. B-cell chronic lymphocytic leukemia may manifest as a proliferation of medium sized lymphocytes with abundant cytoplasm, but these cells usually lack the uniform granulation that is the hallmark of LGL leukemia. Large granulated lymphocytes, which are CD3+, CD4-, CD8+, may be present in the blood of patients with B-cell chronic lymphocytic leukemia but are distinct from the leukemic cell population. B-cell chronic lymphocytic leukemia may be accompanied by neutropenia but it is rarely as severe as in LGL leukemia and is primarily due to bone marrow replacement. Membrane surface markers are definitive and absolutely necessary to establish the diagnosis of LGL leukemia.

LGL leukemia must also be distinguished from a reactive lymphocytosis. This is particularly applicable to young adults. Viral infections such as infectious mononucleosis, are characterized by an increase in reactive lymphocytes in the blood; the major population of these lymphocytes may be morphologically, immunologically, and ultrastructurally identical to those of LGL leukemia and may be accompanied by severe neutropenia. Unlike LGL leukemia, the increase of these lymphocytes in reactive processes is of limited duration. Occasional patients with infectious mononucleosis may have a sustained increase of the CD8+ granulated lymphocytes with an accompanying neutropenia similar to that observed in LGL leukemia. Serologic studies for Epstein-Barr virus should be performed in all cases of large granulated lymphocytosis regardless of the age of the patient.

In some cases, a period of observation may be necessary to establish the diagnosis. Considering the indolent nature of the disease in most patients, this delay in diagnosis does not usually present a problem. Cytogenetics and molecular studies may demonstrate the clonal nature of the lymphocytes in LGL leukemia. Negative results do not absolutely exclude the possibility of a malignant clone. Prolonged observation may be necessary before a definitive diagnosis is established.

As with other lymphoproliferative disorders, the definition of LGL leukemia has been expanded to include disorders that may have some, but not all, of the features of the entity described in the initial reports. The major difficulty relates to what should be viewed as a large granulated lymphocyte. The cell, as identified in the majority of studies, has condensed nuclear chromatin and abundant pale to slightly basophilic cytoplasm that contains numerous coarse azurophilic granules. T-lymphocyte proliferations of larger cells with more immature nuclei and cytoplasmic granules should not be classified as LGL leukemia solely on the basis of the cytoplasmic granulations and immunologic markers if the morphology is at variance with the predominant pattern.

Aggressive forms of node-based T-cell lymphoma in which the lymphoma cells are large with fine nuclear chromatin and distinct nucleoli may have cytoplasmic granules. These lesions are morphologically and clinically distinct from the original concept of LGL leukemia. An aggresive form of large granulated lymphocyte leukemia-lymphoma of NK cell type, primarily occurring in Japanese patients, has been reported (90). The relationship of this entity to other forms of LGL leukemia is unclear.

Treatment and Prognosis. This disorder has an indolent course in most patients. The major problem in LGL leukemia is severe neutropenia with recurrent bacterial infections. These are usually managed with appropriate antibiotic therapy. In patients with severe persistent neutropenia, steroids and cyclosporin A have been used with variable results. Some patients succumb to bacterial infection (73,96). Occasional patients undergo long-term remission (101).

Sézary Syndrome

Definition. A proliferation of helper T lymphocytes that principally involve the skin and blood; the cutaneous involvement is manifest as a generalized pruritic exfoliative erythroderma (111).

Incidence and Clinical Findings. Sézary syndrome is uncommon. Males are affected more than females. The reported average age of onset in women is 55 years; the average age of onset in men is 63 years (127).

The principal clinical finding is a pruritic generalized erythroderma. Lymphadenopathy occurs in 50 to 60 percent of patients and hepatomegaly in approximately 30 percent. Alopecia, onychodystrophy, keratoderma, and palmar and plantar hyperpigmentation may also be present (126,127). Other than the dermatologic problems, many of the patients have a general feeling of well being.

Laboratory Findings. The hemoglobin level and platelet count are normal. There is a lymphocytosis; counts of up to 70×10^9/L have been reported (86). There may be an eosinophilia but it is not marked. Serum IgE may be elevated.

Blood and Bone Marrow Findings. The lymphocytes in Sézary syndrome are atypical helper T lymphocytes, referred to as Sézary cells. These cells have markedly convoluted nuclei. Large and small cell types may be observed (86). The number of lymphocytes that are Sézary cells is usually in excess of 40 percent and may be higher than 80 percent (86).

The most characteristic features of Sézary cells are expressed in the large cell type which is 12 to 25 μm in diameter, has a high nuclear-cytoplasmic ratio, and a nucleus with complex convolutions characterized as cerebriform (fig. 337). The chromatin varies in density and may show a delicate dispersion. Nucleoli are not apparent. The cytoplasm is clear to slightly basophilic; clear vacuoles may be present and are usually PAS positive.

The small cell variant is 8 to 11 μm in diameter. There is a high nuclear-cytoplasmic ratio and the nuclear chromatin is coarse (fig. 338). The characteristic grooving of the nucleus is less readily appreciated than in the large cell type and these cells may be difficult to distinguish from normal small lymphocytes. Some of the small cells may contain numerous cytoplasmic vacuoles which form a "necklace" around the nucleus and stain with PAS (fig. 338).

Histopathologic Findings. Bone marrow sections show preservation of normal hematopoiesis. The involvement by the Sézary cells is usually minimal and characterized by subtle infiltrates scattered in the interstitium and in the sinusoids; small focal aggregates may occur (108). Involvement of the marrow is more readily appreciated from examination of marrow smears than marrow sections.

The skin biopsy shows acanthosis, parakeratosis, and prominent rete pegs. A dense band of Sézary cells infiltrates the papillary and subpapillary dermis. Exocytosis of Sézary cells into

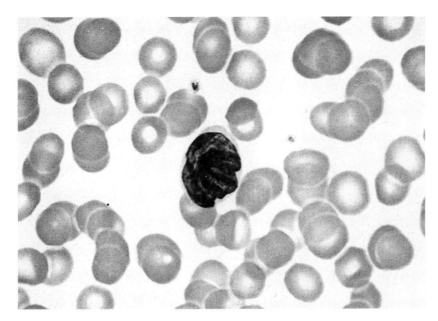

Figure 337
SÉZARY SYNDROME
Sézary cell in a blood smear from a 58-year-old woman with a 2-year history of generalized erythroderma. The nucleus has a "cerebriform" appearance. (Wright-Giemsa stain)

Figure 338
SÉZARY SYNDROME:
SMALL CELL

Three lymphocytes in a blood smear from a 52-year-old male with Sézary syndrome. The nucleus in the cell at the lower left shows delicate creases and folds. The two smaller cells have more condensed nuclear chromatin. The cytoplasm of both these cells contains numerous vacuoles. (Wright-Giemsa stain)

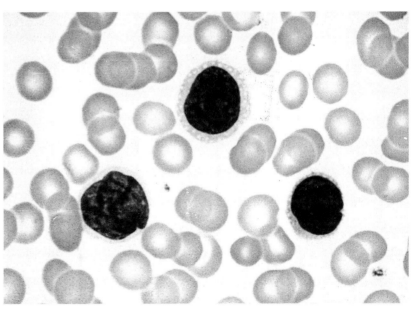

the epidermis is present and Pautrier microabscesses may be observed. A perivascular infiltration occurs. Mitoses are rare. An associated inflammatory cell infiltrate may be present (78).

Involved lymph nodes usually show either partial or focal replacement by mononuclear cells with cerebriform nuclei (110). Uninvolved areas frequently have the findings of dermatopathic lymphadenopathy (105,110).

Cytochemical Findings. The cytoplasmic vacuoles are usually PAS positive. Sézary cells show a positive reaction for beta-glucuronidase in the form of distinct large granules. The cells also react with acid phosphatase; both tartrate-sensitive and tartrate-resistant results have been reported.

Ultrastructural Findings. On ultrastructural study, the large Sézary cell characteristically has a markedly convoluted or serpentine nuclear outline; there is a dense margin of chromatin at the nuclear border (fig. 339) (97). A prominent nucleolus may be present. The cytoplasm frequently

313

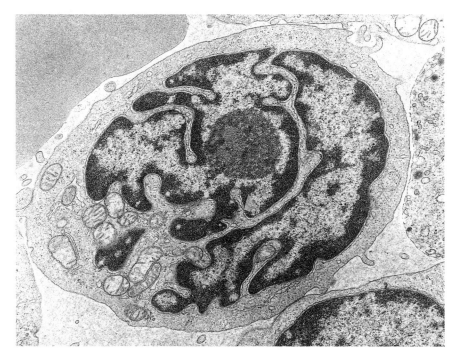

Figure 339
SÉZARY SYNDROME: ULTRASTRUCTURE
Electron micrograph of a Sézary cell from a patient with Sézary syndrome. The nucleus is markedly irregular. A single prominent nucleolus is present. (Uranyl acetate–lead citrate stains, X20,000)

contains large bundles of microfilaments and granules, rare profiles of rough endoplasmic reticulum, occasional mitochondria, and an inconspicuous Golgi region. The small cell variant has a very convoluted nucleus with hypercondensed chromatin. A mixture of large and small cell types is usually present (97).

Immunologic Findings. The Sézary cells are of helper cell phenotypes, CD3+, CD4+, and CD8- and are TdT-negative. They are generally HLA-DR and CD25 negative (76,84,86).

Cytogenetic Findings. The large Sézary cells typically have a tetraploid DNA content and near tetraploid chromosomes (91,112). The small cell type has a diploid or hyperdiploid chromosome number. Various numerical and structural abnormalities are reported but the findings lack specificity (91).

Differential Diagnosis. The cytologic features of the large Sézary cells are so unique that it is difficult to misinterpret them in well-prepared blood smears. The occurrence of these cells in a patient with edematous erythroderma is virtually diagnostic of Sézary syndrome.

The small cell variant is more problematic because the degree of nuclear irregularity may not be substantially different from that found in lymphocytes from normal individuals or in some cases of chronic lymphocytic leukemia. Immunologic markers are necessary to identify the helper T-cell nature of the cells. Proliferations of TdT-negative helper T lymphocytes occurs in a limited number of uncommon disorders including adult T-cell leukemia-lymphoma and T-prolymphocytic leukemia. Adult T-cell leukemia-lymphoma is excluded by HTLV-1 positivity. The white blood cell count in T-prolymphocytic leukemia is usually much higher than in Sézary syndrome. Although cutaneous involvement may occur in T-prolymphocytic leukemia, it is not of the edematous erythrodermic type.

Many patients with dermatosis of various types have atypical lymphocytes in the blood; these cells may have irregularly shaped nuclei and, occasionally, cytoplasmic vacuoles that are PAS positive. Although these cells may be difficult to distinguish from the small cell variant of the Sézary syndrome, the nuclear pattern is not cerebriform. In equivocal cases, buffy coat pellets

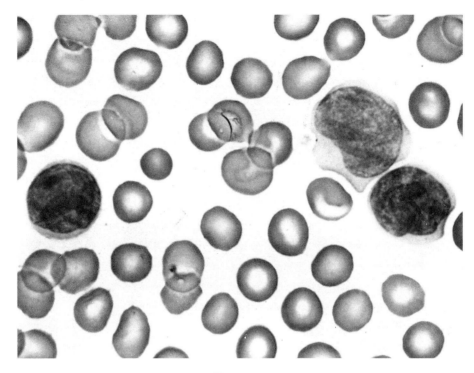

Figure 340
SÉZARY CELLS IN A PATIENT WITHOUT ERYTHRODERMA
Blood smear from a 62-year-old woman showing three lymphocytes with nuclear features of Sézary cells. These lymphocytes were CD3+ and CD4+; there was a progressive increase in these cells over 3 years. The patient had no clinical evidence of erythroderma during this period. (Wright-Giemsa stain)

of the blood can be embedded in plastic. The cerebriform features of the Sézary cell nucleus are readily appreciated.

Uncommonly, lymphocytes that have the morphologic and immunologic features of Sézary cells may be observed in individuals without cutaneous disease (fig. 340). Cells resembling Sézary cells have also been reported in blood smears from normal individuals, but these observations have been disputed (84).

The similarities between Sézary syndrome and mycosis fungoides may present difficulties in the interpretation of blood and marrow specimens. The problem is in part conceptual. Some observers consider Sézary syndrome and mycosis fungoides to be essentially the same disorder (123). Others view them as two disorders of cutaneous T-cell lymphoma with similarities in membrane markers, cytomorphology, and histopathology. The lymphoma cells in the blood and marrow from patients with mycosis fungoides have cytologic features more similar to poorly differentiated lymphoma, with a high nuclear-cytoplasmic ratio, condensed nuclear chromatin, and polymorphic nuclear outline (figs. 341, 342). Large numbers of these cells may be present in blood smears but this finding is uncommon. Also, extensive involvement of the bone marrow may occur in mycosis fungoides, in contrast to Sézary syndrome (fig. 343).

Treatment and Prognosis. Treatment for Sézary syndrome is directed toward the erythroderma (78,126,127). Several therapeutic modalities including long wave ultraviolet light, topical chemotherapy, radiotherapy, electron beam radiotherapy, topical and systemic corticosteroids, and extracorporeal photophoresis have been used with some degree of success. Combinations of alkylating agents such as chlorambucil and steroids have been successful in achieving remission in some patients. Patients with Sézary syndrome may achieve complete remission and long-term survival is reported (127).

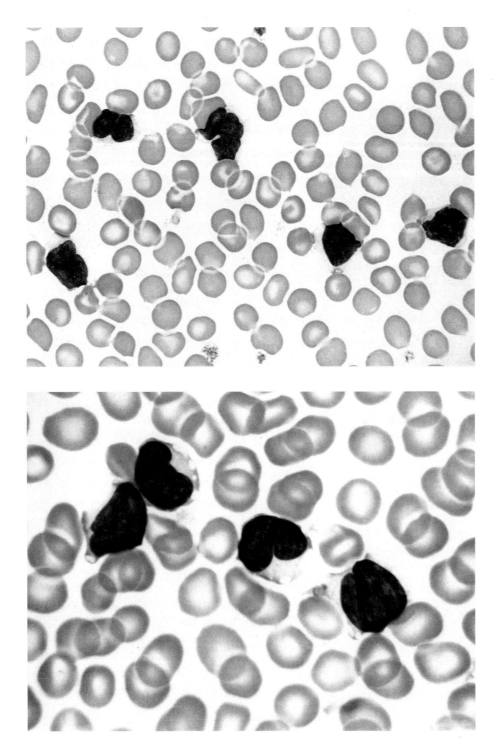

Figure 341

MYCOSIS FUNGOIDES

Top: Five abnormal lymphocytes in a blood smear from a patient with mycosis fungoides. The cells have irregular nuclear contours; the chromatin is clumped. These lymphocytes expressed CD3, CD4, and CD5. They were negative for CD8 and TdT. (Wright-Giemsa stain)

Bottom: Four cells in a blood smear from the same patient. Several of the cells contain cytoplasmic vacuoles, which were PAS positive. Approximately 60 percent of the lymphocytes were of the type illustrated. The nuclei of these lymphocytes are irregular but distinct from the cerebriform nuclear pattern in the Sézary cell shown in figure 337. (Wright-Giemsa stain)

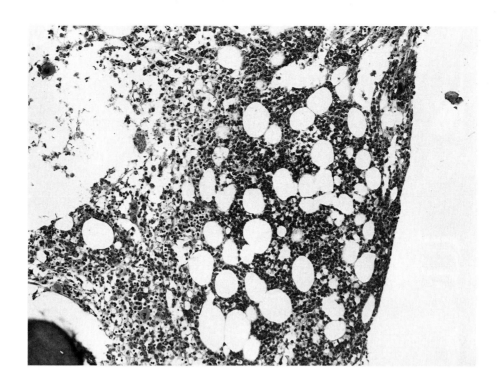

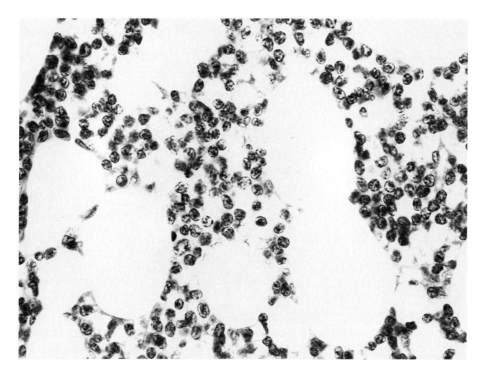

Figure 342
MYCOSIS FUNGOIDES

Top: Focus of cells in a bone marrow biopsy from the patient whose blood is illustrated in figure 341. This was the only lesion in the marrow biopsy. (Hematoxylin and eosin stain)

Bottom: High magnification of the same specimen showing a monomorphous population of lymphocytes. Some of the nuclei have an irregular, somewhat cerebriform appearance. (Hematoxylin and eosin stain)

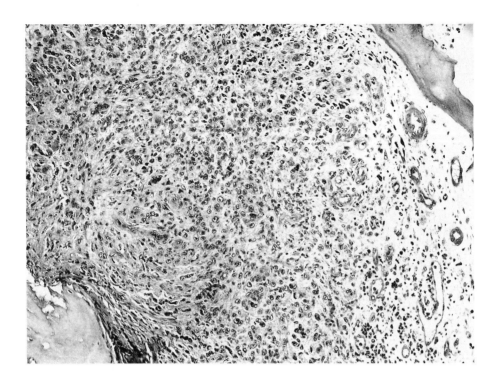

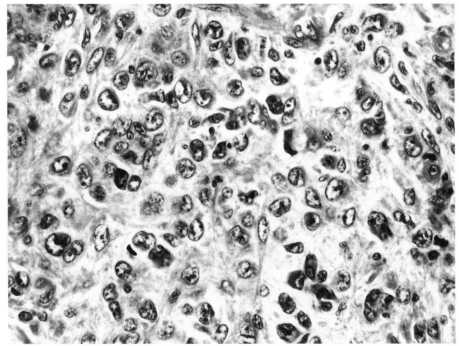

Figure 343
MYCOSIS FUNGOIDES

Top: Bone marrow biopsy from the patient whose blood smear and bone marrow biopsy are illustrated in figures 341 and 342, 3 years following the first biopsy. The marrow at this time showed extensive infiltration by a pleomorphic population of lymphoma cells. The lymphoma cells have a moderate amount of cytoplasm and round to irregular nuclear outlines. The nuclear chromatin is dispersed; multiple nucleoli are present. (Hematoxylin and eosin stain)

Bottom: High magnification of the same specimen. The lymphoma cells vary in size and numerous large cells with prominent nucleoli are present. There is an associated increase in vascular structures and connective tissue. (Hematoxylin and eosin stain)

REFERENCES

B-Cell Small Lymphocytic Leukemias

1. Bain B, Matutes E, Robinson D, et al. Leukaemia as a manifestation of large cell lymphoma. Br J Haematol 1991;77:301–10.

2. Bartl R, Frisch B, Hill W, Burkhardt R, Sommerfeld W, Sund M. Bone marrow histology in hairy cell leukemia. Identification of subtypes and their prognostic significance. Am J Clin Pathol 1983;79:531–45.

3. Batata A, Shen B. Immunophenotyping of subtypes of B-chronic (mature) lymphoid leukemia. A study of 242 cases. Cancer 1992;70:2436–43.

4. Bearman RM, Pangalis GA, Rappaport H. Prolymphocytic leukemia: clinical, histopathological, and cytochemical observations. Cancer 1978;42:2360–72.

5. Bennett JM, Catovsky D, Daniel MT, et al. Proposals for the classification of chronic (mature) B and T lymphoid leukemias. French-American-British (FAB) Cooperative Group. J Clin Pathol 1989;42:567–84.

6. Binet JL, Auquier A, Dighiero G, et al. A new prognostic classification of chronic lymphocytic leukemia derived from a multivariate survival analysis. Cancer 1981;48:198–206.

7. Bouroncle BA. Leukemic reticuloendotheliosis (hairy cell leukemia). Blood 1979;53:412–36.

8. _____. Unusual presentations and complications of hairy cell leukemia. Leukemia 1987;1:288–93.

9. Brunning RD, Parkin JL, Hanson CA. Hematopoietic and lymphoreticular neoplasms. In: Azar HA, ed. Pathology of human neoplasms: an atlas of diagnostic electron microscopy and immunohistochemistry. New York: Raven Press, 1988:221–303.

10. Burke JS. The value of the bone-marrow biopsy in the diagnosis of hairy cell leukemia. Am J Clin Pathol 1978;70:876–84.

11. _____, Byrne GE Jr, Rappaport H. Hairy cell leukemia (leukemic reticuloendotheliosis). I. A clinical pathologic study of 21 patients. Cancer 1974;33:1399–410.

12. _____, Rappaport H. The diagnosis and differential diagnosis of hairy cell leukemia in bone marrow and spleen. Semin Oncol 1984;11:334–6.

13. Carlsson M, Hassan IB, Paul G, Sundström C, Nilsson K, Totterman TH. Hairy cell leukemia (HCL) associated antigen B-ly 7 is an activation /differentiation-associated antigen on HCL and normal B cells but not on B-type chronic lymphocytic leukemia (B-CLL) cells. Leukemia and Lymphoma 1992;6:133–43.

14. Cawley JC, Burns GF, Hayhoe FJ. A chronic lymphoproliferative disorder with distinctive features: a distinct variant of hairy-cell leukemia. Leuk Res 1980;4:547–59.

15. Cheson BD. Recent advances in the treatment of B-cell chronic lymphocytic leukemia. Oncology 1990;4:71–84.

16. Chow KC, Nacilla JQ, Witzig TE, Li CY. Is persistent polyclonal B lymphocytosis caused by Epstein-Barr virus? Study with polymerase chain reaction and in situ hybridization. Am J Hematol 1992;41:270–5.

17. Cleary ML, Wood GS, Warnke R, Chao J, Sklar J. Immunoglobulin gene rearrangements in hairy cell leukemia. Blood 1984;64:99–104.

18. De Oliveira MS, Jaffe ES, Catovsky D. Leukaemic phase of mantle zone (intermediate) lymphoma: its characterisation in 11 cases. J Clin Pathol 1989;42:962–72.

19. Diez Martin JL, Li CY, Banks PM. Blastic variant of hairy-cell leukemia. Am J Clin Pathol 1987;87:576–83.

20. Dighiero G, Travade P, Chevret S, Fenaux P, Chastang C, Binet JL. B-cell chronic lymphocytic leukemia: present status and future directions. French Cooperative Group on CLL. Blood 1991;78:1901–14.

21. Enno A, Catovsky D, O'Brien M, Cherchi M, Kumaran TO, Galton DA. Prolymphocytoid transformation of chronic lymphocytic leukaemia. Br J Haematol 1979; 41:9–18.

22. Flandrin G, Sigaux F, Sebahoun G, Bouffette P. Hairy cell leukemia: clinical presentation and follow-up of 211 patients. Semin Oncol 1984;11(4 Suppl 2):458–78.

23. Freedman AS. Immunobiology of chronic lymphocytic leukemia. Hematol Oncol Clin North Am 1990;4:405–29.

24. Galton DA, Goldman JM, Wiltshaw E, Catovsky D, Henry K, Goldenberg GJ. Prolymphocytic leukaemia. Br J Haematol 1974;27:7–23.

25. Geisler CH, Larsen JK, Hansen NE, et al. Prognostic importance of flow cytometric immunophenotyping of 540 consecutive patients with B-cell chronic lymphocytic leukemia. Blood 1991;78:1795–802.

26. Gordon DS, Jones BM, Browning SW, Spira TJ, Lawrence DN. Persistent polyclonal lymphocytosis of B lymphocytes. N Engl J Med 1982;307:232–6.

27. Han T, Ozer H, Bloom M, Sagawa K, Minowada J. The presence of monoclonal cytoplasmic immunoglobulins in leukemic B cells from patients with chronic lymphocytic leukemia. Blood 1982;59:435–8.

28. Hanson CA, Gribbin TE, Schnitzer B, Schlegelmilch JA, Mitchell BS, Stoolman LM. CD11c (Leu-M5) expression characterizes a B-cell chronic lymphoproliferative disorder with features of both chronic lymphocytic leukemia and hairy cell leukemia. Blood 1990;76:2360–7.

29. _____, Ward PC, Schnitzer B. A multilobular variant of hairy cell leukemia with morphologic similarities to T-cell lymphoma. Am J Surg Pathol 1989;13:671–9.

30. Henderson ES, Han T. Current therapy of acute and chronic leukemia in adults. CA Cancer J Clin 1986;36:322–50.

31. Hounieu H, Chittal SM, al Saati T, et al. Hairy cell leukemia. Diagnosis of bone marrow involvement in paraffin-embedded sections with monoclonal antibody DBA.44. Am J Clin Pathol 1992;98:26–33.

32. International Workshop on Chronic Lymphocytic Leukemia. Chronic lymphocytic leukemia: recommendations for diagnosis, staging, and response criteria. Ann Intern Med 1989;110:236–8.

33. Juliusson G, Oscier DG, Fitchett M, et al. Prognostic subgroups in B-cell chronic lymphocytic leukemia defined by specific chromosomal abnormalities. N Engl J Med 1990;323:720–4.

34. Katayama I, Hirashima K, Maruyama K, et al. Hairy cell leukemia in Japanese patients: a study with monoclonal antibodies. Leukemia 1987;1:301–5.

35. Kjeldsberg CR, Marty J. Prolymphocytic transformation of chronic lymphocytic leukemia. Cancer 1981;48:2447–57.

35a. Lampert I, Catovsky D, Marsh GW, Child JA, Galton DAG. The histopathology of prolymphocytic leukaemia with particular reference to the spleen: a comparison with chronic lymphocytic leukaemia. Histopathology 1980;4:3–19.

36. Lipshutz MD, Mir R, Rai KR, Sawitsky A. Bone marrow biopsy and clinical staging in chronic lymphocytic leukemia. Cancer 1980;46:1422–7.

37. Litz CE, Arthur DC, Gajl-Peczalska KJ, et al. Transformation of chronic lymphocytic leukemia to small non-cleaved lymphoma: a cytogenetic, immunological, and molecular study. Leukemia 1991;11:972–8.

38. Lush CJ, Vora AJ, Campbell AC, Wood JK. Polyclonal CD5+ B-lymphocytosis resembling chronic lymphocytic leukaemia. Br J Haematol 1991;79:119–20.

39. Melo JV, Catovsky D, Galton DA. The relationship between chronic lymphocytic leukaemia and prolymphocytic leukaemia. I. Clinical and laboratory features of 300 patients and characterization of an intermediate group. Br J Haematol 1986;63:377–87.

40. _____, Catovsky D, Galton DA. The relationship between chronic lymphocytic leukaemia and prolymphocytic leukaemia. II. Patterns of evolution of "prolymphocytoid" transformation. Br J Haematol 1986; 64:77–86.

41. _____, Catovsky D, Gregory WM, Galton DA. The relationship between chronic lymphocytic leukaemia and prolymphocytic leukaemia. IV. Analysis of survival and prognostic features. Br J Haematol 1987;65:23–9.

42. _____, Hegde U, Parreira A, Thompson I, Lampert IA, Catovsky D. Splenic B cell lymphoma with circulating villous lymphocytes: differential diagnosis of B cell leukaemias with large spleens. J Clin Pathol 1987;40:642–51.

43. Mercieca J, Matutes E, Moskovic E, et al. Massive abdominal lymphadenopathy in hairy cell leukaemia: a report of 12 cases. Br J Haematol 1992;82:547–54.

44. Mulligan SP, Catovsky D. Splenic lymphoma with villous lymphocytes. Leukemia and Lymphoma 1992;6:97–105.

45. Nanba K, Soban EJ, Bowling MC, Berard CW. Splenic pseudosinuses and hepatic angiomatous lesions. Distinctive features of hairy cell leukemia. Am J Clin Pathol 1977;67:415–26.

46. Nathwani BN, Mohrmann BL, Brynes RK, Taylor C, Hansmann ML, Sheibani K. Monocytoid B-cell lymphomas. Hum Pathol 1992;23:1061–71.

47. Neiman RS, Sullivan AL, Jaffe R. Malignant lymphoma simulating leukemic reticuloendotheliosis: a clinicopathologic study of ten cases. Cancer 1979;43:329–42.

48. Oscier D, Matutes E, Gardiner A, et al. Cytogenetic studies in splenic lymphoma with villous lymphocytes [Abstract]. Blood 1991;78:113A.

49. Owens MR, Strauchen JA, Rowe JM, Bennett JM. Prolymphocytic leukemia: histologic findings in atypical cases. Hematol Oncol 1984;2:249–57.

50. Paoletti M, Bitter MA, Vardiman JW. Hairy-cell leukemia. Morphologic, cytochemical, and immunologic features. Clin Lab Med 1988;8:179–95.

51. Pianezze G, Gentilini I, Casini M, Fabris P, Coser P. Cytoplasmic immunoglobulins in chronic lymphocytic leukemia B cells. Blood 1987;69:1011–4.

51a. Pinto A, Zagonel V, Carbone A, Del Vechio L. Expression of myeloid associated antigens in chronic lymphocytic leukemia. Br J Haematol 1992;82:173–5.

52. Piro LD, Carrera CJ, Carson DA, Beutler E. Lasting remissions in hairy-cell leukemia induced by a single infusion of 2-chlorodeoxyadenosine. N Engl J Med 1990;322:1117–21.

53. Pugh WC, Manning JT, Butler JJ. Paraimmunoblastic variant of small lymphocytic lymphoma/leukemia. Am J Surg Pathol 1988;12:907–17.

54. Rai KR, Sawitsky A, Cronkite EP, Chanana AD, Levy RN, Pasterack BS. Clinical staging of chronic lymphocytic leukemia. Blood 1975;46:219–34.

55. Richter MN. Generalized reticular cell sarcoma of lymph nodes associated with lymphocytic leukemia. Am J Pathol 1928;4:285–92.

56. Ries LA, Hankey BF, Miller BA, Hartman AM, Edwards BK. Cancer statistics review 1973–1988. Bethesda, Maryland: National Cancer Institute, NIH Pub. No. 91–2789, 1991.

56a. Robbins BA, Ellison DJ, Spinosa JC, et al. Diagnostic application of two-color flow cytometry in 161 cases of hairy cell leukemia. Blood 1993;82:1277–87.

57. Rozman C, Montserrat E, Rodriguez-Fernandez JM, et al. Bone marrow histologic pattern—the best single prognostic parameter in chronic lymphocytic leukemia: a multivariate survival analysis of 329 cases. Blood 1984;64:642–8.

58. Sacker A, Suwanjindar P, Braziel R. Molecular genetic analysis of polyclonal B-cell lymphocytosis [Abstract]. Mod Pathol 1993;6:99A.

59. Sadamori N, Han T, Block AW, Sandberg AA. Cytogenetic studies of stimulated lymphocytes in hairy cell leukemia. Cancer Genet Cytogenet 1985;17:69–74.

60. Sainati L, Matutes E, Mulligan S, et al. A variant form of hairy cell leukemia resistant to alpha-interferon: clinical and phenotypic characteristics of 17 patients. Blood 1990;76:157–62.

61. Schrek R, Donnelly WJ. "Hairy" cells in blood in lymphoreticular neoplastic disease and "flagellated" cells of normal lymph nodes. Blood 1966;27:199–211.

62. Shivdasani RA, Hess JL, Skarin AT, Pinkus GS. Intermediate lymphocytic lymphoma: clinical and pathologic features of a recently characterized subtype of non-Hodgkin's lymphoma. J Clin Oncol 1993;11:802–11.

63. Sonnier JA, Buchanan GR, Howard-Peebles PN, Rutledge J, Smith RG. Chromosomal translocation involving the immunoglobulin kappa-chain and heavy-chain loci in a child with chronic lymphocytic leukemia. N Eng J Med 1983;309:590–4.

64. Spiers AS, Moore D, Cassileth PA, et al. Remissions in hairy-cell leukemia with pentostatin (2'-deoxycoformycin). N Engl J Med 1987;316:825–30.

65. Stone RM. Prolymphocytic leukemia. Hematol Oncol Clin North Am 1990;4:457–71.

66. Trump DL, Mann R, Phelps R, Roberts H, Conley CL. Richter's syndrome: diffuse histiocytic lymphoma in patients with chronic lymphocytic leukemia. Am J Med 1980;68:539–48.

67. Wick MR, Li CY, Ludwig J, Levitt R, Pierre RV. Malignant histiocytosis as a terminal condition in chronic lymphocytic leukemia. Mayo Clin Proc 1980;55:108–12.

68. Wormsley SB, Baird SM, Gadol N, Rai KR, Sobol RE. Characteristics of CD11c+, CD5+ chronic B-cell leukemias and the identification of novel peripheral blood B-cell subsets with chronic lymphoid leukemia immunophenotypes. Blood 1990;76:123–30.

69. Yam LT, Janckila AJ, Li CY, Lam WK. Cytochemistry of tartrate-resistant acid phosphatase: 15 years' experience. Leukemia 1987;1:285–8.

70. Zukerberg LR, Medeiros J, Ferry JA, Harris NL. Diffuse low grade B-cell lymphomas: four clinically distinct subtypes defined by a combination of morphologic and immunophenotypic features. Am J Clin Pathol 1993;100:373–85.

T-Cell Small Lymphocytic Proliferations

71. Agnarsson BA, Loughran TP Jr, Starkebaum G, Kadin ME. The pathology of large granular lymphocyte leukemia. Hum Pathol 1989;20:643–51.

72. Bennett JM, Catovsky D, Daniel MT, et al. The French-American-British (FAB) Cooperative Group: proposals for the classification of chronic (mature) B and T lymphoid leukaemias. J Clin Pathol 1989;42:567–84.

73. Berliner N. T gamma lymphocytosis and T cell chronic leukemias. Hematol Oncol Clin North Am 1990;4:473–87.

74. Brito-Babapulle V, Pomfret M, Matutes E, Catovsky D. Cytogenetic studies on prolymphocytic leukemia. II. T cell prolymphocytic leukemia. Blood 1987;70:926–31.

75. Broder S, Bunn PA Jr, Jaffe ES, et al. T-cell lymphoproliferative syndrome associated with human T-cell leukemia/lymphoma virus. Ann Intern Med 1984;100:543–57.

76. Brouet JC, Flandrin G, Seligmann M. Indications of the thymus-derived nature of the proliferating cells in six patients with Sézary's syndrome. N Engl J Med 1973;289:341–4.

77. Brunning RD. T Prolymphocytic leukemia [Editorial]. Blood 1991;78:3111–3.

78. Buechner SA, Winkelmann RK. Sézary syndrome. A clinicopathologic study of 39 cases. Arch Dermatol 1983;119:979–86.

79. Cabrera ME, Gray AM, Cartier L, et al. Simultaneous adult T-cell leukemia/lymphoma and subacute polyneuropathy in a patient from Chile. Leukemia 1991;5:350–3.

80. Case records of the Massachusetts General Hospital. Weekly clinicopathological exercises. Case 36–1989. A 34-year-old Jamaican man with fever, hepatic failure, diarrhea, and a progressive gait disorder. N Engl J Med 1989;321:663–75.

81. Catovsky D, Galetto J, Okos A, Galton DA, Wiltshaw E, Stathopoulos G. Prolymphocytic leukaemia of B and T cell type. Lancet 1973;2:232–4.

82. _____, Greaves MF, Rose M, et al. Adult T-cell lymphoma-leukaemia in Blacks from the West Indies. Lancet 1982;1:639–43.

83. Chan WC, Link S, Mawle A, Check I, Brynes RK, Winton EF. Heterogeneity of large granular lymphocyte proliferations: delineation of two major subtypes. Blood 1986;68:1142–53.

84. Chu AC, Morris JF. Sézary cell morphology induced in peripheral blood lymphocytes: re-evaluation. Blood 1989;73:1603–7.

85. Eimoto T, Mitsui T, Kikuchi M. Ultrastructure of adult T-cell leukemia/lymphoma. Virchows Arch [Cell Pathol] 1981;38:189–208.

86. Flandrin G, Brouet JC. The Sézary cell: cytologic, cytochemical, and immunologic studies. Mayo Clin Proc 1974;49:575–83.

87. Foon KA, Gale RP. Is there a T-cell form of chronic lymphocytic leukemia? Leukemia 1992;6:867–8.

88. Gallo RC, Kalyanaraman VS, Sarngadharan MG, et al. Association of the human type C retrovirus with a subset of adult T-cell cancers. Cancer Res 1983;43:3892–9.

89. Galton DA, Goldman JM, Wiltshaw E, Catovsky D, Henry K, Goldenberg GJ. Prolymphocytic leukaemia. Br J Haematol 1974;27:7–23.

90. Imamura N, Kusunoki Y, Kawa-Ha K, et al. Aggressive natural killer cell leukaemia/lymphoma: report of four cases and review of the literature. Br J Haematol 1990;75:49–59.

91. Johnson GA, Dewald GW, Strand WR, Winkelmann RK. Chromosome studies in 17 patients with Sézary syndrome. Cancer 1985;55:2426–33.

92. Kamada N, Sakurai M, Miyamoto K, et al. Chromosome abnormalities in adult T-cell leukemia/lymphoma: a karyotype review committee report. Cancer Res 1992;52:1481–93.

93. Kawano F, Yamaguchi K, Nishimura H, Tsuda H, Takatsuki K. Variation in the clinical courses of adult T-cell leukemia. Cancer 1985;55:851–6.

94. Kinoshita K, Kamihira S, Ikeda S, et al. Clinical, hematologic, and pathologic features of leukemic T-cell lymphoma. Cancer 1982;50:1554–62.

95. Kiyokawa T, Yamaguchi K, Takeya M, et al. Hypercalcemia and osteoclast proliferation in adult T-cell leukemia. Cancer 1987;59:1187–91.

96. Loughran TP Jr. Clonal diseases of large granular lymphocytes. Blood 1993;82:1–14.

97. Lutzner MA, Jordan HW. The ultrastructure of an abnormal cell in Sézary's syndrome. Blood 1968;31:719–26.

98. Lymphoma Study Group (1984–1987). Major prognostic factors of patients with adult T-cell leukemia-lymphoma. A cooperative study. Leuk Res 1991;15:81–90.

99. Matutes E, Brito-Babapulle V, Swansbury J, et al. Clinical and laboratory features of 78 cases of T-prolymphocytic leukemia. Blood 1991;78:3269–74.

100. _____, Garcia Talavera J, O'Brien M, Catovsky D. The morphological spectrum of T-prolymphocytic leukaemia. Br J Haematol 1986;64:111–24.

101. McKenna RW, Arthur DC, Gajl-Peczalska KJ, Flynn P, Brunning RD. Granulated T cell lymphocytosis with neutropenia: malignant or benign chronic lymphoproliferative disorder? Blood 1985;66:259–66.

102. Neely SM. Adult T-cell leukemia-lymphoma. West J Med 1989;150:557–61

103. Oshimi K. Granular lymphocyte proliferative disorders: report of 12 cases and review of the literature. Leukemia 1988;2:617–27.

104. Pandolfi F, De Rossi G, Ranucci A, et al. Tac-positive, HTLV-negative, T helper phenotype chronic lymphocytic leukemia cells. Blood 1985;65:1531–7.

105. Rappaport H. Tumors of the hematopoietic system. Atlas of Tumor Pathology, 1st Series, Fascicle 8. Washington, D.C.: Armed Forces Institute of Pathology, 1966:347.

106. Reynolds CW, Foon KA. Tγ-lymphoproliferative disease and related disorders in humans and experimental animals: a review of the clinical, cellular, and functional characteristics. Blood 1984;64:1146–58.

107. Sadamori N. Cytogenetic implication in adult T-cell leukemia. A hypothesis of leukemogenesis. Cancer Genet Cytogenet 1991;51:131–6.

108. Salhany KE, Greer JP, Cousar JB, Collins RD. Marrow involvement in cutaneous T-cell lymphoma. A clinicopathologic study of 60 cases. Am J Clin Pathol 1989;92:747–54.

109. Sanada I, Tanaka R, Kumagai E, et al. Chromosomal aberrations in adult T cell leukemia: relationship to the clinical severity. Blood 1985;65:649–54.

110. Scheffer E, Meijer CJ, van Vloten WA, Willemze R. A histologic study of lymph nodes from patients with the Sézary syndrome. Cancer 1986;57:2375–80.

111. Sézary A, Bouvrain Y. Erythrodermie avec présence de cellules monstrueuses dans le derme et le sang circulant. Bull Soc Fr Dermatol Syph 1938;45:254–60.

112. Shah-Reddy I, Mayeda K, Mirchandani I, Koppitch FC. Sézary syndrome with a 14:14(q12;q31) translocation. Cancer 1982;49:75–9.

113. Shimamoto Y, Ono K, Sano M, et al. Differences in prognostic factors between leukemia and lymphoma type of adult T-cell leukemia. Cancer 1989;63:289–94.

114. _____, Suga K, Shimojo M, et al. Comparison of CHOP versus VEPA therapy in patients with lymphoma type of adult T-cell leukemia. Leukemia and Lymphoma 1990;2:335–40.

115. _____, Yamaguchi M, Miyamoto Y, et al. The differences between lymphoma and leukemia type of adult T-cell leukemia. Leukemia and Lymphoma 1990;1:101–12.

116. Shimoyama M, Abe T, Miyamoto K, et al. Chromosome aberrations and clinical features of adult T cell leukemia-lymphoma not associated with human T cell leukemia virus type I. Blood 1987;69:984–9.

117. _____, Minato K, Saito H, et al. Comparison of clinical, morphologic and immunologic characteristics of adult T-cell leukemia-lymphoma and cutaneous T-cell lymphoma. Jpn J Clin Oncol 1979;9:357–72.

118. Tajima K. The T- and B-cell Malignancy Study Group. The 4th nation-wide study of adult T-cell leukemia/lymphoma (ATL) in Japan: estimates of risk of ATL and its geographical and clinical features. Int J Cancer 1990;45:237–43.

119. Takatsuki K, Uchiyama T, Ueshima Y, Hattori T. Adult T-cell leukemia: further clinical observations and cyto-genetic and functional studies of leukemic cells. Jpn J Clin Oncol 1979;9:317–24.

120. _____, Yamaguchi K, Kawano F, et al. Clinical diversity in adult T-cell leukemia-lymphoma. Cancer Res 1985;45(Suppl 9):4644–5S.

121. Teshima T, Akashi K, Shibuya T, et al. Central nervous system involvement in adult T-cell leukemia/lymphoma. Cancer 1990;65:327–32.

122. Uchiyama T, Yodoi J, Sagawa K, Takatsuki K, Uchino H. Adult T-cell leukemia: clinical and hematologic features of 16 cases. Blood 1977;50:481–92.

123. Variakojis D, Rosas-Uribe A, Rappaport H. Mycosis fungoides: pathologic findings in staging laparotomies. Cancer 1974;33:1589–600.

124. Volk JR, Kjeldsberg CR, Eyre HJ, Marty J. T-cell prolymphocytic leukemia. Clinical and immunological characterization. Cancer 1983;52:2049–54.

125. Watanabe T, Yamaguchi K, Takatsuki K, Osame M, Yoshida M. Constitutive expression of parathyroid hormone-related protein gene in human T cell leukemia virus type 1 (HTLV-I) carriers and adult T cell leukemia patients that can be trans-activated by HTLV-I tax gene. J Exp Med 1990;172:759–65.

126. Wieselthier JS, Koh HK. Sézary syndrome: diagnosis, prognosis, and critical review of treatment options. J Am Acad Dermatol 1990;22:381–401.

127. Winkelmann RK. Clinical studies of T-cell erythroderma in the Sézary syndrome. Mayo Clin Proc 1974; 49:519–25.

128. Yamada Y. Phenotypic and functional analysis of leukemic cells from 16 patients with adult T-cell leukemia/lymphoma. Blood 1983;61:192–9.

129. Yamaguchi K, Nishimura H, Kohrogi H, Jono M, Miyamoto Y, Takatsuki K. A proposal for smoldering adult T-cell leukemia: a clinicopathologic study of five cases. Blood 1983;62:758–66.

❖❖❖

PLASMA CELL DYSCRASIAS AND RELATED DISORDERS

The plasma cell dyscrasias are a group of disorders having in common the proliferation of a single clone of immunoglobulin-producing cells generally recognizable as plasma cells or lymphocytes. These cells produce a single class of immunoglobulin, or a polypeptide subunit of a single immunoglobulin, that is detectable in the serum or urine as a monoclonal spike (M protein) on electrophoresis; there is frequently a decrease in the level of normal polyclonal immunoglobulins. The term monoclonal gammopathy refers to only one of the manifestations of the plasma cell dyscrasias, the production of a monoclonal immunoglobulin, which may be found in both neoplastic and reactive disorders.

Several classifications of the plasma cell dyscrasias have been proposed. The most commonly recognized types are: plasma cell myeloma, monoclonal gammopathy of undetermined significance, Waldenström macroglobulinemia (lymphoplasmacytoid lymphoma), heavy chain disease, and primary amyloidosis.

PLASMA CELL MYELOMA (MULTIPLE MYELOMA)

Definition. A neoplastic clonal proliferation of plasma cells characterized by the production of a monoclonal immunoglobulin. The bone marrow is the site of origin of nearly all myelomas and in most cases there is disseminated marrow involvement. Other organs may be secondarily involved.

Incidence and Clinical Findings. The incidence of plasma cell myeloma in the United States in 1989 was 3.9 cases per 100,000 population; it remained stable for the 16 years between 1973 and 1988 (54). Myeloma accounts for about 1 percent of malignant tumors and 10 percent of hematologic malignancies (38). Males are affected more than females by a ratio of approximately 3 to 2. The disease is twice as common in black Americans than in whites. Myeloma is not found in children and rarely reported in individuals less than 35 years of age; the incidence increases with age thereafter. The highest incidence is in individuals in the ninth decade of life.

The most frequent presenting symptom is bone pain in the back or extremities due to lytic lesions or generalized osteoporosis. In advanced cases vertebral collapse may cause a loss of height. Weakness and tiredness, often related to anemia, are also common presenting symptoms. Infections, bleeding, or symptoms of renal failure and hypercalcemia are first manifestations in some patients. Rarely, neurologic symptoms due to spinal cord compression are the reason for seeking medical attention. Mass disease or organomegaly due to extramedullary plasmacytomas or amyloidosis may be early findings in a few cases. Occasionally, asymptomatic individuals are diagnosed with plasma cell myeloma following discovery of a serum monoclonal immunoglobulin spike on routine protein electrophoresis.

Physical findings are nonspecific or lacking in most patients. Pallor is most common followed by organomegaly. Palpable plasmacytomas are rare but tenderness and swelling over the site of a pathologic fracture or plasmacytoma may be observed. Skin lesions due to plasma cell infiltrates or purpura are present in a few patients.

Laboratory Findings. The laboratory studies used to diagnose plasma cell myeloma include serum and urine protein electrophoresis, protein immunoelectrophoresis or immunofixation, serum and urine protein quantitation, radiographic skeletal survey, and bone marrow examination.

The extent to which these evaluations are performed is determined by the degree of suspicion of the diagnosis. The data obtained from these studies form the basis for several clinicopathologic systems for diagnosis of plasma cell myeloma (17,21,38,39).

The requirements for diagnosis are increased abnormal bone marrow plasma cells or a plasmacytoma together with a monoclonal gammopathy in the serum or urine or lytic bone lesions recognized by radiographic studies. The recommended minimum percentage of plasma cells and quantity of monoclonal protein necessary for diagnosis varies for different diagnostic systems (17,21,39). In most, at least 10 percent bone marrow plasma cells and 3 g/dL of monoclonal serum protein or more than 1 g/day of kappa or lambda light chains in the urine are required for diagnosis (38,39).

A monoclonal spike is found on serum protein electrophoresis in the majority of cases. The total gammaglobulin is usually increased because of the monoclonal protein but normal immunoglobulins are commonly decreased. A serum protein electrophoresis spike is usually not detected in cases with low levels of monoclonal protein, as commonly seen in IgD and light chain myelomas; hypogammaglobulinemia may be the only finding. Urine protein electrophoresis on a concentrated 24-hour urine specimen supplements the studies on serum. Monoclonal light chains (Bence Jones protein) are found in some patients without a detectable monoclonal protein in the serum.

Serum and urine immunoelectrophoresis or immunofixation are the preferred methods for characterizing a monoclonal immunoglobulin and for detection of small quantities of monoclonal protein. With these techniques, a monoclonal immunoglobulin will be identified in the serum or urine in 99 percent of cases of myeloma (38). A summary of the frequency with which various monoclonal proteins are seen in plasma cell myeloma, as compiled from several large series of cases, is shown in Table 31.

The kappa light chain is more common than the lambda for all immunoglobulin types of myeloma except IgD. Monoclonal light chains are found in the urine by immunoelectrophoresis in 75 percent of cases; the light chain is kappa in two thirds of these.

The serum monoclonal protein level varies from undetectable to more than 10 g/dL. The median is approximately 5 g/dL for IgG myeloma and 3.5 g/dL for IgA. In cases of light chain plasma cell myeloma, the serum monoclonal protein is very low or undetectable; the 24-hour urine protein level may be mildly to markedly increased but is usually more than 1 g/24 hours. The monoclonal protein level in IgD and IgE myelomas is always low. Uninvolved polyclonal immunoglobulins vary from normal in a minority of cases to markedly reduced.

Radiographic skeletal surveys reveal abnormalities in nearly 75 percent of cases of plasma cell myeloma (42). These may be lytic lesions, pathologic fractures, or generalized osteoporosis. In some cases all of these are present. The vertebrae, pelvis, skull, ribs, femurs, and proximal humeri are most often affected. Computerized tomography (CT) and magnetic resonance imaging (MRI) are

Table 31

MONOCLONAL IMMUNOGLOBULINS IN PLASMA CELL MYELOMA*

Monoclonal Immunoglobulin	Approximate Percent of Cases
IgG	55
IgA	22
Light chain only	18
IgD	2
Biclonal	2
Nonsecretory	1
IgE	<1
IgM	<1

*Data compiled from references 36, 40, and 53.

useful for detecting small bone lesions and extramedullary plasma cell infiltrates (42).

The plasma cell labeling index by tritiated thymidine incorporation or by immunofluorescence labeling is increased in overt plasma cell myeloma and normal in monoclonal gammopathy of undetermined significance and reactive plasmacytosis (17,27,30). A markedly elevated labeling index is a poor prognostic sign. Serum beta-2 microglobulin levels are variably increased in myeloma. Elevated levels reflect increased plasma cell mass, deteriorating renal function, or both (27).

Hypercalcemia is present in approximately one sixth of patients, creatinine is elevated in one third (42), and hyperuricemia is found in more than half (40). Hypoalbuminemia is observed in patients with advanced disease and is a strong indicator of poor prognosis (17).

Blood and Bone Marrow Findings. Anemia is present in about 60 percent of patients at the time of diagnosis (40). Red blood cell indices are usually normocytic and normochromic. Leukopenia and thrombocytopenia are found in less than 20 percent of patients at presentation but frequently evolve during the course of the disease (40). Occasional patients present with leukocytosis or thrombocytosis.

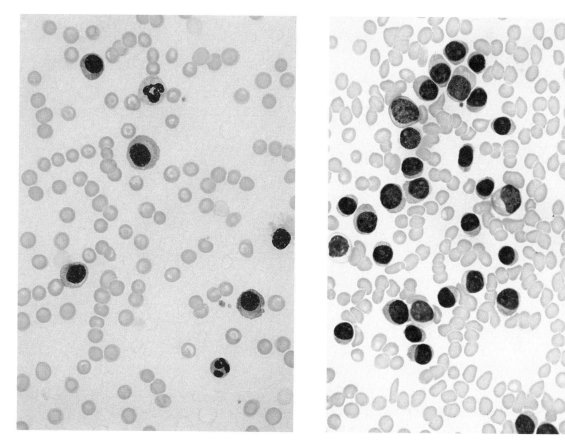

Figure 344
PLASMA CELL LEUKEMIA

Left: A blood smear from a 59-year-old man with plasma cell leukemia. The total blood leukocyte count was slightly elevated. There were 50 percent plasma cells. The monoclonal protein in this case was IgG kappa. (Wright-Giemsa stain)

Right: A blood smear from a 47-year-old female with plasma cell leukemia. The blood leukocyte count was 24.0×10^9/L and 90 percent were plasma cells. Many of the plasma cells have a "lymphoid" feature. The monoclonal protein was IgG kappa. (Wright-Giemsa stain)

The most striking feature on the blood smear is a marked increase in rouleaux formation. The degree of rouleaux is directly related to the quantity and type of monoclonal immunoglobulin and generally parallels the elevation of the erythrocyte sedimentation rate. Circulating plasma cells may be found in approximately 15 percent of cases, usually in low numbers. They are more commonly observed in the terminal stages of the disease. A marked plasmacytosis is present in cases of plasma cell leukemia.

Plasma cell leukemia (PCL) is a myeloma in which the number of plasma cells in the blood is greater than 20 percent of the total leukocytes or the absolute plasma cell count exceeds 2.0×10^9/L (34,49). PLC may be primary, present at the time of initial diagnosis, or secondary, evolving during the course of the disease (34,49,60). Primary PCL is found in approximately 2 percent of cases of plasma cell myeloma (34,49).

Anemia is present in 80 percent of cases of PCL and thrombocytopenia in 50 percent (34,49). Nucleated red blood cells are frequently observed in blood smears. The total leukocyte count may be in the normal range but is usually elevated and may be as high as 100×10^9/L. The cytologic characteristics of the leukemic plasma cells span most of the morphologic spectrum of myelomas but large and pleomorphic plasma cells are unusual (figs. 344, 345). The leukemic cells vary from normal appearing to some that are barely recognizable as plasma cells. In a number of cases the plasma cells are small, with relatively little cytoplasm, and resemble plasmacytoid

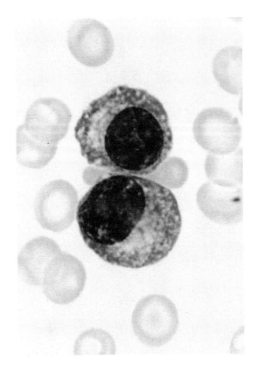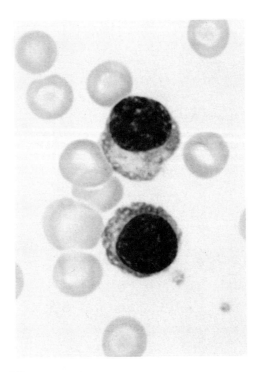

Figure 345
PLASMA CELL LEUKEMIA
A high magnification of plasma cells in a case of plasma cell leukemia. There was a morphologic spectrum in this case from relatively typical-appearing plasma cells on the left to small plasma cells with lymphoid features on the right. (Wright-Giemsa stain)

lymphocytes. Cases with these features may be difficult to distinguish from a peripheralized lymphoma or chronic lymphocytic leukemia.

Monoclonal immunoglobulins of virtually all types have been reported in PCL. IgG is the most common, followed by light chain only and IgA (49). PCL is found in approximately 20 percent of cases of the rare IgE myeloma (32,34).

Most of the usual clinical and laboratory abnormalities associated with myeloma are found in patients with PCL, however, there are several distinguishing features. The median age at diagnosis is younger in patients with PCL. Lymphadenopathy and organomegaly are significantly more common and bone lesions less common. Renal failure is more common at diagnosis. Patients with PCL have more aggressive disease, poorer response to therapy, and a significantly shorter survival time (about 6 months) than patients with more typical myeloma (about 30 to 36 months) (34,49).

The bone marrow examination is the most important element in the diagnosis of plasma cell myeloma; the diagnosis is made from the marrow findings alone in many cases (fig. 346) (15). A bone marrow examination is nearly always required to confirm the diagnosis even when there is substantial supportive immunologic or radiographic evidence. The bone marrow study also provides prognostic information and is helpful in following patients for response to therapy and in identifying recurrent disease. The marrow is the major source of tissue for special studies such as immunophenotyping and thymidine labeling indices.

Aspirate smears and trephine biopsy sections are both necessary for an adequate evaluation. They are independently diagnostic in most cases but in some patients it is a combination of findings in the two preparations that leads to the diagnosis. The diagnostic yield of trephine biopsies is often directly related to their size and number. Focal lesions may be irregularly distributed and widely spaced. Sometimes, there is one focus of myeloma cells in a trephine biopsy and no evidence of a plasma cell infiltrate in the remainder of the sections or in specimens from the contralateral posterior iliac spine. When the

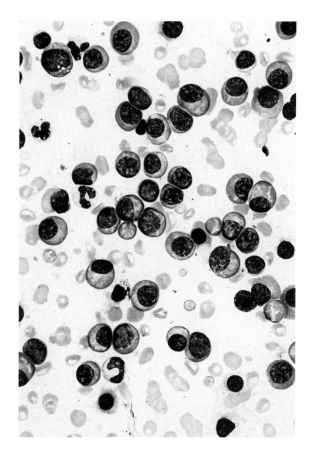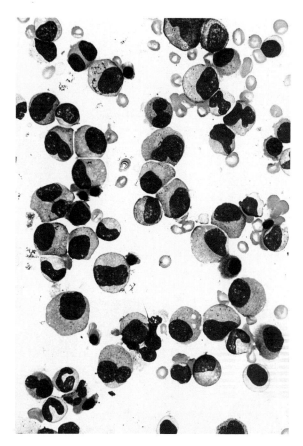

Figure 346
PLASMA CELL MYELOMA
Bone marrow aspirate smears from two patients with plasma cell myeloma and extensive marrow replacement. In both cases the diagnosis of myeloma can be made on the basis of extensive marrow plasmacytosis. (Wright-Giemsa stain)

clinical and laboratory evidence are consistent with a diagnosis of plasma cell myeloma, repeat biopsies may be indicated if the initial study is not diagnostic.

The plasma cells average 20 to 36 percent in the aspirate smears (40,53). They vary from normal appearing with mature features to blast-like cells barely recognizable as plasma cells. The atypical features that characterize plasma cells in cases of myeloma encompass changes in both the nucleus and cytoplasm. The cells are often larger than normal plasma cells, but may be normal sized or small. Moderate to abundant basophilic cytoplasm is usual. An array of cytoplasmic changes are observed. These include fraying of the cytoplasmic borders, cytoplasmic shedding, and the presence of vacuoles, granules, hyaline inclusions, and small or large crystalline

inclusions. The nucleus is larger than normal in most cases and the nuclear chromatin is less condensed; nucleoli are variably prominent.

Myelomas have been classified into mature, intermediate, immature, and plasmablastic cytologic types (figs. 347–351) (29). Patients with plasmablastic myeloma have a median survival period of 10 months compared to 35 months for the other types. There appears to be no significant difference in survival among the other three types. Other classifications include three or six cytologic types (5,11).

Attempts to relate morphologic characteristics to monoclonal immunoglobulin type have been largely unsuccessful except for a small number of cases of IgA myeloma (53). The plasma cells in this group are markedly pleomorphic and include large multinucleated plasma cells, flaming plasma cells,

Figure 347
MATURE-TYPE
MYELOMA

A bone marrow aspirate smear from a 64-year-old woman with plasma cell myeloma. The plasma cells have cytologic features of a mature-type myeloma. (Wright-Giemsa stain)

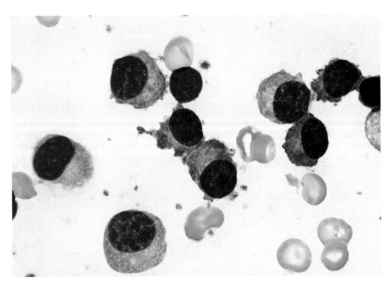

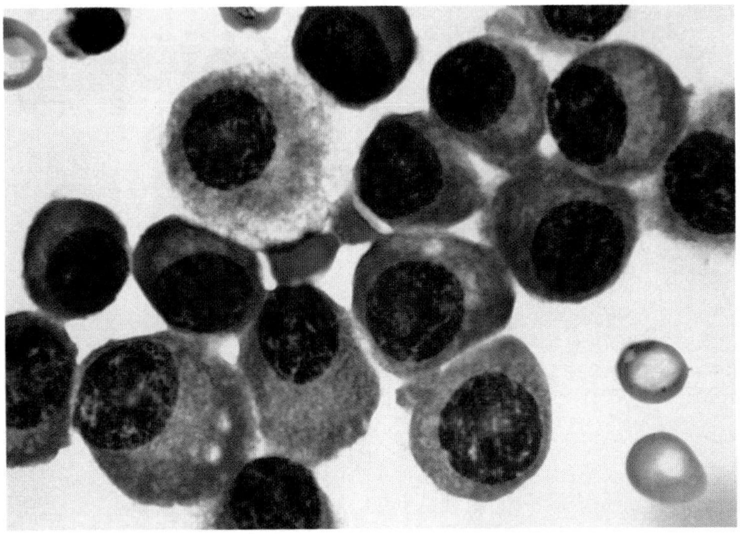

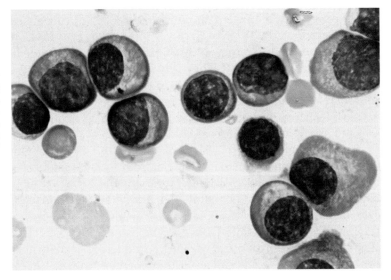

Figure 348
MATURE- TO
INTERMEDIATE-TYPE
MYELOMA

A bone marrow smear from a patient with extensive marrow involvement by plasma cell myeloma. Several of the plasma cells show features of a mature-type myeloma. Others have less dense chromatin and visible nucleoli, features of an intermediate-type myeloma. (Wright-Giemsa stain) (Fig. 35A from McKenna RW. Disorders of bone marrow. In: Sternberg SS, ed. Diagnostic surgical pathology. 2nd ed. New York: Raven Press, 1994:623–72.)

Figure 349
INTERMEDIATE-TYPE MYELOMA

A high magnification of the bone marrow smear illustrated in figure 346, left showing features of intermediate-type myeloma. The plasma cells have moderately dispersed chromatin, occasional nucleoli, and generally less cytoplasm (higher nuclear-cytoplasmic ratio) than in the cases illustrated in figures 347 and 348. (Wright-Giemsa stain)

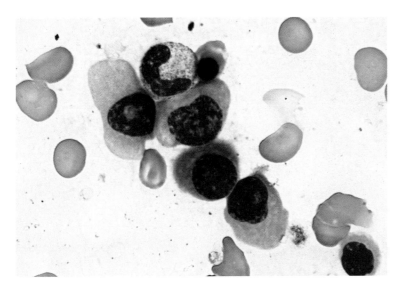

Figure 350
IMMATURE-TYPE MYELOMA
The plasma cells in this bone marrow smear are immature. They have prominent nucleoli and less dense chromatin than those in figures 348 and 349. (Wright-Giemsa stain)

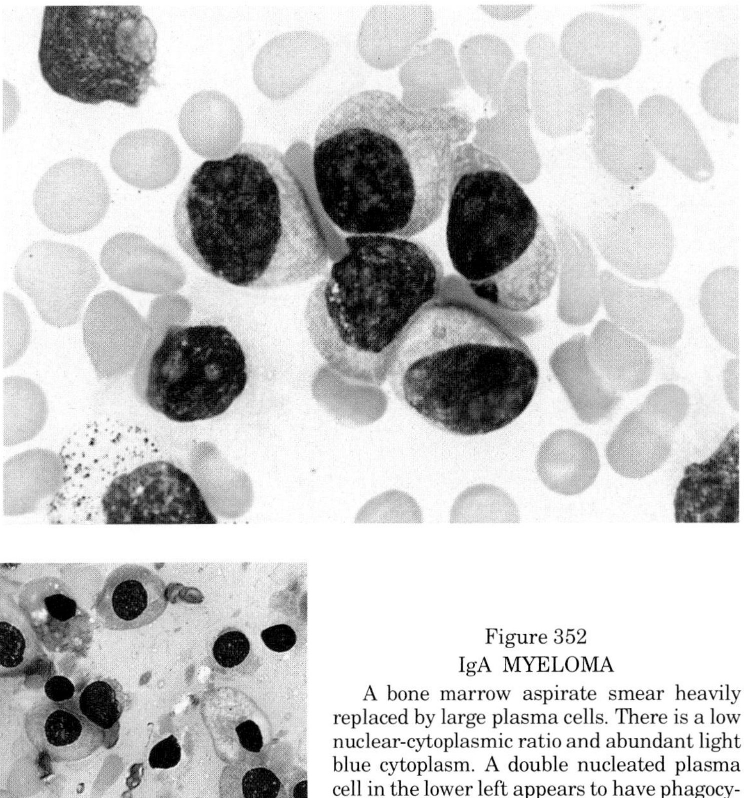

Figure 351
PLASMABLASTIC-TYPE MYELOMA
A bone marrow aspirate from a patient with plasma cell myeloma. There is a relatively high nuclear-cytoplasmic ratio. The nuclei have less dense chromatin than previous examples and contain nucleoli. The plasma cells show features of immature- to plasmablastic-type myeloma. (Wright-Giemsa stain)

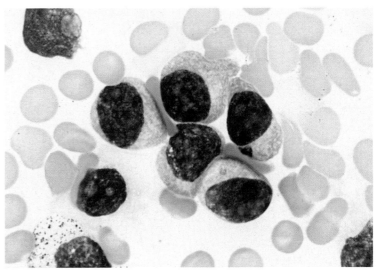

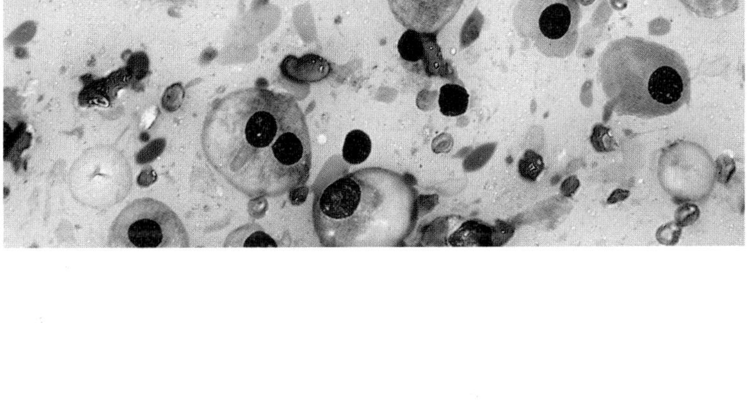

Figure 352
IgA MYELOMA
A bone marrow aspirate smear heavily replaced by large plasma cells. There is a low nuclear-cytoplasmic ratio and abundant light blue cytoplasm. A double nucleated plasma cell in the lower left appears to have phagocytized an erythrocyte. Numerous cytoplasmic fragments are scattered throughout the smear. The patient had a large IgA serum monoclonal spike. (Wright-Giemsa stain)

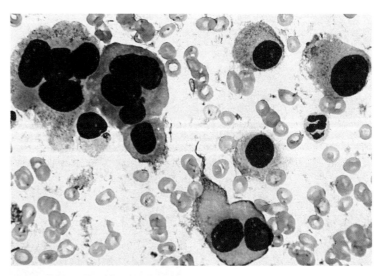

Figure 353
IgA MYELOMA
A bone marrow aspirate showing large pleomorphic multinucleated plasma cells with red-staining cytoplasmic inclusion material (flaming plasma cells). Fragments of red cytoplasm are present at the edges of the cells and scattered about the smear. These distinct morphologic features are strongly associated with IgA myeloma. (Wright-Giemsa stain)

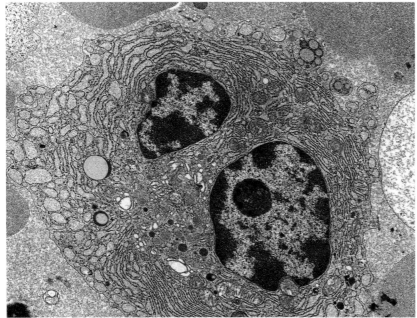

Figure 354
IgA MYELOMA
An electron micrograph showing a large pleomorphic plasma cell from a patient with IgA myeloma. There is nuclear-cytoplasmic asynchrony, with the cytoplasm containing abundant dilated profiles of rough endoplasmic reticulum and a nucleus containing a prominent nucleolus. The endoplasmic reticulum near the peripheral edge of the cytoplasmic border is particularly dilated and contains amorphous pale material, most likely representing immunoglobulin. Flaming plasma cells were abundant on light microscopy. (Uranyl acetate-lead citrate stain, X9,000)

and cells with pale, frayed and fragmented cytoplasm (figs. 352–354). Intranuclear inclusions are found in about 20 percent of cases of IgA myeloma, far more frequently than for other immunologic types (figs. 355, 356) (53).

Approximately 2 percent of myelomas are distinguished by marked nuclear lobulation and contortion, giving them a monocytoid configuration (53,61). In some instances these cells are mixed with other easily recognizable plasma cells, but in other cases they comprise a relatively uniform population and may be difficult to recognize as myeloma cells (figs. 357, 358). Small plasma cells predominate in some cases with occasional giant bizarre plasma cells (fig. 359). In approximately 5 percent of cases of myeloma, the plasma cells have a distinctly lymphoid appearance characterized by small size and slight to moderate amounts of cytoplasm evenly distributed around the nucleus (fig. 360). In one study, 20 percent of cases with "lymphoid" morphology were IgD myelomas (53).

Various types of cytoplasmic and nuclear inclusions are observed in myeloma cells. Large crystalline structures may distort the cytoplasm (figs. 361–363). Cytoplasmic crystals are a common

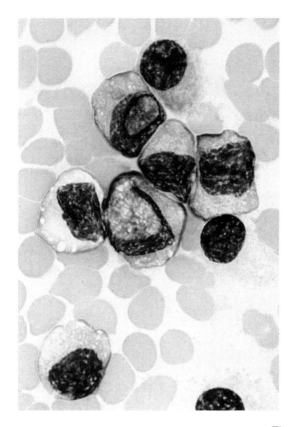
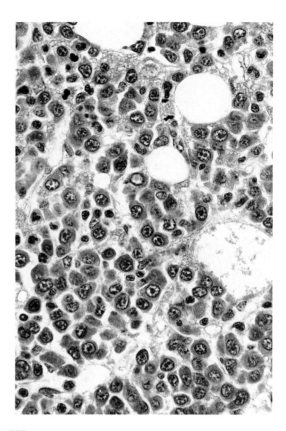

Figure 355
IgA MYELOMA WITH INTRANUCLEAR INCLUSIONS

Left: Bone marrow smear from a patient with IgA myeloma. Large nuclear inclusions (Dutcher bodies) are present in two of the plasma cells. (Wright-Giemsa stain)

Right: A trephine biopsy section from the same patient shows extensive replacement of the marrow. A large nuclear inclusion is present in one of the plasma cells near the center of the field. (Hematoxylin and eosin stain)

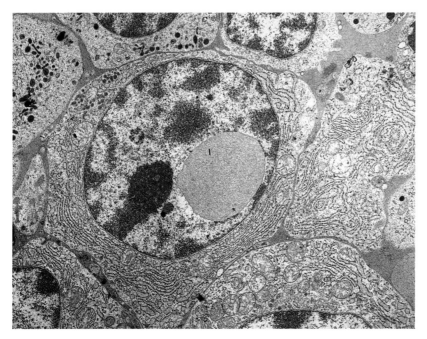

Figure 356
PLASMA CELL WITH INTRANUCLEAR INCLUSION

Electron micrograph of a bone marrow plasma cell from a patient with IgA myeloma illustrating a large nuclear inclusion. The cytoplasm contains abundant profiles of rough endoplasmic reticulum and a cluster of small electron-dense granules. (Uranyl acetate-lead citrate stain, X12,000). (Fig. 3 from Reed M, McKenna RW, Bridges R, Parkin J, Frizzera G, Brunning RD. Morphologic manifestations of monoclonal gammopathies. Am J Clin Pathol 1981;76:8–23.)

Figure 357
IgE MYELOMA
WITH PLEOMORPHIC
PLASMA CELLS

A bone marrow aspirate smear from a patient with IgE myeloma. The plasma cells are large, pleomorphic, and have markedly lobulated nuclei. Less than 1 percent of cases of myeloma are IgE type. (Wright-Giemsa stain)

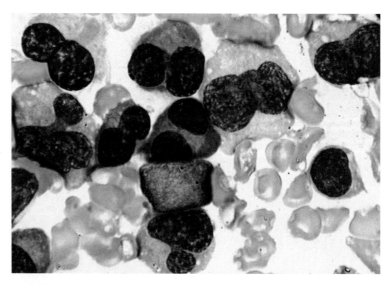

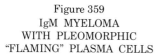

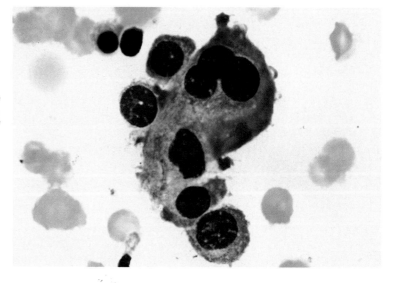

Figure 358
LIGHT CHAIN
MYELOMA WITH
LOBULATED NUCLEI

A bone marrow smear from a patient with light chain myeloma. The nuclei of the plasma cells show striking irregularity and convolution. Most of the plasma cells in this case manifested these lobulated or monocytoid-type nuclei. The neoplastic cells in myelomas of this type may be difficult to recognize as plasma cells. (Wright-Giemsa stain)

Figure 359
IgM MYELOMA
WITH PLEOMORPHIC
"FLAMING" PLASMA CELLS

Plasma cells in a bone marrow aspirate smear from a patient with IgM myeloma. Fewer than 1 percent of cases of myeloma are IgM type. (Wright-Giemsa stain)

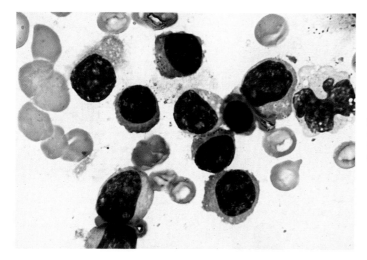

Figure 360
IgD MYELOMA WITH "LYMPHOID"
PLASMA CELLS
The plasma cells in this case of IgD myeloma are small with coarse chromatin. Nucleoli are present in several cells. The plasma cells have a distinctly "lymphoid" appearance, a feature found in some cases of IgD myeloma. (Wright-Giemsa stain)

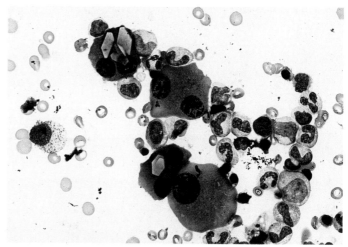

Figure 361
PLASMA CELL MYELOMA WITH
CYTOPLASMIC CRYSTALS
Bone marrow aspirate smear from a 68-year-old man with IgG myeloma showing four large pleomorphic plasma cells. Two of the cells contain large cytoplasmic crystals. (Wright-Giemsa stain)

Figure 362
PLASMA CELL MYELOMA
WITH CYTOPLASMIC
CRYSTALS
Bone marrow trephine biopsy section from a patient with plasma cell myeloma. Many of the plasma cells contain cytoplasmic crystalline inclusions. (Hematoxylin and eosin stain) (Fig. 34B (bottom) from McKenna RW. Disorders of bone marrow. In: Sternberg SS, ed. Diagnostic surgical pathology. 2nd ed. New York: Raven Press, 1994:623–72.)

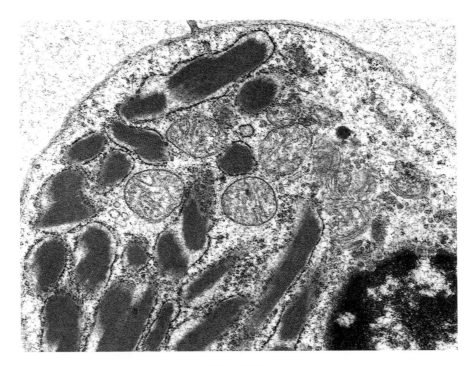

Figure 363
PLASMA CELL WITH CRYSTALLINE INCLUSIONS
An electron micrograph of a plasma cell from a patient with myeloma. The rough endoplasmic reticulum contains multiple crystalline inclusions with a distinct periodicity. (Uranyl acetate-lead citrate stain, X22,000)

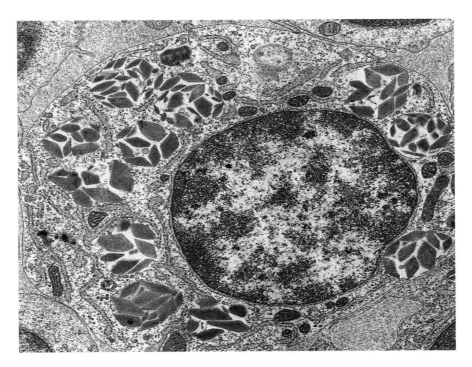

Figure 364
PLASMA CELL WITH CYTOPLASMIC CRYSTALS
An electron micrograph of a plasma cell from a patient with myeloma associated with Fanconi syndrome. There are numerous clusters of crystals in the cytoplasm surrounded by a smooth membrane. (Uranyl acetate-lead citrate stain, X15,000)

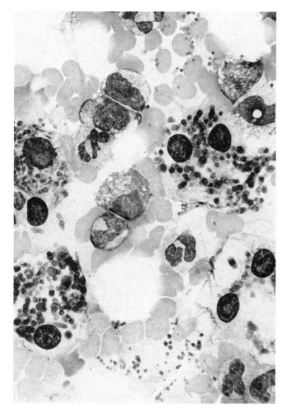

Figure 365
PLASMA CELLS WITH CYTOPLASMIC INCLUSIONS
A bone marrow smear from a patient with plasma cell myeloma. The plasma cells are large with abundant cytoplasm containing multiple inclusions. (Wright-Giemsa stain)

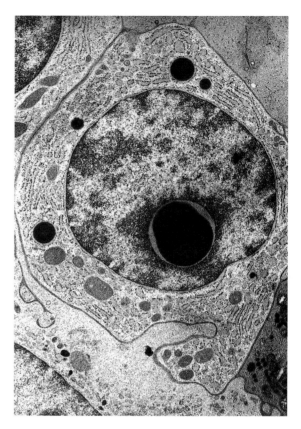

Figure 366
PLASMA CELL WITH CYTOPLASMIC
INCLUSIONS (RUSSELL BODIES)
Electron micrograph of a bone marrow plasma cell from a patient with IgG myeloma. There are several electron-dense inclusions (Russell bodies) in the rough endoplasmic reticulum of the cytoplasm and a large inclusion in the perinuclear envelope invaginating the nucleus. Note the rim of clumped chromatin completely encircling the nuclear inclusion. (Uranyl acetate-lead citrate stain, X13,000)

finding in myelomas occurring in patients with the adult Fanconi syndrome (fig. 364) (46). Other than in the adult Fanconi syndrome, which is invariably associated with kappa light chain immunoglobulins, crystals seem to have no specific relationship to immunologic type. The substructure of the crystalline inclusions is described in the section on ultrastructure.

Multiple large, dark-staining cytoplasmic inclusions are observed in rare cases of myeloma (fig. 365). These are often associated with large pleomorphic plasma cells. Russell body–type intracytoplasmic and intranuclear inclusions are relatively common findings. They usually have a hyaline appearance, are multiple, and small (fig. 366). In contrast, Dutcher-type intranuclear inclusions are pale staining, single, and generally large (see fig. 355). In some cases cytoplasmic inclusions resembling Chinese letters are observed. These

resemble the Buhot plasma cells in patients with mucopolysaccharidosis (fig. 367).

Phagocytic plasma cells are observed in occasional cases of myeloma. Rarely, the erythrophagocytosis is striking (fig. 368) (23). Phagocytized red blood cells may resemble hyaline cytoplasmic inclusions.

Histopathologic Findings. In trephine biopsy sections the pattern of the plasma cell infiltrate may be interstitial, focal, or diffuse (figs. 369–373) (5,53). The extent of bone marrow involvement varies from a small increase in plasma cells in a normocellular marrow to hypercellularity with complete marrow replacement. The pattern of involvement is directly related to the extent of

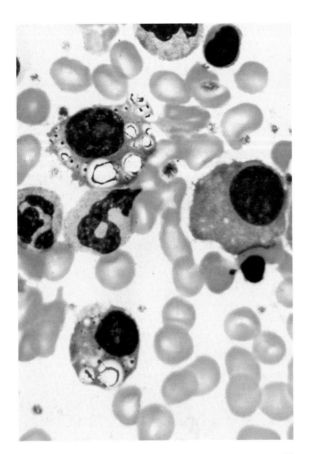
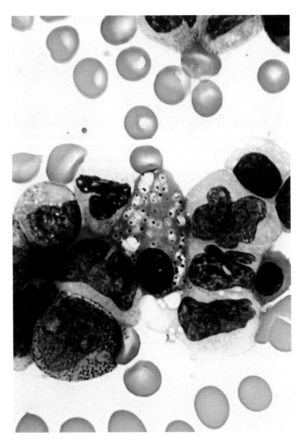

Figure 367
PLASMA CELLS WITH CYTOPLASMIC INCLUSIONS IN MYELOMA AND MUCOPOLYSACCHARIDOSIS
Left: The plasma cells in this case of myeloma contain cytoplasmic inclusions that resemble Chinese letters. Inclusions of this type may be observed in plasma cells in some patients with mucopolysaccharidosis (Buhot cells).
Right: A bone marrow smear from a patient with type III mucopolysaccharidosis (San Filippo disease). A plasma cell is depicted in the center of the field with multiple basophilic inclusions encircled by large clear areas (Buhot cells). (Wright-Giemsa stain)

Figure 368
PHAGOCYTIC
PLASMA CELLS

Plasma cells from the bone marrow of a patient with myeloma. The inclusions in the cytoplasm of two of the myeloma cells are phagocytized red blood cells. Erythrophagocytosis is found in occasional cases of myeloma. In rare cases, it is a striking feature. (Wright-Giemsa stain)

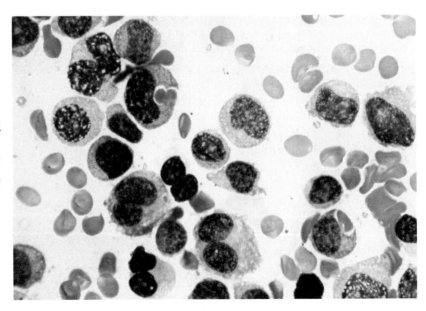

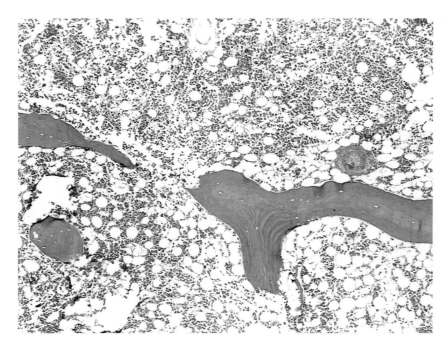

Figure 369
INTERSTITIAL BONE MARROW INVOLVEMENT WITH MYELOMA
A bone marrow trephine biopsy section from an elderly male with myeloma shows an interstitial pattern of bone marrow involvement. (Hematoxylin and eosin stain) (Fig. 34B (top) from McKenna RW. Disorders of bone marrow. In: Sternberg SS, ed. Diagnostic surgical pathology. 2nd ed. New York: Raven Press, 1994:623–72.)

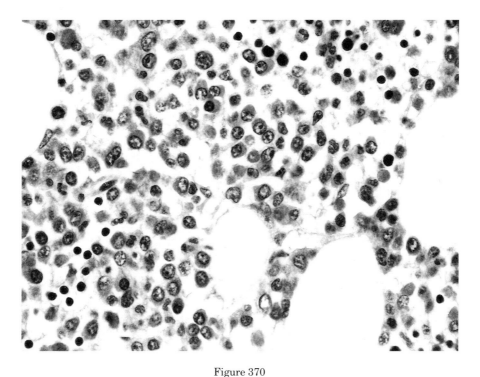

Figure 370
INTERSTITIAL BONE MARROW INVOLVEMENT WITH MYELOMA
A high magnification of an interstitial myeloma cell infiltrate. The plasma cells are in clusters and as single cells mixed with normal hematopoietic cells. The bone marrow was normocellular with preservation of the marrow architecture. (Hematoxylin and eosin stain)

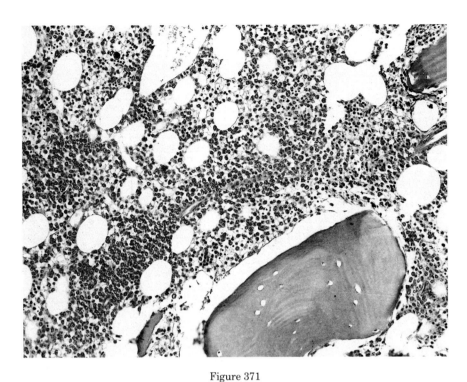

Figure 371
FOCAL AND INTERSTITIAL BONE MARROW INVOLVEMENT WITH MYELOMA
Focal bone marrow aggregates and interstitial infiltration of plasma cells are present in this case of myeloma. (Hematoxylin and eosin stain)

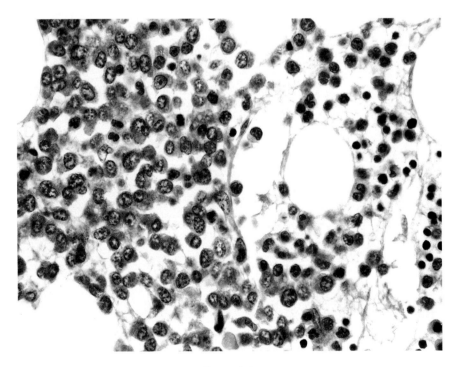

Figure 372
FOCAL BONE MARROW PLASMA CELL INFILTRATE
A higher magnification of the section depicted in figure 371 shows a focus of myeloma plasma cells on the left with normoblasts on the right. (Hematoxylin and eosin stain)

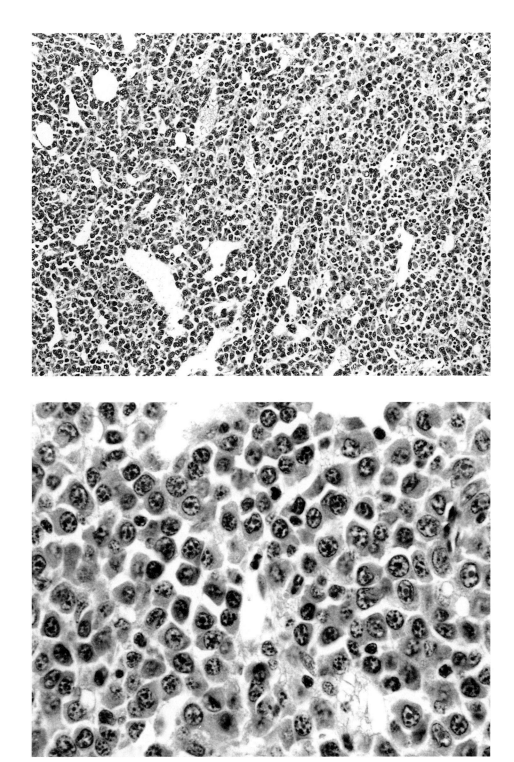

Figure 373
DIFFUSE BONE MARROW INVOLVEMENT WITH MYELOMA

Top: A bone marrow biopsy from a patient with stage III plasma cell myeloma. There is diffuse and extensive marrow involvement and no identifiable normal hematopoiesis in this section. (Hematoxylin and eosin stain)

Bottom: A high magnification of the section illustrated on top. The field consists entirely of immature-appearing plasma cells. (Hematoxylin and eosin stain)

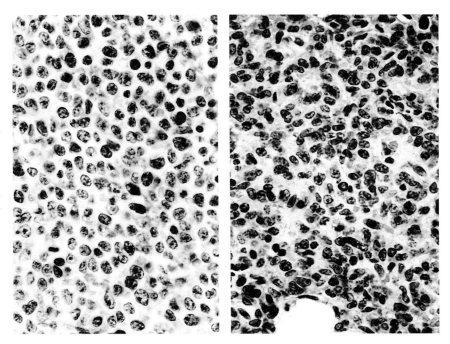

Figure 374
POORLY
DIFFERENTIATED
MYELOMA
Examples of trephine biopsy sections from two cases of atypical myeloma. It is difficult to recognize these as plasma cell infiltrates in routine sections. Cases with atypical morphology of this type must be differentiated from malignant lymphoma. (Hematoxylin and eosin stain)

disease. With the interstitial and focal patterns, there is often considerable marrow sparing and preservation of normal hematopoiesis. With diffuse involvement, expansive areas of the marrow are replaced and hematopoiesis may be markedly suppressed. There is typically progression from interstitial and focal disease in early myeloma to diffuse involvement in advanced stages (5).

A histologic staging system has been proposed based on the plasma cell burden in marrow trephine biopsies (5). In stage I, less than 20 percent of the marrow is replaced by myeloma; stage II, 20 to 50 percent; and stage III, more than 50 percent. There is good correlation between histologic stage and the clinical stage of the disease and prognosis (5).

Myelomas with atypical plasma cell morphology may be difficult to recognize in trephine biopsies. These include plasmablastic myeloma and some cases of myeloma with lymphoid-appearing plasma cells, plasma cells with lobulated nuclei, or markedly pleomorphic plasma cells (figs. 374–376). Cytologic examination of the cells in aspirate smears is often essential for diagnosis in these cases. Occasionally, cytoplasmic inclusions in the myeloma cells are the most striking feature on the bone marrow section (figs. 362, 377–379). The inclusions are often found in large plasma cells that appear distorted by crystalline or globular material (figs. 362, 377–380). The globular inclusions are often strongly positive with the periodic acid–Schiff (PAS) stain (fig. 379).

In approximately 9 percent of cases of myeloma the bone marrow lesions show reticulin fibrosis (figs. 377, 381, 382) (35,53). In many of these the fibrosis is extensive (figs. 381, 382). A disproportionate number of fibrotic myelomas produce monoclonal light chains only (35). Coarse fibrosis is strongly correlated with extensive diffuse marrow involvement and aggressive disease (5).

Cytochemical and Immunohistochemical Findings. There are no cytochemical stains that are specific for plasma cells on bone marrow aspirate smears. Most myeloma plasma cells stain positively for acid phosphatase and often for nonspecific esterase (NSE). They are strongly positive with the methyl green pyronine stain and many of the cytoplasmic and nuclear inclusions stain positively with PAS (fig. 379).

Enzyme immunohistochemical stains with antibodies to plasma cell–associated antigens may be applied to frozen sections or paraffin-embedded sections of bone marrow by an immunoperoxidase or immunoalkaline phosphatase technique. The immunoperoxidase stain for kappa and lambda light chains is the most useful immunohistochemical technique for characterization of malignant

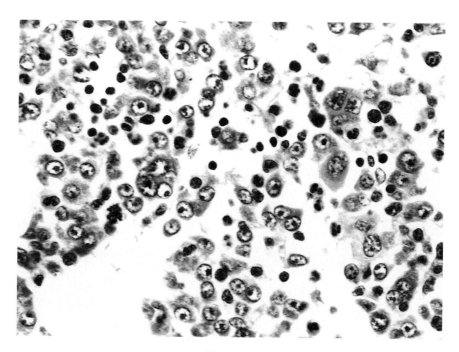

Figure 375
POORLY DIFFERENTIATED MYELOMA

A trephine biopsy section from a patient with plasma cell myeloma with plasmablastic features. There are prominent nucleoli in most of the plasma cells. This type of myeloma must be differentiated from an immunoblastic lymphoma and metastatic tumors such as anaplastic carcinoma and malignant melanoma. (Hematoxylin and eosin stain)

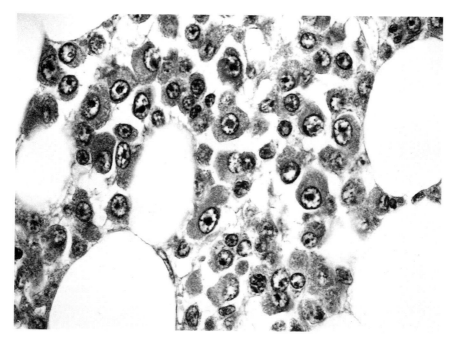

Figure 376
IMMATURE-TYPE MYELOMA

A high magnification of a section of bone marrow from a patient with myeloma showing vesicular eccentrically placed nuclei, large eosinophilic nucleoli, and abundant cytoplasm. (Hematoxylin and eosin stain) (Fig. 23-65 from Brunning RD. Bone marrow. In: Rosai J, ed. Ackerman's surgical pathology. 7th ed. St. Louis: CV Mosby, 1989:1379–453.)

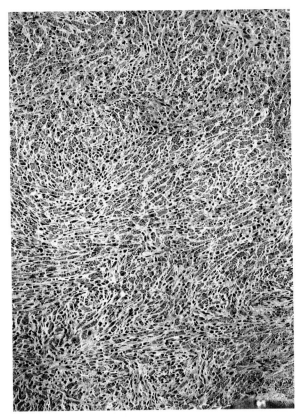

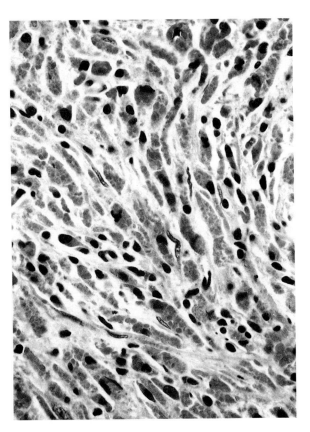

Figure 377
ATYPICAL MYELOMA

A bone marrow biopsy section from a patient with an unusual morphologic presentation of myeloma. The marrow is diffusely infiltrated with atypical plasma cells. There is increased reticulin separating individual and small groups of cells. (Hematoxylin and eosin stain)

Figure 378
ATYPICAL MYELOMA WITH
CYTOPLASMIC INCLUSIONS

A higher magnification of the section illustrated in figure 377 showing large elongated plasma cells filled with cytoplasmic inclusion material. (Hematoxylin and eosin stain)

Figure 379
PLASMA CELLS WITH
PAS-POSITIVE
CYTOPLASMIC INCLUSIONS

The plasma cells in this case of lymphoplasmacytoid lymphoma are large, round, and have abundant cytoplasm. Many are filled with PAS-positive cytoplasmic inclusions. (Periodic acid–Schiff stain) (Fig. 23-70B from Brunning RD. Bone marrow. In: Rosai J, ed. Ackerman's surgical pathology. 7th ed. St. Louis: CV Mosby, 1989:1379–453.)

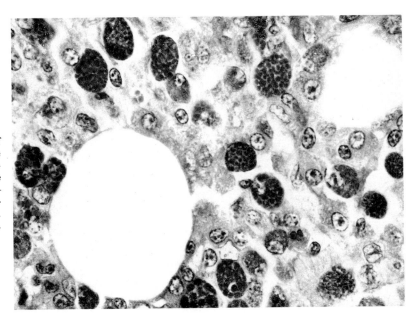

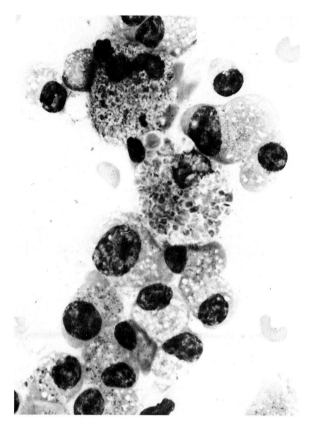

Figure 380
PLASMA CELLS WITH CYTOPLASMIC INCLUSIONS
A bone marrow aspirate smear from a patient with atypical-appearing myeloma. There are numerous cytoplasmic inclusions in many of the plasma cells; others have a vacuolated appearance. (Wright-Giemsa stain)

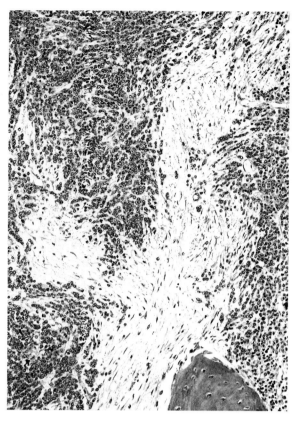

Figure 381
MYELOMA WITH EXTENSIVE
BONE MARROW FIBROSIS
A trephine biopsy section from a patient with plasma cell myeloma. There is a striking desmoplastic reaction. Fibrosis of this degree is an uncommon finding in myeloma. An aspirate was not obtainable in this case. (Hematoxylin and eosin stain)

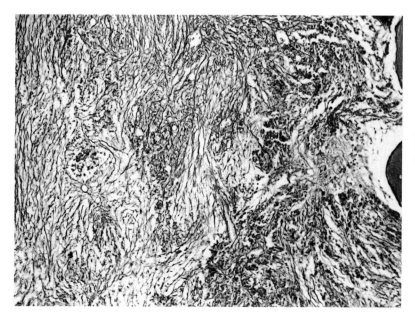

Figure 382
MYELOMA WITH
BONE MARROW FIBROSIS
A reticulin stain from the same case as illustrated in figure 381. There are abundant reticulin fibers. (Wilder reticulin stain)

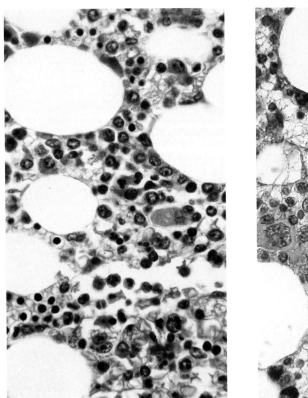
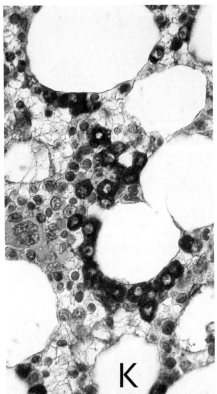

Figure 383
MYELOMA WITH MINIMAL BONE MARROW INVOLVEMENT

A trephine biopsy section from a man with interstitial bone marrow involvement with plasma cell myeloma.
Left: The plasma cell infiltrate is barely noticeable in this field. (Hematoxylin and eosin stain)
Right: An immunoperoxidase stain with an antikappa antibody shows numerous kappa-positive plasma cells. (Immunoperoxidase-antikappa stain)

plasma cell proliferations on trephine sections. Normal and myeloma plasma cells are rich in cytoplasmic immunoglobulin and will generally react strongly with antibodies to kappa or lambda light chains. In cases of myeloma, the plasma cells express a monoclonal pattern of reactivity with either kappa or lambda antibodies (figs. 383, 384) (51,59). In normal bone marrow and in reactive plasma cell proliferations, there is a mixture of kappa- and lambda-reacting plasma cells. A light chain staining ratio of 16 to 1 or higher has been used to distinguish myeloma from a monoclonal gammopathy of undetermined significance (figs. 385, 386) (51). This technique is particularly useful in cases with a low percentage of bone marrow plasma cells and a relatively small monoclonal spike (fig. 383). In addition to identifying neoplastic and reactive plasma cell proliferations, the technique is often

helpful in the differential diagnosis of myeloma from other hematopoietic neoplasms and occasionally from metastatic tumors.

Monoclonal antibody MB2, which recognizes a cytoplasmic antigen in B lymphocytes, may be useful in distinguishing a monoclonal gammapathy of undetermined significance from myeloma and in identifying aggressive myelomas. Immunoperoxidase studies with MB2 on trephine biopsy sections have shown a differential staining pattern, with the plasma cells in most myelomas expressing MB2 and those in most cases of monoclonal gammapathy of undetermined significance staining negatively. Among the myelomas, only a small group of clinically aggressive cases with plasmablastic morphology lacked expression of MB2 (13).

Ultrastructural Findings. Electron microscopy is generally not necessary for the diagnosis of plasma cell myeloma except in a few cases

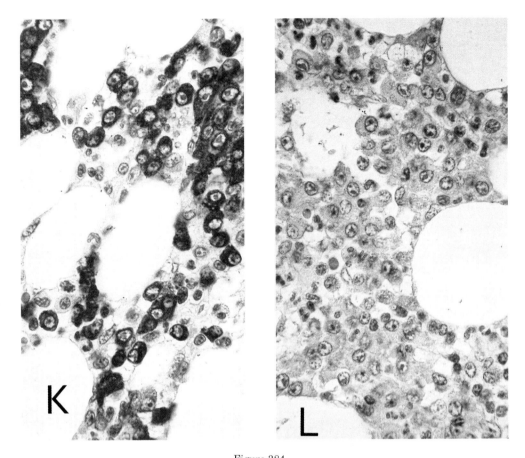

Figure 384
MYELOMA PLASMA CELLS WITH MONOCLONAL STAINING PATTERN
Immunoperoxidase stains of the same case illustrated in figure 383 showing a monoclonal staining pattern.
Left: Antikappa strong reactivity. (Immunoperoxidase stain)
Right: Antilambda negative. (Immunoperoxidase stain)

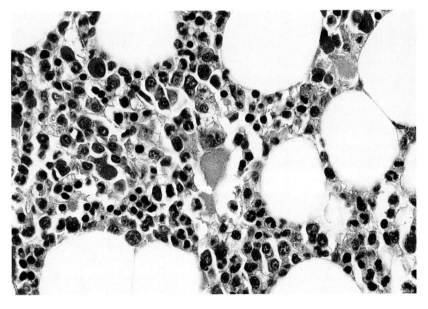

Figure 385
MONOCLONAL GAMMOPATHY
OF UNDETERMINED
SIGNIFICANCE

A bone marrow trephine biopsy section from a 74-year-old female with a 1.3 g/dL serum IgG monoclonal spike. The section shows a moderate interstitial plasma cell infiltrate. (Hematoxylin and eosin stain)

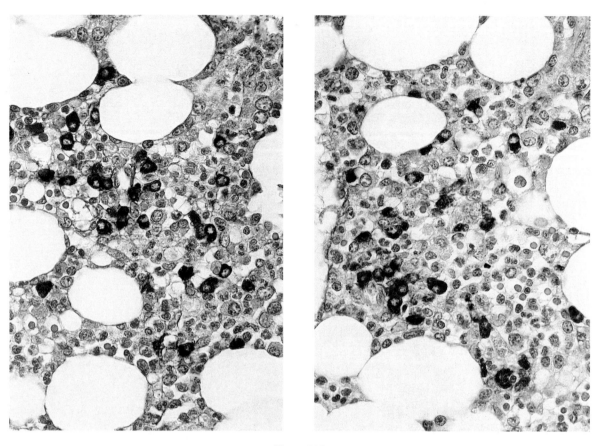

Figure 386
BONE MARROW PLASMACYTOSIS WITH POLYCLONAL STAINING PATTERN
Immunoperoxidase stains for kappa (left) and lambda (right) on the same biopsy as depicted in figure 385. There are approximately equal numbers of plasma cells reacting with antikappa and antilambda antibodies, indicative of a polyclonal plasma cell proliferation. (Immunoperoxidase, antikappa (left) and antilambda (right) stain)

associated with amyloidosis. Ultrastructural abnormalities are present in most cases, however, and electron microscopy is often useful in characterizing the many types of inclusion bodies observed in the plasma cells.

Ultrastructural criteria for the diagnosis of myeloma are based primarily on nuclear-cytoplasmic asynchrony (8). The degrees of asynchrony are defined by the level of nuclear immaturity in relation to the maturation of the rough endoplasmic reticulum (RER) (see figs. 354, 356) (8). In addition to nuclear-cytoplasmic asynchrony, plasma cells in myeloma are typified by cellular pleomorphism and a variety of nuclear and cytoplasmic inclusions. In most cases there is abundant cytoplasm with a prominent Golgi region containing numerous vesicles and clusters of granules. The cytoplasm is filled

with a RER that is usually dilated and may appear as parallel stacked cisternae or as rounded profiles (see figs. 354, 356) (10,45). Most RER cisternae contain amorphous material which represents immunoglobulin produced by the myeloma plasma cell (see fig. 354).

A variety of pale or electron-dense globular and crystalline inclusions may be observed (9). They usually are located within the cisternae of the RER. Electron-dense inclusions correspond to the hyaline-like inclusions observed in light microscopy; they are PAS negative (see fig. 366). The pale globular inclusions are PAS positive by light microscopy. Crystalline inclusions have a distinct periodicity that differs from case to case (see figs. 363, 364) (24); these are common in cases of myeloma associated with adult renal Fanconi syndrome. This condition may precede a plasma cell dyscrasia in some patients and is possibly a manifestation of a latent form of myeloma. The monoclonal immunoglobulin type in these cases is kappa light chain. Crystalline inclusions may be found in plasma cells and macrophages in the marrow and in the renal tubular epithelium (46), and, in contrast to the usual location in the RER of plasma cells, are contained by smooth membranes (see fig. 364).

Nuclear inclusions may also be observed. They are identical to the globular inclusions in the cytoplasm. Most of them are not actually intranuclear but are located in the perinuclear cisterna and invaginate the nucleus, giving the appearance of being intranuclear (see figs. 356, 366) (9).

Some ultrastructural features are associated with, but not specific for, a particular immunoglobulin type of myeloma. These include large, pale, amorphous nuclear inclusions in some IgA myelomas, small lymphoid-appearing plasma cells with heavily condensed chromatin in many cases of IgD myeloma, and large cytoplasmic crystalline inclusions in light chain myeloma (see figs. 356, 363, 364) (10).

The ultrastructural features of the neoplastic cells in plasma cell leukemia are similar to those of other myelomas. In addition, large bundles of microfilaments may be present in the cytoplasm of a high percentage of the leukemic plasma cells (50).

Immunologic Findings. Plasma cell myeloma is a mature B-cell neoplasm that expresses monoclonal cytoplasmic immunoglobulin (CIg) but not surface immunoglobulin (SIg). There is mounting evidence, however, that plasma cell myeloma actually results from an early hematopoietic stem cell disorder that is manifested at a mature stage of B cell development (4,52). Monoclonal blood lymphocytes that are immunophenotypically and immunogenotypically related to the neoplastic bone marrow plasma cells have been identified in all cases of myeloma that have been analyzed (52).

Plasma cells lack several B-lymphocyte antigens that are found on normal peripheral blood B lymphocytes and most B-cell lymphomas. These include HLA-DR, CD19, CD20, CD22, and CD24 (7). They are also CD25 negative. The lack of expression of these antigens is useful in distinguishing them from B-cell lymphomas with plasmacytoid features and other B-lymphoproliferative disorders (7,31).

Both normal and neoplastic plasma cells express CD38 and the mature B-cell antigens PCA-1 and PC-1. They may manifest asynchronous expression of CD10 in cases of aneuploid myeloma (1,4,7,18,22). The combination of monoclonal cytoplasmic immunoglobulin and CD38 expression is virtually diagnostic of myeloma (7). Myelomonocytic antigens are found on myeloma plasma cells in some cases (22). Their expression or expression of CD10 has been associated with an aggressive disease course by some investigators (4,18). Others have found coexpression of CD10 and cytoplasmic immunoglobulin a favorable prognostic indicator (4). Recent studies on normal bone marrow plasma cells have identified a heterogeneous pattern of surface antigen expression. Myeloid specific antigens CD33 and CD13 and the early B-cell antigen CD10 are expressed on a proportion of normal plasma cells (55).

Cytogenetic Findings. Chromosomal abnormalities are detected in 24 to 54 percent of cases of plasma cell myeloma; they are found in nearly all cases of plasma cell leukemia (12,14,26,44,57). The abnormal cytogenetic findings are variable but complex rearrangements and hyperdiploidy are most common. Nearly every chromosome has been involved. Both numerical and structural abnormalities are present in most cases. Rearrangements of chromosome 1 appear to be the most frequent; often there are large marker chromosomes involving the long arm of chromosome 1 (12,57). Abnormalities involving chromosome 14q32 are frequent, most commonly t(11;14)(p13;q32) (12,14,44,57). Abnormalities of chromosomes 5, 9, 11, and 12 are also common. Breakpoints on chromosomes involved in structural rearrangements correlate with known fragile sites and oncogene locations (12).

The relationship of chromosome abnormalities to survival in plasma cell myeloma is controversial. Some investigators report no relationship, others associate the presence of cytogenetic rearrangements with aggressive disease (14,44). Hypodiploidy has been reported to occur mainly in patients with light chain myeloma and those resistant to therapy (26). It is generally true that patients whose bone marrow shows no growth of metaphases have a favorable prognosis (44). There appears to be no reproducible association between abnormal karyotype and type of monoclonal serum immunoglobulin (44).

Myeloma Variants. There are four variants of plasma cell myeloma that have clinical and biologic characteristics that differ from other myelomas. These are plasma cell leukemia, smoldering myeloma, solitary plasmacytoma of bone, and osteosclerotic myeloma. Plasma cell leukemia was discussed in the section on blood findings.

Smoldering Myeloma. This is a rare clinical variant in which the criteria for the diagnosis of plasma cell myeloma are present but the disease shows no progression for 5 years or more without any form of therapeutic intervention (28,43). Approximately 2 percent of cases of myeloma are smoldering myelomas (43). In one study of six cases the monoclonal protein ranged from 3.0 to 3.6 g/dL; five were IgG and one IgA. Five of the six had Bence Jones proteinuria and all had a decrease of normal polyclonal immunoglobulins (43). Patients have more than 10 percent plasma cells in the bone marrow. The plasma cells are morphologically atypical in bone marrow aspirate smears. Focal aggregates, interstitial infiltration of plasma cells, or both are found in trephine biopsy sections. The plasma cells have a low thymidine labeling index relative to most myelomas (17). Patients have no evidence of underlying disease and there are no lytic lesions, anemia, hypercalcemia, renal failure, or other manifestations of myeloma. Clinically the cases behave like monoclonal gammopathy of undetermined significance (MGUS) but fulfill the diagnostic criteria for myeloma (38).

Solitary Plasmacytoma of Bone. This is a localized plasma cell tumor of cytologically mature or immature plasma cells. The spine, pelvis, and femurs are the most common sites of involvement. The criteria for diagnosis include the presence of a single bone lesion with the histology consistent with a plasma cell tumor, absence of a plasma cell infiltrate in random bone marrow biopsies, no evidence of other bone lesions by radiographic examination, and absence of renal failure, hypercalcemia, and anemia that could be attributable to myeloma (16,58).

About 5 percent of patients with plasma cell myeloma present with a solitary plasmacytoma in the form of a single painful bone lesion (16). Seventy percent of patients are male and the median age is younger than for plasma cell myeloma, 50 to 55 years (6). Less than half of the patients have a detectable monoclonal protein level in the serum or urine, reflecting the small size of the plasma cell proliferation; the monoclonal protein may disappear with removal or irradiation of the tumor. Uninvolved immunoglobulins are quantitatively normal.

In most patients there is eventual evolution to plasma cell myeloma (6,16,58). The usual course is progression of disease within 2 to 10 years. New bone lesions, generalized marrow plasmacytosis, and increasing monoclonal protein levels evolve as the disease progresses. Approximately one third of patients remain disease free for more than 10 years (16). Even in many of the patients that develop generalized plasma cell myeloma, the disease has a relatively indolent course. The median survival period for patients presenting with a solitary plasmacytoma exceeds 10 years.

Solitary extramedullary plasmacytomas are most common in the mucous membranes of the upper air passages. They infrequently evolve to plasma cell myeloma (6,58).

Osteosclerotic Myeloma. This myeloma is a component of a rare syndrome that includes polyneuropathy, organomegaly, endocrinopathy, monoclonal gammopathy, and skin lesions (POEMS)(2,48). Males are most often affected and the process may have its onset at a relatively young age. There may be single or multiple sclerotic bone lesions (fig. 387). The monoclonal protein level is quantitatively low and either IgG or IgA. Almost all patients have lambda light chains; Bence Jones proteinuria is common. The bone marrow away from the osteosclerotic plasmocytomas generally contains less than 5 percent plasma cells (48).

Differential Diagnosis. The most common problem in the diagnosis of the plasma cell dyscrasias is the distinction of early and smoldering myeloma from a monoclonal gammopathy of undetermined significance (MGUS) or a secondary reactive bone marrow plasmacytosis. The monoclonal gammopathies of undetermined significance and the characteristics that distinguish them from myeloma are detailed elsewhere in this chapter and will not be repeated here. Reactive bone marrow plasmacytosis in excess of 10 percent may occasionally occur in several conditions including viral infections, immune reactions to drugs, autoimmune disorders such as systemic lupus erythematosus, acquired immune deficiency syndrome, and Hodgkin disease (fig. 388). The plasma cells in these conditions are generally mature in appearance. They may be

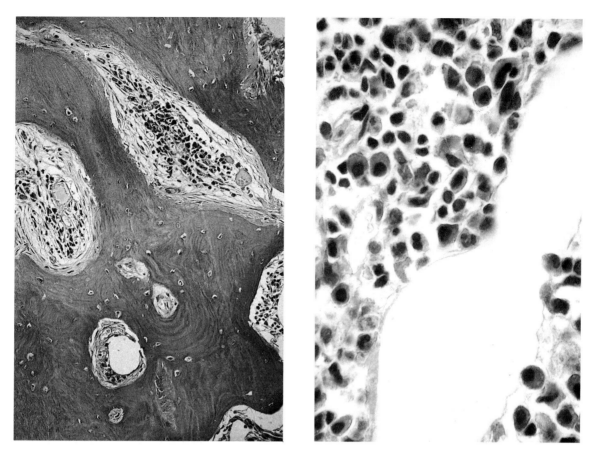

Figure 387
OSTEOSCLEROTIC MYELOMA

Left: A bone marrow biopsy section from a patient with POEMS syndrome. The osteosclerotic changes are typical of myelomas in this syndrome. (Hematoxylin and eosin stain)

Right: A high magnification of osteosclerotic myeloma showing a marrow sinus and several plasma cells. (Hematoxylin and eosin stain)

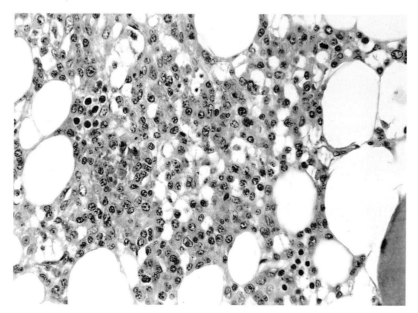

Figure 388
REACTIVE PLASMA
CELL LESION

An aggregate of plasma cells in a post-chemotherapy trephine biopsy section from a 39-year-old male with acute myeloid leukemia. Increased polyclonal (reactive) plasma cells, sometimes in clusters, are found in several conditions as well as some postchemotherapy marrow specimens. (Hematoxylin and eosin stain)

distinguished from myeloma by the lack of a monoclonal protein in the serum or urine. Immunoperoxidase stains for kappa and lambda light chains on marrow sections show a polyclonal plasma cell staining pattern in reactive plasmacytosis and a monoclonal pattern in myeloma.

Occasionally myeloma must be distinguished from a lymphoplasmacytoid lymphoma, immunoblastic lymphoma, or a metastatic tumor. Any of these may potentially show morphologic similarities and be associated with a monoclonal protein. At least some of the diagnostic criteria for myeloma are lacking in these tumors. Careful morphologic study of both bone marrow sections and smears usually distinguishes these lesions. In particularly problematic cases, immunophenotyping using antibodies to lymphocyte and plasma cell–associated antigens, and immunoperoxidase stains for cytoplasmic immunoglobulin on biopsy sections will often help clarify the diagnosis. Solitary plasmacytomas may be more problematic in the differential diagnosis of lymphoma and metastatic tumors. Cases of plasma cell leukemia in which the plasma cells have features of plasmacytoid lymphocytes must be differentiated from peripheralized lymphoplasmacytoid lymphoma, small lymphocytic lymphoma, and chronic lymphocytic leukemia. The findings in the bone marrow and the character of the monoclonal protein usually distinguish these processes.

Treatment and Prognosis. Patients with asymptomatic plasma cell myeloma are generally followed without treatment until symptoms develop or the serum monoclonal protein shows significant elevation. Individuals with solitary plasmacytomas may be treated with local field radiation. The standard treatment for symptomatic generalized plasma cell myeloma is alkylating agent chemotherapy. Melphalan or cyclophosphamide are used as single agents, combined with steroids, or as components of multidrug combination chemotherapy regimens. Objective responses are observed in 50 to 60 percent of patients and complete remission is achieved occasionally. These alkylating agents have improved the median survival period to approximately 30 to 36 months from diagnosis (20,21).

The introduction of alpha-interferon with alkylating agents or combination chemotherapy has increased response rates, increased complete remission, and delayed relapse (41). The use of alpha-interferon in maintenance therapy significantly prolongs remission and survival (47). The combination of VAD (vincristine-doxorubicin-dexamethasone) has been effective in many alkylating agent–resistant myelomas but does not appear to extend survival in previously untreated patients (3,4).

Autologous and allogeneic bone marrow transplantation are being used in an increasing number of patients (3,25,33,41). Age and suitable donors are limiting factors for allogeneic transplants. Almost 40 percent of patients succumb to complications but approximately 40 percent can expect a 5-year disease-free survival (3,25). The long-term disease-free survival for autologous transplantation is less, but age and donor availability are not restricting factors and transplant-related death is only approximately 5 percent (3,33,41).

Response to therapy and detection of relapse or progression of disease may be monitored most effectively by serial serum beta-2 microglobulin levels and periodic quantitative assessment of serum or urine monoclonal proteins. Monitoring bone marrow plasma cell percentage and radiographic changes are less precise.

In most cases plasma cell myeloma is a progressive disease that infrequently enters complete remission. The median survival period is approximately 3 years. Many patients survive less than 1 year. Approximately 10 percent of patients have a chronic course and survive for 10 years or more (3). Many of these patients have smoldering or indolent myeloma (17,28,37,43). The newer treatment modalities discussed above have improved the complete remission and survival rates for many patients in the last few years.

Survival is closely related to the clinical stage of the disease at the time of diagnosis. Staging systems are based on laboratory parameters that are indicators of extent of disease. The studies used in staging generally include hemoglobin level, serum calcium level, size of the monoclonal immunoglobulin spike, and bone radiographic findings. Three stages have been defined based on these criteria (stages I, II, and III). Subgroups of these stages (A and B) are determined by renal function based on serum creatinine levels (17,19). Survival and response to treatment are directly related to the stage of disease at diagnosis; stage III carries the worst prognosis (17).

Other indicators of poor response to therapy and shortened survival are a plasmablastic morphology, greater extent of bone marrow replacement, high plasma cell labeling index, high serum beta-2 microglobulin levels, low serum albumin levels, hypodiploidy, aneuploidy, and very low polyclonal (normal) serum immunoglobulins (5,17,27,56).

The combination of serum beta-2 microglobulin and serum albumin levels appears to provide prognostic information comparable to clinical staging and may lead to de-emphasis of staging in the future (17). A serum beta-2 microglobulin level of more than 6 μg/mL, particularly when associated with a serum albumin of less than 3 g/dL, is strongly associated with poor prognosis (17).

The most common cause of death is infection which may result from a combination of factors including markedly reduced normal immunoglobulins, granulocytopenia from bone marrow replacement by tumor, and immunosuppression by chemotherapeutic drugs. Renal failure is a cause of, or a contributing factor to, death in many cases.

MONOCLONAL GAMMOPATHY OF UNDETERMINED SIGNIFICANCE

Definition. The designation for a monoclonal immunoglobulin spike in the serum or urine of a patient in whom there is no evidence of plasma cell myeloma, amyloidosis, other lymphoproliferative disorder, or any other disease known to produce monoclonal immunoglobulins. The term monoclonal gammopathy of undetermined significance (MGUS) is preferable to the once commonly used designation of benign monoclonal gammopathy since a significant number of cases will evolve in time to a malignant plasma cell dyscrasia (64,65).

Incidence and Clinical Findings. Monoclonal gammopathies are found in at least 3 percent of individuals over the age of 70 years, with no evidence of a plasma cell dyscrasia (64,65). If very sensitive methods of detection are used, 5 percent to more than 8 percent of individuals over 20 years of age will have at least small monoclonal immunoglobulin bands (68,71). In one series using routine methods of detection, 63 percent of monoclonal gammopathies identified in a large laboratory were MGUS; plasma cell myeloma accounted for only 12 percent (64).

The incidence of MGUS is twice as high in blacks than in whites (71). Nearly 60 percent of individuals are male. MGUS is rare in patients less than 40 years old and increases with age through the eighth decade. Because of the frequently advanced age at recognition, many patients have underlying health problems such as cardiovascular diseases, cancer, inflammatory disorders, and neurologic diseases. The monoclonal gammopathy is often identified in the course of evaluation of one of these disorders (65). There is no association with any specific disease process and no specific symptoms or physical findings related to MGUS.

Transient oligoclonal and monoclonal gammopathies have been described in patients following renal and allogeneic bone marrow transplants (66,70). There is a correlation with graft versus host disease in bone marrow transplant recipients (66).

Laboratory Findings. Abnormal laboratory findings in individuals with a MGUS usually reflect a coexisting disease process. Other than the monoclonal gammopathy and a mild increase in bone marrow plasma cells in some cases, there are no consistent or specific laboratory findings. The abnormalities associated with a neoplastic plasma cell dyscrasia are not observed.

A monoclonal spike of variable size is found on serum protein electrophoresis in most cases. In patients with a very small quantity of monoclonal immunoglobulin an M spike is not detected by routine serum protein electrophoresis. Immunoelectrophoresis and immunofixation are required for detection of small spikes and for characterizing the monoclonal protein. The monoclonal protein varies from less than 0.3 to more than 3 g/dL; the median is 1.7 g/dL (65). In more than 95 percent of cases the monoclonal protein is less than 3 g/dL (65,70).

The distribution of monoclonal heavy and light chain types in MGUS is generally reflective of the normal quantitative distribution of immunoglobulin-producing cells except for a disproportionate increase in the frequency of IgM. In 67 to 75 percent of cases the monoclonal heavy chain is gamma; the light chain is kappa in 54 to 63 percent. Monoclonal μ heavy chains are found in 15 percent of cases and alpha in 10 to 14 percent (65,70). Only rare cases of IgD MGUS have been reported and monoclonal protein consisting of light chain only is rare (67). In 2 to 3 percent of cases there is a biclonal gammopathy (65,70).

Light chains (Bence Jones protein) are present in the urine in small quantities in up to 28 percent of cases; in most the quantity of urinary protein is less than 1 g/24 hours. Normal serum polyclonal immunoglobulins are decreased in nearly 30 percent of cases (65,70).

Blood and Bone Marrow Findings. There are no specific blood findings associated with MGUS. Rouleaux formation may be increased in patients with relatively high levels of monoclonal protein. When blood count abnormalities or changes in blood smears are found, they are usually related to a coexisting disease process.

The proportion of plasma cells in bone marrow aspirate smears varies from 1 to 10 percent, with a median of 3 percent (64,70). Approximately half of the patients with MGUS have a mild increase in plasma cells. The plasma cell morphology is usually normal but mild changes, including cytoplasmic inclusions and nucleoli, may be observed in some cases.

Histopathologic Findings. In trephine biopsy sections the marrow is generally normocellular. Plasma cells may be evenly scattered throughout the marrow or found in small groups, often around blood vessels (see fig. 385). Clustering of plasma cells is most common in cases with an increased percentage of these cells.

Cytochemical and Immunohistochemical Findings. The cytochemical characteristics of the plasma cells in MGUS are the same as those in myeloma. Enzyme immunohistochemical staining for kappa and lambda light chains in trephine biopsy sections show variable staining patterns. In the majority of cases there is a polyclonal staining pattern with both kappa- and lambda-positive plasma cells in normal or near normal ratios (see figs. 385, 386). In a minority of cases there is a monoclonal pattern with either kappa- or lambda-staining plasma cells (69).

Ultrastructural Findings. There are no specific ultrastructural features of the plasma cells in MGUS. Electron microscopy is noncontributory to the diagnosis. See ultrastructure in the section Plasma Cell Myeloma.

Cytogenetic Findings. There are no cytogenetic abnormalities described for MGUS.

Differential Diagnosis. The differential diagnosis considerations are confined to neoplastic plasma cell dyscrasias, usually myeloma. In most cases the distinction between myeloma and MGUS is not difficult since myeloma is diagnosed by well-defined criteria, which are lacking in MGUS. Patients with MGUS generally have a serum monoclonal protein of less than 3 g/dL, small amounts or no protein in the urine, less than 5 percent plasma cells in the bone marrow, and no anemia, hypercalcemia, renal failure, or osteolytic lesions. With this combination of findings, a diagnosis of myeloma would generally not be considered. Only in cases of MGUS in which there is an unusually high monoclonal spike or significantly increased bone marrow plasma cells is the diagnosis problematic.

In most cases immunoperoxidase stains for kappa and lambda light chains in the cytoplasm of plasma cells can distinguish myeloma and MGUS (69). There is a light chain staining excess exceeding a ratio of 16 to 1 in the vast majority of cases of myeloma (see fig. 384). In MGUS the ratio is less than 16 to 1 in more than 90 percent of cases (see fig. 386) (69). Patients with MGUS and a monoclonal staining pattern appear to be more likely to progress to overt myeloma. The expression of MB2 may also be useful in differentiating myeloma and MGUS (63) (see differential diagnosis, Plasma Cell Myeloma). Cytogenetic studies, thymidine labeling index, flow cytometric DNA analysis, and the beta-2 microglobulin assay may be useful in some cases (62,72).

Differentiation of MGUS from early myeloma and Waldenström macroglobulinemia may not be possible at the time of initial evaluation. Close observation and monitoring for evidence of progression to overt malignancy must be continued indefinitely.

Treatment and Prognosis. Treatment for MGUS is unnecessary. Only in cases with evolution to a neoplastic plasma cell dyscrasia is therapy required, and then only when there is unequivocal evidence of overt, symptomatic disease.

The clinical course in the majority of individuals is stable with no increase in monoclonal protein or other evidence of progression to a malignant plasma cell dyscrasia. In a minority of cases, however, there is eventual evolution to an overt plasma cell myeloma, amyloidosis, macroglobulinemia, or other malignant lymphoproliferative disorder. In one large study with a median follow-up of 22 years, 47 percent of patients died of unrelated causes without progression of their monoclonal gammopathy; another 19 percent were living with no substantial increase in monoclonal protein; 10 percent had a serum monoclonal protein value of 3 g/dL or more but did not require chemotherapy and were without other changes in clinical status; and 24 percent developed a malignant plasma cell dyscrasia or lymphoproliferative disease (64). By actuarial analysis, the conversion of MGUS to a malignant plasma cell dyscrasia was 17 percent at 10 years and reached 33 percent at 20 years. The mean interval from diagnosis of MGUS to evolution of malignant lymphoplasmacytic disease was 10 years, with a range of 2 to 29 years, after detection of the monoclonal protein. The development of malignancy was either gradual or abrupt following a long interval of stability. The diagnosis was plasma cell myeloma in 66 percent of cases, macroglobulinemia in 12 percent, and amyloidosis in 14 percent; 8 percent had lymphoma or chronic lymphocytic leukemia. Patients with IgM (37 percent) and IgA (32 percent) MGUS are more apt to have progression of their gammopathy than those with IgG (21 percent) (65). Increasing size of the serum monoclonal protein spike is the most reliable parameter for predicting progression of MGUS to a malignant plasma cell dyscrasia (65).

WALDENSTRÖM MACROGLOBULINEMIA (LYMPHOPLASMACYTOID LYMPHOMA)

In hospital populations, up to 19 percent of monoclonal gammopathies are found in patients with lymphoproliferative disorders (87). Monoclonal gammopathies have been reported in nearly all types of B-cell tumors but are most common in lymphoplasmacytoid lymphoma and other small lymphocyte proliferations (76,80,82,84,87). The monoclonal protein is IgM in approximately 60 percent of cases, IgG in 30 percent, and IgA or biclonal in 5 percent; gammopathies of light or heavy chains only are rare (76,87). In the majority of cases the monoclonal protein is an incidental finding in a patient with known lymphoproliferative disease and is without clinical significance. In some patients with IgM gammopathy, the monoclonal protein is a major factor in the pathophysiology of the disease and produces a clinico-pathologic syndrome usually designated as macroglobulinemia or Waldenström macroglobulinemia.

Definition. Waldenström macroglobulinemia is a lymphoplasmacytoid lymphoma or other neoplastic small lymphocyte proliferation associated with IgM monoclonal gammopathy. In most cases the disease is disseminated and involves several tissues including the bone marrow. A hyperviscosity syndrome may be present.

Incidence and Clinical Findings. Reliable data on the incidence of Waldenström macroglobulinemia is not available. Approximately 16 percent of all monoclonal gammopathies are IgM (80). Nearly 60 percent of these are MGUS; the remainder are mostly associated with malignant lymphoproliferative disorders. About 17 percent have the features of Waldenström macroglobulinemia (80).

The median age at diagnosis is approximately 60 years, with a range of 30 to over 90 years; two thirds of patients are males. The most frequent symptoms are weakness, tiredness, weight loss, and bleeding problems. Some patients present with neurologic symptoms related to the hyperviscosity syndrome. Raynaud syndrome may be seen in patients with a serum cryoglobulin.

Lymphadenopathy and organomegaly are common physical findings. The fundus of the eye may show tortuous and dilated retinal vessels and retinal hemorrhages. Bruising and purpura are found in some patients.

The hyperviscosity syndrome is a serious and potentially fatal clinical manifestation of macroglobulinemia. It results from an increase in blood viscosity due to elevated levels of plasma monoclonal protein. Its development is related to the quantity, size, and structure of the immunoglobulin molecule. Although most common in IgM monoclonal gammopathies, hyperviscosity is also seen occasionally in IgG and IgA gammopathies (88). Manifestations include headache, bleeding diatheses, focal and generalized central nervous system impairment, hypervolemia, and congestive heart failure. Progression to coma and death may occur unless there is aggressive therapeutic intervention.

Laboratory Findings. Serum protein electrophoresis shows a monoclonal protein spike in essentially all cases with symptomatic disease. The spike is usually in the gamma region and is characterized as IgM by immunoelectrophoresis. The light chain is kappa in three fourths of patients. The size of the spike varies from 3 to more than 8 g/dL (median 4.3 g/dL) (80). Normal uninvolved immunoglobulins are reduced in approximately half of the patients. Light chains are present in the urine in 80 percent (80). Serum viscosity is increased in about 90 percent of patients, markedly so in 30 percent (80). Cryoglobulins are detected in a small number of patients.

The bleeding time is prolonged and platelet function studies are abnormal in most patients with significant elevations of IgM. Coagulation factors are sometimes decreased. Serum creatinine levels are elevated in approximately one third of cases. Hypercalcemia and radiographic skeletal lesions are rare.

Blood and Bone Marrow Findings. Anemia is a common presenting finding and partially related to the dilutional effects of an expanded plasma volume. Leukopenia or thrombocytopenia are less common. In blood smears rouleaux formation is often marked and the background of the smear may have a slightly purplish color due to the increased serum protein. There is a leukemic blood picture in approximately 30 percent of cases. The cytologic features of the leukemic lymphocytes are typical of chronic lymphocytic leukemia or lymphoplasmacytoid lymphoma. These have been described in detail elsewhere in this text.

The bone marrow is involved in 85 percent of cases of Waldenström macroglobulinemia. In marrow smears the percentage of lymphocytes varies from normal to more than 90 percent. They have the cytologic features of well-differentiated lymphocytes and plasmacytoid lymphocytes (figs. 389, 390). Plasma cells, mast cells, and histiocytes are increased in most patients; in rare cases plasma cells predominate. Intranuclear inclusions (Dutcher bodies) may be observed in some of the lymphocytes (fig. 390).

Histopathologic Findings. In trephine biopsy sections the pattern of bone marrow involvement varies but is usually typical for the type of lymphoproliferative disorder (see chapter Bone Marrow Lymphoma). In cases of lymphoplasmacytoid lymphoma and small lymphocytic lymphoma/chronic lymphocytic leukemia, the pattern may be interstitial, focal nonparatrabecular, or diffuse (fig. 391). In the rare cases of macroglobulinemia in follicular small cleaved cell lymphoma, the pattern is focal and paratrabecular (fig. 392). The extent of involvement varies from a few focal lesions to extensive bone marrow replacement.

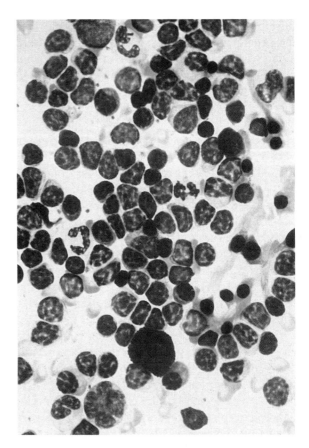

Figure 389
WALDENSTRÖM MACROGLOBULINEMIA

A bone marrow smear from a 72-year-old man with a lymphoplasmacytoid lymphoma and a 4.3 g IgM monoclonal spike. The patient manifested symptoms of Waldenström macroglobulinemia. There are numerous lymphocytes and plasmacytoid lymphocytes. A plasma cell and mast cell are present near the bottom of this field; both were increased in this patient's bone marrow. (Wright-Giemsa stain)

The cytologic characteristics of the cells are usually typical of small lymphocytic and lymphoplasmacytoid lymphomas (figs. 393, 394). In some cases there are numerous plasma cells containing abundant cytoplasm inclusions that stain intensely with PAS (figs. 379, 395, 396). These cells may resemble histiocytes.

Intranuclear inclusions (Dutcher bodies) are commonly observed and may be numerous (figs. 390, 397). Their presence is suggestive of Waldenström macroglobulinemia but is not pathognomonic. They are found in some cases of plasma cell myeloma, other lymphoproliferative diseases, and in reactive conditions.

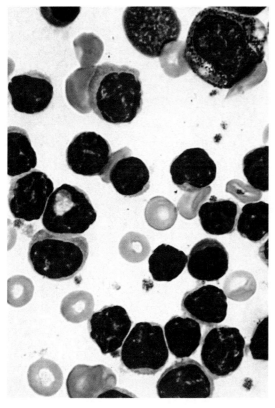

Figure 390
SMALL LYMPHOCYTIC LYMPHOMA WITH
INTRANUCLEAR INCLUSIONS

A bone marrow smear from a 59-year-old man with a small lymphocytic lymphoma and an IgM spike. There is an intranuclear inclusion (Dutcher body) in a lymphocyte at the left of center of the field. (Wright-Giemsa stain)

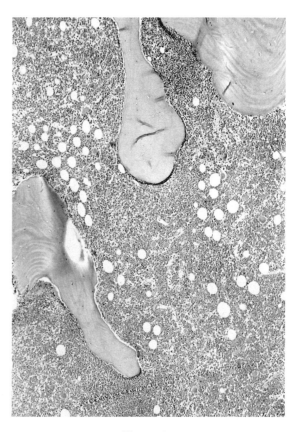

Figure 391
LYMPHOPLASMACYTOID LYMPHOMA
AND MACROGLOBULINEMIA

A trephine biopsy section from a patient with lymphoplasmacytoid lymphoma and an IgM monoclonal spike. There is diffuse marrow infiltration. (Hematoxylin and eosin stain)

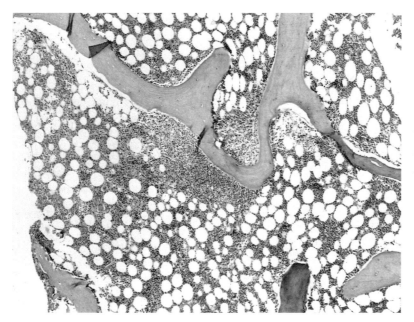

Figure 392
SMALL
CLEAVED CELL LYMPHOMA
AND MACROGLOBULINEMIA

Trephine biopsy section from a patient with focal paratrabecular involvement with small cleaved cell lymphoma. The patient had an IgM monoclonal gammopathy. (Hematoxylin and eosin stain)

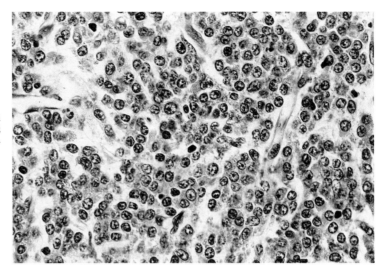

Figure 393
LYMPHOPLASMACYTOID LYMPHOMA
AND MACROGLOBULINEMIA
A trephine biopsy section showing a lymphoplasmacytoid lymphoma in a patient with Waldenström macroglobulinemia. (Hematoxylin and eosin stain)

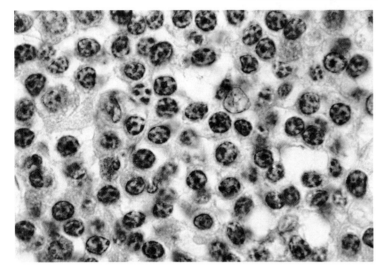

Figure 394
LYMPHOPLASMACYTOID LYMPHOMA
AND MACROGLOBULINEMIA
A high magnification of a lymphoplasmacytoid lymphoma from a patient with Waldenström macroglobulinemia. (Hematoxylin and eosin stain)

Figure 395
LYMPHOPLASMACYTOID
LYMPHOMA AND
MACROGLOBULINEMIA
A bone marrow section from a patient with lymphoplasmacytoid lymphoma and a serum monoclonal IgM spike. There are numerous plasma cells intermixed with small lymphocytes. The plasma cells have abundant eosinophilic cytoplasm; some appear to have inclusion material. (Hematoxylin and eosin stain)

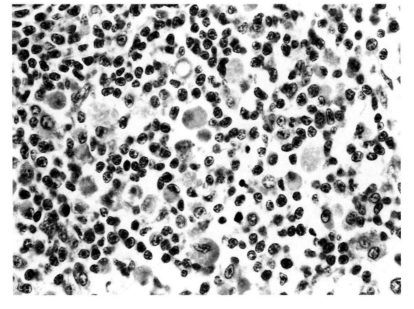

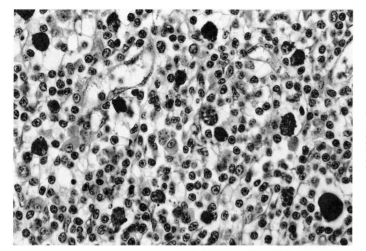

Figure 396
WALDENSTRÖM
MACROGLOBULINEMIA

A bone marrow section from a patient with Waldenström macroglobulinemia shows a lymphoplasmacytoid lymphoma with numerous large plasma cells. Similar to the case illustrated in figure 395, the plasma cells contain abundant PAS-positive material. (Periodic acid–Schiff stain)

Figure 397
SMALL CLEAVED
CELL LYMPHOMA AND
MACROGLOBULINEMIA

A bone marrow section and smear from a patient with a small cleaved cell lymphoma and a serum monoclonal IgM spike. Intranuclear inclusions (Dutcher bodies) (arrows) were easily found in both sections and smears in this case. (Left: Hematoxylin and eosin stains; right: Wright-Giemsa stain)

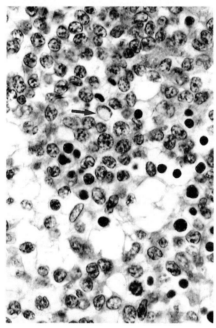

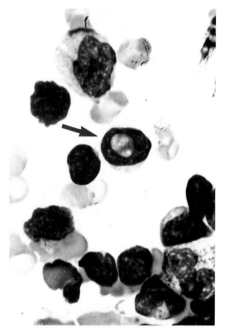

In a minority of cases there is eventual transformation to an aggressive large cell lymphoma. This phenomenon is analogous to the Richter transformation in chronic lymphocytic leukemia.

Cytochemical and Immunohistochemical Findings. There are no cytochemical stains specific for Waldenström macroglobulinemia. Most nuclear and cytoplasmic inclusions stain strongly with PAS. The plasmacytoid lymphocytes react with various B-cell antibodies by immunoperoxidase methods on trephine biopsy sections; there is heterogeneity in staining patterns among cases (79). The plasmacytoid lymphocytes and plasma cells stain monoclonally for cytoplasmic immunoglobulin (77,85).

Ultrastructural Findings. Electron microscopy rarely contributes to the diagnosis. In Waldenström macroglobulinemia the cells generally have a moderate amount of cytoplasm that contains free ribosomes, polyribosomes, a large Golgi region, and abundant rough endoplasmic reticulum (75). Ribosome-lamella complexes are found in the cytoplasm in a small percentage of cases (75). The nuclei are round to slightly indented, with coarsely condensed chromatin and small nucleoli. Nuclear and cytoplasmic inclusions similar to those in the plasma cells in some cases of myeloma are commonly observed in macroglobulinemia. Globular inclusions composed of

357

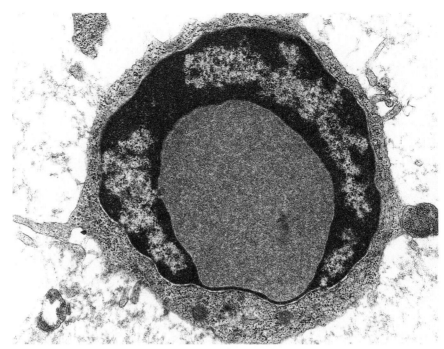

Figure 398
INTRANUCLEAR
INCLUSION
Electron micrograph of a lymphocyte from the bone marrow of a patient with lymphoplasmacytoid lymphoma. There is a large intranuclear inclusion (Dutcher body). (Uranyl acetate-lead citrate stain, X20,000)

pale amorphous substance are located in the rough endoplasmic reticulum. The Dutcher body–type intranuclear inclusions are invaginations of the nuclear envelope. They appear membrane bound and contain pale amorphous material similar to the globular cytoplasmic inclusions (fig. 398) (74).

Immunologic Findings. The plasmacytoid lymphocytes in Waldenström macroglobulinemia coexpress the immunophenotypic characteristics of mature B cells and plasma cells (73,75). They react with monoclonal antibodies to some of the pan–B-cell antigens, such as HLA-DR, CD19, CD20, and CD22. They also contain cytoplasmic immunoglobulin and usually react with plasma cell monoclonal antibodies (MoAbs), PCA-1 and PC-1 (75). Large numbers of monoclonal blood lymphocytes expressing CD9 and CD24 are identified in some cases (86).

Cytogenetic Findings. Cytogenetic abnormalities are identified in approximately half of the cases of Waldenström macroglobulinemia. Multiple rearrangements have been described (78,81,83). There are no cytogenetic changes that are specific. Abnormalities involving chromosome 14 at band q32, similar to the rearrangements in plasma cell myeloma, and trisomy 12, a common

finding in chronic lymphocytic leukemia, have been reported in some cases (78,81,83).

Differential Diagnosis. The differential diagnosis of Waldenström macroglobulinemia is limited. The combination of a lymphoplasmacytoid lymphoma and an IgM monoclonal protein is diagnostic in most cases. A plasma cell myeloma with lymphoid cytologic features may resemble lymphoplasmacytoid lymphoma. The distinction is made by the clinical features and the type of monoclonal protein.

Treatment and Prognosis. Treatment is aimed at control of the primary malignant lymphoproliferative disease and reduction of the monoclonal protein. Alkylating agent chemotherapy alone or in combination with other drugs is the standard treatment. Reduction in tumor mass and monoclonal protein is seen in many cases. In patients with hyperviscosity syndrome plasmapheresis is effective in reducing symptoms.

The course in macroglobulinemia is usually chronic and slowly progressive. The median survival period is 5 years from diagnosis. The cause of death is related to complications of the monoclonal gammopathy (hyperviscosity, infection, hemorrhage) or progression to a refractory lymphoproliferative disorder.

HEAVY CHAIN DISEASES

Definition. A group of syndromes characterized by the production of a monoclonal immunoglobulin that is composed of incomplete heavy chains of IgG, IgA, or IgM and no light chains. The protein abnormality is usually associated with a lymphocyte or plasma cell proliferation, or a combination of both (95). The bone marrow is involved in some cases.

Incidence. There are no reliable data on incidence but all of the heavy chain diseases are extremely rare. Alpha chain disease is the most common, at least three times more common than gamma chain disease and 10 times more common than mμ chain disease. Less than 100 cases of gamma chain disease and fewer than 30 of mμ chain disease have been reported.

Gamma Chain Disease. The median age at diagnosis of gamma chain disease is 61 years (93). Weakness, fatigue, and fever are the most common presenting symptoms. Hepatomegaly, splenomegaly, and lymphadenopathy are each found in about 60 percent of patients (90,93). Serum protein studies may show hypogammaglobulinemia and a monoclonal protein consisting of an incomplete gamma chain (93). Urine protein is usually less than 1 g/24 hours (93). Anemia is present in 80 percent of cases; leukopenia and thrombocytopenia are also common. Atypical lymphocytes and plasma cells may be found on blood smears.

The bone marrow is involved in two thirds of patients (90,93). Approximately 40 percent have a malignancy similar to Waldenström macroglobulinemia. Plasma cells predominate in about 15 percent of cases. Occasionally, gamma chain disease is associated with chronic lymphocytic leukemia or a large cell lymphoma. In some cases there is no evidence of a lymphoproliferative disorder (90,93).

Mμ Chain Disease. The median age at diagnosis is 48 years (89,91). The majority of patients have a long history of chronic lymphocytic leukemia. Mμ chain disease differs from most cases of chronic lymphocytic leukemia by the high frequency of hepatosplenomegaly and the rarity of lymphadenopathy. Occasionally, patients present with a lymphoma, an immunoblastic transformation of chronic lymphocytic leukemia, myeloma, or amyloidosis. Two thirds of patients have characteristic vacuolated plasma cells in the bone marrow (fig. 399).

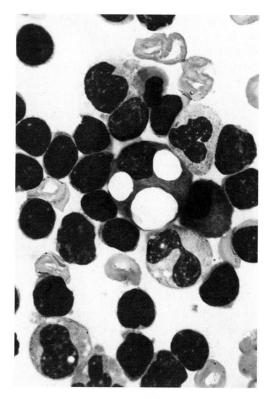

Figure 399
VACUOLATED PLASMA CELL
A bone marrow smear from a patient with a small lymphocytic lymphoma. A vacuolated plasma cell is illustrated in the center of the field. Similar plasma cells have been described in patients with mμ heavy chain disease. (Wright-Giemsa stain)

In more than half of the patients the proliferative cells produce monoclonal light chains that do not assemble with the heavy chain. The light chains are excreted in the urine as Bence Jones protein.

Alpha Chain Disease. This disease primarily affects young individuals; the peak incidence is in the second and third decades of life. The lymphoproliferative disorder associated with alpha chain disease involves the gastrointestinal tract, mainly the small intestine and mesenteric lymph nodes. The lamina propria is heavily infiltrated with lymphoid cells, mostly plasma cells. There is a remarkably uniform clinical picture of severe malabsorption, chronic diarrhea, and abdominal pain and distention (92,94,95). Enlarged mesenteric lymph nodes can often be palpated. Hepatosplenomegaly and lymphadenopathy are rare. The bone marrow is usually normal but alpha chain secreting plasma cells may be identified.

PRIMARY AMYLOIDOSIS

Definition. A plasma cell dyscrasia in which the fibril amyloid protein is produced by monoclonal plasma cells and consists of whole or fragments of immunoglobulin light chains (AL amyloid). The amyloid is deposited in various tissues, accumulates, and leads to organ dysfunction. Primary amyloidosis is associated with plasma cell myeloma in approximately 20 percent of cases (104). In the remaining cases the diagnostic criteria for myeloma are lacking but a moderate monoclonal increase in plasma cells is usually present in the bone marrow.

Classification. Systemic amyloidosis consists of three major categories: *primary* or *light chain (AL) amyloidosis, secondary (AA) amyloidosis,* and *familial (AF) amyloidosis*. Secondary and familial amyloidosis consist of several variants, none of which are associated with plasma cell dyscrasias. They will not be considered further in this discussion nor will the local amyloidoses associated with aging, endocrinopathy, or hemodialysis patients.

AL amyloid is composed of intact immunoglobulin light chains or fragments of light chains that include the amino-terminal (V) region and part of the constant region of the light chain (96). In some cases both intact light chains and fragments are present. Most light chain V-region subgroups are potentially amyloidogenic, however, V-lambda VI is clearly the single most commonly encountered in AL fibril protein (96).

Incidence and Clinical Findings. Primary amyloidosis is a rare disease and there is little published information on its incidence or prevalence in the United States. The reported incidence in one region of the country was approximately one case per 100,000 population per year between 1970 and 1988 (107). The incidence appears to have been relatively stable in the last 40 years (107). Approximately 10 percent of patients with plasma cell myeloma have amyloidosis and 20 percent of patients with primary amyloidosis have myeloma (105,107).

The median age at diagnosis is 64 to 70 years; more than 95 percent of patients are over 40 years of age (104). Sixty to 65 percent of patients are male (106,107). The most common presenting symptoms are fatigue and weight loss (104). Carpal tunnel syndrome or pain related to a peripheral neuropathy are the first signs of disease in some cases. Hemorrhagic manifestations are found in approximately one fifth of cases. Symptoms referable to congestive heart failure, nephrotic syndrome, or malabsorption syndrome are all relatively common.

Physical findings include hepatomegaly in approximately 30 percent of patients and macroglossia in 10 to 22 percent (104,105). Purpura are relatively common. Splenomegaly and lymphadenopathy are uncommon. Edema is often present in patients with congestive heart failure or nephrotic syndrome (104).

Laboratory Findings. A monoclonal immunoglobulin is found in the serum or urine by immunoelectrophoresis in more than 80 percent of patients (104). The monoclonal protein is more often present in cases of amyloidosis with myeloma (100 percent) than without (about 75 percent) and found slightly more often in urine than serum (104). Normal polyclonal serum immunoglobulins are decreased in approximately 30 percent of patients (104).

Proteinuria is identified at diagnosis in over 80 percent of patients by standard urinalysis methods. Evidence of nephrotic syndrome is present in approximately 35 percent. Serum creatinine is above 2.0 mg/dL in 20 to 25 percent of patients (104). Hypercalcemia is occasionally found, most often in patients with myeloma. Liver function studies are abnormal in a minority of cases.

Coagulation studies are important in patients with amyloidosis because of the frequently associated bleeding problems. Hemorrhagic manifestations may result from factor X deficiency due to binding of factor X to amyloid proteins. Bleeding may also be caused by deficiency of vitamin K–dependent clotting factors, fibrinolysis, disseminated intravascular coagulation, and loss of vascular integrity due to amyloid deposition (104).

Bone radiographs are normal in most cases. Osteolytic lesions of bone are confined to patients with myeloma.

The usual method of diagnosis of amyloidosis is by demonstration of amyloid deposition in a tissue biopsy section. The amyloid is most commonly found in the wall of blood vessels. A Congo red stain is the simplest and most practical technique for confirming the presence of amyloid. In primary amyloidosis, subcutaneous fat aspiration and rectal biopsy are each diagnostic in approximately 80 percent of cases when adequate tissue is obtained (96,109). Bone marrow biopsies and skin biopsies are diagnostic in approximately half of the cases; gingival biopsy is less commonly positive (96,110). Renal biopsy is diagnostic in well over 90 percent of cases but carries greater risk than the other procedures and is usually unnecessary. Similarly, liver biopsy is diagnostic in most cases but should be avoided if possible because of associated bleeding complications. Cardiac involvement can be documented by endomyocardial biopsy in a high percentage of cases (110).

A promising method for diagnosing and following patients with amyloidosis is scintigraphy with iodine labeled serum amyloid P component (SAP) (103). SAP has specific binding affinity for amyloid fibrils. Iodine labeled SAP is rapidly localized to amyloid deposits in vivo and is useful in identifying and quantitating amyloid deposition (103).

Blood and Bone Marrow Findings. Blood counts are often normal at the time of diagnosis. Abnormal blood counts, mostly cytopenias, are more frequent in patients with amyloidosis and myeloma. Anemia is the most common abnormality but severe anemia is unusual. Leukocytosis, leukopenia, and thrombocytopenia are rare. Thrombocytosis is found in approximately 7 percent of cases (104). Blood smear findings are usually nonspecific; increased rouleaux formation may be present in cases with a large monoclonal protein spike. Circulating plasma cells are sometimes observed but substantial numbers are found only in the rare cases of amyloidosis associated with plasma cell leukemia.

The bone marrow is usually diagnostic in cases of amyloidosis associated with myeloma but less than half of the nonmyeloma cases are diagnosed by marrow examination. In many cases bone marrow amyloid deposition is minimal and the percentage of plasma cells low. Despite the lower diagnostic yield than for other techniques, the bone marrow biopsy should be routinely performed when amyloidosis is a considered diagnosis. The procedure is easily performed, diagnostic in many cases, and necessary to identify patients with myeloma.

In the marrow aspirate smears there are less than 10 percent plasma cells in the majority of cases; the median is approximately 8 percent (104). Most patients with more than 20 percent plasma cells have overt myeloma. The plasma cells may be morphologically normal, or any of

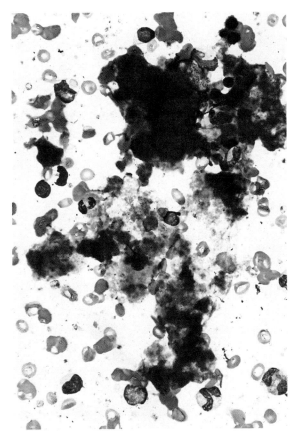

Figure 400
AMYLOIDOSIS
A bone marrow aspirate smear from a patient with amyloidosis. The marrow was heavily replaced with amyloid which is present in large clumps on the marrow smear. (Wright-Giemsa stain)

the spectrum of changes described for cases of plasma cell myeloma may be observed. Vacuolated plasma cells resembling those often found in mμ heavy chain disease are present in some cases (fig. 399) (111). When there is extensive amyloid deposition in the bone marrow, lightly eosinophilic to basophilic proteinaceous material may be scattered on the smears in variously sized clumps (fig. 400).

Histopathologic Findings. Trephine biopsy sections vary from having no identifiable pathologic changes to extensive replacement of the hematopoietic bone marrow with amyloid or overt myeloma with markedly increased plasma cells (fig. 401). The most common finding is a mild increase in plasma cells. If adequately sized vessels are included in the biopsy section, amyloid

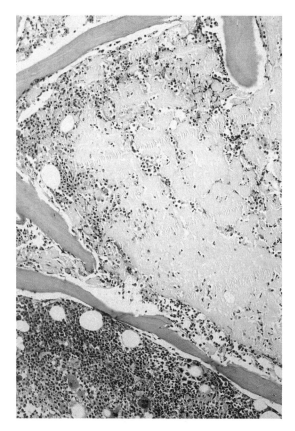

Figure 401
AMYLOIDOSIS
A trephine biopsy section from a patient with amyloidosis. There are large deposits of amyloid replacing extensive portions of bone marrow. (Hematoxylin and eosin stain)

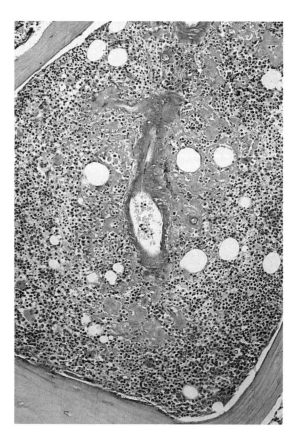

Figure 402
AMYLOIDOSIS
A trephine biopsy section from a patient with amyloidosis. The wall of the blood vessel in the center of the field is thickened by amyloid. There is heavy perivascular amyloid deposition. (Periodic acid–Schiff stain)

may be recognized in a thickened vessel. In cases with amyloid deposits outside a vessel wall, the distribution may be perivascular or have no association with vessels (figs. 401, 402). Occasionally, the entire bone marrow biopsy is replaced with amyloid.

Amyloid is found in many other tissues and organs including kidney, heart, liver, gastrointestinal tract, and peripheral nerves. Blood vessel walls and basement membranes are most commonly affected. Organ parenchyma may become massively replaced by amyloid deposits as the disease progresses.

Histochemical and Immunohistochemical Findings. Amyloid is moderately PAS positive (fig. 402), stains metachromatically with crystal violet and methyl violet, and is fluorescent when reacted with thioflavin T (100,104). The most useful cytochemical procedure in the diagnosis of amyloidosis is the Congo red stain,

which under polarized light produces a characteristic apple-green birefringence (fig. 403). AL and AA amyloid may be distinguished by preincubation of biopsy sections with potassium permanganate followed by Congo red staining; AL amyloid retains its apple-green birefringence but Congo red staining of AA is lost (100). The technique must be interpreted with care, however, because in some cases of primary amyloidosis Congo red staining is reduced after permanganate treatment (104).

The bone marrow plasma cells may show a monoclonal or polyclonal staining pattern with antikappa and antilambda light chain antibodies. The majority show a monoclonal pattern regardless of whether there is evidence of myeloma (100,112,113). Monoclonal lambda staining is most common.

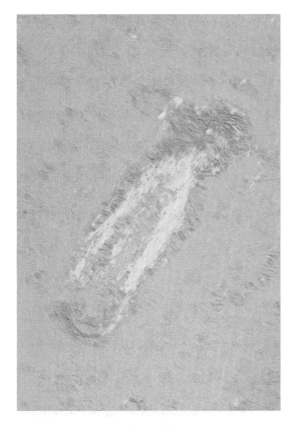

Figure 403
AMYLOIDOSIS

A Congo red stain on a bone marrow section from a patient with amyloidosis shows the typical apple-green birefringence in the vessel wall under polarized light. (Congo red stain)

Immunohistochemical techniques using anti-amyloid fibril antibodies to AL kappa and lambda are useful in characterizing AL amyloid and in distinguishing primary and secondary amyloidosis (100,104,108).

Ultrastructural Findings. The electron microscopic findings are specific and confirm the diagnosis. The ultrastructure of amyloid protein consists of rigid, linear, nonbranching, aggregated fibrils. The fibrils vary from 7 to 10 nm in width, have hollow cores, and are of indeterminate length (100,102,104). There appears to be no consistent ultrastructural differences between primary and secondary amyloidosis (98,104).

Cytogenetic Findings. The cytogenetic rearrangements reported in primary amyloidosis are similar to those in plasma cell myeloma. Abnormalities of chromosomes 1 and 14q+ are the most common (99).

Differential Diagnosis. The differential diagnosis of amyloidosis in the bone marrow is quite limited. The coexistence of myeloma with amyloidosis is determined by the overall clinical picture, including the serum immunoglobulin studies, radiographic findings, and the percentage of plasma cells in the bone marrow.

Amyloid in vessel walls is unlikely to be confused with any other process in the bone marrow and can usually be confirmed by the Congo red stain. In cases with extensive extra-vessel deposits of amyloid, the histopathology may resemble serous atrophy of fat. The Congo red stain, clinical history, and laboratory findings should readily distinguish these two processes.

Treatment and Prognosis. Treatment of primary amyloidosis is aimed at controlling amyloid production and deposition in tissues. Alkylating agents, primarily melphalan, combined with steroids, is the standard chemotherapy regimen. Response rates have been generally disappointing. Improvement in clinical status is achieved in some patients but there is minimal impact on survival. Colchicine is used to inhibit amyloid deposition. It has been effective in cases of amyloidosis in patients with familial Mediterranean fever and appears to extend survival in primary amyloidosis as well (97). Supportive and symptomatic treatment for congestive heart failure, renal failure, and other manifestations related to amyloid deposition are important aspects of therapy (104,106).

The median survival period is approximately 12 months from diagnosis. Shorter survival is usual for patients who present with congestive heart failure (about 4 months). For patients whose only presenting clinical manifestation is peripheral neuropathy, the median survival time is approximately 50 months (106). Patients with myeloma and amyloidosis have a shorter survival period than those without myeloma (104). Parameters that have been associated with poor prognosis are elevated urine creatinine, hepatomegaly, major weight loss, and excretion of lambda light chains in the urine (versus kappa light chains or no monoclonal protein) (101,106). The single most frequent cause of death is cardiac disease (about 40 percent) (106). Other less common causes of death include renal failure, infection, hemorrhage, intestinal obstruction, liver failure, and respiratory failure.

REFERENCES

Plasma Cell Myeloma (Multiple Myeloma)

1. Anderson KC, Park EK, Bates MP, et al. Antigens on human plasma cells identified by monoclonal antibodies. J Immunol 1983;130:1132–8.

2. Bardwick PA, Zvaifler NJ, Gill GN, et al. Plasma cell dyscrasia with polyneuropathy, organomegaly, endocrinopathy, M protein and skin changes: the POEMS syndrome. Report on two cases and review of the literature. Medicine (Baltimore) 1980;59:311–22.

3. Barlogie B. Toward a cure for multiple myeloma? [Editorial] N Engl J Med 1991;325:1304–6.

4. _____, Epstein J, Selvanayagam P, Alexanian R. Plasma cell myeloma—new biological insights and advances in therapy. Blood 1989;73:865–79.

5. Bartl R, Frisch B, Fateh-Moghadam A, Kettner G, Jaeger K, Sommerfeld W. Histologic classification and staging of multiple myeloma. A retrospective and prospective study of 674 cases. Am J Clin Pathol 1987; 87:342–55.

6. Bataille R. Localized plasmacytomas. Clin Haematol 1982;11:113–22.

7. Bennett JM, Catovsky D, Daniel MT, et al. Proposals for the classification of chronic (mature) B and T lymphoid leukemias. French-American-British (FAB) Cooperative Group. J Clin Pathol 1989;42:567–84.

8. Bernier GM, Graham RC Jr. Plasma cell asynchrony in myeloma: correlation of light and electron microscopy. Semin Hematol 1976;13:239–45.

9. Brunning RD, Parkin J. Intranuclear inclusions in plasma cells and lymphocytes from patients with monoclonal gammopathies. Am J Clin Pathol 1976;66:10–21.

10. _____, Parkin J, Hanson CA. Hematopoietic and lymphoreticular neoplasms. In: Azar HA, ed. Pathology of human neoplasms: an atlas of diagnostic and electron microscopy and immunohistochemistry. New York: Raven Press, 1988:221–303.

11. Carter A, Hocherman I, Linn S, Cohen Y, Tatarsky I. Prognostic significance of plasma cell morphology in multiple myeloma. Cancer 1987;60:1060–5.

12. Chen KC, Bevan PC, Matthews JG. Analysis of G banded karyotypes in myeloma cells. J Clin Pathol 1986;39:260–6.

13. Dehou MF, Schots R, Lacor P, et al. Diagnostic and prognostic value of the MB2 monoclonal antibody in paraffin-embedded bone marrow sections of patients with multiple myeloma and monoclonal gammopathy of undetermined significance. Am J Clin Pathol 1990;94:287–91.

14. Dewald GW, Kyle RA, Hicks GA, Greipp PR. The clinical significance of cytogenetic studies in 100 patients with multiple myeloma, plasma cell leukemia or amyloidosis. Blood 1985;66:380–90.

15. Dick FR. Plasma cell myeloma and related disorders with monoclonal gammopathy. In: Koepke JA, ed. Laboratory hematology. New York: Churchill-Livingstone, 1984:445–81.

16. Dimopoulos MA, Moulopoulos A, Delasalle K, Alexanian R. Solitary plasmacytoma of bone and asymptomatic multiple myeloma. Hematol Oncol Clin North Am 1992;6:359–69.

17. Durie BG. Staging and kinetics of multiple myeloma. Semin Oncol 1986;13:300–9.

18. _____, Grogan TM. CALLA-positive myeloma: an aggressive subtype with poor survival. Blood 1985; 66:229–32.

19. _____, Salmon SE. A clinical staging system for multiple myeloma. Correlations of measured myeloma cell mass with presenting clinical features, response to treatment, and survival. Cancer 1975;36:842–54.

20. _____, Salmon SE. The current status and future prospects of treatment for multiple myeloma. Clin Haematol 1982;11:181–210.

21. _____, Salmon SE. Multiple myeloma, macroglobulinemia and monoclonal gammopathies. In: Hoffbrand AV, Brain MC, Hirsh J, eds. Recent advances in haematology. New York: Churchill Livingstone, 1977.

22. Epstein J, Xiao HQ, He XY. Markers of multiple hematopoietic-cell lineages in multiple myeloma. N Engl J Med 1990;322:664–8.

23. Fitchen JH, Lee S. Phagocytic myeloma cells. Am J Clin Pathol 1979;71:722–3.

24. Gabriel L, Escribano L, Perales J, Bellas C, Odriozola J, Navarro JL. Multiple myeloma with crystalline inclusions in most hemopoietic cells. Am J Hematol 1985; 18:405–11.

25. Gahrton G, Tura S, Ljungman P, et al. Allogeneic bone marrow transplantation in multiple myeloma. European Group for Bone Marrow Transplantation. N Engl J Med 1991;325:1267–73.

26. Gould J, Alexanian R, Goodacre A, Pathak S, Hecht B, Barlogie B. Plasma cell karyotype in multiple myeloma. Blood 1988;71:453–6.

27. Greipp PR, Katzmann JA, O'Fallon WM, Kyle RA. Value of beta 2-microglobulin level and plasma cell labeling indices as prognostic factors in patients with newly diagnosed myeloma. Blood 1988;72:219–23.

28. _____, Kyle RA. Clinical, morphological and cell kinetic differences among multiple myeloma, monoclonal gammopathy of undetermined significance, and smoldering multiple myeloma. Blood 1983;62:166–71.

29. _____, Raymond NM, Kyle RA, O'Fallon WM. Multiple myeloma: significance of plasmablastic subtype in morphological classification. Blood 1985; 65:305–10.

30. _____, Witzig TE, Gonchoroff NJ, et al. Immunofluorescence labeling indices in myeloma and related monoclonal gammopathies. Mayo Clin Proc 1987; 62:969–77.

31. Harris NL, Bhan AK. B-cell neoplasms of the lymphocytic, lymphoplasmacytoid, and plasma cell types: immunohistologic analysis and clinical correlation. Hum Pathol 1985;16:829–37.

32. Hegewisch S, Mainzer K, Braumann P. IgE myelomatosis. Presentation of a new case and summary of literature. Blut 1987;55:55–60.

33. Jagannath S, Barlogie B, Dicke K, et al. Autologous bone marrow transplantation in multiple myeloma: identification of prognostic factors. Blood 1990;76:1860–6.

34. Kosmo MA, Gale RP. Plasma cell leukemia. Semin Hematol 1987;24:202–8.

35. Krzyzaniak RL, Buss DH, Cooper MR, Wells HB. Marrow fibrosis and multiple myeloma. Am J Clin Pathol 1988;89:63–8.

36. Kyle RA. "Benign" monoclonal gammopathy—after 20 to 35 years of follow-up. Mayo Clin Proc 1993;68:26–36.

37. _____. "Benign" monoclonal gammopathy. A misnomer? JAMA 1984;251:1849–54.
38. _____. Diagnostic criteria of multiple myeloma. Hematol Oncol Clin North Am 1992;6:347–58.
39. _____. Monoclonal gammopathy of undetermined significance (MGUS). A review. Clin Haematol 1982;11:123–50.
40. _____. Multiple myeloma: review of 869 cases. Mayo Clin Proc 1975;50:29–40.
41. _____. Newer approaches to the therapy of multiple myeloma [Editorial]. Blood 1990;76:1678–9.
42. _____, Greipp PR. Multiple myeloma and other plasma cell disorders. In: Conn RB, ed. Current diagnosis 8. Philadelphia: WB Saunders, 1991:593–7.
43. _____, Greipp PR. Smoldering multiple myeloma. N Eng J Med 1980;302:1347–9.
44. Lisse IM, Drivsholm A, Christoffersen P. Occurrence and type of chromosome abnormalities in consecutive malignant monoclonal gammopathies: correlation with survival. Cancer Genet Cytogenet 1988;35:27–36.
45. Maldonado JE, Brown AL Jr, Bayrd ED, Pease GL. Ultrastructure of the myeloma cell. Cancer 1966;19: 1613–27.
46. _____, Velosa JA, Kyle RA, Wagoner RD, Holley KE, Salassa RM. Fanconi syndrome in adults. A manifestation of latent form of myeloma. Am J Med 1975; 58:354–64.
47. Mandelli F, Avvisati G, Amadori S, et al. Maintenance treatment with recombinant interferon alpha-2b in patients with multiple myeloma responding to conventional induction chemotherapy. N Engl J Med 1990;322:1430–4.
48. Miralles GD, O'Fallon JR, Talley NJ. Plasma-cell dyscrasia with polyneuropathy. The spectrum of POEMS syndrome. N Engl J Med 1992;327:1919–23.
49. Noel P, Kyle RA. Plasma cell leukemia: an evaluation of response to therapy. Am J Med 1987;83:1062–8.
50. Parreira A, Robinson DS, Melo JV, et al. Primary plasma cell leukemia: immunological and ultrastructural studies in 6 cases. Scand J Haematol 1985;35:570–8.
51. Peterson LC, Brown BA, Crosson JT, Mladenovic J. Application of the immunoperoxidase technic to bone marrow trephine biopsies in the classification of patients with monoclonal gammopathies. Am J Clin Pathol 1986;85:688–93.
52. Pilarski LM, Jensen GS. Monoclonal circulating B cells in multiple myeloma. A continuously differentiating, possibly invasive, population as defined by expression of CD45 isoforms and adhesion molecules. Hematol Oncol Clin North Am 1992;6:297–322.
53. Reed M, McKenna RW, Bridges R, Parkin J, Frizzera G, Brunning RD. Morphologic manifestations of monoclonal gammopathies. Am J Clin Pathol 1981;76:8–23.
54. Ries LA, Hankey BF, Miller BA, Hartman AM, Edwards BK. Cancer statistics review 1973–88. National Cancer Institute. NIH Pub. No. 91–2789, 1991.
55. Terstappen LW, Johnsen S, Segers-Nolten IM, Loken MR. Identification and characterization of plasma cells in normal human bone marrow by high-resolution flow cytometry. Blood 1990;76:1739–47.
56. Tienhaara A, Pelliniemi TT. Flow cytometric DNA analysis and clinical correlations in multiple myeloma. Am J Clin Pathol 1992;97:322–30.
57. Ueshima Y, Fukuhara S, Nagai K, Takatsuki K, Uchino H. Cytogenetic studies and clinical aspects of patients with plasma cell leukemia and leukemic macroglobulinemia. Cancer Res 1983;43:905–12.
58. Wiltshaw E. The natural history of extramedullary plasmacytoma and its relation to solitary myeloma of bone and myelomatosis. Medicine (Baltimore) 1976;55:217–38.
59. Wolf BC, Brady K, O'Murchadha MT, Neiman RS. An evaluation of immunohistologic stains for immunoglobulin light chains in bone marrow biopsies in benign and malignant plasma cell proliferations. Am J Clin Pathol 1990;94:742–6.
60. Woodruff RK, Malpas JS, Paxton AM, Lister TA. Plasma cell leukemia (PCL): a report on 15 patients. Blood 1978;52:839–45.
61. Zukerberg LR, Ferry JA, Conlon M, Harris NL. Plasma cell myeloma with cleaved, multilobated and monocytoid nuclei. Am J Clin Pathol 1990;93:657–61.

Monoclonal Gammopathy of Undetermined Significance

62. Boccadoro M, Durie BG, Frutiger Y, et al. Lack of correlation between plasma cell thymidine labeling index and serum beta-2-microglobulin in monoclonal gammopathies. Acta Haematol 1987;78:239–42.
63. Dehou MF, Schots R, Lacor P, et al. Diagnostic and prognostic value of the MB2 monoclonal antibody in paraffin-embedded bone marrow sections of patients with multiple myeloma and monoclonal gammopathy of undetermined significance. Am J Clin Pathol 1990;94:287–91.
64. Kyle RA. "Benign" monoclonal gammopathy—after 20 to 35 years of follow-up. Mayo Clin Proc 1993;68:26–36.
65. _____. "Benign" monoclonal gammopathy. A misnomer? JAMA 1984;251:1849–54.
66. Mitus AJ, Stein R, Rappeport JM, et al. Monoclonal and oligoclonal gammopathy after bone marrow transplantation. Blood 1989;74:2764–8.
67. O'Connor ML, Rice DT, Buss DH, Muss HB. Immunoglobulin D benign monoclonal gammopathy. A case report. Cancer 1991;68:611–6.
68. Papadopoulos NM, Elin RJ, Wilson DM. Incidence of gamma-globulin banding in a healthy population by high-resolution electrophoresis. Clin Chem 1982;28:707–8.
69. Peterson LC, Brown BA, Crosson JT, Mladenovic J. Application of the immunoperoxidase technic to bone marrow trephine biopsies in the classification of patients with monoclonal gammopathies. Am J Clin Pathol 1986;85:688–93.
70. Reed M, McKenna RW, Bridges R, Parkin J, Frizzera G, Brunning RD. Morphologic manifestations of monoclonal gammopathies. Am J Clin Pathol 1981;76:8–23.
71. Singh J, Dudley AW Jr, Kulig KA. Increased incidence of monoclonal gammopathy of undetermined significance in blacks and its age-related differences with whites on the basis of a study of 397 men and one woman in a hospital setting. J Lab Clin Med 1990;116:785–9.
72. Tienhaara A, Pelliniemi TT. Flow cytometric DNA analysis and clinical correlations in multiple myeloma. Am J Clin Pathol 1992;97:322–30.

Waldenström Macroglobulinemia (Lymphoplasmacytoid Lymphoma)

73. Bennett JM, Catovsky D, Daniel MT, et al. Proposals for the classification of chronic (mature) B and T lymphoid leukemias. French-American-British (FAB) Cooperative Group. J Clin Pathol 1989;42:567–84.

74. Brunning RD, Parkin J. Intranuclear inclusions in plasma cells and lymphocytes from patients with monoclonal gammopathies. Am J Clin Pathol 1976;66:10–21.

75. _____, Parkin J, Hanson CA. Hematopoietic and lymphoreticular neoplasms. In: Azar HA, ed. Pathology of human neoplasms: an atlas of diagnostic electron microscopy and immunohistochemistry. New York: Raven Press, 1988:221–303.

76. Dick FR. Plasma cell myeloma and related disorders with monoclonal gammopathy. In: Koepke JA, ed. Laboratory hematology. New York: Churchill-Livingstone, 1984:445–81.

77. Feiner HD, Rizk CC, Finfer MD, et al. IgM monoclonal gammopathy/Waldenström's macroglobulinemia: a morphological and immunophenotypic study of the bone marrow. Mod Pathol 1990;3:348–56.

78. Han T, Sadamori N, Takeuchi J, et al. Clonal chromosome abnormalities in patients with Waldenström's and CLL-associated macroglobulinemia: significance of trisomy 12. Blood 1983;62:525–31.

79. Harris NL, Bhan AK. B-cell neoplasms of the lymphocytic, lymphoplasmacytoid, and plasma cell types: immunohistologic analysis and clinical correlation. Hum Pathol 1985;16:829–37.

80. Kyle RA, Garton JP. The spectrum of IgM monoclonal gammopathy in 430 cases. Mayo Clin Proc 1987; 62:719–31.

81. Nishida K, Taniwaki M, Misawa S, Abe T. Nonrandom rearrangement of chromosome 14 at band q32.33 in human lymphoid malignancies with mature B-cell phenotype. Cancer Res 1989;49:1275–81.

82. Noel P, Kyle RA. Monoclonal proteins in chronic lymphocytic leukemia. Am J Clin Pathol 1987;87:385–8.

83. Palka G, Spadana A, Geraci L, et al. Chromosome changes in 19 patients with Waldenström's macroglobulinemia. Cancer Genet Cytogenet 1987;29:261–9.

84. Pangalis GA, Nathwani BN, Rappaport H. Malignant lymphoma, well differentiated lymphocytic: its relationship with chronic lymphocytic leukemia and macroglobulinemia of Waldenström. Cancer 1977;39:999–1010.

85. Peterson LC, Brown BA, Crosson JT, Mladenovic J. Application of the immunoperoxidase technic to bone marrow trephine biopsies in the classification of patients with monoclonal gammopathies. Am J Clin Pathol 1986;85:688–93.

86. Pilarski LM, Andrews EJ, Serra HM, Ledbetter JA, Ruether BA, Mant MJ. Abnormalities in lymphocyte profile and specificity repertoire of patients with Waldenström's macroglobulinemia, multiple myeloma, and IgM monoclonal gammopathy of undetermined significance. Am J Hematol 1989;30:53–60.

87. Reed M, McKenna RW, Bridges R, Parkin J, Frizzera G, Brunning JD. Morphologic manifestations of monoclonal gammopathies. Am J Clin Pathol 1981;76:8–23.

88. Tursz T, Brouet JC, Flandrin G, Danon F, Clauvel JP, Seligmann M. Clinical and pathologic features of Waldenström's macroglobulinemia in seven patients with serum monoclonal IgG or IgA. Am J Med 1977; 63:499–502.

Heavy Chain Diseases

89. Brouet JC, Seligmann M, Danon F, Belpomme D, Fine JM. Mu-chain disease. Report of two new cases. Arch Intern Med 1979;139:672–4.

90. Fermand JP, Brouet JC, Danon F, Seligmann M. Gamma heavy chain "disease": heterogeneity of the clinicopathologic features. Report of 16 cases and review of the literature. Medicine (Baltimore) 1989;68:321–35.

91. Franklin EC. Mu-chain disease. Arch Intern Med 1975;135:71–2.

92. Galian A, Lecestre MJ, Scotto J, Bognel C, Matuchansky C, Rambaud JC. Pathological study of alpha-chain disease, with special emphasis on evolution. Cancer 1977;39:2081–101.

93. Kyle RA, Greipp PR, Banks PM. The diverse picture of gamma heavy-chain disease. Report of seven cases and review of literature. Mayo Clin Proc 1981;56:439–51.

94. Price SK. Immunoproliferative small intestinal disease: a study of 13 cases with alpha heavy-chain disease. Histopathology 1990;17:7–17.

95. Seligmann M, Mihaesco E, Preud'homme JL, Danon F, Brouet JC. Heavy chain diseases: current findings and concepts. Immunol Rev 1979;48:145–67.

Primary Amyloidosis

96. Buxbaum J. Mechanisms of disease: monoclonal immunoglobulin deposition. Amyloidosis, light chain deposition disease, and light and heavy chain deposition disease. Hematol Oncol Clin North Am 1992;6:323–46.

97. Cohen AS, Rubinow A, Anderson JJ, et al. Survival of patients with primary (AL) amyloidosis. Colchicine-treated cases from 1976 to 1983 compared with cases seen in previous years (1961–1973). Am J Med 1987;82:1182–90.

98. _____, Shirahama T. Electron microscopic analysis of isolated amyloid fibrils from patients with primary, secondary and myeloma-associated disease. A study utilizing shadowing and negative staining techniques. Isr J Med Sci 1973;9:849–56.

99. Durie BG. Cellular and molecular genetic features of myeloma and related disorders. Hematol Oncol Clin North Am 1992;6:463–77.

100. Feiner HD. Pathology of dysproteinemia: light chain amyloidosis, non-amyloid immunoglobulin deposition disease, cryoglobulinemia syndromes and macroglobulinemia of Waldenström. Hum Pathol 1988;19:1255–72.

101. Gertz MA, Kyle RA. Prognostic value of urinary protein in primary systemic amyloidosis (AL). Am J Clin Pathol 1990;94:313–7.

102. Glenner GG. Amyloid deposits and amyloidosis. The beta-fibrilloses (first of two parts). N Engl J Med 1980;302:1283–92.

103. Hawkins PN, Lavender JP, Pepys MB. Evaluation of systemic amyloidosis by scintigraphy with 123I-labeled serum amyloid P component. N Engl J Med 1990;323:508–13

104. Kyle RA, Greipp PR. Amyloidosis (AL). Clinical and laboratory features in 229 cases. Mayo Clin Proc 1983; 58:665–83.

105. _____, Greipp PR. Multiple myeloma and other plasma cell disorders. In: Conn R, ed. Current diagnosis 8. Philadelphia: WB Saunders, 1991:593–7.

106. _____, Greipp PR, O'Fallon WM. Primary systemic amyloidosis: multivariate analysis for prognostic factors in 168 cases. Blood 1986;68:220–4.

107. _____, Linos A, Beard CM, et al. Incidence and natural history of primary systemic amyloidosis in Olmsted County, Minnesota, 1950 through 1989. Blood 1992;79:1817–22.

108. Linke RP, Nathrath WB, Eulitz M. Classification of amyloid syndromes from tissue sections using antibodies against various amyloid fibril proteins: report of 142 cases. In: Glenner GG, Osserman EF, Benditt EP, Calkins E, Cohen AS, Zucker-Franklin D, eds. Amyloidosis. New York: Plenum Press, 1986:599.

109. Orfila C, Giraud P, Modesto A, Suc JM. Abdominal fat tissue aspirate in human amyloidosis: light, electron, and immunofluorescence microscopic studies. Hum Pathol 1986;17:366–9.

110. Pellikka PA, Holmes DR Jr, Edwards WD, Nishimura RA, Tajik AJ, Kyle RA. Endomyocardial biopsy in 30 patients with primary amyloidosis and suspected cardiac involvement. Arch Intern Med 1988;148:662–6.

111. Reed M, McKenna RW, Bridges R, Parkin J, Frizzera G, Brunning RD. Morphologic manifestations of monoclonal gammopathies. Am J Clin Pathol 1981;76:8–23.

112. Wolf BC, Kumar A, Vera JC, Neiman RS. Bone marrow morphology and immunology in systemic amyloidosis. Am J Clin Pathol 1986;86:84–8.

113. Wu SS, Brady K, Anderson JJ, et al. The predictive value of bone marrow morphologic characteristics and immunostaining in primary (AL) amyloidosis. Am J Clin Pathol 1991;96:95–9.

BONE MARROW LYMPHOMAS

The lymphomas are a heterogeneous group of neoplastic lymphoproliferative disorders arising primarily in lymph nodes and less commonly in lymphatic tissues in other organs. The lymphocytes in most lymphomas express immunophenotypic characteristics of intermediate to mature stages of B-cell or T-cell development. The lymphomas generally involve the bone marrow as a secondary process but occasional examples of primary bone marrow lymphoma are reported.

This discussion will focus specifically on the manifestations of lymphomas in the bone marrow. The details of morphologic and immunologic classification and methods of diagnosis as they apply to lymph nodes and other tissues are found in the upcoming Fascicle, Tumors of the Lymph Nodes and Spleen.

HODGKIN DISEASE

Incidence and Clinical Findings. The incidence of Hodgkin disease in the United States in 1988 was 2.8 cases per 100,000 population. There was a slight decrease in incidence between 1973 and 1988. The incidence is higher for males than females and for whites than blacks. Approximately 7,400 cases were diagnosed in 1991 (23). Hodgkin disease is rare in children less than 10 years of age. The incidence increases in the early teens and peaks between ages 20 and 30. It then declines until the late forties, then gradually increases again. In young children, the disease is more common in males than females; in the late teens and early twenties, it is more common in females; and in later years, it is more common in males (23).

Bone marrow involvement is present at the time of diagnosis in approximately 10 to 15 percent of cases (2,18,20,24). Bone marrow disease is most common in males who have constitutional symptoms and are older than average for Hodgkin disease; median age is 45 to 50 years (2,11,18,20). Patients generally present in an advanced clinical stage. Symptoms include weight loss, fever, and night sweats. Organomegaly and lymphadenopathy may be present. Occasionally, patients present with infectious manifestations secondary to altered immune function.

Laboratory Findings. There are no laboratory findings that are unique for Hodgkin disease. The most frequent changes at diagnosis are alteration in blood counts, described below. In advanced disease, biochemical abnormalities similar to those encountered in other types of disseminated neoplasms may occur.

Classification. The most widely used classification of Hodgkin disease in the United States and the one used in this Fascicle is the Rye Modification of the Lukes-Butler Classification (14). This classification and the original proposal of Lukes and Butler are shown in Table 32 (13,14). The Rye Classification system identifies distinct clinical and prognostic groups. Its clinical relevance remains but the therapy response rate and survival differences between categories is considerably less with present day treatment protocols.

Blood and Bone Marrow Findings. Blood counts may be normal or decreased. Neutropenia, thrombocytopenia, and pancytopenia are highly indicative of bone marrow involvement in newly diagnosed patients (7,20). Leukemoid and exudative reactions are sometimes observed and have been associated with a poor prognosis. Lymphocytopenia is also an indicator of poor prognosis in patients with advanced stage disease (2,25). Neutrophilia, eosinophilia, thrombocytosis, and anemia are relatively common findings in Hodgkin

Table 32

HISTOPATHOLOGIC CLASSIFICATIONS OF HODGKIN DISEASE

Lukes-Butler*	Rye Modification**
Lymphocytic-histiocytic Nodular Diffuse	Lymphocyte predominance
Nodular sclerosis	Nodular sclerosis
Mixed cellularity	Mixed cellularity
Diffuse fibrosis	Lymphocyte depletion
Reticular	Lymphocyte depletion

* From reference 13.
** From reference 14.

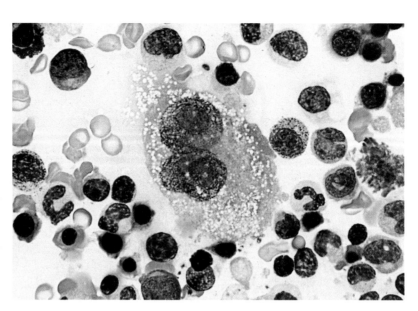

Figure 404
REED-STERNBERG CELL IN
BONE MARROW ASPIRATE
A R-S cell in a bone marrow aspirate smear from a man with advanced Hodgkin disease. R-S cells are rarely encountered in aspirate smears. Reticulin fibrosis in Hodgkin lesions generally prevents their aspiration. (Wright-Giemsa stain) (Fig. 37.7 (right) from McKenna RW. The bone marrow manifestations of Hodgkin's disease, the non-Hodgkin's lymphomas, and lymphoma-like disorders. In: Knowles DM, ed. Neoplastic hematopathology. Baltimore: Williams & Wilkins, 1992:1135–80.)

disease and are not reliable indicators of bone marrow involvement or prognosis (18,24). Reed-Sternberg cells are not found on blood smears.

Involvement of the bone marrow by Hodgkin disease may result from disseminated disease or direct extension from contiguously involved lymph nodes. Most commonly, bone marrow involvement is a manifestation of disseminated disease and is detected in random iliac crest trephine biopsies. Direct extension to the marrow from the lymph nodes in otherwise localized Hodgkin disease is rare but has been observed in cases with large periaortic lymph node masses extending into the vertebral column. Lesions of this type are usually recognized radiographically (17).

Bone marrow examination is commonly used to define the extent of disease during initial staging, to assess response to chemotherapy, and to follow previously treated patients for recurrence. In some instances the primary diagnosis is made from a bone marrow biopsy.

Hodgkin disease is rarely found in aspiration smears because the fibrosis that is invariably associated with the lesions prevents adequate aspiration (figs. 404, 405). When marrow disease is extensive, attempts at aspiration may yield a "dry tap." The trephine biopsy is the best procedure for identifying Hodgkin tissue in the marrow. Bilateral posterior iliac crest biopsies provide more tissue for examination than a single biopsy and increase the yield of demonstrable disease (fig. 406) (3).

Histopathologic Findings. Histopathologic criteria for diagnosing bone marrow involvement in patients with proven Hodgkin disease on a lymph node biopsy were recommended by the Committee on Histopathological Criteria Contributing to Staging of Hodgkin Disease at the Ann Arbor Symposium in 1971 (22). A summary of the committee's recommendations is shown below.

1. Hodgkin disease may be diagnosed when typical Reed-Sternberg cells (R-S cells) or their mononuclear variants are found in the bone marrow in one of the characteristic cellular environments of Hodgkin disease.
2. The presence of atypical histiocytes that lack the nuclear features of R-S cells in one of the characteristic polycellular environments of Hodgkin disease or in focal or diffuse areas of fibrosis, is strongly suggestive of bone marrow involvement.
3. Fibrosis or necrosis alone should be considered suspicious for Hodgkin disease in a previously diagnosed patient.

In the majority of cases, R-S cells can be identified in bone marrow lesions when adequate biopsy material is available for study (fig. 407) (20). These cells are found in a stromal reaction characteristic of Hodgkin disease and not in areas of otherwise normal marrow. Rarely, normal hematopoietic cells and R-S cells may be intermixed at the edge of a lesion (fig. 408). The trephine biopsy should be repeated in cases with lesions suspicious for Hodgkin disease in which

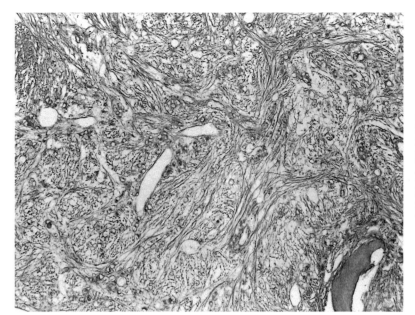

Figure 405
RETICULIN FIBROSIS
IN HODGKIN DISEASE

A reticulin stain on a trephine biopsy from a patient with diffuse bone marrow replacement by Hodgkin disease. Reticulin is markedly increased. (Wilder reticulin stain) (Fig. 37.7 (left) from McKenna RW. The bone marrow manifestations of Hodgkin's disease, the non-Hodgkin's lymphomas, and lymphoma-like disorders. In: Knowles DM, ed. Neoplastic hematopathology. Baltimore: Williams & Wilkins, 1992:1135–80.)

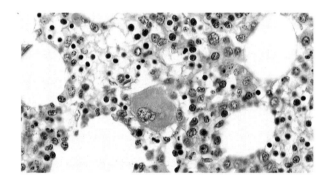

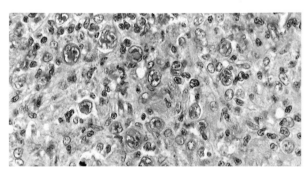

Figure 406
BILATERAL ILIAC CREST TREPHINE BIOPSIES
IN HODGKIN DISEASE

Bilateral posterior iliac crest trephine biopsies from a patient with mixed cellularity Hodgkin disease. The biopsy from the left iliac crest (top) was negative for Hodgkin disease and normocellular. The biopsy from the right iliac crest (bottom) was diffusely infiltrated with Hodgkin tissue. (Hematoxylin and eosin stain) (Fig. 37.1 from McKenna RW. The bone marrow manifestations of Hodgkin's disease, the non-Hodgkin's lymphomas, and lymphoma-like disorders. In: Knowles DM, ed. Neoplastic hematopathology. Baltimore: Williams & Wilkins, 1992:1135–80.)

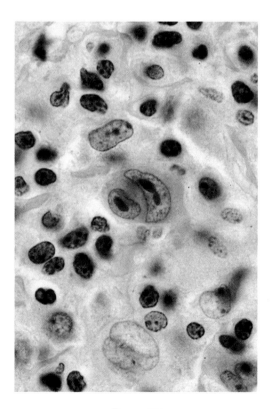

Figure 407
REED-STERNBERG CELL

A typical R-S cell in a trephine biopsy section from a 27-year-old female with Hodgkin disease. (Hematoxylin and eosin stain)

371

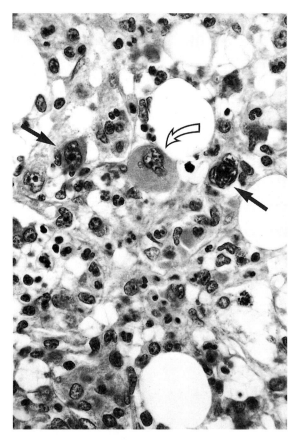

Figure 408
REED-STERNBERG CELLS
ADJACENT TO A MEGAKARYOCYTE

Two R-S cells (dark arrows) are illustrated adjacent to a megakaryocyte (clear arrow) on the edge of a focal bone marrow Hodgkin lesion. It is unusual to find R-S cells admixed with normal hematopoietic cells in bone marrow sections. (Hematoxylin and eosin stain)

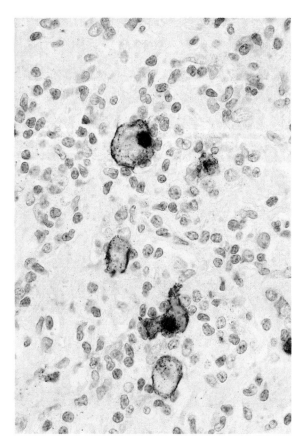

Figure 409
CD15 (LEU-M1) IMMUNOPEROXIDASE
REACTION IN REED-STERNBERG CELLS

A bone marrow biopsy from an 11-year-old boy with lymphocyte depletion Hodgkin disease. The differential diagnosis included anaplastic large cell lymphoma. A typical pattern of reactivity of R-S cells with an antibody to CD15 (Leu-M1) is illustrated. The reaction is at the cell membrane. There is often a block of perinuclear staining. The large neoplastic cells were negative for expression of T-cell or B-cell restricted antigens. (Immunoperoxidase, anti-CD15 stains)

typical R-S cells or variants are not identified in serial sections, unless there is other unequivocal evidence of pathologic stage IV disease.

In some cases the initial diagnosis is made from a bone marrow biopsy taken for evaluation of cytopenias, a fever of unknown origin, or organomegaly. A primary diagnosis in the bone marrow is most likely in lymphocyte depletion or mixed cellularity Hodgkin disease; rarely, the initial diagnosis of nodular sclerosis Hodgkin disease is made by a bone marrow biopsy. In these cases it is essential that typical R-S cells are identified and that other characteristic histologic features of Hodgkin disease are present. Enzyme immunohistochemical studies using a panel of an-

tibodies to antigens expressed by R-S cells, such as CD15 (Leu-M1) and CD30 (Ber-H2), and others expressed by B and T lymphocytes may aid in the diagnosis (fig. 409) (1,12,29).

Caution must be exercised when interpreting bone marrow lesions that resemble Hodgkin disease histologically but lack typical R-S cells. Some non-Hodgkin lymphomas, particularly peripheral T-cell lymphomas, and other bone marrow lesions such as granulomas, polymorphous reactive lymphoid infiltrates, myelofibrosis, systemic mastocytosis, angioimmunoblastic lymphadenopathy, and histiocytic proliferative disorders

Table 33

**FREQUENCY OF
BONE MARROW INVOLVEMENT
BY HISTOLOGIC CATEGORY
OF HODGKIN DISEASE**

Lymph Node Classification	Cases with Marrow Involvement at Diagnosis
Lymphocyte predominance	rare (< 5%)
Nodular sclerosis	5–10%
Mixed cellularity	20–25%
Lymphocyte depletion	50–75%
All types	10–15%

may mimic Hodgkin disease histologically (4,6,10). R-S–like cells have been described in some of these disorders (27).

The highest incidence of bone marrow involvement is found with lymphocyte depletion and mixed cellularity Hodgkin disease (Table 33) (19,20). Less than 10 percent of patients with nodular sclerosis Hodgkin disease have bone marrow involvement at diagnosis and only rare cases of lymphocyte predominance involve the bone marrow (20,24).

The extent of bone marrow involvement in trephine biopsy specimens varies from small lesions occupying less than one third of the marrow space to complete replacement. The pattern of infiltration may be diffuse or focal. Diffuse involvement is observed in 70 to 80 percent of cases. Diffuse lesions occupy entire areas between bone trabeculae and usually replace large contiguous portions of bone marrow. The cellular infiltrate in diffuse lesions may be uniformly distributed or localized between broad areas of sparsely cellular loose or dense connective tissue (figs. 410–412). Focal involvement is found in 20 to 30 percent of cases and is characterized by small isolated lesions that are completely encircled by normal marrow tissue or are paratrabecular in location; a polycellular infiltrate with a uniform mixture of cells throughout the lesion is most common (fig. 413) (20). Both diffuse and focal lesions may be found in the same biopsy.

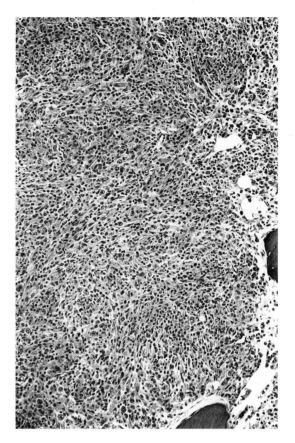

Figure 410
DIFFUSE BONE MARROW INVOLVEMENT
WITH HODGKIN DISEASE
A staging trephine biopsy section from a man with Hodgkin disease. The marrow is diffusely replaced with Hodgkin tissue. The lesion is composed of a pleomorphic cell population including several R-S cells and variants. (Hematoxylin and eosin stain)

Reticulin or collagen is always present in bone marrow lesions. Fibrosis is most prominent with extensive diffuse involvement (see fig. 405) (20).

All of the various histologic patterns of the infiltrate that are found in the lymph nodes may also be observed in bone marrow lesions. The infiltrate is often polycellular with large and small lymphocytes, benign histiocytes, plasma cells, eosinophils, neutrophils, and R-S cells or variants (figs. 414, 415). In some cases a relatively uniform cellular proliferation consisting of lymphocytes or histiocytes is observed (fig. 416). R-S cells and mononuclear variants are the predominant cell types in some cases (figs. 406, 417); in others serial sections are required to find a single example.

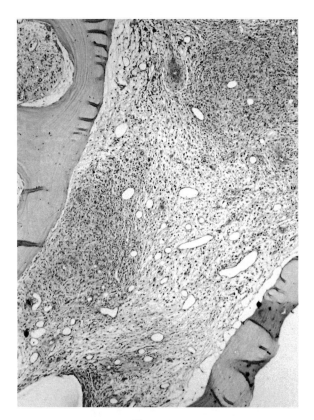

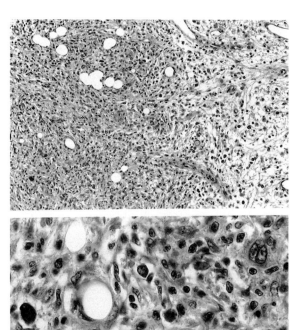

Figure 411
DIFFUSE BONE MARROW INVOLVEMENT
WITH HODGKIN DISEASE

A trephine biopsy from a man with stage IV Hodgkin disease shows diffuse marrow involvement. The lesion is composed of loose fibrous connective tissue and a polycellular infiltrate. Foci of increased cellularity are present; R-S cells are rare. (Hematoxylin and eosin stain)

Figure 412
BONE MARROW HODGKIN DISEASE

Higher magnification of the lesion shown in figure 411 shows a marked increase in vascularity and loose fibrous connective tissue. A polycellular infiltrate and occasional R-S cells are present. (Hematoxylin and eosin stain) (Top: Fig. 37.6 (right) from McKenna RW. The bone marrow manifestations of Hodgkin's disease, the non-Hodgkin's lymphomas, and lymphoma-like disorders. In: Knowles DM, ed. Neoplastic hematopathology. Baltimore: Williams & Wilkins, 1992:1135–80.)

Figure 413
FOCAL BONE MARROW
INVOLVEMENT WITH
HODGKIN DISEASE

This trephine biopsy section shows focal involvement with Hodgkin disease. The lesion is encircled by normal hematopoietic tissue. (Hematoxylin and eosin stain) (Fig. 13–69 (left) from McKenna RW. Bone marrow. In: Dehner LP, ed. Pediatric surgical pathology. 2nd ed. Baltimore: Williams & Wilkins, 1987:838–68.)

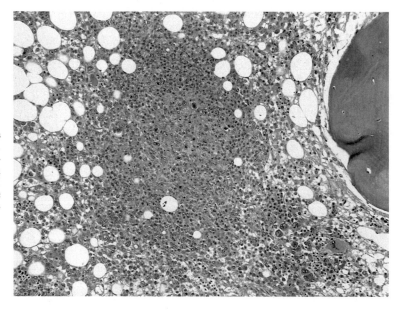

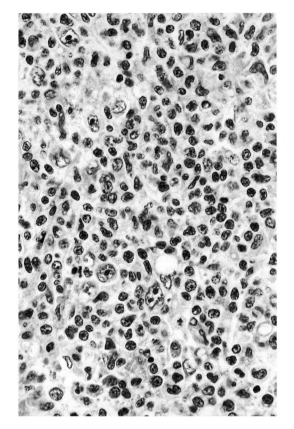

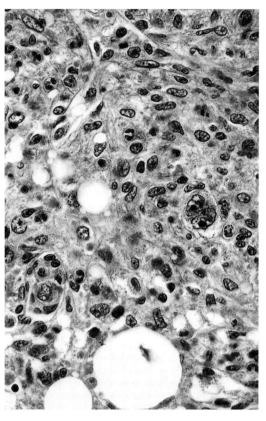

Figure 414
BONE MARROW HODGKIN DISEASE
A trephine biopsy section from a man with Hodgkin disease shows a heteromorphous population of lymphocytes, plasma cells, occasional histiocytes, and small vessels. Typical and mononuclear R-S cells are present. (Hematoxylin and eosin stain)

Figure 415
POLYCELLULAR BONE MARROW
INFILTRATE IN HODGKIN DISEASE
Bone marrow trephine biopsy from a patient with stage IV Hodgkin disease shows a polycellular infiltrate consisting of small and large lymphocytes, histiocytes, plasma cells, and typical and variant R-S cells. (Hematoxylin and eosin stain)

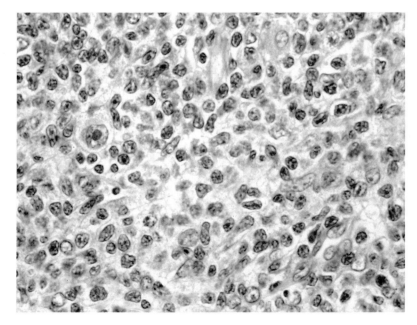

Figure 416
BONE MARROW
HODGKIN DISEASE
A Hodgkin lesion in a bone marrow section, consisting mostly of lymphocytes. There is a single mononuclear R-S cell variant. (Hematoxylin and eosin stain) (Fig. 37.4 from McKenna RW. The bone marrow manifestations of Hodgkin's disease, the non-Hodgkin's lymphomas, and lymphoma-like disorders. In: Knowles DM, ed. Neoplastic hematopathology. Baltimore: Williams & Wilkins, 1992:1135–80.)

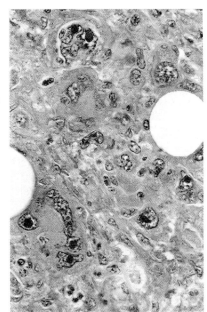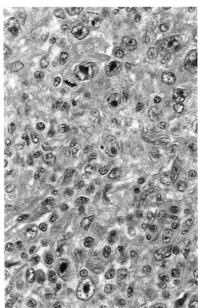

Figure 417
REED-STERNBERG CELLS
IN BONE MARROW

Left: This biopsy from a patient with stage IV Hodgkin disease shows numerous R-S cells and depletion of lymphocytes. (Hematoxylin and eosin stain) (Fig. 37.5 (right) from McKenna RW. The bone marrow manifestations of Hodgkin's disease, the non-Hodgkin's lymphomas, and lymphoma-like disorders. In: Knowles DM, ed. Neoplastic hematopathology. Baltimore: Williams & Wilkins, 1992:1135–80.)

Right: A high magnification of the focal bone marrow lesion illustrated in figure 413. There are numerous mononuclear R-S cell variants. (Hematoxylin and eosin stain)

It is inadvisable to attempt to classify Hodgkin disease with only a bone marrow biopsy. The small size of the marrow biopsy restricts evaluation of the histologic pattern; nodular sclerosis Hodgkin disease will often have the appearance of lymphocyte depletion. In addition, the histopathology may differ significantly in the lymph nodes and bone marrow from the same patient.

The areas of bone marrow adjacent to Hodgkin tissue often show nonspecific changes such as hypoplasia or granulocytic hyperplasia (19,20). Hypoplasia may be particularly prominent in lymphocyte depletion Hodgkin disease (19). Increased plasma cells, erythroid hyperplasia, and eosinophilic and granulocytic hyperplasia may be observed in Hodgkin disease patients without marrow involvement (28). These nonspecific changes are not related to pathologic stage of disease or other prognostic factors.

Post-Treatment Biopsies. The histopathology of post-treatment residual disease and relapse is generally similar to that of pretreatment lesions. Evolution to a more aggressive histopathology occurs in some cases. Posterior iliac crest trephine biopsies taken from patients who have received radiotherapy to the iliac lymph nodes are usually markedly hypocellular or aplastic in appearance. These changes persist even several years after therapy.

Necrosis of Hodgkin tissue is often observed in patients on chemotherapy (20). Usually only part of the Hodgkin tissue is necrotic; patches of amorphous eosinophilic material with karyorrhectic and karyolytic cells may be found (fig. 418). The pattern of the cellular infiltrate of the non-necrotic tissue is otherwise similar to pretreatment lesions. The myelofibrotic component of Hodgkin tissue is reversible with successful chemotherapy and often shows complete resolution (18). Occasionally, granulomas secondary to opportunistic infections such as cryptococcosis are observed separately or in association with Hodgkin lesions (fig. 419).

Immunohistochemical Findings. R-S cells typically express CD15 (Leu-M1), CD30 (Ki-1/Ber-H2), and CD74 (LN-2) by immunohistochemical techniques on bone marrow sections (see fig. 409) (5). These reactions, combined with the usual negative reactivity with antibodies to B-cell and T-cell antigens and lack of expression of CD45 (leukocyte common antigen) and epithelial membrane antigen, may be diagnostic of Hodgkin disease in histologically equivocal cases (5).

Ultrastructural Findings. Ultrastructural examination has no practical utility in diagnosis and classification of Hodgkin disease in the bone marrow.

Differential Diagnosis. Non-Hodgkin lymphomas may simulate Hodgkin disease in bone marrow sections. Peripheral T-cell lymphomas

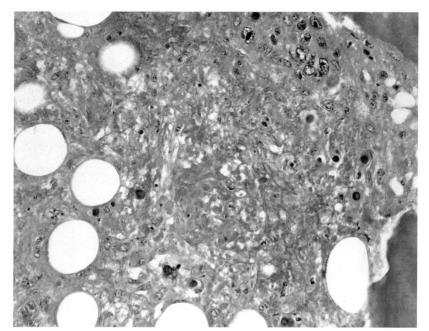

Figure 418
BONE MARROW NECROSIS
IN HODGKIN DISEASE

A postchemotherapy trephine biopsy from a patient with stage IV
Hodgkin disease shows residual
Hodgkin tissue and focal areas of
necrosis. (Hematoxylin and eosin
stain) (Fig. 11 from Brunning RD,
McKenna RW. Bone marrow manifestations of malignant lymphoma
and lymphoma-like conditions.
Pathol Annu 1979;14(Pt 1):1–59.)

Figure 419
INFECTIOUS GRANULOMA
(CRYPTOCOCCOSIS)
IN BONE MARROW

Left: A granuloma in a bone
marrow section from a patient
with treated Hodgkin disease.
There are several large histiocytes. Clear, round inclusions
are present in the cytoplasm of
some of the cells, suggesting en-
capsulated yeast forms. (Hematoxylin and eosin stain)

Right: A PAS reaction
stained the intracytoplasmic inclusions. Bone marrow cultures
grew *Cryptococcus neoformans*.
(Periodic acid–Schiff stain)

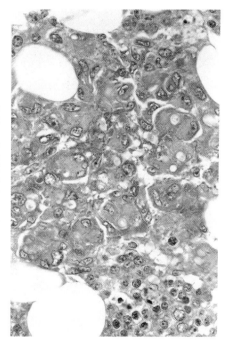

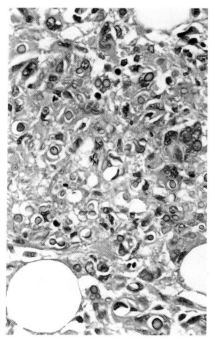

with a polymorphous cell proliferation and epithelioid histiocytes are particularly problematic
(10). Occasionally, the marrow lesions in follicular lymphomas manifest histologic features similar to Hodgkin disease, e.g., fibrosis, histiocyte-
like proliferation, pleomorphic cell population.
R-S–like cells have been observed in the bone

marrow of patients with peripheral T-cell and
follicular lymphomas (10,16). The cytology of the
lymphoma cells on marrow smears or trephine
imprints in non-Hodgkin lymphoma may help
distinguish the process from Hodgkin disease
(10,15,26). Immunohistochemical stains with a
panel of antibodies may clarify the diagnosis in

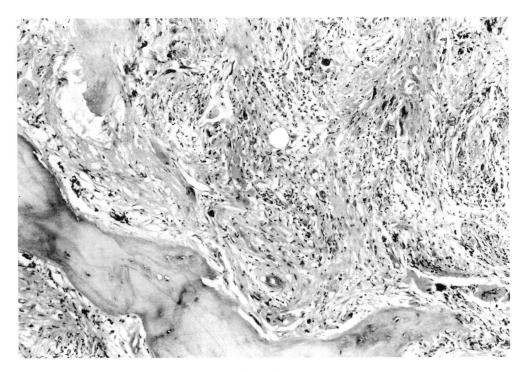

Figure 420
IDIOPATHIC MYELOFIBROSIS RESEMBLING HODGKIN DISEASE
A bone marrow section from a patient with idiopathic myelofibrosis shows distorted megakaryocytes which could be misinterpreted as R-S cells. (Hematoxylin and eosin stain)

problematic cases (see fig. 409) (1,12,29). In some instances lymph node or other tissue biopsies may be necessary.

Benign lymphocytic aggregates or tubercle-like granulomas are found in bone marrow sections in up to 12 percent of patients with negative-staging bone marrow biopsies (20). These can potentially be misinterpreted as Hodgkin tissue. Other disorders that may resemble the bone marrow lesions of Hodgkin disease include myelofibrosis, prolymphocytic transformation of chronic lymphocytic leukemia (Richter syndrome), angioimmunoblastic lymphadenopathy, eosinophilic granuloma, and systemic mast cell disease (fig. 420). The features that distinguish these lesions are discussed in other sections of this Fascicle.

Secondary myelodysplastic syndromes and acute myeloid leukemias may follow treatment for Hodgkin disease with alkylating agents or radiotherapy. In some cases these secondary processes are associated with myelofibrosis and reactive lymphocytic infiltrates (9). The changes in the marrow biopsies may resemble Hodgkin le-

sions. The absence of R-S cells and the presence of dysplastic changes or increased myeloblasts in blood smears, bone marrow smears, or trephine imprints should alert the pathologist to the correct diagnosis. The giant erythroblasts found in parvovirus B19 infection may infrequently cause a problem in diagnosis. These cells can be confused with R-S cells in bone marrow smears (fig. 421). They are distinguished by their distribution in the bone marrow and the absence of the usual stromal reaction found in Hodgkin disease (fig. 422).

Treatment and Prognosis. Limited (pathologic stages I and II) disease is generally treated with radiation therapy. Long-term disease-free survival can be achieved in approximately 85 percent of patients (8). In patients with localized massive disease or with limited disease below the diaphragm, combined modality radiation and chemotherapy is often used with good results. For most patients with advanced stage disease (stages III and IV), which includes patients with bone marrow involvement, chemotherapy or chemotherapy combined with radiation are the treatments

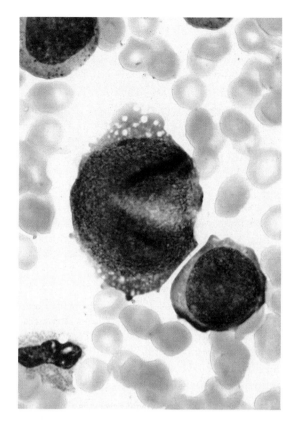

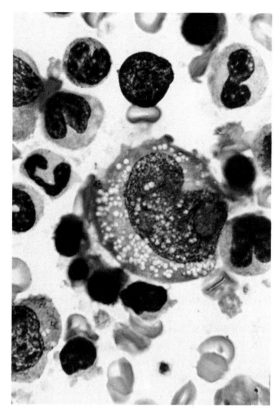

Figure 421
GIANT ERYTHROBLASTS AND A REED-STERNBERG CELL

Left: Giant erythroblasts in a bone marrow smear from a patient with parvovirus B19 infection. The larger of the two cells resembles a R-S cell. The diagnosis of Hodgkin disease was entertained in this patient who also had lymphadenopathy and giant erythroblasts in a lymph node biopsy section.

Right: The R-S cell in the bone marrow from a patient with mixed cellularity Hodgkin disease is similar to the giant erythroblast. (Wright-Giemsa stain)

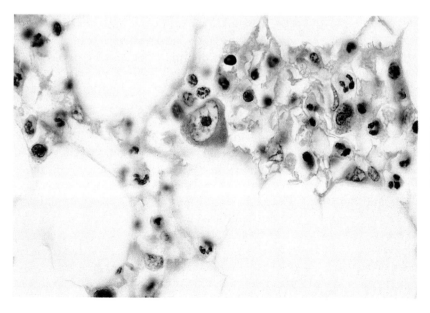

Figure 422
GIANT ERYTHROBLAST

A trephine biopsy section from a patient with a parvovirus B19 infection. The giant erythroblast resembles a mononuclear R-S cell but lacks the appropriate cellular environment of Hodgkin disease. (Hematoxylin and eosin stain)

of choice. Complete remission can be achieved in up to 80 percent of patients and long-term survival or cure in approximately 70 percent (8). The treatment regimens generally consist of nitrogen mustard, vincristine, procarbazine, and prednisone (MOPP); adriamycin, bleomycin, vinblastine, and dacarbazine (ABVD); or a protocol alternating the two. Autologous bone marrow and peripheral blood stem cell transplantation have been used in selected patients. Long-term remission has been achieved in 20 to 40 percent of cases (8).

Long-term complications of therapy are seen in some patients. These include secondary neoplasms, sterility, and other effects of tissue damage by radiation or chemotherapy.

NON-HODGKIN LYMPHOMAS

Incidence and Clinical Findings. Non-Hodgkin lymphomas are approximately five times as common as Hodgkin disease. The incidence in 1988 was 13.6 cases per 100,000 population, an increase of more than 50 percent since 1973. The incidence is nearly 50 percent higher for males than females and for whites than blacks. Approximately 37,000 new cases were diagnosed in the United States in 1991 (91). The overall incidence increases with age but varies for the different categories of non-Hodgkin lymphoma. The majority of lymphomas in children are lymphoblastic or small noncleaved cell, which decrease in frequency with age. Follicular lymphomas and small lymphocytic lymphomas are rare in young people but common in mid-life and increase with age. The overall incidence of bone marrow involvement is 30 to 53 percent and varies widely for the different categories of lymphoma (33,46,50,55,66,67,72,96).

The clinical manifestations in patients with bone marrow involvement with non-Hodgkin lymphoma are more variable than in Hodgkin disease. Many patients with low-grade lymphomas are completely asymptomatic whereas patients with intermediate- and high-grade lymphomas and bone marrow involvement more often have constitutional symptoms and may have blood cytopenias. Organomegaly and/or lymphadenopathy are usually observed.

Laboratory Findings. There are no specific laboratory findings. Similar to Hodgkin disease, the most frequent changes at diagnosis are alterations in blood counts. These are described below. Biochemical abnormalities generally indicate advanced disease and often reflect extranodal organ invasion.

Classification. The International Working Formulation Classification of non-Hodgkin lymphoma shown in Table 34 is used in this discussion (83).

Blood and Bone Marrow Findings. The blood counts may be normal or variable cytopenias may be seen. Autoimmune hemolytic anemia is occasionally present, usually with small lymphocytic lymphomas. Circulating lymphoma cells are found in blood smears in 10 to 25 percent of cases overall and in 40 to 50 percent of those with bone marrow involvement. Blood involvement is rare in cases without bone marrow disease (55,72); the degree of involvement is generally related to the extent of marrow disease (72). The incidence of circulating lymphoma cells is highest for the low-grade lymphomas, small lymphocytic and follicular small cleaved cell, but virtually every category may manifest blood involvement.

Usually, a small or moderate number of lymphoma cells are identified on scanning a blood smear, but the total leukocyte count and differential are unaffected (fig. 423). In some cases of small cleaved cell lymphoma, intermediately differentiated (mantle zone) lymphoma, peripheral T-cell lymphoma (adult T-cell leukemia-lymphoma), and cutaneous T-cell lymphoma (Sézary syndrome), an elevated leukocyte count may be the first recognizable manifestation of the disease. A frankly leukemic picture is encountered in some cases (fig. 424). The blood smear findings must often be distinguished from chronic lymphocytic leukemia (77,95,99). The cytologic features, immunophenotype, and pattern of distribution in the bone marrow usually serve to appropriately characterize the lymphoproliferative disorder. A lymph node biopsy will confirm the diagnosis of follicular small cleaved or mantle zone lymphoma. Patients with low-grade lymphomas may have normal or only slightly decreased hemoglobin levels and platelet and neutrophil counts even with marked lymphocytosis.

The incidence of circulating lymphoma cells is probably higher than has been reported in morphologic studies. A small number of unrecognized circulating lymphoma cells can be identified by flow cytometry or immunogenotypic

Table 34

WORKING FORMULATION CLASSIFICATION FOR NON-HODGKIN LYMPHOMAS*

Low grade
    Malignant lymphoma, small lymphocytic
        Consistent with chronic lymphocytic leukemia
        Plasmacytoid
    Malignant lymphoma, follicular, predominantly small cleaved cell
    Malignant lymphoma, follicular, mixed small cleaved and large cell

Intermediate grade
    Malignant lymphoma, follicular, predominantly large cell
    Malignant lymphoma, diffuse, small cleaved cell
    Malignant lymphoma, diffuse, mixed small and large cell
        Epithelial component
    Malignant lymphoma, diffuse, large cell

High grade
    Malignant lymphoma, large cell immunoblastic
        Plasmacytoid
        Clear cell
        Polymorphous
        Epithelial cell component
    Malignant lymphoma, lymphoblastic
    Malignant lymphoma, small noncleaved cell

Miscellaneous
    True histiocytic lymphoma
    Cutaneous T-cell lymphoma
    Composite lymphoma
    Unclassifiable

* From reference 83.

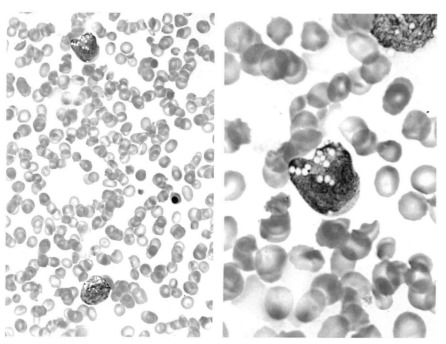

Figure 423
BLOOD INVOLVEMENT IN LARGE CELL LYMPHOMA

Left: Two lymphoma cells are present on this blood smear from a patient with diffuse large cell lymphoma. A nucleated red blood cell is also illustrated. The patient was pancytopenic.

Right: A high magnification of one of the lymphoma cells. The cell is large with a moderate amount of vacuolated cytoplasm, relatively dispersed nuclear chromatin, and three prominent nucleoli. (Wright-Giemsa stain) (Fig. 37.25 from McKenna RW. The bone marrow manifestations of Hodgkin's disease, the non-Hodgkin's lymphomas, and lymphoma-like disorders. In: Knowles DM, ed. Neoplastic hematopathology. Baltimore: Williams & Wilkins, 1992: 1135–80.)

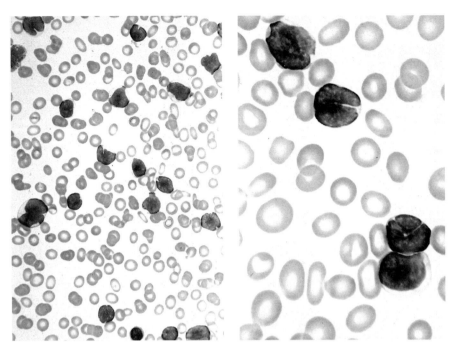

Figure 424

LEUKEMIC BLOOD PICTURE IN FOLLICULAR SMALL CLEAVED CELL LYMPHOMA

Left: There is marked leukocytosis consisting of small cleaved lymphoma cells.

Right: A higher magnification illustrates the typical cytologic features of small cleaved cells. (Wright-Giemsa stain) (Fig. 36.26 from McKenna RW. The bone marrow manifestations of Hodgkin's disease, the non-Hodgkin's lymphomas, and lymphoma-like disorders. In: Knowles DM, ed. Neoplastic hematopathology. Baltimore: Williams & Wilkins, 1992:1135–80.)

analysis in some cases of small lymphocytic and small cleaved cell lymphomas that lack morphologic evidence of blood involvement (52,73,74).

The utility of the bone marrow biopsy in patients with non-Hodgkin lymphoma has been demonstrated in several studies (38,48,50,55,66, 72,96). Its importance in pathologic staging of clinical stage I and II disease and in following patients with advanced disease for response to therapy is well documented (89). However, the bone marrow biopsy findings may not contribute significantly to management decisions or provide prognostic information for patients with advanced clinical stages of follicular predominantly small cleaved cell, diffuse large cell, and diffuse mixed small and large cell lymphomas (34).

The bone marrow examination should include trephine biopsy sections, trephine imprints, aspiration smears, and blood smears (38). A combination of clues obtained from examination of each of the marrow preparations and blood smears often leads to the correct diagnosis when one specimen alone would be equivocal. Trephine biopsies are more often positive for non-Hodgkin lymphoma than aspirate smears, but in the majority of cases disease is found in both the biopsy and aspirate smears. In a minority of cases the aspirate smears are diagnostic when the sections are negative or equivocal (55,62,67, 72). In addition to the morphologic evaluation, the aspirated marrow is the best material for several supplementary studies including immunophenotyping, cytogenetics, and immunogenotypic analysis. These additional studies may provide important prognostic and therapeutic information and help confirm the diagnosis of non-Hodgkin lymphoma in difficult cases.

Hematopoietic bone marrow involvement in malignant lymphoma is usually generalized. However, the lesions are often focal with intervening normal uninvolved marrow. These focal lesions can be missed if the volume of the biopsy specimen is insufficient. Bilateral posterior iliac crest trephine biopsies provide more tissue for examination and samples two separate sites.

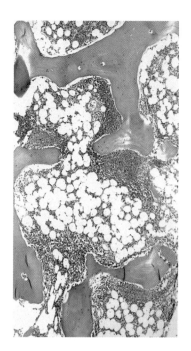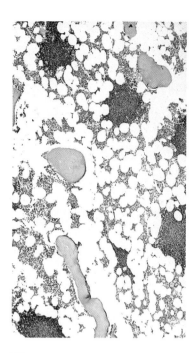

Figure 425
FOCAL BONE MARROW LESIONS IN NON-HODGKIN LYMPHOMA

Left: A bone marrow trephine biopsy section from a patient with follicular small cleaved cell lymphoma shows a focal paratrabecular pattern of involvement. (Hematoxylin and eosin stain)

Right: A bone marrow trephine biopsy section from a patient with a small lymphocytic lymphoma shows focal random (nonparatrabecular) distribution of lesions. (Hematoxylin and eosin stain) (Fig. 37.9 from McKenna RW. The bone marrow manifestations of Hodgkin's disease, the non-Hodgkin's lymphomas, and lymphoma-like disorders. In: Knowles DM, ed. Neoplastic hematopathology. Baltimore: Williams & Wilkins, 1992:1135–80.)

Several reports have addressed the incidence and morphologic features of bone marrow involvement in relation to the Rappaport or Lukes-Collins classifications of non-Hodgkin lymphoma (38,50,55,63,66,75,77,90,96). Studies of bone marrow lymphomas using the International Working Formulation have appeared more recently (72, 76,83). In the following discussion, non-Hodgkin lymphomas that have a high incidence of bone marrow involvement or that may present major diagnostic problems will be emphasized.

The bone marrow is involved most frequently in the low-grade lymphomas comprised primarily of small cells (small lymphocytic and small cleaved cell), high-grade lymphomas of lymphoblastic and small noncleaved cell types, and the various peripheral T-cell lymphomas that span all of the Working Formulation groups (55,59,63). Among B-cell lymphomas, those with a follicular pattern have a greater predilection for marrow involvement than diffuse lymphomas, except for the small lymphocytic category (48,55,76).

Pattern and Extent of Bone Marrow Involvement in Biopsy Sections. There are four major patterns of bone marrow infiltration: focal paratrabecular, focal random (nonparatrabecular), interstitial, and diffuse (figs. 425, 426). Focal lesions are encountered more frequently (about 70 percent of cases) than interstitial or diffuse infiltration (about 30 percent of cases) (55). Paratrabecular focal lesions are slightly more common than randomly distributed ones. In some cases both patterns of focal involvement are present in the same biopsy specimen. The number of lesions varies from a single focus of involvement to several on each section.

Some categories of non-Hodgkin lymphoma have a predilection for a particular pattern of marrow infiltration. For example, the bone marrow lesions of follicular predominantly small cleaved cell and mixed small and large cell lymphomas are predominantly focal and paratrabecular, small lymphocytic lymphomas are usually randomly focal, and small noncleaved cell

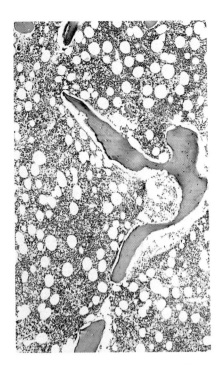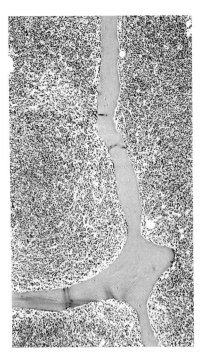

Figure 426

INTERSTITIAL AND DIFFUSE BONE MARROW INVOLVEMENT WITH NON-HODGKIN LYMPHOMA

Left: A bone marrow trephine biopsy showing an interstitial pattern of involvement in a patient with intermediate lymphocytic lymphoma. The marrow is normocellular and the lymphoma infiltrate blends with normal hematopoietic cells at this magnification. (Hematoxylin and eosin stain)

Right: A trephine biopsy section shows diffuse marrow infiltration by small noncleaved cell lymphoma. The hematopoietic marrow and fat are completely replaced. (Hematoxylin and eosin stain) (Fig. 37.10 from McKenna RW. The bone marrow manifestations of Hodgkin's disease, the non-Hodgkin's lymphomas, and lymphoma-like disorders. In: Knowles DM, ed. Neoplastic hematopathology. Baltimore: Williams & Wilkins, 1992:1135–80.)

and lymphoblastic lymphomas generally have an interstitial or diffuse pattern of infiltration (38,50, 55,67,72,76,77).

The degree of bone marrow replacement correlates with the pattern of infiltration. With focal lesions there is often considerable marrow sparing, with less than 30 percent of the marrow space occupied by malignant lymphoma (55). With advanced disease, focal lesions enlarge and may coalesce and occupy a greater portion of the marrow. With interstitial infiltration much of the hematopoietic tissue and marrow fat are spared. Diffuse involvement is associated with extensive replacement of normal bone marrow elements.

Morphologic Discordance of Lymph Node and Bone Marrow Histology. Histologic discordance between the lymph node and bone marrow is noted in 15 to 40 percent of cases (33,46,54,55, 67,70). The more aggressive subtype is usually found in the lymph node. Divergent histology is most common with follicular, diffuse large cell, and diffuse mixed small and large cell lymphomas (33,46,54,55,70). In a typical discordant pattern, the lymph node has a follicular large cell or mixed small and large cell lymphoma while the lesions in the bone marrow show small cleaved cell or small lymphocyte histology (fig. 427) (33,55,70). A low-grade lymphoma in the bone marrow of patients with high- or intermediate-grade large cell lymphoma in the lymph nodes does not negatively impact on prognosis; median survival for these patients is equal to those without marrow involvement (46,54). However, in patients with low- or intermediate-grade lymph node lymphoma a high-grade marrow lymphoma does carry a poorer prognosis (70). In the large majority of cases, the divergent histology in the lymph nodes and bone marrow appears to represent tumor morphologic heterogeneity of the same neoplastic clone (70).

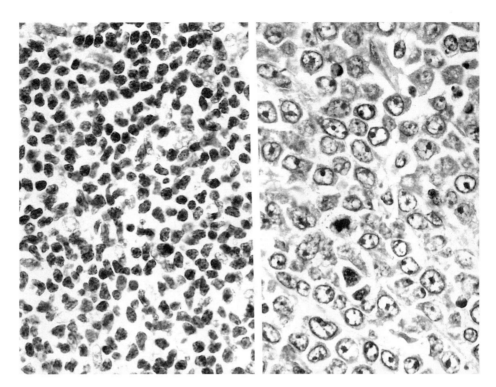

Figure 427
MORPHOLOGIC DISCORDANCE IN FOLLICULAR LYMPHOMA
This figure illustrates morphologic discordance of lymph node and bone marrow lesions from a patient with follicular lymphoma.
Left: The bone marrow trephine biopsy section shows lesions consisting of small cleaved cells. (Hematoxylin and eosin stain)
Right: A lymph node biopsy from the same patient shows follicular predominantly large cell lymphoma. (Hematoxylin and eosin stain) (Fig. 37.11 from McKenna RW. The bone marrow manifestations of Hodgkin's disease, the non-Hodgkin's lymphomas, and lymphoma-like disorders. In: Knowles DM, ed. Neoplastic hematopathology. Baltimore: Williams & Wilkins, 1992:1135–80.)

Low-Grade Lymphomas. *Small Lymphocytic and Lymphoplasmacytoid Lymphomas.* These involve the bone marrow in 80 to 90 percent of cases (55,67). The proliferative lymphocytes are generally cytologically uniform, with mature features. In most cases the pattern of involvement in trephine biopsy sections is randomly focal or interstitial (fig. 428). A diffuse pattern or a combination of focal and interstitial infiltration may be observed with extensive marrow replacement. Focal lesions are round, oval, or irregular in shape with sharply or poorly circumscribed margins. An increase in small lymphocytes may be noted in areas between foci of lymphoma. Considerable preservation of normal marrow is usually observed even with relatively extensive marrow infiltration. The bone marrow smears show a slight to marked increase in mature-appearing lymphocytes, with sparse to moderate cytoplasm and round nuclei with coarse nuclear chromatin; nucleoli are generally lacking (fig. 429).

Small lymphocytic lymphoma and chronic lymphocytic leukemia are distinguished on the basis of the blood lymphocyte count. The proliferative lymphocytes in the two disorders are cytologically and immunologically identical, although clinical and biological differences have been reported (75,86). Chronic lymphocytic leukemia is the preferred diagnosis when the blood lymphocyte count exceeds 10×10^9/L (36).

A monoclonal gammopathy, usually of IgM type, is associated with some cases of small lymphocytic lymphoma with marrow involvement. This is most common in cases of lymphoplasmacytoid lymphoma. The clinical manifestations of Waldenström macroglobulinemia may be present (86).

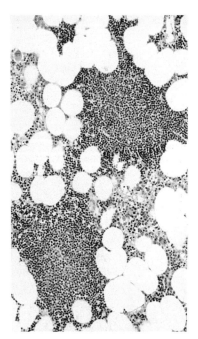

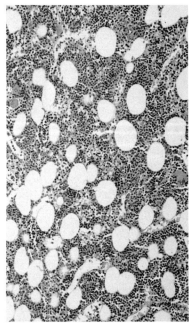

Figure 428
SMALL LYMPHOCYTIC
LYMPHOMA

Left: A trephine biopsy section from a 73-year-old man with a small lymphocytic lymphoma. There is random (nonparatrabecular) focal involvement in the marrow. (Hematoxylin and eosin stain).

Right: A trephine biopsy section from a 50-year-old woman with small lymphocytic lymphoma. There is interstitial infiltration of the bone marrow. (Hematoxylin and eosin stain)

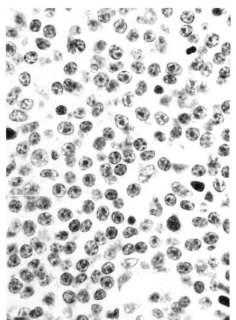

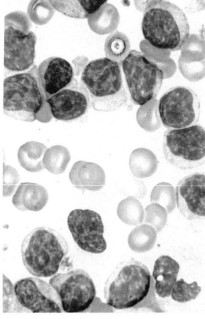

Figure 429
SMALL LYMPHOCYTIC
LYMPHOMA

Left: A high magnification of a focal marrow lesion in a trephine biopsy section from a patient with small lymphocytic lymphoma. (Hematoxylin and eosin stain).

Right: A bone marrow aspirate smear from the same case shows well-differentiated lymphocytes. (Wright-Giemsa stain) (Fig. 37.13 from McKenna RW. The bone marrow manifestations of Hodgkin's disease, the non-Hodgkin's lymphomas, and lymphoma-like disorders. In: Knowles DM, ed. Neoplastic hematopathology. Baltimore: Williams & Wilkins, 1992: 1135–80.)

The large majority of cases of small lymphocytic lymphoma/chronic lymphocytic leukemia are of B-cell type and have a characteristic immunophenotype that includes weak expression of surface immunoglobulin and expression of the CD5 antigen (36). A small number of cases have a T-cell immunophenotype (36). These may be morphologically indistinguishable from B-cell small lymphocytic proliferations or express a significant degree of cytologic heterogeneity and atypia (fig. 430).

Intermediate Lymphocytic and Mantle Zone Lymphomas. These are cytologically and often immunologically "intermediate" between small lymphocytic and small cleaved cell lymphomas and have either a mantle zone or diffuse histologic pattern in the lymph nodes and spleen (37,42,

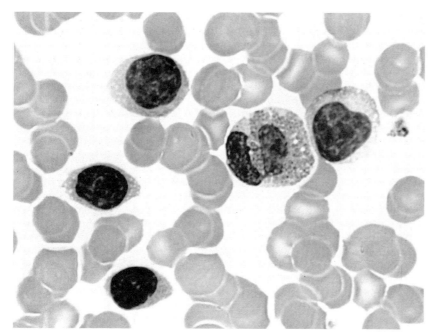

Figure 430
T-CELL SMALL
LYMPHOCYTIC
LEUKEMIA-LYMPHOMA

A blood smear from a patient with T-cell small lymphocytic leukemia-lymphoma. The lymphocytes are mature-appearing with condensed chromatin and lack nucleoli. The nuclei are generally round with occasional cells having slightly convoluted nuclei. The blood picture is similar to B-cell chronic lymphocytic leukemia. (Wright-Giemsa stain) (Fig. 37.14 from McKenna RW. The bone marrow manifestations of Hodgkin's disease, the non-Hodgkin's lymphomas, and lymphoma-like disorders. In: Knowles DM, ed. Neoplastic hematopathology. Baltimore: Williams & Wilkins, 1992:1135–80.)

Figure 431
INTERMEDIATELY
DIFFERENTIATED
LYMPHOCYTIC LYMPHOMA

A trephine biopsy section from a patient with intermediately differentiated lymphocytic lymphoma shows an interstitial pattern of infiltration. (Hematoxylin and eosin stain)

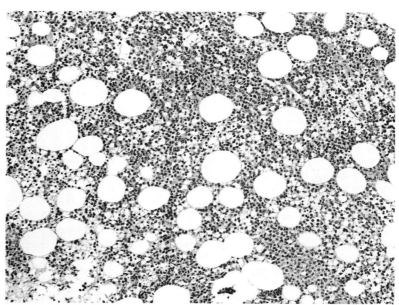

49,65,87). In the bone marrow and blood, intermediate lymphocytic lymphomas resemble small lymphocytic lymphomas (38,50,55,76).

The bone marrow is involved at diagnosis in approximately 65 percent of cases (102). The pattern of involvement is usually randomly focal or interstitial (fig. 431). The major cytologic features that distinguish intermediate lymphocytic lymphomas from other small lymphocytic lymphomas are an irregular nuclear shape or the presence of nucleoli in a portion of the lymphocytes. There is generally a mixture of well-differentiated–appearing lymphocytes and cells with coarsely clumped chromatin and nuclear irregularity or indentation. These cytologic features are apparent on both the trephine biopsy sections and aspirate smears (fig. 432) (50,55). Patients with a mantle zone lymphoma may present with spleen and bone marrow involvement, without peripheral lymphadenopathy. In these

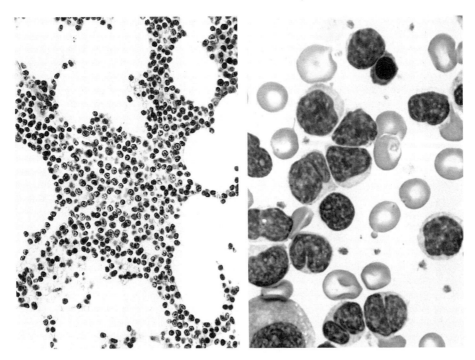

Figure 432
INTERMEDIATELY DIFFERENTIATED LYMPHOCYTIC LYMPHOMA

Left: A section of a trephine biopsy from a patient with intermediate lymphocytic lymphoma shows a focal collection of lymphoma cells in an interstitial infiltrate. The cells have relatively condensed nuclear chromatin similar to small lymphocytic lymphoma but many of the nuclei have irregular borders or cleaved nuclei. (Hematoxylin and eosin stain)

Right: A marrow aspirate smear from the same patient also resembles small lymphocytic lymphoma but many of the lymphocytes have indented or partially cleaved nuclei. (Wright-Giemsa stain) (Fig. 37.15 (right) from McKenna RW. The bone marrow manifestations of Hodgkin's disease, the non-Hodgkin's lymphomas, and lymphoma-like disorders. In: Knowles DM, ed. Neoplastic hematopathology. Baltimore: Williams & Wilkins, 1992:1135–80.)

cases a biopsy of the bone marrow may be the initial diagnostic tissue.

Follicular Predominantly Small Cleaved Cell, and Follicular Mixed Small Cleaved and Large Cell Lymphomas. These have a high incidence (50 to 60 percent) of marrow involvement at diagnosis (55,72,77). In trephine biopsy sections the predominant pattern of marrow infiltration is focal and distinctly paratrabecular, generally with complete sparing of the adjacent bone marrow (fig. 433) (50,77). Even in a heavily infiltrated marrow with coalescence of focal lesions, a paratrabecular concentration of lymphoma cells can still be identified (fig. 434). The lymphoma cells are predominantly small cleaved cells in most cases regardless of the lymph node histology (figs. 435, 436) (55,77). In a minority of cases, a broad morphologic spectrum of lymphocytes is observed including large cleaved and noncleaved cells, small cleaved cells, and small mature-appearing lymphocytes (77). Transforma-

tion of bone marrow lesions from predominantly small cleaved to large cleaved or noncleaved cells may occur after several months or years; lymphoma cells resembling Reed-Sternberg cells are occasionally found (78).

Bone marrow lesions consisting of a central concentration of large cleaved and noncleaved lymphocytes with small cleaved cells at the periphery may resemble a germinal center (fig. 437). Careful examination of the cytology of the lymphocytes usually allows distinction of these lesions from a reactive process. Clusters of histiocytes resembling a granuloma may be found in some follicular lymphomas in the bone marrow (38). Morphologic distinction of these infiltrates from granulomas, Hodgkin disease, or a peripheral T-cell lymphoma may be difficult; immunohistochemical studies on frozen or paraffin-embedded sections may help resolve the issue (30,44).

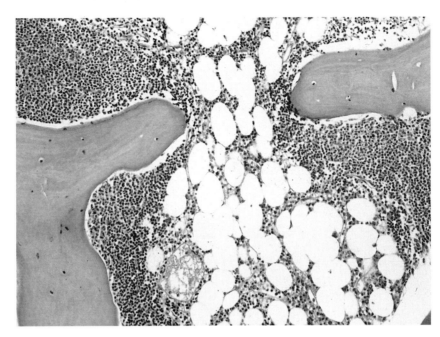

Figure 433
FOLLICULAR SMALL CLEAVED CELL LYMPHOMA
A trephine biopsy section from a patient with follicular small cleaved cell lymphoma. The pattern of involvement is focal and distinctly paratrabecular. There is complete sparing of the marrow between foci of lymphoma. (Hematoxylin and eosin stain) (Fig. 19 from McKenna RW. Disorders of bone marrow. In: Sternberg SS, ed. Diagnostic surgical pathology. New York: Raven Press, 1989:479-513.)

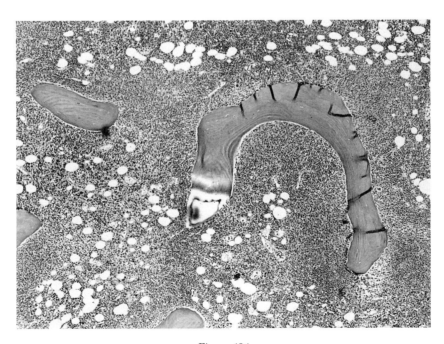

Figure 434
FOLLICULAR SMALL CLEAVED CELL LYMPHOMA
A bone marrow biopsy section from a patient with a follicular small cleaved cell lymphoma. The marrow is heavily infiltrated. A paratrabecular concentration of the lymphoma cells can be appreciated even in this case of advanced bone marrow disease. (Hematoxylin and eosin stain)

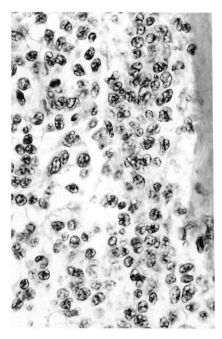
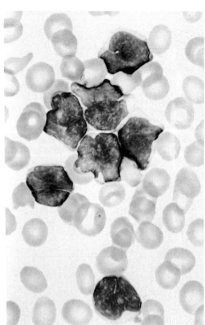

Figure 435
FOLLICULAR SMALL
CLEAVED CELL LYMPHOMA
Left: A trephine biopsy section
from a patient with follicular
small cleaved cell lymphoma.
There is a concentration of small
cleaved cells adjacent to the
trabeculum. (Hematoxylin and
eosin stain)
Right: The bone marrow aspirate smears contained numerous
small cleaved cells. (Wright-
Giemsa stain) (Fig. 37.16 from Mc-
Kenna RW. The bone marrow manifestations of Hodgkin's disease, the
non-Hodgkin's lymphomas, and
lymphoma-like disorders. In:
Knowles DM, ed. Neoplastic
hematopathology. Baltimore: Williams & Wilkins, 1992:1135–80.)

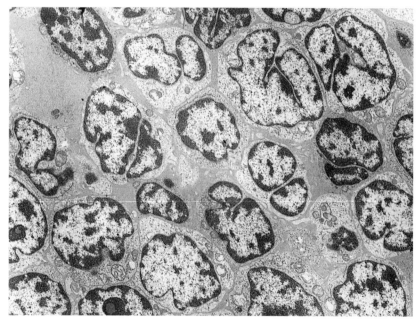

Figure 436
FOLLICULAR
SMALL CLEAVED
CELL LYMPHOMA
An electron micrograph of
small cleaved lymphoma cells
from the blood of a patient presenting with a leukemic blood picture.
Many of the cells have deeply indented or cleaved nuclei; some nuclei appear to be bisected. Nuclear
chromatin is condensed and nucleoli are small. (Uranyl acetate-lead
citrate stain, X9,000)

In many cases a diagnosis of small cleaved cell lymphoma is made from bone marrow aspirate smears (fig. 435). The cytology of the lymphoma cells encompasses a wide morphologic spectrum that includes small cleaved cells, large transformed lymphocytes, and well-differentiated lymphocytes. The predominant cell is usually the small cleaved cell, characterized by sparse or no recognizable cytoplasm and a smooth, uniformly-staining nucleus that is frequently deeply indented or cleaved (50,77,95). Smear preparations often contain few or no obvious lymphoma cells, either because of a sparsity of marrow lesions or because reticulin in the lesions interferes with collection of a representative aspirate.

Monocytoid B-Cell Lymphomas. These lymphomas are not specifically designated in the Working Formulation Classification but are included in

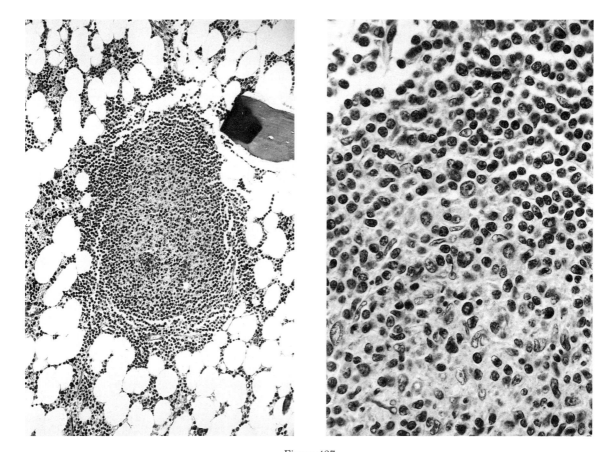

Figure 437
FOLLICULAR LYMPHOMA RESEMBLING A GERMINAL CENTER
Left: A low magnification of a follicular lymphoma resembling a germinal center in a bone marrow biopsy. (Hematoxylin and eosin stain)
Right: A high magnification of the same lesion shows a margin of small lymphoma cells adjacent to larger cells. Only occasional small cells are cleaved. Many of the large cells have angulated nuclei. (Hematoxylin and eosin stain)

the low-grade small lymphocytic lymphomas (94). The incidence of marrow involvement has not been well studied but is thought to be significantly lower than for other low-grade lymphomas (98). A monocytoid B-cell lymphoma registry reports an incidence of blood and bone marrow involvement of approximately 4 percent (98). In some studies, however, the incidence of marrow involvement has been higher (about 40 percent) (82). One reported case with blood and bone marrow disease had an interstitial marrow infiltrate and circulating lymphoma cells with plasmacytoid features and irregular nuclei (41). Others have a paratrabecular pattern of marrow involvement (fig. 438). Patients with marrow involvement appear to have more extensive and aggressive disease and a poorer response to treatment (98).

Intermediate-Grade Lymphomas. Intermediate-grade non-Hodgkin lymphomas have a lower incidence of bone marrow involvement at diagnosis than low-grade lymphomas. Diffuse small cleaved cell, diffuse mixed small and large cell, and most of the follicular and diffuse large cell lymphomas are included in this group. There is no clear correlation between the type of intermediate-grade lymphoma and the pattern of bone marrow involvement.

Diffuse Small Cleaved Cell Lymphomas. These lymphomas have been reported to involve the bone marrow in 30 to 42 percent of cases (87,102). No specific pattern of involvement predominates. With minimal marrow disease the infiltrate may be focal or interstitial. Extensive marrow replacement results from confluence of

391

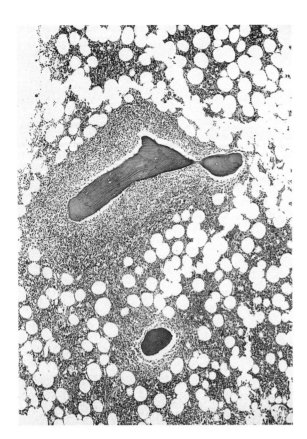

Figure 438
MONOCYTOID B-CELL LYMPHOMA

A trephine biopsy section from a patient with monocytoid B-cell lymphoma shows a distinctly paratrabecular pattern of involvement. (Hematoxylin and eosin stain)

focal lesions or diffuse involvement. Scattered or small clusters of histiocytes may be observed in the lesions. The cytology of the lymphoma cells in bone marrow sections and smears resembles that of follicular predominantly small cleaved cell lymphoma; in some cases the nuclear chromatin is less dense and nucleoli may be more prominent (38). Some of the intermediate lymphocytic lymphomas without mantle zone histology may be included in this category.

Diffuse Mixed Small and Large Cell, and Diffuse Large Cell Lymphomas. A morphologic spectrum of B-cell and T-cell lymphomas are included in these categories. The incidence of marrow involvement for this group varies from 30 to 56 percent (55,72). In marrow biopsies the greatest diagnostic challenges are the *peripheral T-cell lymphomas.* This morphologically diverse group has a common origin in post-thymic lymphocytes (100). Most of the peripheral T-cell lymphomas are in the diffuse mixed small and large cell category but they also encompass some of the high-grade large cell immunoblastic and low-grade small lymphocytic lymphomas (83). They are discussed here because of the high incidence of bone marrow involvement (60 to 75 percent) for all histologic types and the several common and unique features they share (45,59,63). Bone marrow involvement by peripheral T-cell lymphomas is associated with poor prognosis (43,46).

The pattern of marrow involvement of the peripheral T-cell lymphomas is about equally split between diffuse and randomly focal lesions; rarely, focal paratrabecular lesions are encountered (63,103). In mixed small and large cell, and large cell immunoblastic lymphomas, some of the lesions consist of a heteromorphous lymphocyte population and a polycellular infiltrate of eosinophils, plasma cells, neutrophils, endothelial cells, and epithelioid histiocytes (figs. 439–441). There may be prominent vascularity and reticulin fibrosis. The reactive cell component is mixed with the lymphoma cells. Epithelioid histiocytes are often found in clusters and may impart a granulomatous appearance. Reticulin fibrosis is confined to the lymphoma lesions and does not extend to the uninvolved adjacent marrow. Foci of necrosis may be observed primarily in cases of large cell immunoblastic lymphoma.

In some large cell immunoblastic lymphomas, large lymphocytes and immunoblasts predominate and the reactive cell infiltrate is not a prominent feature. The small lymphocytic peripheral T-cell lesions are usually cytologically uniform and resemble either a small lymphocytic lymphoma/chronic lymphocytic leukemia or have the features of adult T-cell leukemia-lymphoma (fig. 442) (63,99). Discordant histology between lymph nodes and bone marrow is rarely encountered in any of the peripheral T-cell lymphomas (59,63).

In some cases of mixed small and large cell, and large cell immunoblastic T-cell lymphomas, diffuse bone marrow infiltrates may blend uniformly with the normal hematopoietic cells. Reticulin fibrosis is generally a component of these lesions and the overall picture may suggest a myeloproliferative disorder (figs. 443, 444) (31,59,63). With this pattern of infiltration, the lymphoma may be difficult to discern even with rather extensive marrow disease. In the absence of a confirmatory lymph node biopsy, the diagnosis can be problematic.

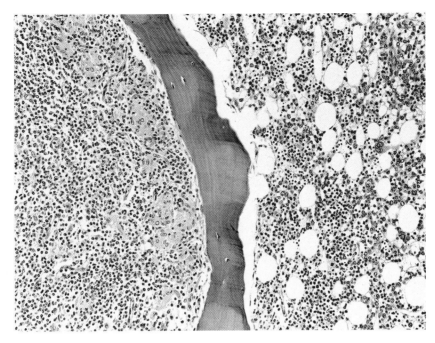

Figure 439
PERIPHERAL T-CELL LYMPHOMA
Bone marrow trephine section from a man with peripheral T-cell lymphoma. A bone trabeculum separates a lymphoma infiltrate (left) from normal hematopoietic tissue. (Hematoxylin and eosin stain) (Fig. 37.17 (left) from McKenna RW. The bone marrow manifestations of Hodgkin's disease, the non-Hodgkin's lymphomas, and lymphoma-like disorders. In: Knowles DM, ed. Neoplastic hematopathology. Baltimore: Williams & Wilkins, 1992:1135–80.)

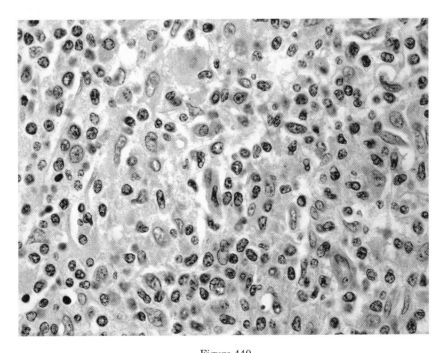

Figure 440
PERIPHERAL T-CELL LYMPHOMA (DIFFUSE MIXED)
A higher magnification of the same biopsy illustrated in figure 439. The lesion is composed of a heteromorphous population of lymphocytes, clusters of epithelioid histiocytes, small vessels, and endothelial cells. (Hematoxylin and eosin stain)

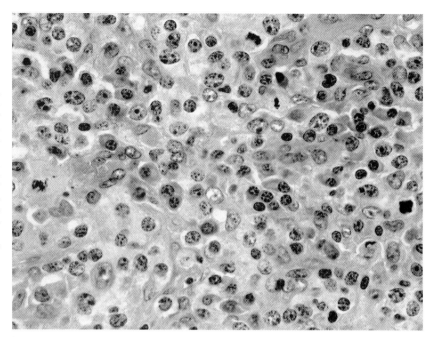

Figure 441
PERIPHERAL
T-CELL LYMPHOMA
A trephine biopsy section from a patient with a peripheral T-cell lymphoma. There was diffuse involvement of the bone marrow in this case. The infiltrate shows a mixture of large lymphoma cells and plasma cells. (Hematoxylin and eosin stain) (Fig. 37.18 from McKenna RW. The bone marrow manifestations of Hodgkin's disease, the non-Hodgkin's lymphomas, and lymphoma-like disorders. In: Knowles DM, ed. Neoplastic hematopathology. Baltimore: Williams & Wilkins, 1992:1135–80.)

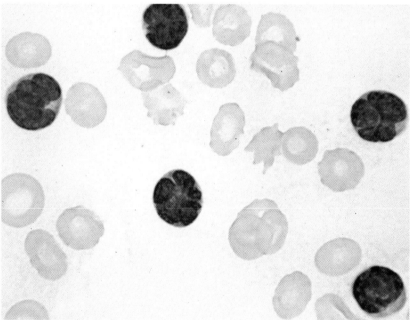

Figure 442
ADULT T-CELL
LEUKEMIA-LYMPHOMA
A blood smear from a patient with adult T-cell leukemia-lymphoma shows the markedly irregular nuclei typical of this disorder. (Wright-Giemsa stain)

Pleomorphic focal lesions are randomly distributed and usually poorly circumscribed. They can be difficult to distinguish from lymphohistiocytic reactive lesions, particularly those commonly found in the bone marrow of patients with AIDS or an autoimmune disease (59,63,68, 80,85). In some cases the marrow histology may be indistinguishable from angioimmunoblastic lymphadenopathy or Hodgkin disease (63).

Immunohistochemistry on bone marrow sections, immunophenotyping of aspirated marrow, and DNA analysis for T-cell receptor gene rearrangements may be helpful in the differential diagnosis (59,103).

A marrow aspirate is often difficult to obtain because of the fibrosis associated with many of the peripheral T-cell lymphomas. Despite this, lymphoma cells are found in aspirate smears in

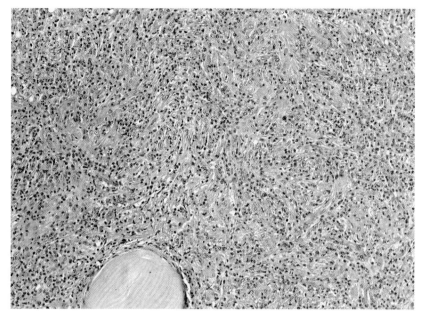

Figure 443
PERIPHERAL
T-CELL LYMPHOMA

A bone marrow trephine biopsy from a patient with peripheral T-cell lymphoma. The bone marrow is diffusely and extensively infiltrated. There is a polycellular infiltrate and reticulin fibrosis. (Hematoxylin and eosin stain) (Fig. 37.19 from McKenna RW. The bone marrow manifestations of Hodgkin disease, the non-Hodgkin's lymphomas, and lymphoma-like disorders. In: Knowles DM, ed. Neoplastic hematopathology. Baltimore: Williams & Wilkins, 1992:1135–80.)

Figure 444
PERIPHERAL
T-CELL LYMPHOMA

A higher magnification of the same biopsy illustrated in figure 443. There is fibrosis and increased vascularity. The lymphoma blends with the normal hematopoietic cells. Peripheral T-cell lymphomas with this pattern of involvement may resemble a myeloproliferative disorder. (Hematoxylin and eosin stain)

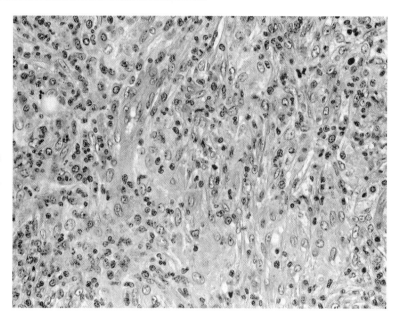

at least half of the cases with bone marrow disease (63). Interpretation of the smears may be difficult because of the heteromorphous lymphocyte population, many of which exhibit cytologic features of mature or reactive lymphocytes (fig. 445) (63). The number of lymphoma cells varies from rare to greater than 90 percent of the bone marrow cells. The morphologic spectrum of cells in the diffuse mixed small and large cell lymphomas generally reflects the heterogeneity of the lesions in the trephine sections (fig. 445).

With large cell immunoblastic lymphomas there are fewer immunoblasts in the aspiration smears than are apparent in the trephine sections (63). The immunoblasts have lightly to deeply basophilic cytoplasm and are sometimes finely vacuolated. The contour of the nucleus varies but is usually convoluted. The chromatin is dispersed and prominent nucleoli are present. The cytoplasm of the small and medium sized lymphocytes ranges from sparse to moderately abundant and is lightly to deeply basophilic. The

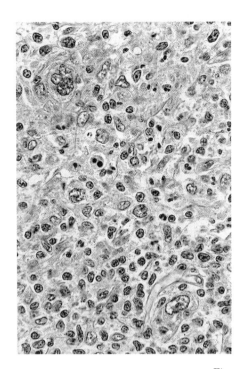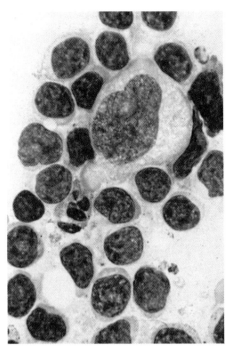

Figure 445
PERIPHERAL T-CELL LYMPHOMA RESEMBLING HODGKIN DISEASE

Left: A high magnification of a trephine biopsy section from a patient with diffuse mixed peripheral T-cell lymphoma. There is a mixture of small and large cells. Some pleomorphic cells resemble R-S cells. (Hematoxylin and eosin stain)

Right: A bone marrow trephine biopsy touch preparation from the same patient. The majority of the lymphoma cells are medium sized with condensed chromatin; some have a slightly irregular nuclear border and/or visible nucleoli. A single large cell comparable to those in the trephine section is present. This cell has condensed chromatin, a prominent nucleolus, and abundant cytoplasm. (Wright-Giemsa stain) (Fig. 37.20 from McKenna RW. The bone marrow manifestations of Hodgkin's disease, the non-Hodgkin's lymphomas, and lymphoma-like disorders. In: Knowles DM, ed. Neoplastic hematopathology. Baltimore: Williams & Wilkins, 1992:1135–80.)

nuclear chromatin is coarse and nucleoli are indistinct; convolution may be less apparent in smear preparations than in sections.

The *intermediate-grade lymphomas of B-cell type* include follicular and diffuse large cell and diffuse mixed small and large cell lymphomas. These have a relatively low incidence of marrow involvement at diagnosis, about 25 percent (46,55). The pattern and extent of bone marrow infiltration in trephine biopsy sections is highly variable, ranging from minimal small foci to virtual total marrow replacement. In some patients with minimal involvement, lymphoma is only detectable by identification of lymphoma cells in smears or imprints.

The lesions in trephine sections are usually readily recognizable by the abnormal cytologic characteristics of the lymphocytes (figs. 446, 447). They may be composed of fairly uniform, large cells with large, round nuclei, prominent nucleoli, and a moderate amount of cytoplasm or there may be striking variability in nuclear size and outline; the cells may have contorted nuclei and abundant cytoplasm. In most instances reticulin is increased and a profound desmoplastic reaction is sometimes observed (50).

The cytology of the large cell lymphomas in smear and imprint preparations is highly variable and generally pleomorphic. The spectrum of cell types includes large lymphocytes with large nuclei and abundant, often vacuolated, cytoplasm. The nucleus may be round or slightly convoluted with delicate reticular chromatin; nucleoli are prominent and may be single or multiple (figs. 446, 447). In some cases extremely large cells with abundant basophilic, vacuolated cytoplasm are observed. Some of these large cells contain fine azurophilic granules; cytoplasmic projections or fragmentation may be present (38,50).

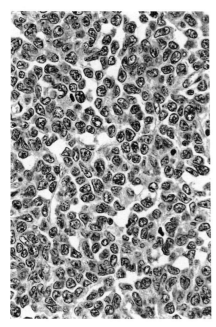

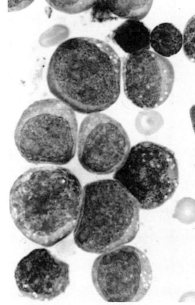

Figure 446
DIFFUSE LARGE
CELL LYMPHOMA

Left: A trephine biopsy section from a patient with extensive marrow replacement by diffuse large cell lymphoma. (Hematoxylin and eosin stain)

Right: The aspirate smears from the same patient consisted primarily of large lymphoma cells with basophilic cytoplasm, coarsely reticular chromatin, and prominent nucleoli. (Wright-Giemsa stain) (Fig. 37.21 from McKenna RW. The bone marrow manifestations of Hodgkin's disease, the non-Hodgkin's lymphomas, and lymphoma-like disorders. In: Knowles DM, ed. Neoplastic hematopathology. Baltimore: Williams & Wilkins, 1992:1135–80.)

Figure 447
FOLLICULAR LARGE
CELL LYMPHOMA

Left: A high magnification of a lesion on a trephine section from a patient with follicular large cleaved cell lymphoma. (Hematoxylin and eosin stain)

Right: Aspirate smear from the same case shows several lymphoma cells. (Wright-Giemsa stain)

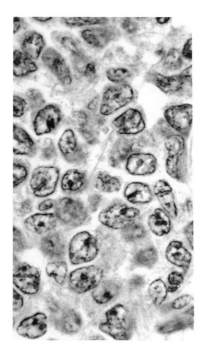

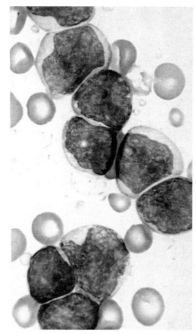

High-Grade Lymphomas. Patients with high-grade non-Hodgkin lymphomas commonly have bone marrow involvement at presentation, especially those with lymphoblastic or small noncleaved cell lymphoma, or large cell immunoblastic lymphoma, polymorphous or with an epithelioid component. The latter was discussed above with the peripheral T-cell lymphomas.

Lymphoblastic Lymphomas. The incidence of marrow involvement by lymphoblastic lymphomas is 50 to 60 percent (55,72). The bone marrow may be the primary tissue available for examination in patients presenting with a mediastinal mass and no peripheral lymphadenopathy. The histologic and cytologic features of lymphoblastic lymphoma are identical to those of acute

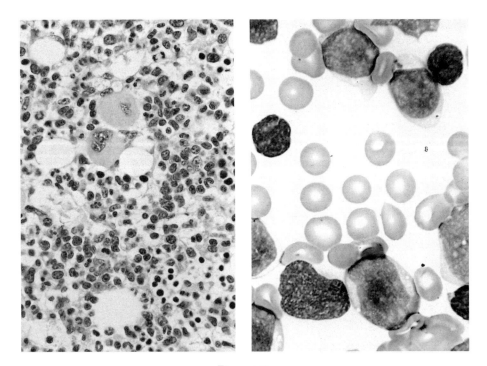

Figure 448
LYMPHOBLASTIC LYMPHOMA
Left: A trephine biopsy section from a patient with lymphoblastic lymphoma shows partial marrow involvement. (Hematoxylin and eosin stain)
Right: A bone marrow aspirate smear from a 15-year-old male with a mediastinal mass and hepatosplenomegaly shows lymphoblasts of two morphologic types. The majority are relatively large with a moderate amount of cytoplasm, reticular chromatin, and nucleoli. A minor population are small hyperchromatic convoluted lymphoblasts. The lymphoblasts expressed a T-cell immunophenotype. (Wright-Giemsa stain) (Fig. 37.22 (right) from McKenna RW. The bone marrow manifestations of Hodgkin's disease, the non-Hodgkin's lymphomas, and lymphoma-like disorders. In: Knowles DM, ed. Neoplastic hematopathology. Baltimore: Williams & Wilkins, 1992:1135–80.)

lymphoblastic leukemia (32,79,81). The distinction is usually based on the percentage of lymphoblasts in the marrow at the time of diagnosis. If greater than 25 percent of the marrow cells are lymphoblasts, a designation of acute lymphoblastic leukemia is usually made. The high incidence of marrow involvement for lymphoblastic lymphoma and the morphologic and immunologic uniformity with acute lymphoblastic leukemia has led to use of the term *lymphoblastic leukemia-lymphoma* in cases of acute lymphoblastic leukemia with mass disease and T-cell immunophenotype (47). The lymphoma cells in approximately 70 percent of cases of lymphoblastic lymphoma express a T-cell immunophenotype and 30 percent a B-cell precursor immunophenotype.

The pattern of marrow infiltration is nearly always interstitial or diffuse in trephine biopsies

(55,72). The degree of involvement varies from occasional lymphoma cells recognizable only in smear preparations to up to 25 percent of the bone marrow cells. Nuclear convolution and a high mitotic rate are prominent features (fig. 448) (32). Nonconvoluted types have round or oval nuclei and are more cytologically uniform (81).

In bone marrow smears the cells are identical to those of acute lymphoblastic leukemia L1 or L2 (35). Those of T-cell immunophenotype may differ subtly from most cases of non–T-cell acute lymphoblastic leukemia by the presence of a minor population of small, markedly hyperchromatic cells that have convoluted nuclei (see section on T-cell acute lymphoblastic leukemia) (fig. 448) (79). The identification of lymphoblasts in smears is essential to the diagnosis when there is minimal involvement not recognizable in the trephine sections.

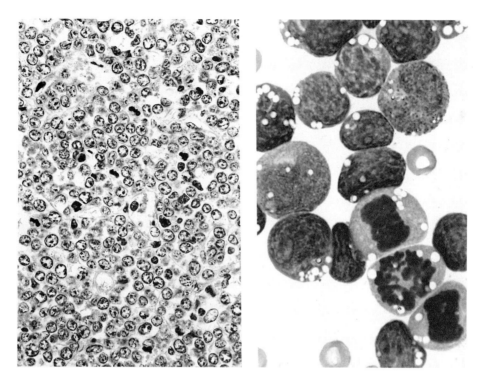

Figure 449
SMALL NONCLEAVED CELL LYMPHOMA (BURKITT TYPE)
Left: A trephine biopsy section from a patient with a small noncleaved cell lymphoma. There is diffuse infiltration of the bone marrow. The lymphoma cells exhibit a high mitotic rate. (Hematoxylin and eosin stain)
Right: A bone marrow aspirate smear shows several lymphoma cells. The cells have coarse nuclear chromatin, one to three nucleoli, and deeply basophilic cytoplasm containing several sharply defined clear vacuoles. The morphology and immunophenotype of small noncleaved cell lymphoma is identical to acute lymphoblastic leukemia L3. (Wright-Giemsa stain) (Fig. 37.23 from McKenna RW. The bone marrow manifestations of Hodgkin's disease, the non-Hodgkin's lymphomas, and lymphoma-like disorders. In: Knowles DM, ed. Neoplastic hematopathology. Baltimore: Williams & Wilkins, 1992:1135–80.)

Small Noncleaved Cell Lymphomas. The incidence of marrow involvement by small noncleaved cell lymphomas varies from 0 to 57 percent in different studies (55,66,96). Many patients without initial involvement manifest marrow invasion later in their disease course. Similar to lymphoblastic lymphoma, the pattern is nearly always diffuse or interstitial and the extent of involvement varies from occasional scattered lymphoma cells to complete replacement of the bone marrow (39,55). Even with extensive involvement, the "starry sky" pattern, commonly observed in lymph nodes, is infrequent (39). There may be small foci or expansive areas of necrosis; in some cases the entire section consists of necrotic tissue. In bone marrow sections, the cells have round or oval nuclei with two to four small nucleoli. There is a distinct rim of cytoplasm and cell borders are sharply defined. Mitotic figures are numerous (fig. 449).

In aspirate smears, the cytology of the lymphoma cells is generally diagnostic. They are medium to large, with a round or oval nucleus containing reticular or slightly condensed chromatin. Nucleoli are generally small but may be multiple. There is a moderate amount of deeply basophilic cytoplasm which in most cases contains a variable number of sharply defined vacuoles (figs. 449, 450). The vacuoles stain with oil red 0.

A diagnosis of acute lymphoblastic leukemia L3 may be appropriate in cases where the bone marrow is the most obvious or only apparent site of involvement. A careful search in these instances will often reveal a tumor mass, usually in the abdominal cavity (39). L3 leukemia is morphologically, immunologically, and biologically identical to small noncleaved cell lymphoma (35) (see section, Acute Lymphoblastic Leukemia L3).

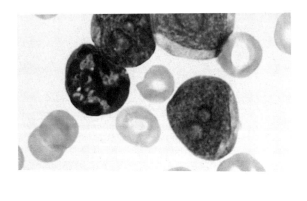

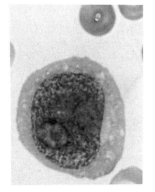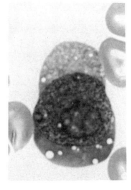

Figure 450
SMALL NONCLEAVED CELL
LYMPHOMA (NON-BURKITT TYPE)

A composite of lymphoma cells from a bone marrow aspirate from a 35-year-old male with AIDS and small noncleaved cell lymphoma (non-Burkitt type) (Wright-Giemsa stain)

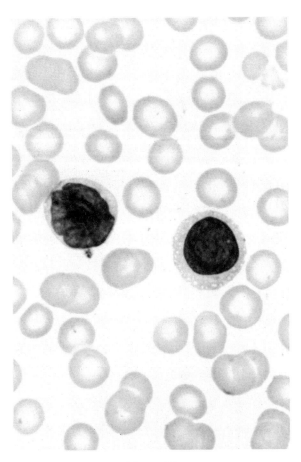

Figure 451
SÉZARY SYNDROME

A blood smear from a patient with Sézary syndrome shows two Sézary cells. (Wright-Giemsa stain)

Miscellaneous Lymphomas. *Cutaneous T-Cell Lymphomas.* These generally spare the bone marrow or manifest minimal involvement. Marrow disease has been identified in trephine biopsy sections in up to 20 percent of cases in one study (93). Nodules or interstitial infiltrates of lymphocytes with cerebriform nuclei are characteristic. The lesions are often subtle, without increased cellularity. Circulating cerebriform lymphocytes are nearly always identified in blood smears in cases with an infiltrative interstitial pattern of bone marrow involvement (figs. 451, 452) (93).

True Histiocytic Lymphomas. These are rare disorders. Most of the neoplasms diagnosed as histiocytic lymphomas in the past are now recognized as large cell anaplastic lymphomas of T or B lymphocytes or reactive histiocytic proliferations (92). Rare examples of malignant histiocytic proliferations in the bone marrow may

exist. These might be more aptly designated malignant histiocytosis. They must be distinguished from reactive histiocytic lesions.

Post-Therapy Bone Marrow and Minimal Residual Disease. Changes following chemotherapy vary for the different types of non-Hodgkin lymphoma. Bone marrow lesions in low-grade lymphomas diminish in size with response to chemotherapy but many do not completely resolve; detection of residual disease is relatively common. With some therapy protocols for follicular predominantly small cleaved lymphoma, the paratrabecular foci of lymphoma become progressively hypocellular and sometimes contain few or no small cleaved cells (84). The presence of these hypocellular paratrabecular foci does not necessarily

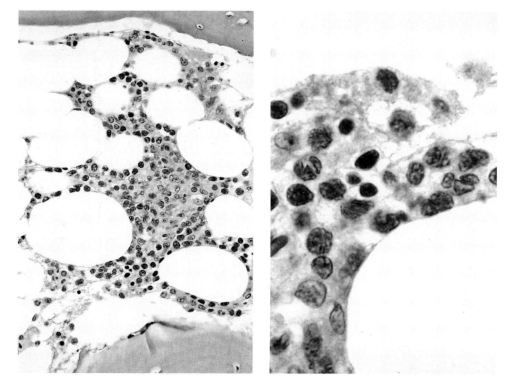

Figure 452
SÉZARY SYNDROME
A trephine biopsy section from a patient with Sézary syndrome. There was extensive organ infiltration and an elevated blood leukocyte count but only a few small foci of convoluted lymphocytes on the bone marrow section. (Hematoxylin and eosin stain)

indicate remission and has no predictive value for longer survival or cure (84). Reticulin fiber content is not significantly decreased in focal lesions even with response to therapy (97).

Complete resolution of bone marrow lesions is observed with response to chemotherapy for high-grade lymphomas. Necrotic tumor may be seen in the marrow biopsy following induction therapy. Repopulation of the marrow with normal hematopoietic tissue follows.

Bone marrow relapse is usually morphologically similar to the original lymphoma, however, transformation to a more aggressive histopathologic type may occur in some low-grade lymphomas. Early relapse or minimal residual marrow disease may be identified prior to morphologic detection by demonstrating clonality using immunophenotyping or immunogenetic analysis (52,59,73). The clinical significance and therapeutic approach for minimal residual disease detected by these techniques have not been clarified.

Immunologic and Immunohistochemical Findings. Immunophenotyping is an integral component of the diagnostic armamentarium for non-Hodgkin lymphoma. Bone marrow and blood specimens lend themselves particularly well to either flow cytometric or enzyme immunohistochemical analysis. These studies are important in establishing a lymphoma lineage as B cell or T cell, in distinguishing lymphomas from metastatic tumors, and in differentiating neoplastic and reactive bone marrow lymphoid lesions. There is presently an array of monoclonal and polyclonal antibodies available for recognizing lymphocyte-restricted and -associated antigens. An appropriate panel, including both B-cell and T-cell antigens, should be used. Numerous reviews of immunophenotyping techniques and the specific findings in non-Hodgkin lymphoma are available (30,40,44,47,48,59,71,103). Immunophenotypic findings in specific lymphoproliferative disorders are described throughout this text and will not be detailed here. The majority of non-Hodgkin lymphomas in the bone marrow express B-cell antigens, a smaller number type as T-cell lymphomas, and rare cases express neither B- or T-cell markers. Both B-cell and T-cell lymphomas may express an aberrant immunophenotype; immunophenotypic aberrancy is particularly common in peripheral T-cell lymphomas (59,63,103).

Ultrastructural Findings. Electron microscopy may occasionally contribute to the diagnosis or classification of bone marrow non-Hodgkin lymphoma. This is most likely when the bone marrow is the primary site of disease or other involved tissues are inaccessible to biopsy. Usually, a diagnosis of lymphoma will have been established; the ultrastructural findings provide additional information about the character of the lymphoma cells. Electron microscopy is of most practical value for characterizing small cell metastatic tumors in the bone marrow and differentiating them from lymphoma.

Low-Grade Lymphomas. The ultrastructural findings of small lymphocytic lymphomas are identical to those of chronic lymphocytic leukemia (40). The cells have round or slightly oval nuclei with condensed nuclear chromatin and inconspicuous nucleoli. The cytoplasm is sparse and contains scattered free ribosomes, a small Golgi region, a few mitochondria, and rare strands of rough endoplasmic reticulum (RER). Cytoplasmic inclusions are found in some cases. In the plasmacytoid variants, nuclear inclusions may be present. These inclusions, when observed by light microscopy, are actually invaginations of the perinuclear envelope. These are illustrated in the section on Waldenström macroglobulinemia, elsewhere in this Fascicle. The cytoplasm of the plasmacytoid lymphomas contains abundant RER, free ribosomes and polyribosomes, and a large Golgi region. Cytoplasmic inclusions of RER-bound globules or ribosome-lamella complexes may be observed (40) (see illustrations in sections, Chronic Lymphocytic and Hairy Cell Leukemias).

Follicular small cleaved cells often have deeply indented or cleaved nuclei and may appear to be bisected in ultrastructural studies (see fig. 436). The nuclear chromatin is condensed and nucleoli are small. Most cells have scant cytoplasm and contain scattered ribosomes and polyribosomes, a poorly developed Golgi area, scant RER, and a

few small granules. Transformed or large lymphoma cells that have round, indented, or cleaved nuclei with peripheral chromatin condensation and prominent nucleoli may be observed. The cytoplasm is more abundant than in the small cleaved cells and contains numerous ribosomes and several large mitochondria (40).

Intermediate-Grade Lymphomas. The diffuse small cleaved cell lymphomas show ultrastructural features similar to those described above for the follicular small cleaved cell lymphomas. The ultrastructure of the follicular and diffuse large cell lymphomas is similar. The lymphoma cells may have profound nuclear indentation and clefting; some appear to be segmented. The chromatin is condensed and peripherally distributed. Nucleoli are generally large and often multiple. In some cases the nuclei are round or oval, have evenly dispersed chromatin, and one or more large prominent nucleoli. The cytoplasm is moderately abundant and contains scattered or numerous mitochondria that may appear swollen, a small Golgi region, free ribosomes and polyribosomes, rare strands of RER, and occasional granules. Large single or scattered lipid vacuoles are observed in some cells and infrequently, cytoplasmic immunoglobulin inclusions are seen. Scattered small cleaved cells are present in many cases.

The ultrastructural features of the diffuse mixed small and large cell lymphomas reflect the variation observed with light microscopy (40). The peripheral T-cell lymphomas included in this category often consist of small, large, and intermediate cells with irregularly indented nuclei and heavily condensed peripheral chromatin with indistinct nucleoli. The cytoplasm contains large mitochondria, rare RER, a small Golgi region, and scattered granules, often with central densities encircled by a pale matrix.

High-Grade Lymphomas. The ultrastructure of the large cell immunoblastic lymphomas is characterized by round or oval nuclei with dispersed or peripherally marginated chromatin and large prominent nucleoli. The cytoplasm is generally abundant and contains free polyribosomes, RER, a prominent Golgi region, and large mitochondria. The cytoplasm in B-cell immunoblastic lymphomas frequently contains large amounts of RER, which may be dilated and contain inclusions; these have been shown to consist of immunoglobulin. Some of these inclusions occupy a large portion of the cytoplasm. Plasma cells and cells manifesting ultrastructural features intermediate between immunoblasts and plasma cells may be observed. T-cell immunoblasts may exhibit more nuclear irregularity, condensed chromatin, and prominent, often multiple, nucleoli.

Some cases of large cell immunoblastic lymphoma have multilobulated nuclei. The cells are very large and have an extremely irregular nuclear border. The chromatin is evenly dispersed and nucleoli are usually small. Nuclear blebing is often prominent. There is a moderate amount of cytoplasm with no distinctive characteristics.

The larger blasts in lymphoblastic lymphomas are characterized by nuclear irregularity, fine nuclear chromatin, and usually a single prominent nucleolus. The cytoplasm contains a large Golgi region, scattered small lysosomal granules, ribosomes, and occasional RER. Smaller lymphoblasts have less nuclear irregularity, peripherally condensed chromatin, and less conspicuous nucleoli. There is less cytoplasm than in the large lymphoblasts and a less prominent Golgi region. (See illustrations in the section, Acute Lymphoblastic Leukemia.)

Small noncleaved cell lymphomas are characterized by uniform ultrastructural features including round or oval nuclei containing moderately condensed chromatin, multiple prominent nucleoli, and a narrow rim of cytoplasm. The cytoplasm contains numerous free ribosomes and polyribosomes, and multiple large lipid vacuoles, corresponding to the cytoplasmic vacuoles observed with light microscopy. (See illustrations in the section, Acute Lymphoblastic Leukemia.)

Differential Diagnosis. Several benign conditions and lesions of undetermined biology may simulate non-Hodgkin lymphoma in the bone marrow. These include reactive lymphoid lesions, increased bone marrow lymphoid progenitor cells (hematogones), granulomas, angioimmunoblastic lymphadenopathy, idiopathic myelofibrosis, Langerhans cell histiocytosis, and mast cell disease. These are discussed in the following chapters. Neoplastic lesions of the bone marrow that may be considered in the differential diagnosis of non-Hodgkin lymphoma include hairy cell leukemia, transformation of chronic lymphocytic leukemia, prolymphocytic leukemia, malig-

nant histiocytosis, plasma cell myeloma, acute lymphoblastic leukemia, and metastatic tumors. Each of these is covered in detail elsewhere in this Fascicle and will be discussed here only in the context of the features that aid in their distinction from bone marrow lymphoma.

A differential diagnosis of hairy cell leukemia and non-Hodgkin lymphoma may arise in adult patients that present with splenomegaly and blood cytopenias. Hairy cell leukemia is most likely to be confused with small lymphocytic, intermediate lymphocytic, or small cleaved cell lymphoma. The diagnosis rests on the distinctive morphologic, cytochemical, and immunologic characteristics discussed in the section on hairy cell leukemia.

Transformation of chronic lymphocytic leukemia (Richter syndrome) may simulate lymphoma in bone marrow (36,53,69). When transformation occurs in a localized anatomic region a diagnosis of diffuse large cell lymphoma or Hodgkin disease may be considered. In some cases focal areas of a bone marrow trephine biopsy section may show transformation, with the remainder of the marrow typical of chronic lymphocytic leukemia (fig. 453). A history of chronic lymphocytic leukemia and its coexistence with a large cell lymphocyte proliferation should first raise suspicion of transformation rather than a second distinct lymphoproliferative disorder. Immunologic marker studies can help confirm a suspected diagnosis of transformation. The immunophenotype closely approximates that of the original chronic lymphocytic leukemia clone in approximately two thirds of cases; minor immunologic evolution may occur (36,53,69). A second clonally distinct lymphoproliferative disorder has been observed in some cases of chronic lymphocytic leukemia.

Prolymphocytic leukemia may infrequently be considered in the differential diagnosis. The presentation of a profoundly elevated leukocyte count and extensive marrow infiltration should distinguish this disorder from non-Hodgkin lymphoma (36,58). Atypical cases of prolymphocytic leukemia with unusually low leukocyte counts or lymphadenopathy may be problematic. A detailed discussion is found in the section on prolymphocytic leukemia.

In malignant histiocytosis the cells may be indistinguishable from the malignant cells of a large cell lymphoma in both biopsy sections and smears

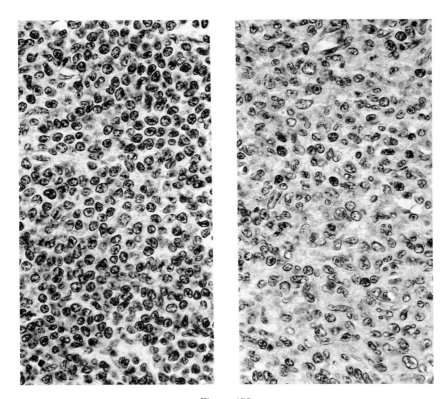

Figure 453
TRANSFORMATION OF CHRONIC LYMPHOCYTIC LEUKEMIA
A bone marrow biopsy section from a patient with a 5-year history of chronic lymphocytic leukemia.
Left: In this field the infiltrate consists of small lymphocytes typical of chronic lymphocytic leukemia.
Right: In this field of the same trephine biopsy section, the cells are larger with more dispersed chromatin. Some of the nuclei are irregular or angulated. Many have large prominent single nucleoli typical of prolymphocytes. (Hematoxylin and eosin stain) (Fig. 37.42 (right) from McKenna RW. The bone marrow manifestations of Hodgkin disease, the non-Hodgkin's lymphomas, and lymphoma-like disorders. In: Knowles DM, ed. Neoplastic hematopathology. Baltimore: Williams & Wilkins, 1992:1135–80.)

(38,64,101). Cytochemical reactions such as nonspecific esterase or immunohistochemical studies for lysosomal enzymes and surface antigens associated with the monocyte-macrophage system may reveal the histiocytic nature of the cells (64).

The bone marrow lesions in plasma cell myeloma are sometimes mistaken for lymphoma. Confusion is most likely when the plasma cell infiltrate is focal, associated with fibrosis, or composed of a very atypical plasma cell or a plasmablastic infiltrate (61) (see the section, Plasma Cell Myeloma). The distinction is made by careful assessment of the cytology of the cells on aspirate smears or trephine imprints and review of the laboratory findings including serum and urine immunoglobulin analysis. Enzyme immunohistochemical studies for immunoglobulin light and heavy chains on trephine biopsy sections show a monoclonal staining pattern in the cytoplasm of the plasma cells in cases of myeloma (88).

Distinguishing acute lymphoblastic leukemia from lymphoblastic lymphoma and small noncleaved cell lymphoma is somewhat arbitrary. In the case of lymphoblastic lymphoma, the designation is usually based on the extent of bone marrow disease and extramedullary tissue masses. If there are less than 25 percent lymphoblasts in the marrow at the time of presentation, lymphoblastic lymphoma is the preferred diagnosis. In cases with greater than 25 percent bone marrow blasts and extensive extramedullary disease, the designation lymphoblastic leukemia-lymphoma is often used. Most of the cases in which the marrow is initially spared or minimally involved have a T-cell immunophenotype. Small noncleaved cell lymphomas correspond cytologically to B-cell (SIg+) acute lymphoblastic leukemia

L3. The designation L3 leukemia is usually reserved for those cases with extensive bone marrow and blood involvement at presentation and relatively minimal extramedullary disease.

Several metastatic tumors may present with bone marrow involvement. Rarely, the initial tissue available for diagnosis is from a bone marrow trephine biopsy and aspirate smear (56,57). The cytologic features of some metastatic solid tissue tumors may resemble lymphoma in marrow smears and occasionally in trephine biopsy sections. In children, the clinical presentation and morphology of neuroblastoma, embryonal rhabdomyosarcoma, retinoblastoma, Ewing sarcoma, and medulloblastoma may simulate lymphoblastic lymphoma or occasionally, small noncleaved cell lymphoma (see section, Metastatic Tumors Involving the Bone Marrow). In adults, small cell carcinoma, melanoma and, less commonly, other carcinomas may resemble lymphoma in marrow biopsies.

The necessity to distinguish one of these tumors from lymphoma usually arises when a primary tissue mass is not identified and the patient is initially evaluated for blood cytopenias or a leukoerythroblastic reaction. In marrow aspirate smears, metastatic tumor cells will generally be found in clumps or clusters; large numbers of damaged tumor cells and bare nuclei may be observed throughout the smear. Occasionally, the neoplastic cells in small cell tumors in children are spread evenly on the smear as single cells with few or no clumps. When this occurs, the morphologic distinction from lymphoma or leukemia may be difficult. The trephine biopsy sections may show histologic features distinctive of the metastatic tumor. In equivocal cases terminal deoxynucleotidyltransferase (TdT) assays, immunophenotyping, electron microscopy, or enzyme immunohistochemistry may be necessary.

Immunohistochemistry using antibodies for the characterization of various metastatic tumors is particularly helpful for distinguishing lymphoma from a solid tissue tumor.

Treatment and Prognosis. Treatment protocols and prognosis differ according to the stage of disease and the lymphoma grades of the Working Formulation Classification (60). The presence of bone marrow involvement always indicates disseminated disease (stage IV). Most patients with low-grade lymphomas present with bone marrow involvement but do not necessarily require therapy if symptomatology is minimal. There appears to be no survival advantage with early chemotherapy in this group. When treatment is indicated, various standard chemotherapy protocols are used and there are minimal differences in survival among them. The median survival period for low-grade lymphomas is 5 to 11 years (60).

Patients with intermediate- or high-grade lymphomas with bone marrow involvement are generally treated with one of an array of available multiagent chemotherapy protocols. Overall, complete remission rates for intermediate-grade and large cell lymphomas are between 72 and 84 percent with newer treatment regimens and long-term survival is achieved in 48 to 65 percent (60). For patients with bone marrow involvement, however, both remission rates and long-term survival are less impressive. Results are also poorer for high-grade lymphomas, but long-term remissions and cures are achieved in some patients. Bone marrow transplantation has been curative in selected patients.

Several prognostic indicators have been identified for non-Hodgkin lymphomas (60). Bone marrow involvement is an unfavorable factor in prognosis and negatively affects survival in all grades of lymphoma.

REFERENCES

Hodgkin Disease

1. Andrade RE, Wick MR, Frizzera G, Gajl-Peczalska KJ. Immunophenotyping of hematopoietic malignancies in paraffin sections. Hum Pathol 1988;19:394–402.

2. Bartl R, Frisch B, Burkhardt R, Huhn D, Pappenberger R. Assessment of bone marrow histology in Hodgkin's disease: correlation with clinical factors. Br J Haematol 1984;51:345–60.

3. Brunning RD, Bloomfield CD, McKenna RW, Peterson LA. Bilateral trephine bone marrow biopsies in lymphoma and other neoplastic diseases. Ann Intern Med 1975;82:365–66.

4. _____, McKenna RW. Bone marrow manifestations of malignant lymphoma and lymphoma-like conditions. Pathol Annual 1979;14(Pt 1):1–59.

5. Burke JS. Hodgkin's disease: histopathology and differential diagnosis. In: Knowles DM, ed. Neoplastic hematopathology. Baltimore: Williams & Wilkins, 1992:497–533.

6. Colon-Otero G, McClure SP, Phyliky RL, White WL, Banks PM. Peripheral T-cell lymphoma simulating Hodgkin's disease with initial bone marrow involvement. Mayo Clin Proc 1986;61:68–71.

7. Ellis ME, Diehl LF, Granger E, Elson E. Trephine needle bone marrow biopsy in the initial staging of Hodgkin's disease: sensitivity and specificity of the Ann Arbor staging procedure criteria. Am J Hematol 1989;30:115–20.

8. Eyre HJ. Hodgkin's disease. In: Lee GR, Bithell TC, Foerster J, Athens JW, Lukens JN, eds. Wintrobe's clinical hematology. 9th ed. Philadelphia: Lea & Febiger, 1993:2054–81.

9. Gottlieb CA, Maeda K, Hawley RC, Abraham JP. Myelodysplasia with bone marrow lymphocytosis and fibrosis mimicking recurrent Hodgkin's disease. Am J Clin Pathol 1989;91:6–11.

10. Hanson CA, Brunning RD, Gajl-Peczalska KJ, Frizzera G, McKenna RW. Bone marrow manifestations of peripheral T-cell lymphoma. A study of 30 cases. Am J Clin Pathol 1986;86:449–60.

11. Jacquillat C, Auclerc G, Auclerc MF, Andrieu JM, Weil M, Bernard J. Hodgkin's disease: characteristics and prognosis of forms with initial bone marrow involvement. Nouv Presse Med 1981;10:95–100.

12. Kubic VL, Brunning RD. Immunohistochemical evaluation of neoplasms in bone marrow biopsies using monoclonal antibodies reactive in paraffin-embedded tissue. Mod Pathol 1989;2:618–29.

13. Lukes RJ, Butler JJ, Hicks EB. The natural history of Hodgkin's disease as related to its pathologic picture. Cancer 1966;19:317–44.

14. _____, Craver LF, Hall TC, Rappaport H, Ruben P. Report of the nomenclature committee. Cancer Res 1966;26:1311.

15. McKenna RW, Bloomfield CD, Brunning RD. Nodular lymphoma: bone marrow and blood manifestations. Cancer 1975;36:428–40.

16. _____, Brunning RD. Reed-Sternberg-like cells in nodular lymphoma involving the bone marrow. Am J Clin Pathol 1975;63:779–85.

17. Musshoff K. Prognostic and therapeutic implications of staging in extranodal Hodgkin's disease. Cancer Res 1971;31:1814–27.

18. Myers CE, Chabner BA, DeVita VT, Gralnick HR. Bone marrow involvement in Hodgkin's disease: pathology and response to MOPP chemotherapy. Blood 1974;44:197–204.

19. Neiman RS, Rosen PJ, Lukes RJ. Lymphocyte-depletion Hodgkin's disease. A clinicopathologic entity. N Engl J Med 1973;288:751–5.

20. O'Carroll DI, McKenna RW, Brunning RD. Bone marrow manifestations of Hodgkin's disease. Cancer 1976;38:1717–28.

21. Osborne BM, Butler JJ. Hypocellular paratrabecular foci of treated small cleaved cell lymphoma in bone marrow biopsies. Am J Surg Pathol 1989;13:382–8.

22. Rappaport H, Berard CW, Butler JJ, Dorfman RF, Lukes RJ, Thomas LB. Report of the Committee on Histopathological Criteria Contributing to Staging of Hodgkin's Disease. Cancer Res 1971;31:1864–5.

23. Ries LA, Hankey BF, Miller BA, Hartman AM, Edwards BK. Cancer statistics review, 1973–1988. National Cancer Institute. NIH Pub. No. 91–2789, 1991.

24. Rosenberg SA. Hodgkin's disease of the bone marrow. Cancer Res 1971;31:1733–6.

25. Specht L, Nissen NI. Prognostic factors in Hodgkin's disease stage IV. Eur J Haematol 1988;41:359–67.

26. Spiro S, Galton DA, Wiltshaw E, Lohmann RC. Follicular lymphoma: a study of 75 cases with special reference to the syndrome resembling chronic lymphocytic leukaemia. Br J Cancer 1975;31(Suppl 2):60–72.

27. Strum SB, Park JK, Rappaport H. Observation of cells resembling Sternberg-Reed cells in conditions other than Hodgkin's disease. Cancer 1970;26:176–90.

28. Te velde J, den Ottolander GJ, Spaander PJ, Van Den Berg C, Hartgrink-Groeneveld CA. The bone marrow in Hodgkin's disease: the non-involved marrow. Histopathology 1978;2:31–46.

29. White DM, Smith AG, Whitehouse JM, Smith JL. Peripheral T cell lymphoma: value of bone marrow trephine immunophenotyping. J Clin Pathol 1989;42:403–8.

Non-Hodgkin Lymphomas

30. Andrade RE, Wick MR, Frizzera G, Gajl-Peczalska KJ. Immunophenotyping of hematopoietic malignancies in paraffin sections. Hum Pathol 1988;19:394–402.

31. Auger MJ, Nash JR, Mackie MJ. Marrow involvement with T cell lymphoma initially presenting as abnormal myelopoiesis. J Clin Pathol 1986;39:134–7.

32. Barcos MP, Lukes RJ. Malignant lymphoma of convoluted lymphocytes: a new entity of possible T-cell type. In: Sinks LF, Godden JO, eds. Conflicts in childhood cancer: an evaluation of current management. New York: Alan R. Liss, 1975:147–78.

33. Bartl R, Hansmann ML, Frisch B, Burkhardt R. Comparative histology of malignant lymphomas in lymph node and bone marrow. Br J Haematol 1988;69:229–37.

34. Bennett JM, Cain KC, Glick JH, Johnson GJ, Ezdinli E, O'Connell MJ. The significance of bone marrow involvement in non-Hodgkin's lymphoma: the Eastern Cooperative Oncology Group experience. J Clin Oncol 1986;4:1462–9.

35. _____, Catovsky D, Daniel MT, et al. Proposals for the classification of the acute leukaemias. French-American-British (FAB) cooperative group. Br J Haematol 1976;33:451–8.

36. _____, Catovsky D, Daniel MT, et al. Proposals for the classification of chronic (mature) B and T lymphoid leukaemias. French-American-British (FAB) Cooperative Group. J Clin Pathol 1989;42:567–84.

37. Berard CW. Reticuloendothelial system: an overview of neoplasia. In: Rebuck JW, Berard CW, Abell MR, eds. The reticuloendothelial system. Baltimore: Williams & Wilkins, 1975:301–17. (International Academy of Pathology Monograph, No. 16).

38. Brunning RD, McKenna RW. Bone marrow manifestations of malignant lymphoma and lymphoma-like conditions. Pathol Annual 1979;14(Pt 1):1–59.

39. _____, McKenna RW, Bloomfield CD, Coccia P, Gail-Peczalska KJ. Bone marrow involvement in Burkitt's lymphoma. Cancer 1977;40:1771–9.

40. _____, Parkin JL, Hanson CA. Hematopoietic and lymphoreticular neoplasms. In: Azar HA, ed. Pathology of human neoplasms: an atlas of diagnostic electron microscopy and immunohistochemistry. New York: Raven Press, 1988:221–303.

41. Carbone A, Gloghini A, Pinto A, Attadia V, Zagonel V, Volpe R. Monocytoid B-cell lymphoma with bone marrow and peripheral blood involvement at presentation. Am J Clin Pathol 1989;92:228–36.

42. _____, Poletti A, Manconi R, et al. Intermediate lymphocytic lymphoma encompassing diffuse and mantle zone pattern variants. A distinct entity among low grade lymphomas? Eur J Cancer Clin Oncol 1989;25:113–21.

43. Caulet S, Delmer A, Audouin J, et al. Histopathological study of bone marrow biopsies in 30 cases of T-cell lymphoma with clinical, biological and survival correlations. Hematol Oncol 1990;8:155–68.

44. Chilosi M, Pizzolo G, Fiore-Donati L, Bofill M, Janossy G. Routine immunofluorescent and histochemical analysis of bone marrow involvement of lymphoma/leukaemia: the use of cryostat sections. Br J Cancer 1983;48:763–75.

45. Colon-Otero G, McClure SP, Phyliky RL, White WL, Banks PM. Peripheral T-cell lymphoma simulating Hodgkin's disease with initial bone marrow involvement. Mayo Clin Proc 1986;61:68–71.

46. Conlan MG, Bast M, Armitage JO, Weisenburger DD. Bone marrow involvement by non-Hodgkin's lymphoma: the clinical significance of morphologic discordance between the lymph node and bone marrow. Nebraska Lymphoma Study Group. J Clin Oncol 1990;8:1163–72.

47. Cossman J, Chused TM, Fisher RI, Magrath I, Bollum F, Jaffe ES. Diversity of immunologic phenotypes of lymphoblastic lymphoma. Cancer Res 1983;43:4486–90.

48. Cousar JB, Glick AD, York JC, Miers M, Collins RD. Peripheral blood and bone marrow involvement by non-Hodgkin's lymphoma: morphological, immunological and cytochemical features. Prog Clin Pathol 1984;9:173–96.

49. De Oliveira MS, Jaffe ES, Catovsky D. Leukaemic phase of mantle zone (intermediate) lymphoma: its characterization in 11 cases. J Clin Pathol 1989;42:962–72.

50. Dick F, Bloomfield CD, Brunning RD. Incidence, cytology and histopathology of non-Hodgkin's lymphomas in the bone marrow. Cancer 1974;33:1382–98.

51. Ellis ME, Diehl LF, Granger E, Elson E. Trephine needle bone marrow biopsy in the initial staging of Hodgkin's disease: sensitivity and specificity of the Ann Arbor staging procedure criteria. Am J Hematol 1989;30:115–20.

52. Ellison DJ, Hu E, Zovich D, Pinter-Brown L, Pattengale PK. Immunogenetic analysis of bone marrow aspirates in patients with non-Hodgkin lymphomas. Am J Hematol 1990;33:160–6.

53. Enno A, Catovsky D, O'Brien M, Cherchi M, Kumaran TO, Galton DA. Prolymphocytoid transformation of chronic lymphocytic leukemia. Br J Haematol 1979;41:9–18.

54. Fisher DE, Jacobson JO, Ault KA, Harris NL. Diffuse large cell lymphoma with discordant bone marrow histology. Clinical features and biological implications. Cancer 1989;64:1879–87.

55. Foucar K, McKenna RW, Frizzera G, Brunning RD. Bone marrow and blood involvement by lymphoma in relationship to the Lukes-Collins classification. Cancer 1982;49:888–97.

56. Frisch B, Bartl R, Mahl G, Burkhardt R. Scope and value of bone marrow biopsies in metastatic cancer. Invasion Metastasis 1984;4(Suppl 1):12–30.

57. Gale PF, McKenna RW. Monitoring metastasis in bone marrow. In: Stoll BA, ed. Screening and monitoring of cancer. Chichester, England: John Wiley and Sons, 1985:265–83.

58. Galton DA, Goldman JM, Wiltshaw E, Catovsky D, Henry K, Goldenberg GJ. Prolymphocytic leukaemia. Br J Haematol 1974;27:7–23.

59. Gaulard P, Kanavaros P, Farcet JP, et al. Bone marrow histologic and immunohistochemical findings in peripheral T cell lymphoma: a study of 38 cases. Hum Pathol 1991;22:331–8.

60. Greer JD, Macon WR, List AF, McCurley TL. Non-Hodgkin's lymphomas (NHL). In: Lee GR, Bithell TC, Foerster J, Athens JW, Lukens JN, eds. Wintrobe's clinical hematology. 9th ed. Philadelphia: Lea and Febiger, 1993:2082–142.

61. Greipp PR, Raymond NM, Kyle RA, O'Fallon WM. Multiple myeloma: significance of plasmablastic subtype in morphological classification. Blood 1985;65:305–10.

62. Haddy TB, Parker RI, Magrath IT. Bone marrow involvement in young patients with non-Hodgkin's lymphoma: the importance of multiple bone marrow samples for accurate staging. Med Pediatr Oncol 1989; 17:418–23.

63. Hanson CA, Brunning RD, Gajl-Peczalska KJ, Frizzera G, McKenna RW. Bone marrow manifestations of peripheral T-cell lymphoma. A study of 30 cases. Am J Clin Pathol 1986;86:449–60.

64. Jaffe ES. Histiocytoses of lymph nodes: biology and differential diagnosis. Semin Diagn Pathol 1988; 5:376–90.

65. _____, Bookman MA, Longo DL. Lymphocytic lymphoma of intermediate differentiation—mantle zone lymphoma: a distinct subtype of B-cell lymphoma. Hum Pathol 1987;18:877–80.

66. Jones SE, Rosenberg SA, Kaplan HS. Non-Hodgkin's lymphomas. I. Bone marrow involvement. Cancer 1972; 29:954–60.

67. Juneja SK, Wolf MM, Cooper IA. Value of bilateral bone marrow biopsy specimens in non-Hodgkin's lymphoma. J Clin Pathol 1990;43:630–2.

68. Karcher DS, Frost AR. The bone marrow in human immunodeficiency virus (HIV)-related disease. Morphology and clinical correlation. Am J Clin Pathol 1991;95:63–71.

69. Kjeldsberg CR, Marty J. Prolymphocytoid transformation of chronic lymphocytic leukemia. Cancer 1981;58:2447–57.

70. Kluin PM, van Krieken JH, Kleiverda K, Kluin-Nelemans HC. Discordant morphologic characteristics of B-cell lymphomas in bone marrow and lymph node biopsies. Am J Clin Pathol 1990;94:59–66.

71. Kubic VL, Brunning RD. Immunohistochemical evaluation of neoplasms in bone marrow biopsies using monoclonal antibodies reactive in paraffin-embedded tissue. Mod Pathol 1989;2:618–29.

72. Lai HS, Tien HF, Hsieh HC, et al. Bone marrow involvement in non-Hodgkin's lymphoma. Taiwan I Hsueh Hui Tsa Chih 1989;88:114–21.

73. Liang R, Chan VV, Chan TK, Todd D, Ho F. Immunoglobulin gene rearrangement in the peripheral blood and bone marrow of patients with lymphomas of the mucosa-associated lymphoid tissues. Acta Haematol 1990;84:19–23.

74. Ligler FS, Smith RG, Kettman JR, et al. Detection of tumor cells in the peripheral blood of nonleukemic patients with B-cell lymphoma: analysis of "clonal excess". Blood 1980;55:792–801.

75. Lukes RJ, Collins RD. A functional classification of malignant lymphomas. In: The reticuloendothelial system. JW Rebuck, CW Berard, MR Abel, eds. Baltimore: Williams & Wilkins, 1975:213–42.

76. McKenna RW. The bone marrow manifestations of Hodgkin's disease, the non-Hodgkin lymphomas, and lymphoma-like disorders. In: Knowles DM, ed. Neoplastic hematopathology. Baltimore: Williams & Wilkins, 1992:1135–80.

77. _____, Bloomfield CD, Brunning RD. Nodular lymphoma: bone marrow and blood manifestations. Cancer 1975;36:428–40.

78. _____, Brunning RD. Reed-Sternberg-like cells in nodular lymphoma involving the bone marrow. Am J Clin Pathol 1975;63:779–85.

79. _____, Parkin J, Brunning RD. Morphological and ultrastructural characteristics of T-cell acute lymphoblastic leukemia. Cancer 1979;44:1290–7.

80. Mead JH, Mason TE. Lymphoma versus AIDS [Letter]. Am J Clin Pathol 1983;80:546–7.

81. Nathwani BN, Kim H, Rappaport H. Malignant lymphoma, lymphoblastic. Cancer 1976;38:964–83.

82. _____, Mohrman BL, Brynes RK, Taylor CR, Hansmann ML, Sheibani K. Monocytoid B-cell lymphomas: an assessment of diagnostic criteria and a perspective on histogenesis. Hum Pathol 1992;23:1061–71.

83. National Cancer Institute sponsored study of classifications of non-Hodgkin's lymphomas: summary and description of a working formulation for clinical usage. The Non-Hodgkin's Lymphoma Pathologic Classification Project. Cancer 1982;49:2112–35.

84. Osborne BM, Butler JJ. Hypocellular paratrabecular foci of treated small cleaved cell lymphoma in bone marrow biopsies. Am J Surg Pathol 1989;13:382–8.

85. _____, Guarda LA, Butler JJ. Bone marrow biopsies in patients with the acquired immunodeficiency syndrome. Hum Pathol 1984;15:1048–53.

86. Pangalis GA, Nathwani BN, Rappaport H. Malignant lymphoma, well differentiated lymphocytic: its relationship with chronic lymphocytic leukemia and macroglobulinemia of Waldenström. Cancer 1977;39:999–1010.

87. Perry DA, Bast MA, Armitage JO, Weisenburger DD. Diffuse intermediate lymphocytic lymphoma. A clinicopathologic study and comparison with small lymphocytic lymphoma and diffuse small cleaved cell lymphoma. Cancer 1990;66:1995–2000.

88. Peterson LC, Brown BA, Crosson JT, Mladenovic J. Application of the immunoperoxidase technic to bone marrow trephine biopsies in the classification of patients with monoclonal gammopathies. Am J Clin Pathol 1986;85:688–93.

89. Pond GD, Castellino RA, Horning S, Hoppe RT. Non-Hodgkin lymphoma: influence of lymphography, CT, and bone marrow biopsy on staging and management. Radiology 1989;170(1 Pt 1):159–64.

90. Rappaport H. Tumors of the hematopoietic system. Atlas of Tumor Pathology, 1st Series, Fascicle 8. Washington, D.C.: Armed Forces Institute of Pathology, 1966.

91. Ries LA, Hankey BF, Miller BA, Hartman AM, Edwards BK. Cancer statistics review, 1973–1988. National Cancer Institute. NIH Pub. No. 91–2789, 1991.

92. Risdall RJ, McKenna RW, Nesbit ME, et al. Virus-associated hemophagocytic syndrome: a benign histiocytic proliferation distinct from malignant histiocytosis. Cancer 1979;44:993–1002.

93. Salhany KE, Greer JP, Cousar JB, Collins RD. Marrow involvement in cutaneous T-cell lymphoma. A clinicopathologic study of 60 cases. Am J Clin Pathol 1989;92:747–54.

94. Sheibani K, Burke J, Swartz W, Nademanee A, Winberg C. Monocytoid B cell lymphoma: clinicopathologic study of 21 cases of a unique type of low grade lymphoma. Cancer 1988;62:1531–8.

95. Spiro S, Galton DA, Wiltshaw E, Lohmann RC. Follicular lymphoma: a study of 75 cases with special reference to the syndrome resembling chronic lymphocytic leukaemia. Br J Cancer 1975;31(Suppl 2):60–72.

96. Stein RS, Ultmann JE, Byrne GE Jr, Moran EM, Golomb HM, Oetzel N. Bone marrow involvement in non-Hodgkin's lymphoma: implications for staging and therapy. Cancer 1976;37:629–36.

97. Thiele J, Langohr J, Skorupka M, Fischer R. Reticulin fibre content of bone marrow infiltrates of malignant non-Hodgkin's lymphomas (B-cell type, low malignancy)—a morphometric evaluation before and after therapy. Virchows Arch [A] 1990;417:485–92.

98. Traweek ST, Sheibani K. Regarding the article entitled "Monocytoid B-cell lymphoma with bone marrow and peripheral blood involvement at presentation" [Letter]. Am J Clin Pathol 1990;94:117–8.

99. Uchiyama T, Yodoi J, Sagawa K, Takatsuki K, Uchino H. Adult T-cell leukemia: clinical and hematologic features of 16 cases. Blood 1977;50:481–92.

100. Waldron JA, Leech JH, Glick AD, Flexner JM, Collins RD. Malignant lymphoma of peripheral T-lymphocyte origin: immunologic, pathologic, and clinical features in six patients. Cancer 1977;40:1604–17.

101. Warnke RA, Kim H, Dorfman RF. Malignant histiocytosis (histiocytic medullary reticulosis). I. Clinicopathologic study of 29 cases. Cancer 1975;35:215–30.

102. Weisenburger DD, Duggan MJ, Perry DA, Sanger WG, Armitage JO. Non-Hodgkin's lymphomas of mantle zone origin. Pathol Annu 1991;26(Pt 1):139–58.

103. White DM, Smith AG, Whitehouse JM, Smith JL. Peripheral T cell lymphoma: value of bone marrow trephine immunophenotyping. J Clin Pathol 1989;42:403–8.

LESIONS SIMULATING LYMPHOMA AND MISCELLANEOUS TUMOR-LIKE LESIONS IN THE BONE MARROW

There are several neoplastic and reactive conditions that may simulate lymphoma in the bone marrow in their clinical presentation and pathologic changes. The neoplastic disorders have been discussed in the section on differential diagnosis of bone marrow lymphoma and detailed in other sections of this Fascicle. This section will deal with benign conditions and lesions of undetermined biology that commonly mimic lymphoma in the bone marrow. These disorders include reactive lymphoid lesions, increased bone marrow lymphocyte progenitor cells (hematogones), granulomas, and angioimmunoblastic lymphadenopathy.

BENIGN-REACTIVE LYMPHOID LESIONS

Definition. Non-neoplastic focal lymphocyte proliferations in the bone marrow. They may be found in association with an array of diseases and in healthy individuals.

Incidence and Clinical Findings. Reactive lymphoid lesions have been identified in 18 to 47 percent of bone marrow biopsy specimens (14,17,18,23). They are particularly common in geriatric patients and increase in frequency after age 50; they are slightly more common in women. They are found in patients with a variety of unrelated disorders as well as in healthy persons (3,22,23). In the geriatric population reactive lymphoid lesions are not associated with any particular disease and are of unknown clinical significance. In young individuals they are often associated with an immune disorder or inflammatory process (22,23).

Laboratory Findings. There are no specific laboratory findings associated with reactive lymphocytic lesions of the bone marrow, but abnormal laboratory studies may point to an underlying disease process in some cases.

Blood and Bone Marrow Findings. There are no changes in blood counts or blood smear morphology specifically related to these lesions. Changes in the blood usually reflect an associated disease process.

Bone marrow aspirate smears may be normal, reflect changes of an underlying disease, or show increased lymphocytes and other reactive cells. The lymphocytes have mature cytologic features. A spectrum of morphology, from relatively uniform, small and medium sized lymphocytes to a more heteromorphous proliferation with reactive lymphocytes, may be observed. Increased histiocytes, mast cells, and plasma cells are present in some cases. The spectrum of lymphocytes and other reactive cells may be best appreciated in particle crush preparations, where sheets of lymphocytes may occupy a large portion of the smear.

Histopathologic Findings. In trephine biopsy sections, reactive lymphoid lesions range from 50 to 1,000 μm in diameter and vary in number from a solitary focus on one section to several on each section. They are randomly distributed in the bone marrow without a paratrabecular predilection. Three general morphologic types have been described: lymphocytic aggregates, polymorphous lymphohistiocytic lesions, and germinal centers.

The most common benign lymphoid lesions in the bone marrow are *lymphocytic aggregates*. These are relatively small, round to oval, well-circumscribed, and clearly demarcated from the surrounding marrow. Small blood vessels or endothelia are often present in these lesions. The cellular components are loosely arranged and consist of well-differentiated lymphocytes of varying size (fig. 454). Histiocytes, plasma cells, mast cells, and eosinophils may be present (1,6,18,23). These lesions are commonly encountered in bone marrow biopsies from older individuals but may be found in all age groups. There is no association with a specific disease process. Their significance is unknown.

Reactive polymorphous lymphohistiocytic lesions are less common and differ from the lymphocytic aggregates described above in several respects. They are polycellular, consisting of a heteromorphous population of lymphocytes including small lymphocytes, transformed lymphocytes, lymphocytes with irregular nuclei,

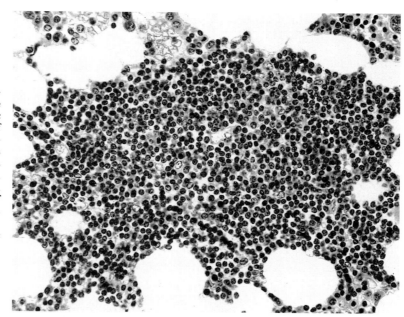

Figure 454
LYMPHOCYTIC AGGREGATE

A trephine biopsy section from a 72-year-old woman with carcinoma of the breast. A well-circumscribed lymphocytic aggregate composed predominantly of well-differentiated lymphocytes is illustrated. Lymphocytic aggregates of this nature are common incidental findings in geriatric patients. (Hematoxylin and eosin stain) (Fig. 37.27 from McKenna RW. The bone marrow manifestations of Hodgkin's disease, the non-Hodgkin's lymphomas, and lymphoma-like disorders. In: Knowles DM, ed. Neoplastic hematopathology. Baltimore: Williams & Wilkins, 1992:1135–80.)

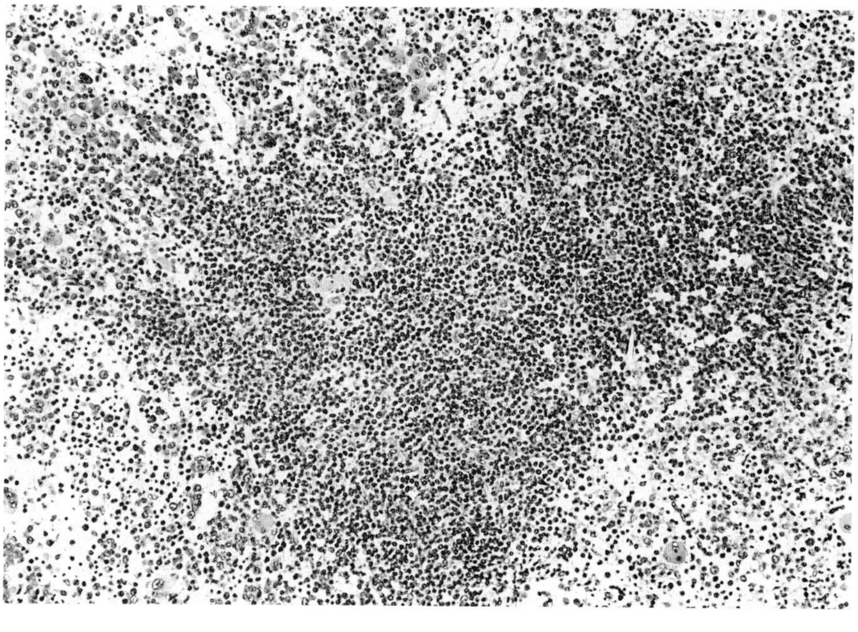

Figure 455
REACTIVE
POLYMORPHOUS
LYMPHOHISTIOCYTIC
LESION

Trephine biopsy section from a 26-year-old male with chronic immune-mediated blood cytopenias. There were several reactive polymorphous lymphohistiocytic lesions in the marrow sections. This lesion is large and has irregular margins. (Hematoxylin and eosin stain) (Fig. 37.29 from McKenna RW. The bone marrow manifestations of Hodgkin's disease, the non-Hodgkin's lymphomas, and lymphoma-like disorders. In: Knowles DM, ed. Neoplastic hematopathology. Baltimore: Williams & Wilkins, 1992:1135–80.)

plasma cells, epithelioid histiocytes, eosinophils, mast cells, and endothelial cells. They may be multiple, have poorly defined margins, and occupy relatively large portions of bone marrow in contradistinction to lymphocytic aggregates (figs. 455, 456) (2,7,13,19,21,24). These florid polymorphous lymphohistiocytic lesions are commonly observed in the bone marrow of patients with immune disorders such as the acquired immune deficiency syndrome (AIDS) and rheumatoid arthritis (2,7,13,19,21–24).

Germinal centers are the least common of the three reactive lymphoid lesions in the bone marrow. They are randomly distributed and are often single on a trephine section. They consist of a mantle of small lymphocytes encircling a distinct germinal center composed of various large transformed lymphocytes, scattered histiocytes, and frequent mitotic figures (fig. 457) (1,9). These are most common in young patients and are often associated with an immune or inflammatory disorder.

410

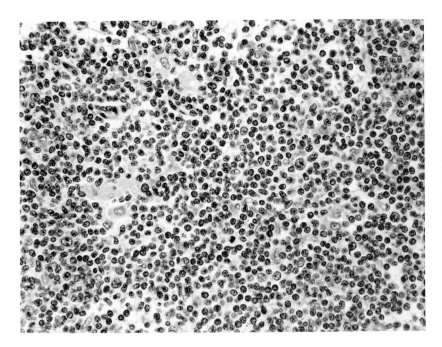

Figure 456
REACTIVE
POLYMORPHOUS
LYMPHOHISTIOCYTIC
LESION

A higher magnification of the lesion illustrated in figure 455 shows predominantly small lymphocytes with scattered transformed lymphocytes, histiocytes, and endothelium. Florid reactive lesions of this type may be mistaken for a malignant lymphoma. (Hematoxylin and eosin stain)

Figure 457
GERMINAL CENTER
IN A REACTIVE
LYMPHOCYTIC LESION

A bone marrow trephine biopsy section from a child with juvenile rheumatoid arthritis. A well-circumscribed reactive lymphoid lesion with a germinal center is illustrated (left). A mantle zone of small lymphocytes encircles the germinal center which consists of large lymphocytes; several are in mitosis (right). (Hematoxylin and eosin stain) (Fig. 37.28 from McKenna RW. The bone marrow manifestations of Hodgkin's disease, the non-Hodgkin's lymphomas, and lymphoma-like disorders. In: Knowles DM, ed. Neoplastic hematopathology. Baltimore: Williams & Wilkins, 1992:1135–80.)

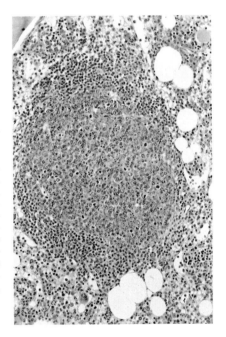
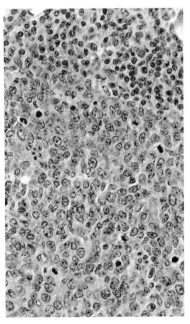

Differential Diagnosis. The reactive lymphoid lesions in the bone marrow are most significant because of their morphologic similarity to some of the malignant lymphomas. In the right clinical context they can be misinterpreted as bone marrow involvement by a lymphoma. This is most problematic in staging biopsies and in following patients with a diagnosis of lymphoma. A serious diagnostic dilemma may occasionally be encountered when florid reactive lymphoid lesions are found in marrow biopsies from patients undergoing evaluation for blood cytopenias, constitutional symptoms, or a poorly accessible tumor. Criteria for distinguishing reactive

Table 35

DISTINCTION BETWEEN BENIGN (REACTIVE) LYMPHOCYTIC LESIONS AND MALIGNANT LYMPHOMA IN BONE MARROW SECTIONS*

Benign	Malignant
Random distribution	Frequently paratrabecular
Usually well circumscribed	Often irregular shape with infiltration into adjacent marrow
Polymorphous cellularity with small lymphocytes, plasma cells, transformed lymphocytes, immunoblasts, histiocytes, and endothelial cells; cellular atypia is less common	Usually homogeneous, may be foci of transformation in small lymphocytic lymphomas; cellular atypia (cleaved or convoluted nuclei, nucleoli, etc.) in small cleaved and mixed lymphomas
Vascularity is frequently prominent	Vascularity is not usually prominent (except in Hodgkin disease and peripheral T-cell lymphomas)
Germinal centers are occasionally present	Germinal centers are not present
No lymphoma cells are present in marrow smears and imprints	Lymphoma cells may be present in smears and imprints

* Table 1 from McKenna RW. Disorders of bone marrow. In: Sternberg SS, ed. Diagnostic surgical pathology, Vol 1. New York: Raven Press, 1989:479–513.

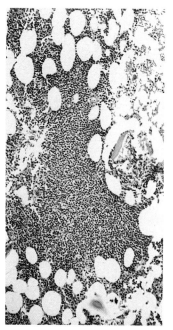 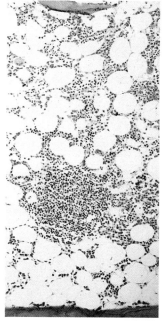

Figure 458
SMALL LYMPHOCYTIC LYMPHOMA CONTRASTED WITH A BENIGN LYMPHOCYTIC AGGREGATE

Trephine biopsy sections contrasting focal involvement with a small lymphocytic lymphoma (left) and a benign lymphoid aggregate (right). Focal lymphoma lesions are usually more abundant, larger, and often irregular in shape and infiltrate the adjacent marrow. The cell composition in lymphoma is usually more homogeneous and compact. (Fig. 21 from McKenna RW. Disorders of bone marrow. In: Sternberg SS, ed. Diagnostic surgical pathology, Vol. 1. New York: Raven Press, 1989:479–513.)

lymphoid lesions from lymphoma are listed in Table 35 (fig. 458). Unfortunately, exceptions to these criteria are relatively common.

Benign-reactive lymphocytic aggregates have been identified in trephine biopsies in 6 and 9 percent, respectively, of cases of Hodgkin disease and non-Hodgkin lymphoma at the time of staging (5,20). When the typical features are present, recognition of lymphocytic aggregates and their

distinction from lymphoma is generally not difficult. The usual small size, well-defined borders, random distribution in the bone marrow, prominent vascularity, and polymorphous cell proliferation serve to distinguish most lymphocytic aggregates from malignant lymphoma. Problems occur when the aggregates are present in large numbers or are of unusually large size. In these cases they may resemble small lymphocytic or follicular

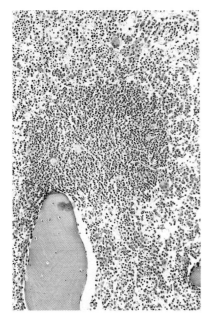

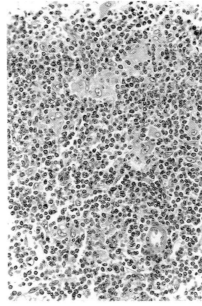

Figure 459
REACTIVE POLYMORPHOUS
LYMPHOHISTIOCYTIC LESION
A trephine biopsy from a patient with acquired immune deficiency syndrome (AIDS) showing a low and high magnification of a reactive polymorphous lymphohistiocytic lesion. The lesion is large but in this instance is relatively well circumscribed. It is composed primarily of various sized lymphocytes and several epithelioid histiocytes. (Hematoxylin and eosin stain) (Figs. 37.30 (left) and 37.31 (left) from McKenna RW. The bone marrow manifestations of Hodgkin's disease, the non-Hodgkin's lymphomas, and lymphoma-like disorders. In: Knowles DM, ed. Neoplastic hematopathology. Baltimore: Williams & Wilkins, 1992:1135–80.)

Figure 460
PERIPHERAL
T-CELL LYMPHOMA
A trephine biopsy showing low and high magnification of a focal lesion in a patient with a peripheral T-cell lymphoma. The cell composition is strikingly similar to the reactive lesion illustrated in figure 459. The differential diagnosis of reactive polymorphous lymphohistiocytic lesions in bone marrow often includes peripheral T-cell lymphoma or Hodgkin disease. (Hematoxylin and eosin stain) (Fig. 37.30 (right) and 37.31 (right) from McKenna RW. The bone marrow manifestations of Hodgkin's disease, the non-Hodgkin's lymphomas, and lymphoma-like disorders. In: Knowles DM, ed. Neoplastic hematopathology. Baltimore: Williams & Wilkins, 1992:1135–80.)

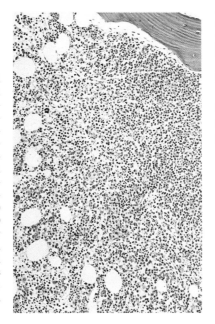

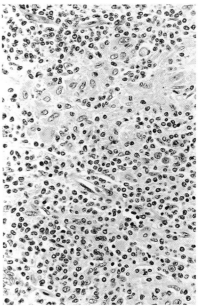

small cleaved cell lymphomas. The florid polymorphous lymphohistiocytic reactive lesions are often large and have poorly defined borders; they may resemble a peripheral T-cell lymphoma or Hodgkin disease.

Caution must be exercised in the interpretation of bone marrow lymphoid infiltrates in patients with immune disorders. The lymphohistiocytic lesions found in marrow sections from patients with AIDS or the AIDS-related complex

may be indistinguishable from peripheral T-cell lymphoma of mixed cell type (figs. 459, 460) (2,11,12,19,21). T-cell lymphomas, however, are rarely encountered in patients with AIDS and the diagnosis should not be made in the absence of a confirmatory lymph node biopsy. Immunophenotyping, cytogenetic studies, or immunogenotypic analysis may be necessary to distinguish florid reactive lymphocytic proliferations from malignant lymphoma (4,8,11,16,25,26).

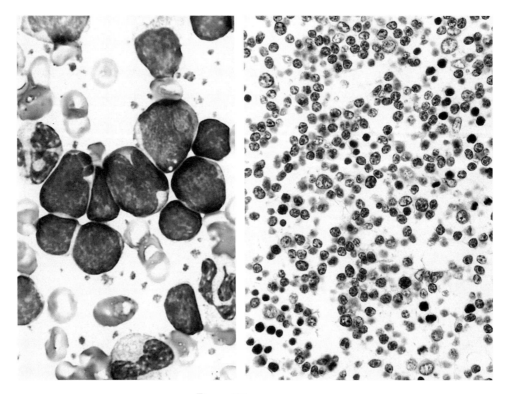

Figure 461
BONE MARROW LYMPHOCYTE PROGENITOR CELLS (HEMATOGONES)
A bone marrow aspirate smear and trephine biopsy section from a 2-year-old male bone marrow transplant donor.
Left: The aspirate smear contains approximately 50 percent lymphocyte progenitor cells (hematogones), some of which resemble lymphoblasts. (Wright-Giemsa stain) (Fig. 37.32 (right) from McKenna RW. The bone marrow manifestations of Hodgkin's disease, the non-Hodgkin's lymphomas, and lymphoma-like disorders. In: Knowles DM, ed. Neoplastic hematopathology. Baltimore: Williams & Wilkins, 1992:1135–80.)
Right: The trephine biopsy section contains a high percentage of lymphoid cells and is nearly 100 percent cellular. A bone marrow with increased numbers of these cells could be mistaken for lymphoblastic lymphoma. (Hematoxylin and eosin stain) (Figures 160 and 163 are from the same patient.)

Treatment and Prognosis. Reactive lymphoid lesions of the bone marrow do not require treatment unless secondary to an underlying treatable inflammatory disorder.

The finding of lymphoid aggregates in bone marrow sections appears to be significantly associated with eventual progression to a neoplastic lymphoproliferative disorder. Histologically and immunophenotypically, benign hyperplastic lymphoid lesions in bone marrow and other sites have been shown to contain a clonal B-lymphocyte expansion by immunogenotypic analysis (15,25). Some of these lesions have progressed to malignant lymphomas (15). In one study, approximately one third of the patients with benign lymphoid aggregates progressed to a lymphoproliferative disease (10).

INCREASED BONE MARROW LYMPHOCYTE PROGENITOR CELLS (HEMATOGONES)

A discussion of the normal lymphocyte progenitor cells commonly observed in large numbers in the bone marrow of children and their distinction from the lymphoblasts of acute lymphoblastic leukemia (ALL) and lymphoblastic lymphoma is found in the chapter Acute Lymphoblastic Leukemia (fig. 461).

BONE MARROW GRANULOMAS

Definition. Collections of epithelioid histiocytes and lymphocytes in the bone marrow. They are similar to granulomas in other tissues.

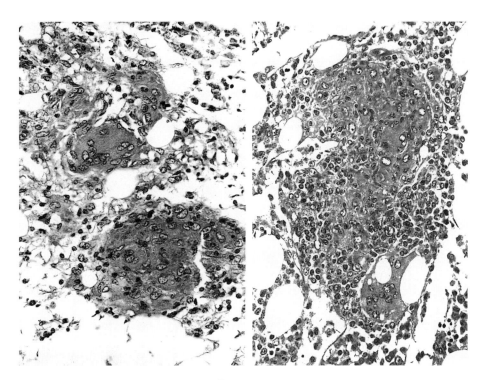

Figure 462
BONE MARROW GRANULOMAS
Bone marrow granulomas in two patients undergoing staging for Hodgkin disease. Nonspecific granulomas may be found in the bone marrow in patients with Hodgkin disease and can be mistaken for Hodgkin tissue. The absence of Reed-Sternberg cells and the presence of Langhans giant cells distinguish the two processes. (Hematoxylin and eosin stain) (Left: Fig. 13.70 from McKenna RW. Bone marrow. In: Dehner LP, ed. Pediatric surgical pathology. 2nd ed. Baltimore: Williams & Wilkins, 1987:838–68. Right: Fig. 2 from McKenna R. Disorders of bone marrow. In: Sternberg SS, ed. Diagnostic surgical pathology, Vol. 1. New York: Raven Press. 1989:479–513.)

Incidence and Clinical Findings. Granulomas may be found in bone marrow biopsies as an incidental finding or in the course of a directed search in patients suspected of having an infectious disease (27,28). The majority of bone marrow granulomas have no demonstrable infectious etiology. They have been observed in the bone marrow in approximately 7 percent of patients whose biopsies were negative for Hodgkin disease at the time of staging and slightly less commonly in patients with non-Hodgkin lymphoma (27–32,35). Patients may be asymptomatic or manifest symptoms and signs related to the underlying disease process.

Laboratory Findings. Laboratory findings may be normal or reflect an underlying infection or neoplastic disease.

Blood and Bone Marrow Findings. Blood smears are usually normal but may exhibit changes secondary to the underlying cause of the bone marrow granulomas. In most cases the bone marrow aspirate smears are also normal but may show secondary changes. Occasionally, clusters or sheets of histiocytes are observed. When the etiology is an infectious agent, histiocytes may contain microorganisms in their cytoplasm.

Histopathologic Findings. In trephine biopsy sections, the granulomas are generally non-necrotic, sarcoid-like and consist of lymphocytes, epithelioid histiocytes, occasional Langhans giant cells, and eosinophils (fig. 462) (29,30,32). They are usually small focal lesions and may be present in only one of two or more trephine biopsy specimens.

Differential Diagnosis. Granulomas may resemble Hodgkin disease or a peripheral T-cell lymphoma when they are unusually large or confluent, lack giant cells, and have a prominent eosinophil component. Granulomas are distinguished from Hodgkin tissue by the usual predominance of epithelioid histiocytes, Langhans

Figure 463
IDIOPATHIC
MYELOFIBROSIS
MIMICKING
HODGKIN DISEASE

A trephine biopsy section from a patient with idiopathic myelofibrosis. The bone marrow is markedly fibrotic and normal hematopoiesis is reduced. Clusters of megakaryocytes are present. Primary myelofibrosis may simulate Hodgkin disease or peripheral T-cell lymphoma. The abnormal megakaryocytes can potentially be misinterpreted as Reed-Sternberg cells in technically poor sections. (Hematoxylin and eosin stain) (Fig. 37.38 from McKenna RW. The bone marrow manifestations of Hodgkin's disease, the non-Hodgkin's lymphomas, and lymphoma-like disorders. In: Knowles DM, ed. Neoplastic hematopathology. Baltimore: Williams & Wilkins, 1992:1135–80.)

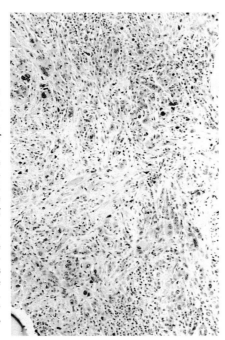 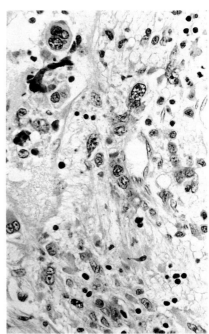

giant cells, and the absence of typical Reed-Sternberg cells or variants. Comparing the cytologic features of the lymphocytes with lymphoma tissue from the lymph nodes is important in distinguishing bone marrow granulomas from peripheral T-cell lymphoma.

The presence of granulomas in the bone marrow should always be considered carefully, particularly in patients receiving immunosuppressive chemotherapy. Appropriate special stains and microbiologic cultures should be performed when bone marrow granulomas are found. Opportunistic infections such as cryptococcosis and histoplasmosis may be first encountered in a bone marrow biopsy. The granulomas in immunosuppressed patients with *Mycobacterium avium* intracellulare may resemble clusters of histiocytes or storage cells. The diagnosis may be missed unless acid fast stains are performed.

Treatment and Prognosis. Treatment is directed toward the underlying cause of the granuloma. In cases of nonspecific or incidental granulomas, no treatment is required. Prognosis for infectious granulomas is related to the underlying causative agent and its response to therapy. The significance and prognostic implications of nonspecific granulomas in patients with a lymphoma is not clear. It has been suggested that the granulomas in Hodgkin disease are a manifestation of altered delayed hypersensitivity (30). However, there is also evidence to suggest that the granulomas reflect a host response to the tumor; their presence may be indicative of a favorable prognosis (33,34). Bone marrow granulomas in some patients with non-Hodgkin lymphoma have been closely associated with lymphoma infiltrates and may represent a direct immune response to the lymphoma (31,35).

IDIOPATHIC BONE MARROW FIBROSIS

The pathology of idiopathic myelofibrosis is discussed in detail in the chapter, Chronic Myeloproliferative Diseases. Myelofibrosis may occasionally resemble Hodgkin disease or peripheral T-cell lymphoma (36–38). The clusters of megakaryocytes in primary myelofibrosis may be misinterpreted as Reed-Sternberg cells in suboptimally prepared trephine sections but should be readily distinguished in technically good preparations (fig. 463). Lymphoid infiltrates are present in some cases and may potentially contribute to diagnostic problems (40). Examination of blood smears for the characteristic abnormalities associated with myelofibrosis and familiarity with the patient's clinical manifestations will aid in the diagnosis (39).

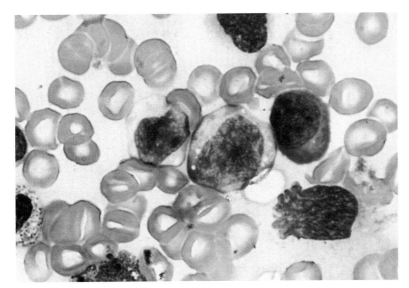

Figure 464
BLOOD INVOLVEMENT IN
ANGIOIMMUNOBLASTIC
LYMPHADENOPATHY
A blood smear from a patient with angioimmunoblastic lymphadenopathy and a markedly elevated leukocyte count. There is reactive lymphocytosis with circulating immunoblasts and plasma cells. Two reactive lymphocytes and a plasma cell are shown. (Wright-Giemsa stain)

ANGIOIMMUNOBLASTIC LYMPHADENOPATHY (IMMUNOBLASTIC LYMPHADENOPATHY)

Definition. An atypical lymphoid hyperplasia of uncertain pathogenesis characterized by proliferation of lymphocytes, plasma cells, immunoblasts, and small vessels.

Incidence and Clinical Findings. Angioimmunoblastic lymphadenopathy (AIL) is an uncommon form of lymph node hyperplasia that involves the bone marrow in approximately 50 percent of cases (49). The clinical signs and symptoms are similar to those of malignant lymphoma. Generalized lymphadenopathy and hepatosplenomegaly are presenting physical findings. In patients with bone marrow involvement, cytopenias and related symptoms may occur.

Laboratory Findings. Patients typically have anemia and hypergammaglobulinemia. A minority of patients present with a Coombs positive hemolytic anemia.

Blood and Bone Marrow Findings. A spectrum of changes in blood counts may be present at diagnosis. These include neutrophilia, eosinophilia, and various cytopenias, particularly lymphocytopenia. Eosinophilia, immunoblasts, plasma cells, and reactive lymphocytes are seen in blood smears in some cases; rarely, there is a profound leukocytosis (fig. 464) (48).

In bone marrow aspirate smears mature lymphocytes are often increased in number and immunoblasts may be observed. Erythroid hyperplasia may be present in patients with immune hemolytic anemia.

Histopathologic Findings. The lesions in trephine biopsy sections vary in their composition but are generally similar to those in lymph nodes. There is a proliferation of immunoblasts, plasmacytoid immunoblasts, and plasma cells. A vascular proliferation of numerous small arborizing vessels and the deposition of amorphous pale eosinophilic interstitial material are usually observed (figs. 465, 466) (41,43,45,48,49). Bone marrow involvement may be focal or diffuse; focal lesions are either paratrabecular or randomly distributed. In addition to immunoblasts and plasma cells, the infiltrate often contains histiocytes, eosinophils, a heteromorphous population of lymphocytes, and occasionally, large multinucleated cells. Reticulin is generally increased and a fibroblastic proliferation replacing large areas of bone marrow has been observed in some cases. Uninvolved marrow is usually hypercellular (48).

Differential Diagnosis. The bone marrow lesions of AIL are not pathognomonic. Similar infiltrates may be observed in marrow biopsies from patients with immune cytopenias, viral infections, AIDS, and occasionally in other conditions associated with lymphocytic hyperplasia. The lesions often resemble malignant lymphoma, particularly Hodgkin disease or a peripheral T-cell lymphoma.

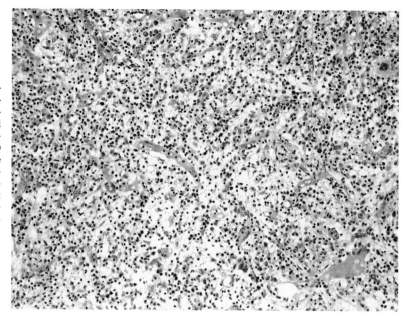

Figure 465
ANGIOIMMUNOBLASTIC
LYMPHADENOPATHY

A trephine biopsy section from a patient with angioimmunoblastic lymphadenopathy. There is diffuse bone marrow involvement with a loosely arranged lymphoid infiltrate and vascular proliferation. (Hematoxylin and eosin stain) (Fig. 37.35 (left) from McKenna RW. The bone marrow manifestations of Hodgkin's disease, the non-Hodgkin's lymphomas, and lymphoma-like disorders. In: Knowles DM, ed. Neoplastic hematopathology. Baltimore: Williams & Wilkins, 1992:1135–80.)

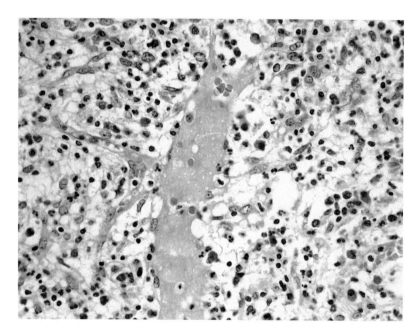

Figure 466
ANGIOIMMUNOBLASTIC
LYMPHADENOPATHY

A higher magnification of the biopsy illustrated in figure 465 shows a pleomorphic cell population consisting of lymphocytes, immunoblasts, and plasma cells. There are numerous small arborizing vessels and amorphous pale eosinophilic interstitial material. (Hematoxylin and eosin stain) (Fig. 37.35 (right) from McKenna RW. The bone marrow manifestations of Hodgkin's disease, the non-Hodgkin's lymphomas, and lymphoma-like disorders. In: Knowles DM, ed. Neoplastic hematopathology. Baltimore: Williams & Wilkins, 1992:1135–80.)

The distribution of AIL lesions in the bone marrow, their polycellular infiltrate, and the presence of reticulin fibrosis are all characteristic of Hodgkin disease. However, the background observed in AIL, consisting of a complete spectrum of lymphocyte size, is not characteristic of Hodgkin disease and typical Reed-Sternberg cells are uncommon (46). In many cases, the distinction of AIL from Hodgkin disease ultimately rests on the lymph node histopathology.

Some of the lymphocytic proliferations that were previously designated as AIL are presently considered to be variants of peripheral T-cell lymphoma (AIL-like T-cell lymphoma) (42,44,46, 50). Infiltrates of AIL-like T-cell lymphoma in the bone marrow may lack the definitive cytologic criteria of neoplasia and be virtually identical to AIL. Distinguishing these two disorders on a marrow biopsy is exceedingly difficult.

Treatment and Prognosis. Patients with AIL are generally treated with prednisone or chemotherapy, or both. The response is variable but temporary complete remission is achieved in over 50 percent of cases. A relatively high percentage of AILs evolve to malignant lymphomas which are the cause of death (46). The median survival time is approximately 2 1/2 years (47). Patients achieving a complete remission have a significantly longer survival period than those failing therapy.

MAST CELL DISEASE

Definition. An abnormal proliferation of mast cells in one or more organs, also termed *mastocytosis*. The most commonly involved organ is the skin and in most instances the disease is limited to the cutaneous tissues. In systemic mastocytosis, occurring in approximately 10 percent of cases, the disease is disseminated and may involve several organ systems (53,76,83,87). The most frequent sites of involvement are the skin, bone marrow, spleen, lymph nodes, and liver. Hematologic manifestations of variable nature and degree are often encountered.

Incidence and Clinical Findings. Systemic mast cell disease is rare. Reliable data regarding its incidence are lacking. The incidence of bone marrow involvement in patients with systemic mast cell disease is greater than 90 percent. The time of diagnosis of the systemic disease ranges from young adulthood to advanced age; median ages have varied in different studies from 48 to 71 years (53,61,63,83,87). The disorder is slightly more common in males than females. Patients who have a history of cutaneous mast cell disease are generally younger (median age 36 to 44) than those without cutaneous manifestations (median age 63 to 75) (53,61,63).

Patients with systemic mast cell disease and urticaria pigmentosa are often otherwise asymptomatic (53,61,76). The severity of the symptoms in those without cutaneous disease is highly variable. Constitutional symptoms are common and include weakness, fatigue, fever, night sweats, and weight loss (87). Most patients manifest effects of the chemical mediators released by the mast cells, most notably histamine. Generalized pruritis, urticaria, episodic flushing, bronchospasm, arthralgia, headache, tachycar-

dia, hypotension, and syncope are mostly attributed to elevated histamine levels. These symptoms may be periodic and in some cases are precipitated by a specific factor such as a drug, a food, or exposure to heat or cold (83). Gastrointestinal manifestations, including abdominal pain, diarrhea, nausea, vomiting, and bleeding, are present in 25 to 80 percent of patients (51,56). Ascites and esophageal varices due to portal hypertension resulting from hepatic fibrosis have been reported (52,78,83). Neurologic and psychiatric manifestations include seizures, alteration in cognitive functions, and affective changes; hypotensive episodes may be the cause of these symptoms (67,74).

Occasionally, the first clinical manifestations are due to tumorous mass disease. Splenomegaly, hepatomegaly, lymphadenopathy, or pathologic fractures due to bone tumors are most common (71). Patients with mast cell leukemia have severe constitutional and gastrointestinal symptoms and extensive organ infiltration (84).

Physical findings in addition to skin manifestations are splenomegaly in approximately 40 to 70 percent of patients, hepatomegaly in 20 to 72 percent, and lymphadenopathy in 10 to 50 percent, (53,61,76,83,87). Organomegaly and lymphadenopathy appear to be more common in patients without urticaria pigmentosa (53,61).

Laboratory Findings. A moderate to marked elevation of mast cell mediators can usually be demonstrated by biochemical measurement of secretory products including histamine, prostaglandin D_2, tryptase, and heparin (72). Tryptase assays often provide the most useful diagnostic information (77). When combined with other studies, biochemical analysis of mast cell mediators may provide important diagnostic information (58).

Between 40 and 84 percent of patients present with hematologic abnormalities (53,63,87). The hematologic findings in patients from four large studies are shown in Table 36.

Radiographic changes due to mass disease or tissue alteration by chemical mediators are common. Evidence of bone lesions is found in more than half of the patients (53,66,76,87). The radiographic changes are varied and include generalized osteoporosis and osteoblastic and osteolytic lesions; any combination of these may coexist in the same patient (55,71). The osteoblastic and osteolytic lesions often simulate metastatic

Table 36

HEMATOLOGIC FINDINGS IN SYSTEMIC MAST CELL DISEASE*

	Study Results (percent with finding)			
	Sager and Even-Paz (76)	Brunning et al. (53)	Travis et al. (83)	Horny et al. (63)
Anemia	42	36	47	26**
Leukopenia	13	21	16	0**
Thrombocytopenia	21	14	16	2**
Pancytopenia	NR+	14	NR	7
Bicytopenia	NR	NR	NR	25‡
Leukocytosis	18	21	19	39
Monocytosis	7	NR	16	25
Lymphocytosis	2	NR	2	0
Eosinophilia	12	43	19	23
Basophilia	2	NR	7	21
Erythrocytosis	NR	NR	NR	2
Thrombocytosis	NR	NR	9	7
Circulating mast cells	16	0	4	7

* Table 82-1 from McKenna RW, Hernandez J, Peterson L. Benign and malignant mast cell disorders. In: Bick RL, ed. Hematology: clinical and laboratory practice. St. Louis: CV Mosby, 1993:1261–72.
**Does not include the patients with bicytopenia or pancytopenia.
+ NR: Not reported.
‡ Most patients with bicytopenia had anemia and thrombocytopenia.

carcinoma or plasma cell myeloma (fig. 467) (53,83). Evidence of pathologic fractures is noted in some cases (53,71). Radiographic changes in the gastrointestinal tract are slightly less common than in bone. Peptic ulcers and mucosal abnormalities are the most frequent (83). Radiographic changes in the gastrointestinal tract, like those in bone, are not pathognomonic for mast cell disease but their recognition is important in directing other diagnostic studies and in defining the extent of the disease (64).

Blood and Bone Marrow Findings. In blood smears cytopenias or leukocytosis are the most frequent abnormalities. Eosinophilia is relatively common and may be marked in cases of mast cell leukemia, occasionally simulating the hypereosinophilic syndrome (fig. 468). Mast cells are infrequently observed except in the rare case of mast cell leukemia. Circulating cells may have typical mast cell cytologic features or appear abnormal with decreased granules and irregularly shaped nuclei (fig. 469). A significant number of patients with systemic mast cell disease present with, or later develop, a chronic myeloproliferative disorder, acute myeloid leukemia, or myelodysplastic syndrome (61,63,79,82,85). In these cases, dysplastic changes in blood cells or increased myeloblasts may be observed.

The bone marrow is the most common site of extracutaneous mast cell disease; involvement is found in approximately 90 percent of cases (53,83). Most often, bone marrow aspirate smears have only a few scattered mast cells. Smears of crushed marrow particles are the most likely to contain larger numbers of mast cells (53). The mast cells vary from normal appearing with round nuclei and densely packed granules to unusually large cells with abundant cytoplasm and scattered fine granules. Small cells with lobulated or spindle shaped nuclei and sparse

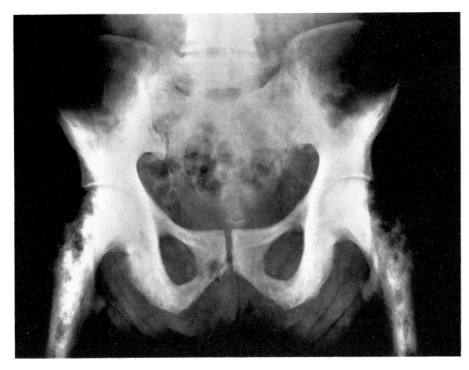

Figure 467
RADIOGRAPHIC BONE
LESIONS IN SYSTEMIC
MAST CELL DISEASE
This X ray of the femurs
and pelvic bones in a pa-
tient with systemic mast
cell disease shows extensive
osteolytic and osteoblastic
lesions. (Fig. 1 from Brunning RD, McKenna RW,
Rosai J, Parkin JL, Risdall
R. Systemic mastocytosis:
extracutaneous manifesta-
tions. Am J Surg Pathol
1983;7:425–38.)

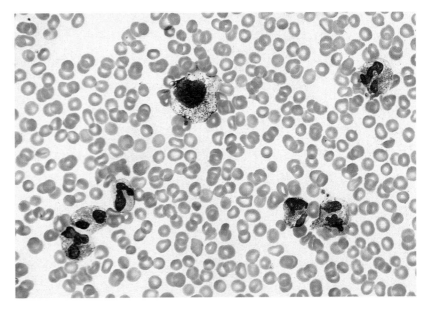

Figure 468
MAST CELL LEUKEMIA AND
EOSINOPHILIA
A blood smear from a young
woman with mast cell leukemia and
marked eosinophilia. There are five
eosinophils, one neutrophil, and a
large atypical-appearing mast cell
with relatively sparse small granules
and a slightly lobulated nucleus.
This patient had eosinophilia as a
presenting feature and was initially
thought to have a hypereosinophilic
syndrome. Eosinophilia is observed
in approximately one third of patients with systemic mast cell disease. (Wright-Giemsa stain)

granulation may be observed in some cases (53). In cases of mast cell leukemia, numerous atypical mast cells are found in aspirate smears (fig. 470) (53,63,76,84,85,87). When there is a concurrent myeloproliferative process, atypical-appearing mast cells may be found in the marrow smears along with increased myeloblasts and dysplastic hematopoietic cells (figs. 471, 472) (61,63,85).

Histopathologic Findings. The pattern of involvement in bone marrow trephine biopsy sections is focal in greater than 80 percent of cases and diffuse in less than 20 percent (53,61,83). The focal lesions may be paratrabecular, perivascular, or randomly distributed; all three types of lesions may be observed in the same biopsy specimen (53). The paratrabecular lesions may marginate

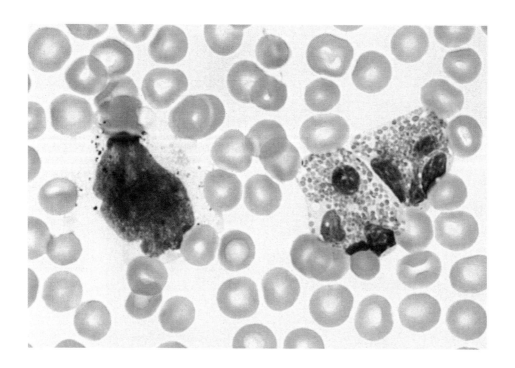

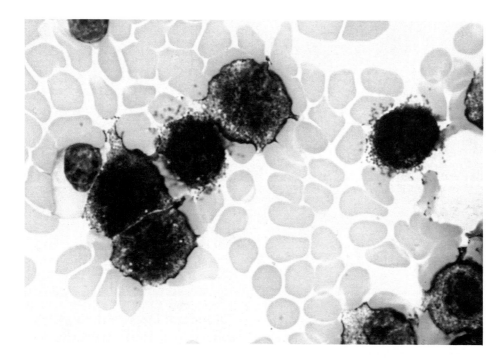

Figure 469
MAST CELL LEUKEMIA

Top: A high magnification of the same blood smear depicted in figure 468 shows an atypical, sparsely granulated mast cell with an irregular nuclear border. Two eosinophils are present in this field. (Wright-Giemsa stain)

Bottom: A blood smear from a man with mast cell leukemia shows several relatively normal-appearing mast cells concentrated at the thin edge of the smear. (Wright-Giemsa stain)

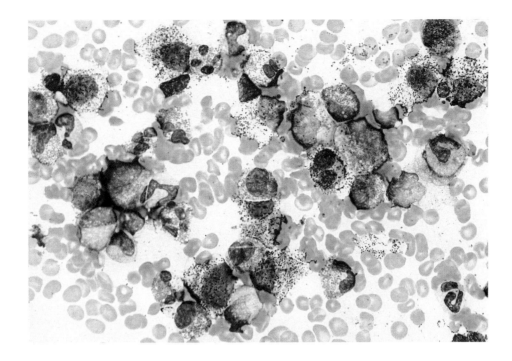

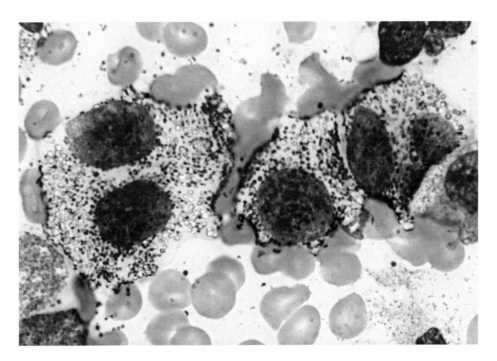

Figure 470
MAST CELL LEUKEMIA

Top: Low magnification of a bone marrow smear from a woman with mast cell leukemia. There are numerous immature, atypical mast cells. Abnormal mast cells were also found in the blood smear in this case (see figures 468, 469). (Wright-Giemsa stain)

Bottom: High magnification of the same bone marrow smear. The mast cells are large with sparse granulation. Many have lobulated nuclei. (Wright-Giemsa stain)

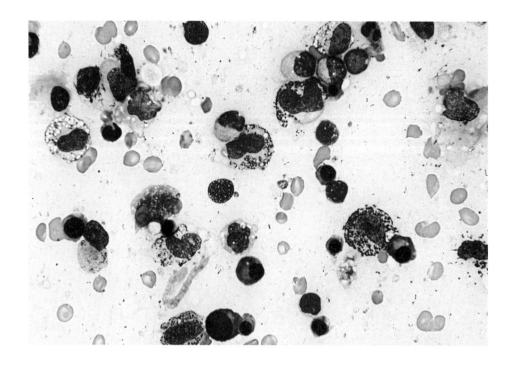

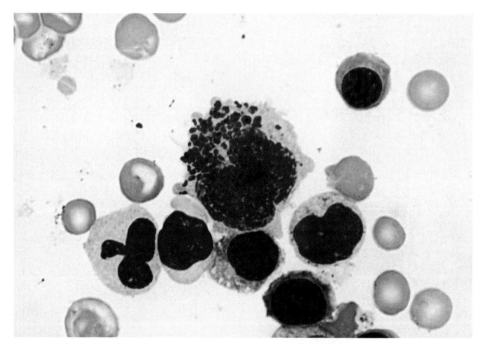

Figure 471
MYELODYSPLASTIC SYNDROME IN A PATIENT WITH SYSTEMIC MAST CELL DISEASE

Top: Bone marrow smear from a patient with systemic mastocytosis and a myelodysplastic syndrome. Several atypical, hypogranular mast cells with oval indented nuclei are present. These findings in bone marrow smears could be misinterpreted as hypergranular promyelocytic leukemia (M3).

Bottom: A dysplastic neutrophil, normoblasts, and an atypical mast cell are illustrated. (Wright-Giemsa stain)

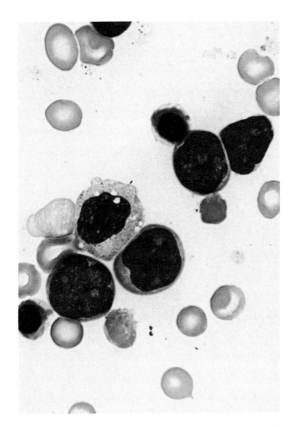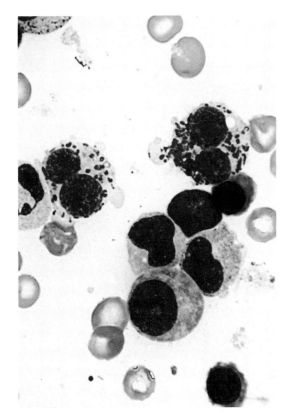

Figure 472

MYELODYSPLASTIC SYNDROME IN A PATIENT WITH SYSTEMIC MAST CELL DISEASE

Left: A bone marrow aspirate smear from a 63-year-old man with systemic mast cell disease and a myelodysplastic syndrome. Several myeloblasts are present in this field. Myeloblasts comprised approximately 15 percent of the bone marrow cells. (Fig. 82-10A from McKenna RW, Hernandez J, Peterson L. Benign and malignant mast cell disorders. In: Bick RL, ed. Hematology: clinical and laboratory practice. St. Louis: CV Mosby, 1993:1261–72.)

Right: Two atypical mast cells with lobulated nuclei and relatively sparse granulation from the same marrow aspirate smear as depicted on the left. (Wright-Giemsa stain)

along the trabecular border or be juxtaposed to the trabeculum. Those that marginate are associated with fibrosis and expansion of the trabeculae (figs. 473, 474). In perivascular lesions there is usually prominent medial and adventitial hypertrophy (fig. 475).

The focal marrow lesions may be polycellular or relatively monocellular (53,60). Polycellular lesions are usually randomly distributed and characterized by a mixture of mast cells, lymphocytes, eosinophils, neutrophils, histiocytes, endothelial cells, and fibroblasts. The various cell types may be randomly distributed but more commonly there is compartmentalization with a central focus of lymphocytes encircled by mast cells or a cluster of mast cells ringed by lymphocytes (figs. 476–478). The mast cells are usually

round or oval with abundant eosinophilic cytoplasm. Eosinophils are scattered among the mast cells, with the greatest concentration at the periphery. The lymphocyte component consists of both T and B cells (60).

The monocellular focal lesions are composed primarily of mast cells, with occasional lymphocytes and eosinophils. The mast cells are frequently elongate or spindle shaped with pale to lightly eosinophilic cytoplasm. The nuclei are round, oval, elongate, or monocytoid in configuration; these mast cells may resemble histiocytes or fibroblasts.

In all types of focal lesions, nucleoli are inconspicuous in the mast cells and mitotic figures absent. The uninvolved portion of the bone marrow may be normocellular or hypercellular with increased granulocytes (53).

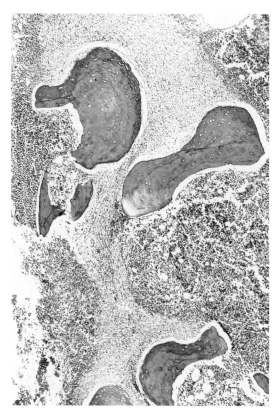
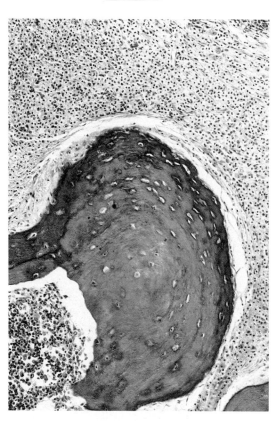

Figure 473
FOCAL PARATRABECULAR MAST CELL LESION

Left: A bone marrow trephine biopsy section from a patient with systemic mast cell disease showing focal paratrabecular involvement. The marrow is fibrotic in this area and the bone trabeculae are mottled, irregular, and thickened.

Right: A high magnification of the lesion seen on the left shows fibrosis and scattered mast cells. Cytochemistry is often required to identify the mast cells in histologic sections. (Hematoxylin and eosin stain)

Figure 474
PARATRABECULAR
MAST CELL LESION
WITH SPINDLE SHAPED NUCLEI

Left: A trephine biopsy section from a 72-year-old man shows a small focal paratrabecular mast cell lesion. There is abnormal thickening and irregularity of the bone trabeculum.

Right: The mast cells have oval to spindle shaped nuclei and resemble fibroblasts. (Hematoxylin and eosin stain)

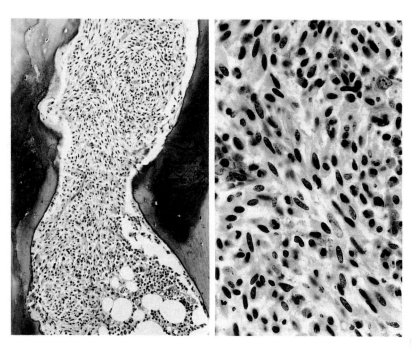

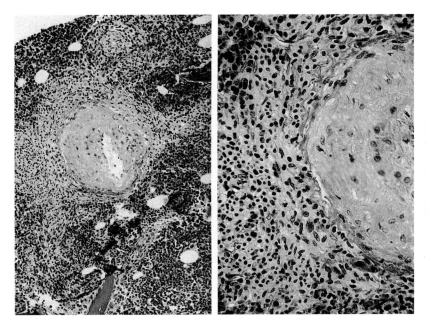

Figure 475
FOCAL PERIVASCULAR
MAST CELL LESION
A bone marrow trephine biopsy section from a patient with systemic mast cell disease. There is a focal perivascular mast cell infiltrate. The vessel wall is thickened and encircled by mast cells. (Hematoxylin and eosin stain) (Fig. 3 from Brunning RD, McKenna RW, Rosai J, Parkin JL, Risdall R. Systemic mastocytosis: extracutaneous manifestations. Am J Surg Pathol 1983;7:425–38.)

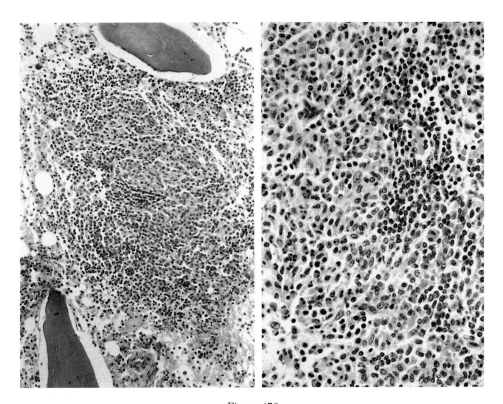

Figure 476
FOCAL POLYMORPHIC MAST CELL LESION

Left: A focal, randomly distributed (nonparatrabecular) polymorphic mast cell lesion.

Right: A higher magnification of this lesion shows a polycellular infiltrate consisting of lymphocytes, mast cells, and eosinophils. The lymphocyte component is encircled by mast cells and eosinophils. The mast cells in this case are round with abundant eosinophilic cytoplasm and resemble histiocytes. (Hematoxylin and eosin stain) (Fig. 37.37 from McKenna RW. The bone marrow manifestations of Hodgkin's disease, the non-Hodgkin's lymphomas, and lymphoma-like disorders. In: Knowles DM, ed. Neoplastic hematopathology. Baltimore: Williams & Wilkins, 1992:1135–80.)

Figure 477
FOCAL POLYMORPHIC
MAST CELL LESION

A high magnification of the lesion depicted in figure 476 shows sheets of mast cells encircling the central core of lymphocytes. Eosinophils are scattered among the mast cells. The mast cells have oval nuclei and a moderate amount of eosinophilic cytoplasm. They resemble histiocytes. This type of mast cell lesion appears to be identical to an eosinophilic fibrohistiocytic lesion. (Hematoxylin and eosin stain)

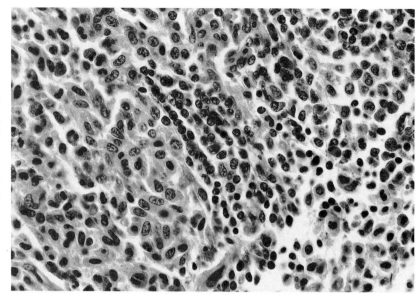

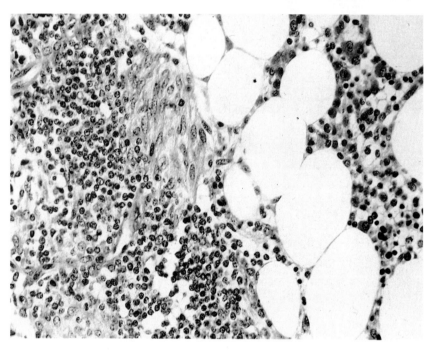

Figure 478
FOCAL MAST CELL LESION

A small, randomly focal bone marrow lesion from a patient with systemic mastocytosis. The mast cells resemble fibroblasts and are partially encircled by lymphocytes. (Hematoxylin and eosin stain) (Fig. 82-5 from McKenna RW, Hernandez J, Peterson L. Benign and malignant mast cell disorders. In: Bick RL, ed. Hematology: clinical and laboratory practice. St Louis: CV Mosby, 1993:1261–72.)

In diffuse lesions the entire marrow space between trabeculae is replaced (fig. 479). The mast cells vary from round to elongate and may resemble fibroblasts. They are frequently intermixed with neutrophils, eosinophils, and macrophages. Moderate to marked fibrosis is present and normal hematopoietic cells are markedly reduced.

Bone changes may occur in both focal and diffuse lesions. Widened, mottled, irregular trabeculae are often observed, particularly with

paratrabecular lesions (figs. 473, 474, 479). In some cases osteoclasts are increased and associated with thinning of trabeculae (53,86).

In mast cell leukemia the bone marrow is markedly hypercellular with replacement of normal hematopoietic cells by immature, atypical-appearing mast cells (fig. 480) (61,84). In patients with a concurrent myeloid leukemia or myelodysplastic syndrome, the bone marrow biopsy shows features of both disorders.

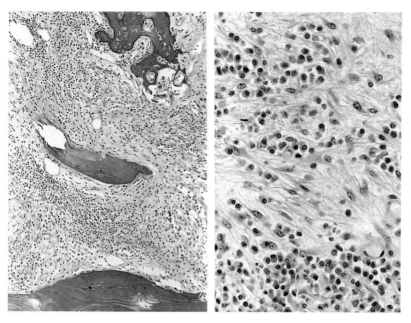

Figure 479
DIFFUSE BONE MARROW
INVOLVEMENT IN SYSTEMIC
MAST CELL DISEASE

Left: A bone marrow trephine biopsy section from a patient with systemic mastocytosis shows diffuse replacement of the marrow. There is striking fibrosis and abnormal bone trabeculae.

Right: A higher magnification shows mast cells that are round or oval, have abundant cytoplasm, and resemble histiocytes or plasma cells. Others are elongate or spindle shaped. (Hematoxylin and eosin stain)

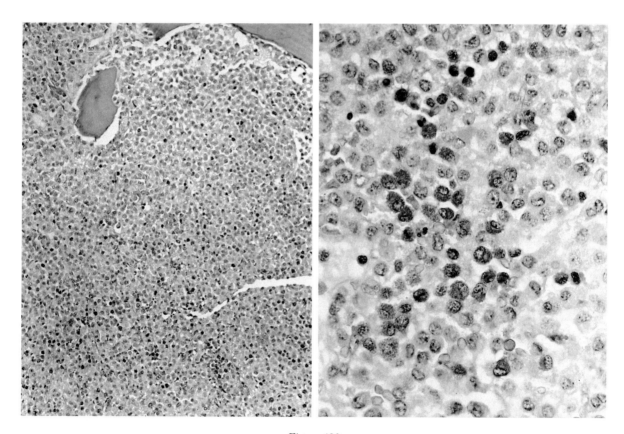

Figure 480
MAST CELL LEUKEMIA

Left: A bone marrow trephine biopsy section from a patient with mast cell leukemia showing diffuse marrow replacement with a uniform-appearing cellular infiltrate. (Hematoxylin and eosin stain)

Right: A high magnification of the biopsy. The mast cells are immature in appearance and diffusely replace the bone marrow. Eosinophils are markedly increased and are scattered among the mast cells. (Hematoxylin and eosin stain)

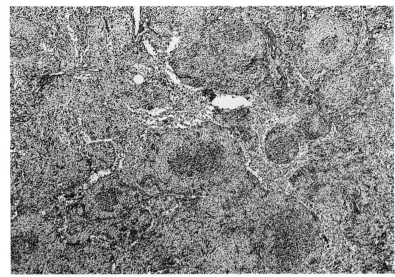

Figure 481
LYMPH NODE INVOLVEMENT
WITH MAST CELL DISEASE

A lymph node biopsy section showing extensive involvement with mastocytosis, with partial preservation of the nodal architecture. There is a prominent perifollicular infiltrate with atrophy of the follicular structures and numerous mast cells in the sinuses. (Hematoxylin and eosin stain) (Fig. 9A from Brunning RD, McKenna RW, Rosai J, Parkin JL, Risdall R. Systemic mastocytosis: extracutaneous manifestations. Am J Surg Pathol 1983;7:425–38.)

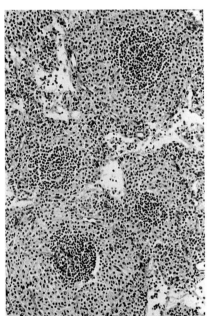
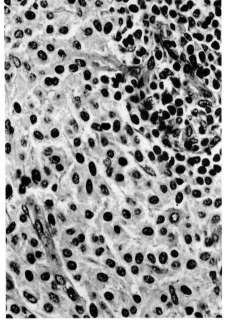

Figure 482
LYMPH NODE
INVOLVEMENT WITH
MAST CELL DISEASE

Left: A higher magnification of the lymph node seen in figure 481 shows a distinct perifollicular mast cell infiltrate. The mast cells encircling the follicles show abundant light staining cytoplasm and centrally located nuclei. The pattern of involvement is similar to that of hairy cell leukemia. (Fig. 9B from Brunning RD, McKenna RW, Rosai J, Parkin JL, Risdall R. Systemic mastocytosis: extracutaneous manifestations. Am J Surg Pathol 1983;7:425–38.)

Right: The mast cells have abundant cytoplasm and round to oval, widely separated nuclei. (Hematoxylin and eosin stain)

The lymph nodes, spleen, and liver are commonly involved in systemic mast cell disease and occasionally the diagnosis is made from a lymph node or liver biopsy or a splenectomy specimen. In the lymph nodes the mast cell infiltration primarily involves the sinuses and paracortex (53,81). A prominent perifollicular mast cell infiltrate is observed in many cases (figs. 481, 482). The cellular composition may be homogeneous or polycellular, similar to the bone marrow lesions. Vascular proliferation and fibrosis may be present.

The most prominent feature of splenic mast cell disease is the marked diffuse or nodular fibrosis involving both the red and white pulp. The mast cell infiltrate is diffuse or focal-perivascular. Eosinophils are often mixed with the mast cells (53,81,87). The mast cells are difficult to recognize when there is extensive fibrosis (fig. 483) (53,81). Cytochemical stains may be required.

In the liver there is moderate to marked portal fibrosis. The mast cell infiltrate may expand the portal tracts and sinusoids (fig. 484) (53,89). A

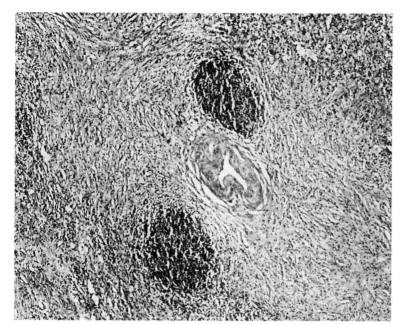

Figure 483
SPLENIC INVOLVEMENT WITH
MAST CELL DISEASE
This section from an enlarged, surgically removed spleen from a patient with systemic mast cell disease shows marked perivascular fibrosis. (Hematoxylin and eosin stain)

Figure 484
LIVER INVOLVEMENT
WITH MAST CELL DISEASE
A section of a liver biopsy from a patient with mastocytosis showing a cluster of mast cells in the portal tract. The mast cells have clear staining cytoplasm. (Hematoxylin and eosin stain) (Fig. 82-13 from McKenna RW, Hernandez J, Peterson L. Benign and malignant mast cell disorders. In: Bick RL, ed. Hematology: clinical and laboratory practice. St Louis: CV Mosby, 1993:1261–72.)

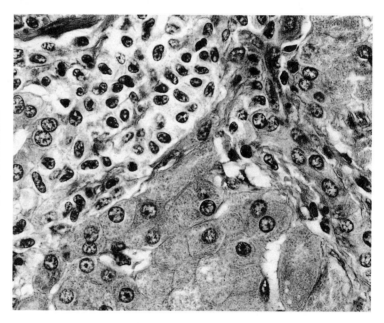

chronic inflammatory cellular infiltration is present with plasma cells, lymphocytes, and eosinophils (89). Kupffer cell hyperplasia is often present. A histologic diagnosis of liver involvement in mast cell disease is difficult without the aid of cytochemistry (89).

Cytochemical and Immunohistochemical Findings. The recognition of a mast cell proliferation in hematoxylin and eosin stained sections of bone marrow or other tissues may be difficult because of their morphologic similarity to histiocytes and fibroblasts. When a diagnosis of mast cell disease is suspected on clinical grounds or by histologic features, cytochemistry may confirm the diagnosis.

The mast cell granules exhibit prominent metachromasia with the Giemsa and toluidine blue stains in both marrow smears and tissue sections (fig. 485) (68). These stains are applicable to decalcified paraffin-embedded tissue processed

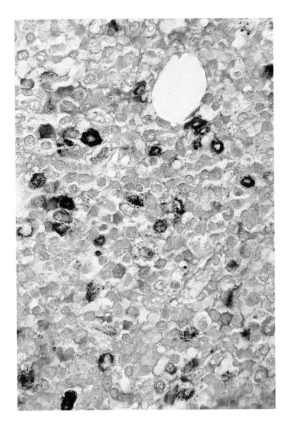 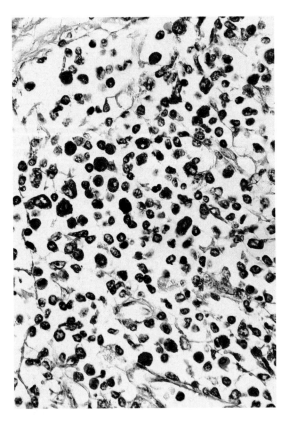

Figure 485
CYTOCHEMISTRY OF MAST CELL LESIONS

Left: A toluidine blue stain of a bone marrow lesion from a patient with systemic mast cell disease. The mast cell granules stain metachromatically. This pattern of staining helps differentiate the lesions in mast cell disease from those of other disorders. (Toluidine blue 0 stain)

Right: A section of spleen from a patient with systemic mast cell disease stained for chloroacetate esterase activity. The mast cells show strong reactivity. (Chloroacetate esterase stain)

with various fixatives. The toluidine blue stain does not appear to be as reliable when applied to tissues fixed with mercurial fixatives such as B5 and Zenker. The chloroacetate esterase (CAE) stain, which reacts with mast cells and neutrophils and their precursors, may be of aid in identifying mast cells in nondecalcified formalin-fixed specimens (fig. 485) (53,83).

Enzyme immunohistochemical studies may be useful in the diagnosis in some cases. Positive staining for vimentin, leukocyte common antigen (LCA), lysozyme, alpha-1-antitrypsin, and alpha-1-antichymotrypsin have been demonstrated in normal mast cells and in cases of systemic mast cell disease (62). Antibodies for several of the chemical mediators produced by mast cells are also available and can be applied by immunoperoxidase methods (62).

Ultrastructural Findings. The mast cells in bone marrow lesions of systemic mast cell disease are round to elongate with extremely irregular and infolded cell margins. The granules are often small and contain scrolls, lamellae, and rope-like material (88). Many of the cells show evidence of degranulation and the cytoplasm is frequently filled with microfilaments (fig. 486) (53,88). Ultrastructural studies rarely contribute to the diagnosis of mast cell disease.

Cytogenetic Findings. There is little available data on cytogenetic changes in mast cell disease. Bone marrow clonal chromosome abnormalities have been identified in a minority of the cases studied (79). No specific chromosome rearrangements have been identified. The abnormalities observed are those commonly found in myeloid leukemias and myelodysplastic syndromes

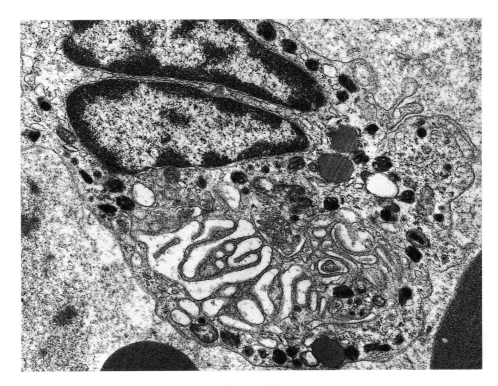

Figure 486
ELECTRON MICROGRAPH OF A MAST CELL FROM THE BONE MARROW
OF A PATIENT WITH SYSTEMIC MAST CELL DISEASE
The cytoplasm is relatively sparsely granulated. (Uranyl acetate-lead citrate stain, X10,000)

(79,84,85). In cases of mast cell disease with a concurrent myeloproliferative disorder, the incidence of cytogenetic changes is higher.

Differential Diagnosis. Four conditions that merit particular consideration in the differential diagnosis of the bone marrow lesions in systemic mast cell disease are primary myelofibrosis, angioimmunoblastic lymphadenopathy, hypergranular promyelocytic leukemia (M3), and eosinophilic fibrohistiocytic lesions. The distinction of mast cell disease from these disorders can generally be accomplished by a combination of clinical features, histopathology, and cytochemical stains.

When there is diffuse marrow involvement, distinguishing mast cell disease from primary myelofibrosis may be problematic. In these cases, the mast cells are often elongated and resemble fibroblasts. They may be uniformly distributed or appear in collections in fibrotic areas. The lesions differ from advanced primary myelofibrosis, which is characterized by a mixture of cells and densely fibrotic areas that frequently contain few cellular elements; megakary-

ocytes may be prominent and found in clusters. The reticulin stain in advanced myelofibrosis is generally characterized by a denser concentration of thicker reticulin fibers than in mast cell disease (53,86). Cytochemical demonstration of mast cells is of critical importance in this differential diagnosis.

Bone marrow involvement in angioimmunoblastic lymphadenopathy may be focal or diffuse and is often paratrabecular (70). The lesions are usually loosely structured and composed of randomly distributed lymphocytes, plasma cells, immunoblasts, and collections of eosinophils. Prominent vascular proliferation may be present. In contrast, the polycellular lesions of mast cell disease are fairly densely packed with specific cell types grouped together; plasma cells and immunoblasts are not an integral part of the lesions and there is usually only minimal vascular proliferation.

Cases of mast cell leukemia and, rarely, a myelodysplastic syndrome occurring concurrently with systemic mast cell disease may be confused with hypergranular promyelocytic leukemia (M3) in bone marrow smears. The overall bone marrow morphologic findings, together with the contrasting cytochemical profiles of the two disorders, distinguish them.

Eosinophilic fibrohistiocytic lesions of bone marrow bear a strong resemblance to mast cell disease (see figs. 476, 477) (53,75,80). The large histiocytic cells described in eosinophilic fibrohistiocytic lesions have been identified as mast cells in some studies (80). In most cases, these lesions appear to represent a benign form of systemic mast cell disease. Their biologic relationship to lesions of symptomatic, generalized mast cell disease is unclear.

Occasionally, mast cell disease must be differentiated from a spectrum of infiltrative disorders of the hematopoietic tissues, including Hodgkin disease and non-Hodgkin lymphoma, granulomatous disease, and hairy cell leukemia. The clinical and laboratory findings and the histopathology of the bone marrow biopsies should distinguish mast cell disease from these disorders (53).

Treatment and Prognosis. Treatment for systemic mast cell disease is largely supportive; there is no cure. Therapy is directed at providing relief from systemic symptoms. Therapeutic agents that block the effects of histamine such as chlorpheniramine, an H_1 histamine antagonist, and cimetidine or ranitidine, H_2 histamine antagonists, have been used alone or in combination (59,69). Aspirin therapy, as an inhibitor of prostaglandin synthesis, in combination with H_1 and H_2 antagonists, has been effective in some patients unresponsive to histamine antagonist therapy alone (73). Aspirin must be used cautiously, however, since it has been implicated in exacerbating clinical symptoms in some patients (54,69). Oral disodium chromoglycate, which inhibits mast cell degranulation, has been effective in some cases (59,69,78). For patients with heparin or prostaglandin E_2-mediated severe osteopenia, inhibitors of bone resorption, such as clodronate, may be partially effective (55). Radiation, steroids, and chemotherapeutic agents have been used in patients with advanced systemic mast cell disease with varying and usually limited success (65,69,83,87). Splenectomy may have beneficial effects in reducing complications from blood cytopenias in patients with aggressive forms of the disease (57).

The clinical course is generally chronic, with slow progression of symptoms. Patients often die from unrelated causes. Males fair less well than females and older individuals often have more aggressive disease (63,83). Clinical factors that have been associated with a poor prognosis include constitutional symptoms, abnormal liver function tests, anemia, thrombocytopenia, other hematologic disorders, and certain bone marrow histologic changes (61,83). Progression to mast cell leukemia is rare but the occurrence of other malignancies is relatively common. The second malignancy is most often a myeloid leukemia but lymphomas and carcinomas have also been reported (53,61,63,68,76,83,84,87). A 37 percent incidence of myeloid, monocytic, and mast cell leukemias was found in one study (68). Patients that present with, or evolve to, mast cell leukemia have a particularly poor prognosis, with a median survival of approximately 5 months (84). The relatively common occurrence of acute myeloid and monocytic leukemia in patients with systemic mast cell disease is probably a reflection of the close relationship of the genesis of mast cells and myeloid hematopoietic cells (53,79,83,85,90).

REFERENCES

Benign-Reactive Lymphoid Lesions

1. Brunning RD, McKenna RW. Bone marrow manifestations of malignant lymphoma and lymphoma-like conditions. Pathol Annu 1979;14(Pt 1):1–59.

2. Castella A, Croxson TS, Mildvan D, Witt OH, Zalusky R. The bone marrow in AIDS. A histologic, hematologic, and microbiologic study. Am J Clin Pathol 1985;84:425–32.

3. Cervantes F, Pereira A, Marti JM, Feliu E, Rozman C. Bone marrow lymphoid nodules in myeloproliferative disorders: association with the nonmyelosclerotic phases of idiopathic myelofibrosis and immunological significance. Br J Haematol 1988;70:279–82.

4. Chilosi M, Pizzolo G, Fiore-Donati L, Bofill M, Janossy G. Routine immunofluorescent and histochemical analysis of bone marrow involvement of lymphoma/leukaemia: the use of cryostat sections. Br J Cancer 1983;48:763–75.

5. Conlan MG, Bast M, Armitage JO, Weisenburger DD. Bone marrow involvement by non-Hodgkin's lymphoma: the clinical significance of morphologic discordance between the lymph node and bone marrow. Nebraska Lymphoma Study Group. J Clin Oncol 1990;8:1163–72.

6. Crocker J, Jones EL, Curran RC. Study of nuclear sizes in the centers of malignant and benign lymphoid follicles. J Clin Pathol 1983;36:1332–4.

7. Danova M, Riccardi A, Brugnatelli S, et al. Bone marrow morphology and proliferative activity in acquired immunodeficiency syndrome. Haematologica 1989;74:365–9.

8. Ellison DJ, Hu E, Zovich D, Pinter-Brown L, Pattengale PK. Immunogenetic analysis of bone marrow aspirates in patients with non-Hodgkin lymphomas. Am J Hematol 1990;33:160–6.

9. Farhi DC. Germinal centers in the bone marrow. Hematol Pathol 1989;3:133–6.

10. Faulkner-Jones BE, Howie AJ, Boughton BJ, Franklin IM. Lymphoid aggregates in bone marrow: study of eventual outcome. J Clin Pathol 1988;41:768–75.

11. Gaulard P, Kanavaros P, Farcet JP, et al. Bone marrow histologic and immunohistochemical findings in peripheral T-cell lymphoma: a study of 38 cases. Hum Pathol 1991;22:331–8.

12. Hanson CA, Brunning RD, Gajl-Peczalska KJ, Frizzera G, McKenna RW. Bone marrow manifestations of peripheral T-cell lymphoma. A study of 30 cases. Am J Clin Pathol 1986;86:449–60.

13. Karcher DS, Frost AR. The bone marrow in human immunodeficiency virus (HIV)-related disease: morphology and clinical correlation. Am J Clin Pathol 1991;95:63–71.

14. Kemona A, Dziecio J, Sulik M, Bernaczyk A, Sulkowski S. Lymphocytic aggregations in the bone marrow: their occurrence and morphologic analysis. Patol Pol 1989;40:219–25.

15. Knowles DM, Athan E, Ubriaco A, et al. Extranodal noncutaneous lymphoid hyperplasias represent a continuous spectrum of B-cell neoplasia: demonstration by molecular genetic analysis. Blood 1989;73:1635–45.

16. Liang R, Chan VV, Chan TK, Todd D, Ho F. Immunoglobulin gene rearrangement in the peripheral blood and bone marrow of patients with lymphomas of the mucosa-associated lymphoid tissues. Acta Haematol 1990;84:19–23.

17. Liu PI, Takanari H, Yatani R, Nelson G. Comparative studies of bone marrow from the United States and Japan. Ann Clin Lab Sci 1989;19:345–51.

18. Maeda K, Hyun BH, Rebuck JW. Lymphoid follicles in bone marrow aspirates. Am J Clin Pathol 1977;67:41–8.

19. Mead JH, Mason TE. Lymphoma versus AIDS [Letter]. Am J Clin Pathol 1983;80:546–7.

20. O'Carroll DI, McKenna RW, Brunning RD. Bone marrow manifestations of Hodgkin's disease. Cancer 1976;38:1717–28.

21. Osborne BM, Guarda LA, Butler JJ. Bone marrow biopsies in patients with the acquired immunodeficiency syndrome. Hum Pathol 1984;15:1048–53.

22. Rosenthal NS, Farhi DC. Bone marrow findings in connective tissue disease. Am J Clin Pathol 1989;92:650–4.

23. Rywlin AM, Ortega RS, Dominguez CJ. Lymphoid nodules of bone marrow: normal and abnormal. Blood 1974;43:389–400.

24. Sandhaus LM, Scudder R. Hematologic and bone marrow abnormalities in pediatric patients with human immunodeficiency virus (HIV) infection. Pediatr Pathol 1989;9:277–88.

25. _____, Voelkerding KV, Dougherty J, Raska K Jr. Combined utility of gene rearrangement analysis and flow cytometry in the diagnosis of lymphoproliferative disease in the bone marrow. Hematol Pathol 1990;4:135–48.

26. Sangster G, Crocker J, Nar P, Leyland MJ. Benign and malignant (B cell) focal lymphoid aggregates in bone marrow trephines shown by means of an immunogold-silver technique. J Clin Pathol 1986;39:453–7.

Granulomas

27. Bhargava V, Farhi DC. Bone marrow granulomas: clinicopathologic findings in 72 cases and review of the literature. Hematol Pathol 1988;2:43–50.

28. Bodem CR, Hamory BH, Taylor HM, Kleopfer L. Granulomatous bone marrow disease. A review of the literature and clinicopathologic analysis of 58 cases. Medicine (Baltimore) 1983;62:372–83.

29. Brincker H. Sarcoid reactions and sarcoidosis in Hodgkin's disease and other malignant lymphomata. Br J Cancer 1972;26:120–3.

30. Kadin ME, Donaldson SS, Dorfman RF. Isolated granulomas in Hodgkin's disease. N Engl J Med 1970;283:859–61.

31. Kahn LB, King H, Jacobs P. Florid epithelial cell and sarcoid-type reaction associated with non-Hodgkin's lymphoma. S Afr Med J 1977;51:341–7.

32. O'Carroll DI, McKenna RW, Brunning RD. Bone marrow manifestations of Hodgkin's disease. Cancer 1976;38:1717–28.

33. O'Connell MJ, Schimpff SC, Kirschner RH, Abt AB, Wiernick PH. Epithelioid granulomas in Hodgkin disease. A favorable prognostic sign? JAMA 1975;233:886–9.

34. Sacks EL, Donaldson SS, Gordon J, Dorfman RF. Epithelioid granulomas associated with Hodgkin's disease: clinical correlations in 55 previously untreated patients. Cancer 1978;41:562–7.

35. Yu NC, Rywlin AM. Granulomatous lesions of the bone marrow in non-Hodgkin's lymphoma. Hum Pathol 1982; 13:905–10.

Idiopathic Bone Marrow Fibrosis

36. Auger MJ, Nash JR, Mackie MJ. Marrow involvement with T cell lymphoma initially presenting as abnormal myelopoiesis. J Clin Pathol 1986;39:134–7.

37. Gaulard P, Kanavaros P, Farcet JP, et al. Bone marrow histologic and immunohistochemical findings in peripheral T-cell lymphoma: a study of 38 cases. Hum Pathol 1991;22:331–8.

38. Hanson CA, Brunning RD, Gajl-Peczalska KJ, Frizzera G, McKenna RW. Bone marrow manifestations of peripheral T-cell lymphoma. A study of 30 cases. Am J Clin Pathol 1986;86:449–60.

39. Hasselbalch H. Idiopathic myelofibrosis: a clinical study of 80 patients. Am J Haematol 1990;34:291–300.

40. Jäger K, Burkhardt R, Bartl R, Frisch B, Mahl G. Lymphoid infiltrates in chronic myeloproliferative disorders (MPD). Verh Dtsch Ges Pathol 1983;67:239–42.

Angioimmunoblastic Lymphadenopathy (Immunoblastic Lymphadenopathy)

41. Brunning RD, McKenna RW. Bone marrow manifestations of malignant lymphoma and lymphoma-like conditions. Pathol Annu 1979;14(Pt 1):1–59.

42. Frizzera G, Kaneko Y, Sakurai M. Angioimmunoblastic lymphadenopathy and related disorders: a retrospective look in search of definitions. Leukemia 1989;3:1–5.

43. _____, Moran EM, Rappaport H. Angio-immunoblastic lymphadenopathy: diagnosis and clinical course. Am J Med 1975;59:803–18.

44. Kaneko Y, Maseki N, Sakurai M, et al. Characteristic karyotypic pattern in T-cell lymphoproliferative disorders with reactive "angioimmunoblastic lymphadenopathy with dysproteinemia-type" features. Blood 1988;72:413–21.

45. Lukes RJ, Tindle BH. Immunoblastic lymphadenopathy. A hyperimmune entity resembling Hodgkin's disease. N Engl J Med 1975;292:1–8.

46. Nathwani BN, Winberg CD, Bearman RM. Angioimmunoblastic lymphadenopathy with dysproteinemia and its progression to malignant lymphoma. In: Jaffe E, ed. Surgical pathology of the lymph nodes and related organs. Philadelphia: WB Saunders, 1985:57–85.

47. Pangalis GA, Moran EM, Nathwani BN, Zelman RJ, Kim H, Rappaport H. Angioimmunoblastic lymphadenopathy. Long-term follow-up study. Cancer 1983;52:318–21.

48. _____, Moran EM, Rappaport H. Blood and bone marrow findings in angioimmunoblastic lymphadenopathy. Blood 1978;51:71–83.

49. Schnaidt U, Vykoupil KF, Thiele J, Georgii A. Angioimmunoblastic lymphadenopathy. Histopathology of bone marrow involvement. Virchows Arch [A] 1980;389:369–80.

50. Suchi T, Lennert K, Tu LY, et al. Histopathology and immunocytochemistry of peripheral T cell lymphomas: a proposal for their classification. J Clin Pathol 1987; 40:995–1015.

Mast Cell Disease

51. Ammann RW, Vetter D, Deyhle P, Tschen H, Sulser H, Schmid M. Gastrointestinal involvement in systemic mastocytosis. Gut 1976;17:107–12.

52. Bonnet P, Smadja C, Szekely AM, et al. Intractable ascites in systemic mastocytosis treated by portal diversion. Dig Dis Sci 1987;32:209–13.

53. Brunning RD, McKenna RW, Rosai J, Parkin JL, Risdall R. Systemic mastocytosis. Extracutaneous manifestations. Am J Surg Pathol 1983;7:425–38.

54. Crawhall JC, Wilkinson RD. Systemic mastocytosis: management of an unusual case with histamine (H1 and H2) antagonists and cyclooxygenase inhibition. Clin Invest Med 1987;10:1–4.

55. Cundy T, Beneton MN, Darby AJ, Marshall WJ, Kanis JA. Osteopenia in systemic mastocytosis: natural history and responses to treatment with inhibitors of bone resorption. Bone 1987;8:149–55.

56. Fishman RS, Fleming CR, Li CY. Systemic mastocytosis with review of gastrointestinal manifestations. Mayo Clin Proc 1979;54:51–4.

57. Friedman BS, Darling G, Norton J, Hamby L, Metcalfe D. Splenectomy in the management of systemic mast cell disease. Surgery 1990;107:94–100.

58. _____, Steinberg SC, Meggs WJ, Kaliner MA, Frieri M, Metcalfe DD. Analysis of plasma histamine levels in patients with mast cell disorders. Am J Med 1989;87:649–54.

59. Frieri M, Alling DW, Metcalfe DD. Comparison of the therapeutic efficacy of cromolyn sodium with that of combined chlorpheniramine and cimetidine in systemic mastocytosis. Results of a double-blind clinical trial. Am J Med 1985;78:9–14.

60. Horny HP, Kaiserling E. Lymphoid cells and tissue mast cells of bone marrow lesions in systemic mastocytosis: a histological and immunohistological study. Br J Haematol 1988;69:449–55.

61. _____, Parwaresch MR, Lennert K. Bone marrow findings in systemic mastocytosis. Hum Pathol 1985;16:808–14.

62. _____, Reimann O, Kaiserling E. Immunoreactivity of normal and neoplastic human tissue mast cells. Am J Clin Pathol 1988;89:335–40.

63. _____, Ruck M, Wehrmann M, Kaiserling E. Blood findings in generalized mastocytosis: evidence of frequent simultaneous occurrence of myeloproliferative disorders. Br J Haematol 1990;76:186–93.

64. Huang TY, Yam LT, Li CY. Radiological features of systemic mast-cell disease. Br J Radiol 1987;60:765–70.

65. Jane SM, Sutherland R, Salem HH. Malignant systemic mastocytosis. Aust N Z J Med 1988;18:610–2.

66. Johnson AC, Johnson S, Lester PD, Halter S, James E Jr. Systemic mastocytosis and mastocytosis-like syndrome: radiologic features of gastrointestinal manifestations. South Med J 1988;81:729–33.

67. Korenblat PE, Wedner HJ, Whyte MP, Frankel S, Avioli LV. Systemic mastocytosis. Arch Intern Med 1984;144:2249–53.

68. Lennert K, Parwaresch MR. Mast cells and mast cell neoplasia: a review. Histopathology 1979;3:349–65.

69. Metcalfe DD. The treatment of mastocytosis: an overview. J Invest Dermatol 1991;96:55–59S.

70. Pangalis GA, Moran EM, Rappaport H. Blood and marrow findings in angioimmunoblastic lymphadenopathy. Blood 1978;51:71–83.

71. Rafii M, Firooznia H, Golimbu C, Balthazar E. Pathologic fracture in systemic mastocytosis. Radiographic spectrum and review of the literature. Clin Orthop 1983;180:260–7.

72. Roberts LJ II, Oates JA. Biochemical diagnosis of systemic mast cell disorders. J Invest Dermatol 1991;96:19–25S.

73. _____, Sweetman BJ, Lewis RA, Austen KF, Oates JA. Increased production of prostaglandin D_2 in patients with systemic mastocytosis. N Eng J Med 1980;303:1400–4.

74. Rogers MP, Bloomingdale K, Murawski BJ, Soter NA, Reich P, Austen KF. Mixed organic brain syndrome as a manifestation of systemic mastocytosis. Psychosom Med 1986;48:437–47.

75. Rywlin AM, Hoffman EP, Ortega RS. Eosinophilic fibrohistiocytic lesion of bone marrow: a distinctive new morphologic finding, probably related to drug hypersensitivity. Blood 1972;40:464–72.

76. Sagher F, Even-Paz Z. Mastocytosis and the mast cell. Chicago: Yearbook Medical Publishers, 1967.

77. Schwartz LB. Tryptase, a mediator of human mast cells. J Allergy Clin Immunol 1990;86(4 Pt 2):594–8.

78. Sumpio BE, O'Leary G, Gusberg RJ. Variceal bleeding, hypersplenism, and systemic mastocytosis. Arch Surgery 1988;123:767–9.

79. Swolin B, Rödjer S, Roupe G. Cytogenetic studies and in vitro colony growth in patients with mastocytosis. Blood 1987;70:1928–32.

80. teVelde J, Vismans FJ, Leenheers-Binnendijk L, Vos CJ, Smeenk D, Bijvoet OL. The eosinophilic fibrohistiocytic lesion of the bone marrow. A mastocellular lesion in bone disease. Virchows Arch [A] 1978; 377:277–85.

81. Travis WD, Li CY. Pathology of the lymph node and spleen in systemic mast cell disease. Mod Pathol 1988;1:4–14.

82. _____, Li CY, Bergstralh EJ. Solid and hematologic malignancies in 60 patients with systemic mast cell disease. Arch Pathol Lab Med 1989;113:365–8.

83. _____, Li CY, Bergstralh EJ, Yam LT, Swee RG. Systemic mast cell disease. Analysis of 58 cases and literature review. Medicine (Baltimore) 1988;67:345–68.

84. _____, Li CY, Hoagland HC, Travis LB, Banks PM. Mast cell leukemia: report of a case and review of the literature. Mayo Clin Proc 1986;61:957–66.

85. _____, Li CY, Yam LT, Bergstralh EJ, Swee RG. Significance of systemic mast cell disease with associated hematologic disorders. Cancer 1988;62:965–72.

86. Udoji WC, Razavi SA. Mast cells and myelofibrosis. Am J Clin Pathol 1975;63:203–9.

87. Webb TA, Li CY, Yam LT. Systemic mast cell disease: a clinical and hematopathologic study of 26 cases. Cancer 1982;49:927–38.

88. Weidner N, Horan RF, Austen KF. Mast-cell phenotype in indolent forms of mastocytosis. Ultrastructural features, fluorescence detection of avidin binding, and immunofluorescent determination of chymase, tryptase, and carboxypeptidase. Am J Pathol 1992; 140:847–57.

89. Yam LT, Chan CH, Li CY. Hepatic involvement in systemic mast cell disease. Am J Med 1986;80:819–26.

90. Zucker-Franklin D. Ultrastructure evidence for the common origin of human mast cells and basophils. Blood 1980;56:534–40.

✧ ✧ ✧

HISTIOCYTIC PROLIFERATIONS OF THE BONE MARROW

Histiocytic proliferations of the bone marrow include several reactive or tumor-like conditions and rare examples of neoplastic diseases. The histiocytic disorders that may involve the bone marrow include storage histiocyte disorders, Langerhans cell histiocytosis, hemophagocytic syndromes, and malignant histiocytosis.

STORAGE HISTIOCYTE DISORDERS

Definition. Disorders resulting from inborn errors of metabolism leading to hyperplasia of the monocyte-macrophage system and accumulation of large amounts of storage material in the cytoplasm of histiocytes. They are a heterogeneous group of diseases having in common an inherited deficiency of a hydrolytic enzyme that is normally present in lysosomes and is essential for normal catabolism. Products that are ordinarily degraded by the affected enzyme remain undigested and accumulate in the cell cytoplasm. Collections of storage histiocytes may form tumor-like lesions in hematopoietic tissues. These are occasionally important in the differential diagnosis of neoplastic disorders of the bone marrow.

Incidence and Clinical Findings. All of the histiocyte lysosomal storage diseases are rare and nearly all are autosomal recessive disorders. The clinical manifestations of different types vary from an asymptomatic course to a severe debilitating illness with death at a young age. The clinical severity often relates to the effects of the enzyme deficiency on cells other than histiocytes, such as the neurons of the central nervous system. Degenerative neurologic changes, seizures, and mental retardation accompany several of the storage disorders; facial and skeletal abnormalities are striking in some cases. The clinical symptoms that result from storage histiocyte proliferation in hematopoietic tissues are manifestations of organomegaly and blood cytopenias. Bone pain is a symptom of tumorous masses in some patients (16).

Laboratory Findings. Cellular enzyme assays are available for many of the storage diseases, including most of those associated with histiocytic proliferations in the bone marrow. These studies detect decreased activity of a particular lysosomal enzyme and provide a definitive diagnosis. Urine and serum may contain excessive quantities of storage material that can be measured by biochemical assays.

Blood and Bone Marrow Findings. Blood cytopenias are present in some of the storage diseases due to hypersplenism and encroachment on the bone marrow by masses of storage histiocytes. Leukocyte inclusions of various types are characteristic of several of the storage disorders. For example, vacuolated lymphocytes are common in Niemann-Pick disease and metachromatic granular inclusions are found in lymphocytes and Alder-Reilly bodies in granulocytes in cases of mucopolysaccharidosis (3).

In several storage diseases, storage histiocytes are present in the bone marrow as tumor-like masses or individual scattered cells. The bone marrow findings in Gaucher disease, Niemann-Pick disease, and the mucopolysaccharidoses are described below.

Gaucher Disease. Gaucher disease is inherited as an autosomal recessive trait. It is the most prevalent lysosomal storage disorder. Patients with Gaucher disease are deficient in glucocerebrosidase, resulting in glucocerebroside accumulation in the lysosomes of histiocytes (1). There are three clinical variants, presumably due to different mutations affecting the same or similar gene loci. *Type II (acute neuronopathic)* and *type III (subacute neuronopathic) Gaucher disease* are serious progressive diseases that result in death at a young age (1). *Type I, non-neuronopathic adult Gaucher disease (glycosylceramide lipidosis)* has a chronic course and is the storage disorder most likely to be diagnosed from a bone marrow biopsy (3,12). Patients with type I Gaucher disease generally present with splenomegaly and blood cytopenias. Hepatomegaly and osteolytic bone lesions are present in some cases (2).

Most patients present with blood cytopenias but there are no specific findings in the blood smears. Gaucher cells in marrow smears or trephine imprints are large, 20 to 100 µm in diameter, and usually have a single small nucleus. The cytoplasm has a striated or fibrillary pattern, like wrinkled tissue paper, and is pale blue to grey in

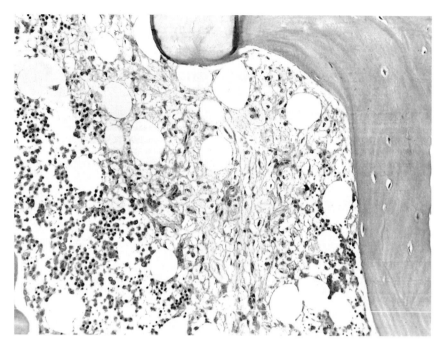

Figure 487
GAUCHER DISEASE
A trephine biopsy section from a 24-year-old woman with splenomegaly and pancytopenia. There is a focal lesion consisting of Gaucher-type histiocytes adjacent to a bone trabeculum. (Hematoxylin and eosin stain) (Fig. 27 from McKenna RW. Disorders of bone marrow. In: Sternberg SS, ed. Diagnostic surgical pathology, Vol. 1. New York: Raven Press, 1989:479–513.)

Wright-Giemsa stained preparations (3,9,11). In some cases, bone marrow smears are devoid of Gaucher cells even when there is an abundance of storage histiocytes on the trephine biopsy sections.

The histopathology of trephine biopsy sections varies from small focal lesions to near total replacement of the marrow with Gaucher cells (fig. 487). The striated or fibrillary cytoplasm of the histiocytes is usually easily recognized in biopsy sections (fig. 488). Hemosiderin pigment is often present in the cytoplasm. Reticulin fibrosis may be prominent in areas of Gaucher cell proliferation. The uninvolved marrow is hypercellular. Bone necrosis due to vascular alterations induced by Gaucher cell proliferation occurs in the spine and long bones in some patients (9). Necrosis is rarely encountered in posterior iliac crest trephine biopsies. Increased bone marrow plasma cells, a monoclonal gammopathy, and plasma cell myeloma are occasionally associated with Gaucher disease (6). The significance of this association is unclear.

Cytochemically, Gaucher cells react strongly to enzyme cytochemical stains for tartrate-resistant acid phosphatase and nonspecific esterase (NSE) (11). They are often intensely positive with the periodic acid–Schiff (PAS) reaction (3).

Ultrastructurally, the cytoplasmic storage material is composed of membrane-bound structures containing hollow tubules measuring 250 to 725 Ångström units in diameter (3,11).

The morphologic differential diagnosis of Gaucher disease in the bone marrow includes other disorders in which histiocytes are increased and found in clusters in trephine biopsy sections. These include other storage disorders, Langerhans cell histiocytosis, infection-associated hemophagocytic syndrome, and infectious granulomas. All of these disorders and their defining morphologic features are described elsewhere in the text. Myelofibrosis and hairy cell leukemia may mimic type I Gaucher disease clinically but the morphologic features in the blood and bone marrow are distinctive.

Cells cytologically similar to Gaucher cells are observed in small numbers in marrow smears from patients with chronic myelogenous leukemia and have been reported in acute leukemia

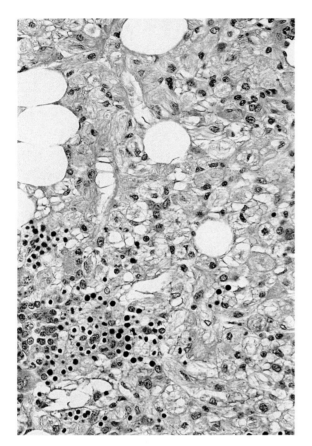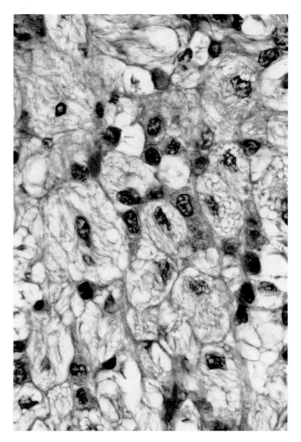

Figure 488
GAUCHER DISEASE
Left: There is extensive replacement of normal hematopoietic tissue by Gaucher histiocytes. A focus of normal hematopoietic cells is present in the lower left of the field. (Hematoxylin and eosin stain)
Right: A higher magnification of the figure on the left shows large histiocytes with striated-appearing cytoplasm typical of Gaucher disease. (Hematoxylin and eosin stain)

and congenital dyserythropoietic anemia (5,14, 15). In the appropriate clinical setting, however, the distinctive cytologic features of Gaucher histiocytes are virtually diagnostic.

Niemann-Pick Diseases. The Niemann-Pick diseases (sphingomyelin-cholesterol lipidoses) include two major types of storage disorders, each with several clinical forms (13). The disorders are characterized by the accumulation of sphingomyelin, cholesterol, glycosphingolipid, and bis (monoacyl-glycero)-phosphate in various body tissues due to a deficiency of sphingomyelinase. Hepatosplenomegaly and foamy histiocytes in the bone marrow, spleen, and lymph nodes are common features of all variants (13). Niemann-Pick diseases typically cause severe physical and mental symptoms at an early age. Death usually occurs in early childhood.

The disease may resemble acute neuropathic (type II) Gaucher disease in its clinical features.

In blood smears, lymphocytes with numerous sharply defined lipid vacuoles may be observed. Large histiocytes, 20 to 50 μm in diameter, are often found in abundance near the thin edge of bone marrow smears (3). They contain a single, centrally or eccentrically located nucleus and finely vacuolated cytoplasm (fig. 489). Occasionally, sea blue histiocytes filled with many large homogeneous blue or blue-green granules are present.

A diffuse pattern of involvement with variable marrow replacement is most common in trephine biopsy sections; scattered or large clusters of foamy histiocytes may be observed.

The presence of foamy histiocytes in the bone marrow is suggestive, but not pathognomonic, of

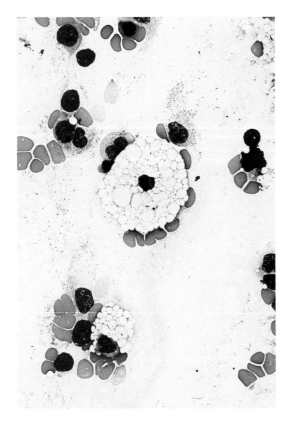

Figure 489
NIEMANN-PICK HISTIOCYTE
Bone marrow aspirate smear from a child with Niemann-Pick disease. A large foamy histiocyte typical of this disorder is illustrated. (Wright-Giemsa stain)

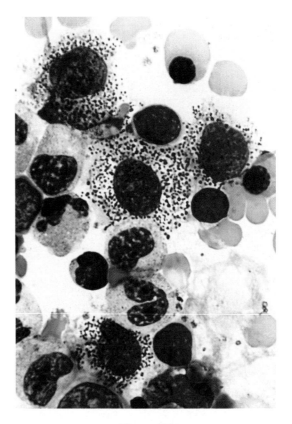

Figure 490
MUCOPOLYSACCHARIDOSIS
A bone marrow aspirate smear from a child with type III mucopolysaccharidosis (Sanfilippo disease). Four histiocytes containing metachromatic granules are present in this field. (Wright-Giemsa stain)

Niemann-Pick disease. The differential diagnosis may include other histiocytoses, particularly those with foamy histiocytes. Similar cells are present in other conditions in which lipids accumulate in the cytoplasm of histiocytes, such as the hyperlipidemias. A presumptive diagnosis of Niemann-Pick disease can be made on the basis of the marrow infiltration and the presence of hepatosplenomegaly. The diagnosis is confirmed by documentation of decreased sphingo-myelinase activity in tissue samples, leukocyte extracts, or cultured skin fibroblasts (13).

Mucopolysaccharidoses. These are a rare group of autosomal recessive disorders caused by a deficiency of the lysosomal enzymes needed for the stepwise degradation of glycosaminoglycans (mucopolysaccharides) (10). There are about 10 variants of this disorder that share many clinical features. Mental retardation is characteristic of

several, including Hurler, Hunter, and San-filippo syndromes. There is wide variation in clinical severity among the different mucopoly-saccharidoses and within any single type (10). The diagnosis is made by enzyme assays using fibroblasts, leukocytes, or serum.

Blood smears in several variants show abnormal leukocyte granules and cytoplasmic inclusions. The most commonly observed abnormality is dark basophilic granules surrounded by a clear halo in the cytoplasm of lymphocytes (3). The number and size of these inclusions varies. The granules stain metachromatically with the toluidine blue 0 stain. Alder-Reilly granulation is present in the granulocytes in some cases (3).

In bone marrow smears, variable numbers of large histiocytes packed with basophilic inclusions of various size are observed (fig. 490). These cells resemble mast cells; like mast cells the granules stain metachromatically with toluidine blue 0. In some cases, plasma cells contain numerous cytoplasmic inclusions identical to those in histiocytes (see fig. 367) (3).

In trephine biopsy sections, the histiocytes are generally scattered among other hematopoietic cells. Small clusters may be observed, but mass proliferations are not encountered. In most cases, the obvious clinical symptomatology and the characteristic morphology of the storage histiocytes eliminates consideration of other storage diseases or a neoplastic or reactive histiocyte disorder.

Treatment and Prognosis. Treatment is largely symptomatic and supportive. Experimental trials of enzyme replacement therapy and renal and splenic transplants for some storage diseases have had limited success (4,7). Bone marrow transplantation offers the potential for effective metabolic correction in selected storage disorders (8).

The prognosis varies according to the effect and severity of the enzyme deficiency. Most patients with severe forms of storage disease, e.g., type II Gaucher disease and most of the Niemann-Pick diseases, have an aggressive degenerative course and die in childhood. Those with less severe disease, e.g., type I Gaucher disease, may have a chronic progressive course or be asymptomatic.

LANGERHANS CELL HISTIOCYTOSIS

Definition. A localized or disseminated proliferation of Langerhans cells (21). The disease is of unknown etiology but is often associated with abnormalities of the immune system (20). There is no definitive evidence that Langerhans cell histiocytosis (LCH) is a neoplastic disorder. Three clinical variants are recognized: *eosinophilic granuloma, multifocal eosinophilic granulomas (Hand-Schüller-Christian disease)*, and *progressive disseminated LCH (Letterer-Siwe disease)* (20,21). These three variants differ in clinical severity but have common histopathologic features (19).

Incidence and Clinical Findings. Langerhans cell histiocytosis is rare, with an estimated incidence in the United States of 0.2 to 0.5 cases per 100,000 children per year (24). The clinical manifestations vary from asymptomatic to severe constitutional symptoms and progressive disease. In the most common form, eosinophilic granuloma, symptoms usually are referable to a lytic bone lesion and include pain and swelling in the affected area. With multifocal eosinophilic granulomas, several lytic bone lesions and often other organ system involvement are present; rarely, the syndrome of lytic lesions, exophthalmos, and diabetes insipidus is encountered. Lymphadenopathy and hepatosplenomegaly are uncommon except in the most severe cases. The disseminated aggressive form of LCH, Letterer-Siwe disease, is an acute illness with constitutional symptoms, bone and pulmonary lesions, organomegaly, extensive rash, and blood cytopenias.

Laboratory Findings. Lytic radiographic lesions of bone are the most common findings. The skull, femurs, ribs, pelvis, vertebrae, and mandible are the most frequent sites of involvement (20,21,24,27).

Blood and Bone Marrow Findings. There are no pathognomonic blood findings. In the most severe forms of the disease, blood cytopenias may evolve from bone marrow infiltration and splenomegaly. Langerhans cells are rarely, if ever, encountered in blood smears.

The initial diagnosis of LCH is rarely made from a bone marrow needle biopsy but marrow examination is routinely performed to identify the extent of the disease and for assessment of blood cytopenias. Isolated radiographic bone lesions are the most common initial findings and although the ilium is involved in some cases, it is unusual to capture a solitary lesion in a random bone marrow needle biopsy. Lesions identified radiographically are usually removed by open biopsy rather than needle biopsy. Posterior iliac crest marrow biopsies often contain diagnostic tissue in cases of multifocal or generalized bone marrow involvement.

The bone marrow aspirate smears are usually not diagnostic but in some cases increased histiocytes are observed in clusters or as scattered single cells near the thin edge of the smear. The histiocytes have folded, indented, or elongated nuclei and lightly basophilic cytoplasm (fig. 491).

Histopathologic Findings. On trephine biopsy sections the lesions are focal and randomly distributed or large and confluent, occupying most of the marrow space (fig. 492) (25). The lesions may consist predominantly of Langerhans histiocytes or be polymorphous with mixtures of Langerhans cells, multinucleated giant cells, neutrophils, eosinophils, plasma cells, and lymphocytes (figs. 492–495). Lesions may contain

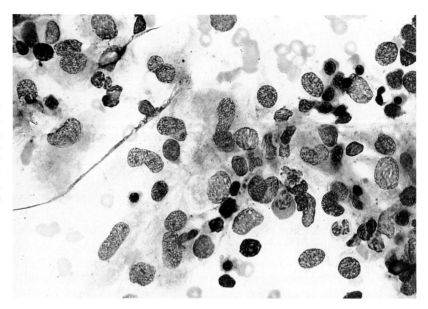

Figure 491
LANGERHANS
CELL HISTIOCYTOSIS

A bone marrow aspirate smear from a young child with Langerhans cell histiocytosis. Several histiocytes are present in a cluster near the edge of the smear; some have folded or indented nuclei. Bone marrow aspirate smears are rarely diagnostic in this disorder. (Wright-Giemsa stain)

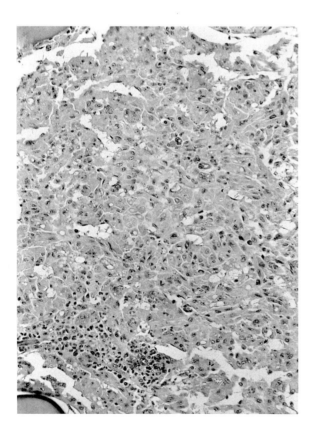

Figure 492
LANGERHANS CELL HISTIOCYTOSIS

A trephine biopsy from a child with Langerhans cell histiocytosis shows a lesion spanning the area between two trabeculae. Langerhans histiocytes are the predominant cell type in this lesion. (Hematoxylin and eosin stain)

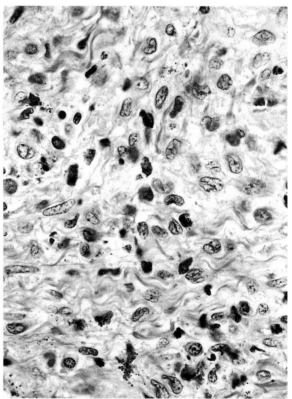

Figure 493
LANGERHANS CELL HISTIOCYTOSIS

A trephine biopsy section from a patient with Langerhans cell histiocytosis. There is fibrosis associated with the Langerhans cell proliferation. The histiocytes are interspersed with eosinophils, fibroblasts, and plasma cells. (Hematoxylin and eosin stain)

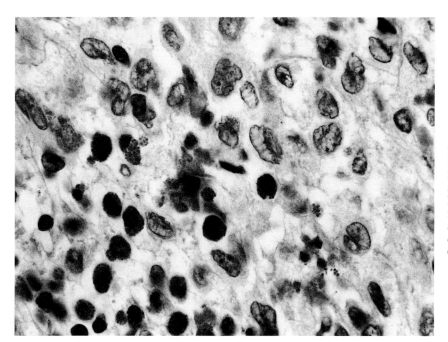

Figure 494
LANGERHANS CELL
HISTIOCYTOSIS
(EOSINOPHILIC
GRANULOMA)

A trephine biopsy from a patient with an eosinophilic granuloma shows typical Langerhans histiocytes. The histiocyte nuclei are grooved and folded and exhibit irregular margins; cytoplasmic margins are indistinct. There are numerous eosinophils at the center and lower left of the field. (Hematoxylin and eosin stain)

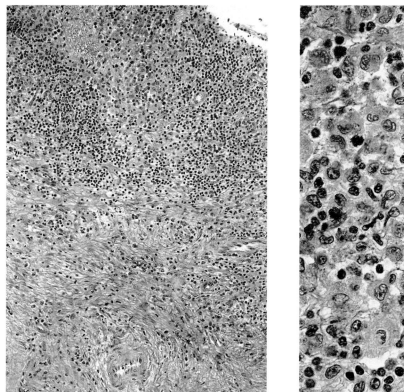

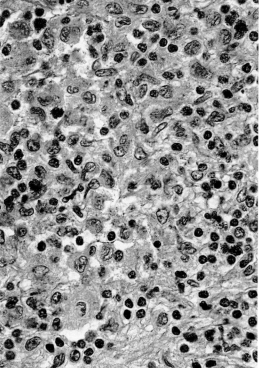

Figure 495
LANGERHANS CELL HISTIOCYTOSIS (EOSINOPHILIC GRANULOMA)

Left: A low-power view of a bone marrow section from a patient with eosinophilic granuloma. The lesion is polycellular with considerable fibrosis and patches rich in lymphocytes. (Hematoxylin and eosin stain)

Right: A high-power view of the bone marrow section on the left. The higher magnification shows typical nuclear morphology of Langerhans histiocytes and scattered eosinophils. (Hematoxylin and eosin stain)

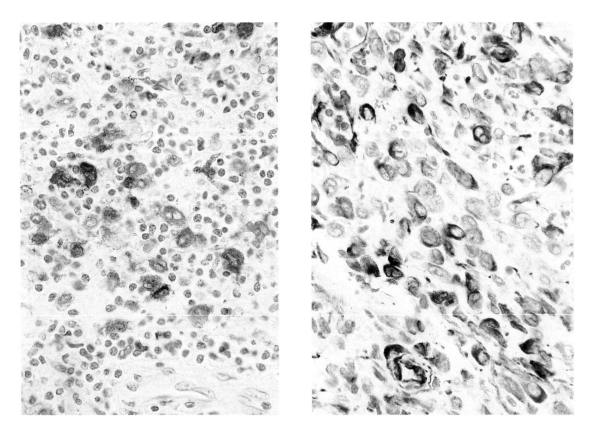

Figure 496
LANGERHANS CELL HISTIOCYTOSIS (EOSINOPHILIC GRANULOMA)

Left: An immunoperoxidase stain of the lesion shown in figure 495. The histiocytes show a strong reaction with antibodies to S-100 protein.

Right: An immunoperoxidase stain of the lesion shown in figure 495. The histiocytes are strongly positive when reacted with an antibody to vimentin.

considerable fibrous tissue and large collections of eosinophils that produce an abscess-like appearance (figs. 493, 495) (19).

The Langerhans cells are mature-appearing histiocytes measuring 15 to 25 µm in diameter, with a centrally located nucleus. The nucleus is characteristically indented or grooved and contains delicate chromatin and inconspicuous nucleoli (figs. 493–495) (19). The cytoplasm is eosinophilic and may contain hemosiderin granules. The marrow adjacent to the lesions is normocellular or hypercellular. Bone trabeculum are normal in appearance in small lesions but may be displaced when large portions of the bone marrow are involved.

Cytochemical and Immunohistochemical Findings. Langerhans cells are differentiated from other histiocytes by their cytochemical and immunohistochemical profile. In contrast to

phagocytic histiocytes, Langerhans cells react negatively for nonspecific esterase and alpha-1-antichymotrypsin. They express a positive reaction with S-100 neuroprotein and vimentin antibodies (fig. 496) (19,22,26). They also express HLA-DR and CD1 antigens and react with peanut lectin and mannosidase antibodies (20).

Ultrastructural Findings. Langerhans cells are large with abundant cytoplasm and irregularly shaped nuclei. The cytoplasm contains rough endoplasmic reticulum, mitochondria, and primary lysosomes. Secondary lysosomes and lipid inclusions are present in some cases (19). The ultrastructural feature that is of most value in the diagnosis of LCH is the Birbeck granule, a cytoplasmic rod-like pentilaminar body often attached to the cell membrane. Identification of this structure is essentially diagnostic of Langerhans cells (22,26).

Differential Diagnosis. In most cases, the clinical presentation, other tissue biopsies, and the characteristic histopathology in the bone marrow are diagnostic of LCH. In rare cases, other histiocytoses or other polycellular lesions in bone marrow such as granulomas, Hodgkin disease, and mast cell disease may be considered. The characteristic nuclear indentation of the histiocytes, lack of prominent nucleoli, and the lipid and pigment in the cytoplasm should identify cases of LCH. When the histopathology is equivocal, the immunohistochemical profile and the presence of Birbeck granules by electron microscopy are diagnostic.

Treatment and Prognosis. Treatment of localized bone disease is aimed at complete removal of the lesion, usually by curettage. Irradiation may be effective for eradicating inoperable lesions. For generalized disease, chemotherapy is usually indicated. Corticosteroids, vinblastine, and 6-mercaptopurine are the agents most often used (23). Radiotherapy may be used for lesions in weight-bearing bones. Treatment for generalized disease is aimed at control but not necessarily total eradication of disease.

The extent of disease, as determined by the number of affected organs and the degree of dysfunction, appears to be the most important indicator of prognosis (17–19). The prognosis for localized disease is excellent. Most patients are cured by removal or radiation of the lesion. In the more aggressive forms of multisystem or generalized disease, control of morbidity and prevention of death are often possible with chemotherapy but a significant number of patients progress and succumb to fulminant disease.

INFECTION-ASSOCIATED HEMOPHAGOCYTIC SYNDROME

Definition. A systemic reactive proliferation of phagocytic histiocytes induced by an infection, usually of viral origin. Infection-associated hemophagocytic syndrome (IAHS) was initially described as virus-associated hemophagocytic syndrome (VAHS) (38). Although the large majority of cases are related to a viral infection, it has become apparent that infectious agents other than viruses, including some bacteria and fungi, may be associated with a similar hemophagocytic syndrome. The term IAHS allows for inclusion of the occasional case of non-viral etiology.

Pathogenesis. The pathogenesis of this disorder is poorly understood but hemophagocytic syndromes usually occur in patients with an immune deficiency (35). The immune deficit may be inherited, acquired, or iatrogenic due to immunosuppressive drugs (31–33,35,36,38,39). Aberrant cytokine production by normal or neoplastic T lymphocytes has been suggested as the etiology of the histiocytic hyperplasia and hemophagocytosis (31,40). The bone marrow, lymph nodes, spleen, and liver are the major sites of histiocytic proliferation. The process may mimic a malignant histiocytic proliferation.

IAHS shares clinical and morphologic features with a rare autosomal recessive disease, *familial erythrophagocytic lymphohistiocytosis (FEL)* (30, 34,35). The two may be clinically indistinguishable. The pathogenic relationship between IAHS and FEL is controversial (35). The morphologic changes in both disorders are virtually identical and will be considered together (32,34).

Incidence and Clinical Findings. There is no available data on the incidence of IAHS but it is clearly uncommon. The disorder is probably underdiagnosed because of its association with other serious diseases and the difficulty in documenting the diagnosis in some cases. De novo IAHS, occurring in patients not receiving immunosuppressive therapy, appears to be most common in children. There is often a history of a recent viral-like illness. The onset of IAHS is manifested by an abrupt change in clinical course characterized by high fever, severe constitutional symptoms, organomegaly, and pancytopenia. Hepatosplenomegaly is usually present and lymphadenopathy, rash, and diffuse pulmonary infiltrates are common.

Patients with FEL are diagnosed in the first 2 years of life in 80 percent of cases; there is often a family history of the disorder. Failure to thrive, fever, weight loss, hepatosplenomegaly, and a maculopapular rash are the most common manifestations.

Laboratory Findings. Abnormal liver function studies indicative of hepatocellular injury and abnormal coagulation parameters are present in most patients and reflect the systemic nature of the disease. The coagulopathy appears to be partially related to liver failure but disseminated

Figure 497
INFECTION-ASSOCIATED
HEMOPHAGOCYTIC SYNDROME

A bone marrow aspirate smear from a child with infection-associated hemophagocytic syndrome secondary to an Epstein-Barr virus infection. On this field there are several large histiocytes. Phagocytosis of nucleated red blood cells, neutrophils, and platelets is evident. The histiocytes have the appearance of reactive cells and should be readily distinguishable from neoplastic histiocytes. (Wright-Giemsa stain)

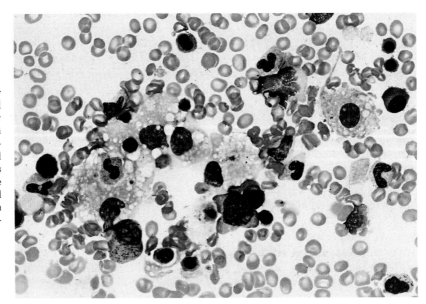

intravascular coagulation (DIC) with hypofibrinogenemia and increased fibrin degradation products is a prominent feature. Hypogammaglobulinemia has been identified in occasional patients and a positive Coombs test has been reported in a minority. In patients with FEL, hypertriglyceridemia is a relatively constant finding and is also found in some patients with IAHS (32,34,38).

Evidence of an acute viral infection is present in most patients who are thoroughly evaluated for viral disease. Viruses of the herpes group, Epstein-Barr virus (EBV) or cytomegalovirus (CMV), have been implicated most frequently but other viruses have also been identified (38). Findings similar to those described above may be seen in patients severely immunosuppressed by drugs, such as renal transplant recipients. In these patients the onset of the IAHS may occur within a few weeks or several months after beginning immunosuppressive therapy. The clinical and morphologic manifestations are similar to those in patients without a history of immunosuppression.

Blood and Bone Marrow Findings. Blood cytopenias are invariably present. Most patients have a severe pancytopenia or bicytopenia, usually anemia and thrombocytopenia. Atypical lymphocytes are present in most cases, but are generally not a prominent feature. Occasionally, a more striking lymphocytosis may occur in FEL or IAHS. Rare histiocytes may be observed in blood smears.

The most striking morphologic feature in the bone marrow is histiocytic hyperplasia with prominent phagocytosis of the red blood cells, platelets, and nucleated hematopoietic cells (figs. 497, 498). Both intact and degenerating phagocytized cells are observed. The cytoplasm of some of the histiocytes is filled with ingested elements while others contain primarily vacuoles of varying size. The histiocytes are mature in appearance with a low nuclear-cytoplasmic ratio, abundant cytoplasm, relatively condensed-appearing nuclear chromatin, and inconspicuous nucleoli. Histiocytic hyperplasia is most evident in buffy coat smears of the aspirate specimens, where the histiocytes are concentrated at the thin edge (38).

Histopathologic Findings. In trephine biopsies, histiocytes may be found in clusters and individually dispersed throughout the marrow section. Granulomatous lesions or reactive lymphocytic aggregates are present in some cases. In the most severe cases, there is extensive destruction of normal marrow elements and marked histiocytic hyperplasia (fig. 499). The bone marrow is usually hypocellular with decreased granulopoiesis and erythropoiesis; megakaryocytes are increased or normal in number (figs. 499, 500). In the early stages, the bone marrow may lack diagnostic specificity and appear hypercellular without obvious histiocytic hyperplasia or hemophagocytosis. Serial marrow biopsies may be required for diagnosis. In

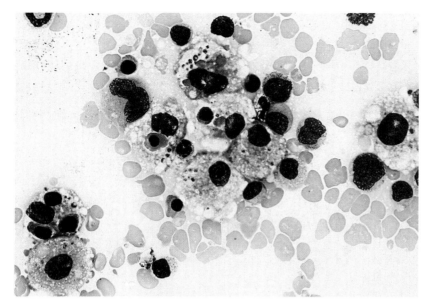

Figure 498
INFECTION-ASSOCIATED
HEMOPHAGOCYTIC SYNDROME
A large cluster of reactive histio-cytes is illustrated near the thin edge of a bone marrow smear. They show marked hemophagocytosis. The pa-tient is a child with the typical clini-cal features of an infection-associ-ated hemophagocytic syndrome. (Wright-Giemsa stain)

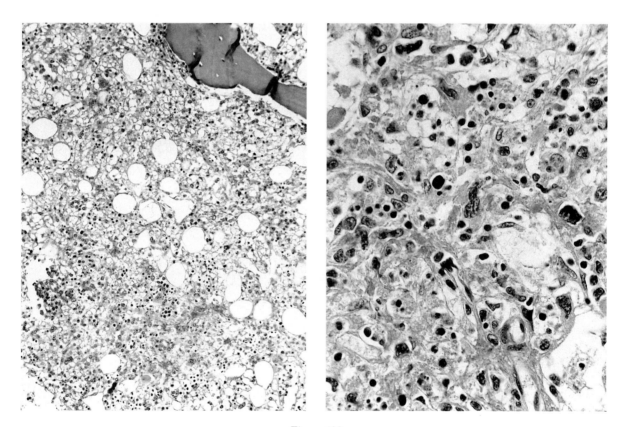

Figure 499
INFECTION-ASSOCIATED HEMOPHAGOCYTIC SYNDROME
Left: A trephine biopsy from a child with Epstein-Barr virus–associated hemophagocytic syndrome (VAHS) shows a striking decrease in hematopoietic cells and multiple foci of necrosis. (Hematoxylin and eosin stain)
Right: A higher magnification of the section shown on the left. There is marked histiocytic hyperplasia with hemophagocyto-sis and a reduction in hematopoiesis. Bone marrow destruction of this nature is common in advanced VAHS. (Hematoxylin and eosin stain) (Fig. 44 from McKenna RW. Disorders of bone marrow. In: Sternberg SS, ed. Diagnostic surgical pathology, Vol. 1. 2nd ed. New York: Raven Press, 1994:623–72.)

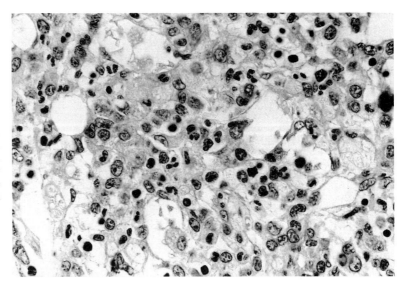

Figure 500
INFECTION-ASSOCIATED
HEMOPHAGOCYTIC SYNDROME

A section of bone marrow from a 3-year-old male with virus-associated hemophagocytic syndrome. There is marked histiocytic hyperplasia and hemophagocytosis. Hematopoietic cells are markedly reduced but bone marrow destruction is not as obvious as in the case illustrated in figure 499. (Hematoxylin and eosin stain)

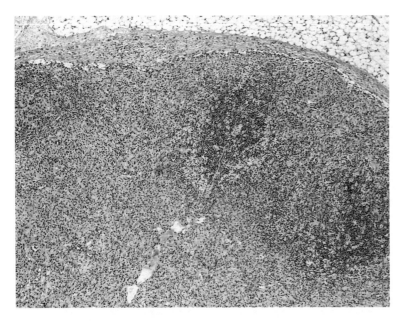

Figure 501
INFECTION-ASSOCIATED
HEMOPHAGOCYTIC SYNDROME

A lymph node section from a 5-year-old boy with virus-associated hemophagocytic syndrome. The general architecture of the lymph node is intact. Residual follicles are present but germinal centers are atrophic; lymphocytes are depleted. Sinuses appear compressed in some areas but the subcapsular sinuses are open. (Hematoxylin and eosin stain)

some patients sequential loss of the granulocytic and erythrocytic marrow compartments is observed in serial bone marrow examinations.

Histiocytic hyperplasia is also evident in other reticuloendothelial tissues. In lymph nodes the general architecture is usually intact. Histiocytes are increased and distributed in the sinusoids, cortex, and paracortex (fig. 501). Lymphocyte depletion is often striking and burned-out germinal centers may be evident. Increased immunoblasts and plasma cells are seen in some cases. Vascular proliferation is prominent (fig. 502) (29,38).

In the liver the histiocytic proliferation involves the portal tracts and sinusoids; hepatocellular necrosis is often present. Histiocyte proliferation is observed in the splenic red pulp and occasionally in the leptomeninges. Cytomegalic inclusions have been identified in various tissues in cases associated with CMV infections.

Differential Diagnosis. It is important to distinguish IAHS from malignant histiocytosis (Table 37). The most important distinguishing features are the cytologic characteristics of the proliferative histiocytes in the two processes. In IAHS the histiocytes have cytologic features of

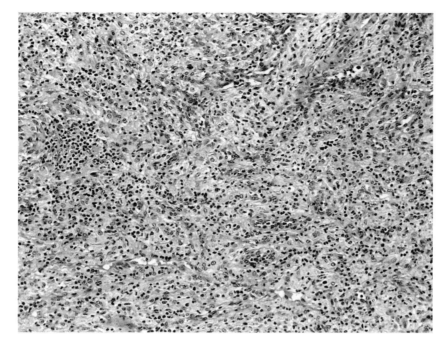

Figure 502
INFECTION-ASSOCIATED
HEMOPHAGOCYTIC
SYNDROME
A higher magnification of the paracortex of the lymph node illustrated in figure 501. Lymphocytes are depleted, vascularity appears increased, and large numbers of histiocytes are present. (Hematoxylin and eosin stain)

Table 37

DIFFERENTIATING FEATURES OF INFECTION-ASSOCIATED HEMOPHAGOCYTIC SYNDROME (IAHS) AND MALIGNANT HISTIOCYTOSIS (MH)*

	IAHS	MH
Bone marrow involvement	Moderate to marked	Absent to moderate
Lymph node involvement	Minimal to marked	Moderate to marked
Blood cytopenias	Marked	Mild or absent
Coagulopathy	Marked	Absent
Hepatitis	Marked	Absent to mild
Proliferative histiocytes	Mature with benign (reactive) cytologic characteristics	Immature with neoplastic cytologic characteristics
Mitotic activity	Low	High
Hemophagocytosis by proliferative histiocytes	Marked	Minimal or absent in malignant cells
Cytochemistry-immunocytochemistry		
Acid phosphatase	Strong positivity	Moderate to strong positivity
Nonspecific esterase	Strong positivity	Moderate to strong positivity
Alpha-1-antichymotrypsin	Strong positivity	Moderate to strong positivity

*From Risdall et al. (37) and Risdall et al. (38)

mature cells. Marked hemophagocytosis is invariably present. Cells with neoplastic cytologic characteristics are not observed. The diagnosis is usually made from examination of the bone marrow. In malignant histiocytosis the diagnosis is most often established from examination of the lymph nodes, spleen, or liver (37,38). The proliferative histiocytes have cytologic characteristics of neoplastic cells, including a high nuclear-cytoplasmic ratio, large nuclei with reticular chromatin, and usually, a prominent nucleolus. The cytoplasm is basophilic and phagocytosis is only rarely demonstrable (29,38). At diagnosis, the bone marrow is often uninvolved, or only minimally involved, with a few neoplastic histiocytes found scattered in the marrow smears, often with no recognizable infiltrate in trephine biopsy sections.

Treatment and Prognosis. IAHS is potentially reversible with appropriate supportive therapy. In patients on immunosuppressive agents, the drugs must be discontinued or reduced to halt progression of the disease. Chemotherapeutic agents are usually not indicated and may further suppress the immune response. However, in severe cases, epipodophyllotoxin VP16 alone or in combination with steroids and other agents, has been effective in temporarily suppressing the histiocytic hyperplasia and hemophagocytosis; the syndrome often recurs when the drug is withdrawn. Bone marrow transplant has been effective in reversing the disease in some children with FEL and has treatment potential for patients with irreversible IAHS (28).

Many patients with IAHS have a fulminant clinical course. The mortality rate is 30 to 40 percent during the acute illness. Patients surviving the acute manifestations usually recover in 1 to 8 weeks. Recurrence is rare. In very young children, particularly those with FEL, the disease is usually fatal in a relatively short period of time.

MALIGNANT HISTIOCYTOSIS

Definition. A neoplastic proliferation of cells of monocyte/macrophage lineage at a stage of differentiation intermediate between monoblasts and mature histiocytes (41,43). The neoplastic cells express morphologic, immunologic, and enzymatic features of phagocytic histiocytes (47). Malignant histiocytosis (MH) and *true histiocytic lymphoma* are generally considered to be neoplasms of similar cell types, differing only in their presentation as disseminated (MH) or localized (true histiocytic lymphoma) tumors (43,44,47).

Incidence and Clinical Findings. Malignant histiocytosis is a rare neoplasm. Accurate data concerning incidence is not available but clearly MH accounts for fewer than 1 percent of the malignant neoplasms of hematopoietic tissues. Most of the disorders that were considered MH in the past are now recognized as reactive hemophagocytic syndromes or anaplastic large cell lymphomas of T-cell or B-cell type. These findings have greatly reduced the reported incidence of MH and histiocytic lymphoma.

Age at diagnosis ranges from childhood to the ninth decade (48,51,52). Males predominate by as much as 2 to 1 in some series (48). Patients present with the clinical spectrum common to the non-Hodgkin lymphomas (47). Fever and lymphadenopathy are the most frequent presenting manifestations. Hepatosplenomegaly is present at diagnosis or occurs as the disease progresses. Symptoms related to infiltration of the gastrointestinal tract, skin, and soft tissues are present in some cases. The disease is most often disseminated (stage IV) at diagnosis (48,51,52).

Laboratory Findings. There are no specific laboratory findings. Abnormal liver function studies are often found in patients with liver involvement. Blood cytopenias are occasionally present at diagnosis and generally reflect advanced disease.

Blood and Bone Marrow Findings. Circulating malignant histiocytes may be identified on blood smears from patients in the late stages of disease. In bone marrow aspirate smears there is usually good preservation of normal hematopoiesis. Malignant histiocytes are scattered among the normal hematopoietic cells. They vary in size but are generally larger than any of the other bone marrow cells except megakaryocytes. They have a large nucleus and a relatively high nuclear-cytoplasmic ratio. The nucleus is round, oval, or folded. Nuclear borders may be smooth or irregular. The chromatin is coarsely reticular and usually one or more prominent nucleoli are present. The cytoplasm is basophilic and often contains sharply defined vacuoles and, occasionally, scattered azure granules (fig. 503). Hemophagocytosis is rarely observed. Even with very

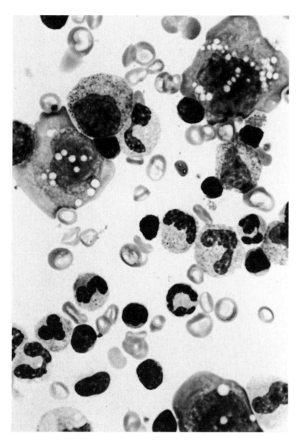

Figure 503
MALIGNANT HISTIOCYTOSIS
A bone marrow smear from a patient with a diagnosis of malignant histiocytosis. There are three large neoplastic cells in this field. (Wright-Giemsa stain) (Fig. 37.45 from McKenna RW. The bone marrow manifestations of Hodgkin's disease, the non-Hodgkin's lymphomas, and lymphoma-like disorders. In: Knowles DM, ed. Neoplastic hematopathology. Baltimore: Williams & Wilkins, 1992:1135–80.)

minimal marrow disease, the malignant histiocytes can usually be recognized in aspirate smears by their distinctive cytologic characteristics.

Histopathologic Findings. In trephine biopsy sections involvement by MH may be focal or diffuse. Extensive bone marrow disease is rare except in advanced and terminal stages. Recognition of bone marrow disease in trephine sections is difficult in cases with minimal infiltration by scattered malignant histiocytes. The malignant histiocytes are large and have abundant, lightly eosinophilic cytoplasm, often with distinct cytoplasmic membranes. The nucleus is large and may have round to markedly irregular nuclear bor-

ders; one or more prominent eosinophilic nucleoli are usually present. Occasionally, very large cells with multilobulated nuclei are present. In many cases, reactive phagocytic histiocytes may be scattered among the malignant histiocytes. Hemophagocytosis by the neoplastic cells may be observed but is rare (42–44,49,50).

Cytochemical and Immunohistochemical Findings. Malignant histiocytes generally manifest the cytochemical characteristics of phagocytic histiocytes. They are uniformly NSE and acid phosphatase positive but there is heterogeneity among cases in reactivity for lysozyme, alpha-1-antitrypsin, and alpha-1-antichymotrypsin; alpha-1-antichymotrypsin appears to be the most sensitive marker (47,49). Anticathepsin B antibodies also appear to have a high sensitivity for marking MH (47).

Monoclonal antibodies applied to frozen sections may be useful in the differential diagnosis. The malignant histiocytes generally express CD11c, CD14, and CD68. Expression of these antigens in the absence of expression of T- and B-cell–associated antigens is strong evidence for a histiocytic lineage (47).

Ultrastructural Findings. Electron microscopic examination of malignant histiocytes shows no specific diagnostic features. The cells usually have an irregularly shaped nucleus with dispersed chromatin and one to three nucleoli. There is abundant cytoplasm containing a prominent Golgi region, numerous polyribosomes, mitochondria, endoplasmic reticulum, cytoplasmic vesicles, abundant lysosomes, and often numerous lipid droplets (49). Microtubules and microfilaments are observed in some cases. Phagocytized nuclear debris may be present (49).

Differential Diagnosis. MH must be distinguished from anaplastic large cell lymphomas, monoblastic leukemia (M5A), and reactive hemophagocytic syndromes. Anaplastic large cell lymphomas are usually characterized by expression of CD30, and T-cell or, less often, B-cell antigens. The neoplastic cells in many cases of anaplastic large cell lymphomas have a specific bone marrow chromosome rearrangement, t(2;5) (45, 46). Occasionally, poorly differentiated monocytic (monoblastic) leukemia (M5A) may be mistaken for MH, especially when extramedullary tissue infiltration is the primary manifestation and the bone marrow is only partially involved.

The distinctive cytologic features of the monoblasts and promonocytes are recognizable in Wright-Giemsa stained smears or touch preparations. The cytochemical profile of MH and monoblastic leukemia may be identical. In most cases, extensive bone marrow and blood involvement evolves over a brief period of time and the process is identified as leukemia. The distinctive features of MH and the reactive histiocytoses were discussed in the section on infection-associated hemophagocytic syndrome.

Treatment and Prognosis. Multiagent chemotherapy, alone or in combination with radiotherapy, is the usual treatment. The results vary in different studies, probably reflecting the heterogeneity of cases diagnosed as MH. Treatment results are generally poorer than for intermediate grade non-Hodgkin lymphoma. In some series, fewer than half of the patients with MH enter a complete remission (48). In other studies, more than two thirds achieve complete remission, many for prolonged periods (51,52). Patients with localized disease treated with radiation combined with chemotherapy appear to have the best results.

The prognosis is poor for patients who fail treatment; the median survival is less than 1 year (48). For patients that enter complete remission, overall 2-year disease-free survival is approximately 40 percent.

REFERENCES

Storage Histiocyte Disorders

1. Barranger JA, Ginns EI. Glucosylceramide lipidoses: Gaucher disease. In: Scriver CR, Beaudet AL, Sly WS, Valle D, eds. The metabolic basis of inherited disease, Vol. 2. 6th ed. New York: McGraw-Hill, 1989:1677–98.
2. Beutler E. Gaucher's disease. N Engl J Med 1991;325:1354–60.
3. Brunning RD. Morphologic alterations in nucleated blood and marrow cells in genetic disorders. Hum Pathol 1970;1:99–124.
4. Desnick SJ, Desnick RJ, Brady RO, et al. Renal transplantation in Type II Gaucher disease. In: Bergsma D, ed. Enzyme therapy in genetic diseases. Baltimore: Williams and Wilkins, 1973:109–19.
5. Dosik H, Rosner F, Sawitsky A. Acquired lipidosis: Gaucher-like cells and "blue cells" in chronic granulocytic leukemia. Semin Hematol 1972;9:309–16.
6. Garfinkel D, Sidi Y, Ben-Bassat M, Salomon F, Hazaz B, Pinkas J. Coexistence of Gaucher's disease and multiple myeloma. Arch Intern Med 1982;142:2229–30.
7. Groth CG, Blomstrand R, Hagenfeldt L, Öckerman PA, Samuelsson K, Svennerholm L. Metabolic changes following splenic transplantation in a case of Gaucher's disease. In: Volk BW, Aronson SM, eds. Sphingolipids, sphingolipidoses and allied disorders. New York: Plenum Press, 1972:633–9.
8. Hobbs JR, Hugh-Jones K, Barrett AJ, et al. Reversal of clinical features of Hurler's disease and biochemical improvement after treatment by bone-marrow transplantation. Lancet 1981;2:709–12.
9. Lee RE. The pathology of Gaucher disease. In: Desnick RJ, Gatt S, Grabowski GA, eds. Gaucher disease: a century of delineation and research. New York: Alan R. Liss, 1982:177–217. (Progress in clinical and biological research, Vol. 95).
10. Neufeld EF, Muenzer J. The mucopolysaccharidoses. In: Scriver CR, Beaudet AL, Sly WS, Valle D, eds. The metabolic basis of inherited disease, Vol 2. 6th ed. New York: McGraw-Hill, 1989:1565–88.
11. Parkin JL, Brunning RD. Pathology of the Gaucher cell. In: Desnick RJ, Gatt S, Grabowski GA, eds. Gaucher disease: a century of delineation and research. New York: Alan R. Liss, 1982:151–75. (Progress in clinical and biological research, Vol. 95).
12. Peters SP, Lee RE, Glew RH. Gaucher's disease: a review. Medicine (Baltimore) 1977;56:425–42.
13. Spence MW, Callahan JW. Sphingomyelin-cholesterol lipidoses: the Niemann-Pick group of diseases. In: Scriver CR, Beaudet Al, Sly WS, Valle D, eds. The metabolic basis of inherited disease, Vol 2. 6th ed. New York: McGraw-Hill, 1989:1655–76.
14. Van Dorpe A, Broeckaert-van Orshoven A, Desmet V, Verwilghen RL. Gaucher-like cells and congenital dyserythropoietic anemia, type II (HEMPAS). Br J Haematol 1973;25:165–70.
15. Witzleben CL, Drake WL Jr, Sammon J, Mohabbat OM. Gaucher's cells in acute leukemia of childhood. J Pediatr 1970;76:129–31.
16. Yosipovitch Z, Katz K. Bone crisis in Gaucher disease—an update. Isr J Med Sci 1990;26:593–5.

Langerhans Cell Histiocytosis

17. Berry DH, Gresik MV, Humphrey GB, et al. Natural history of histiocytosis X: a Pediatric Oncology Group study. Med Pediatr Oncol 1986;14:1–5.
18. Broadbent V. Favourable prognostic features in histiocytosis X: bone involvement and absence of skin disease. Arch Dis Child 1986;61:1219–21.
19. Dehner LP. Morphologic findings in the histiocytic syndromes. Semin Oncol 1991;18:8–17.
20. Favara BE. Langerhans' cell histiocytosis pathobiology and pathogenesis. Semin Oncol 1991;18:3–7.
21. _____, McCarthy RC, Mierau GW. Histiocytosis X. Hum Pathol 1983;14:663–76.

22. Ide F, Iwase T, Saito I, Umemura S, Nakajima T. Immunohistochemical and ultrastructural analysis of the proliferating cells in histiocytosis X. Cancer 1984;53:917–21.
23. Komp DM. Concepts in staging and clinical studies for treatment of Langerhans' cell histiocytosis. Semin Oncol 1991;18:18–23.
24. Ladisch S, Jaffe ES. The histiocytoses. In: Pizzo PA, Poplack DG, eds. Principles and practice of pediatric oncology. Philadelphia: JB Lippincott, 1989:491–504.
25. Mclain K, Ramsay NK, Robison L, Sundberg RD, Nesbit M Jr. Bone marrow involvement in histiocytosis X. Med Pediatr Oncol 1983;11:167–71.
26. Mierau GW, Favara BE. S-100 protein immunohistochemistry and electron microscopy in the diagnosis of Langerhans' cell proliferative disorders: a comparative assessment. Ultrastruct Pathol 1986;10:303–9.
27. Nauert C, Zornoza J, Ayala A, Harle TS. Eosinophilic granuloma of bone: diagnosis and management. Skeletal Radial 1983;10:227–35.

Infection-Associated Hemophagocytic Syndromes

28. Blanche S, Caniglia M, Girault D, Landman J, Griscelli C, Fischer A. Treatment of hemophagocytic lymphohistiocytosis with chemotherapy and bone marrow transplantation: a single-center study of 22 cases. Blood 1991;78:51–4.
29. Dehner LP. Morphologic findings in the histiocytic syndromes. Semin Oncol 1991;18:8–17.
30. Farquhar JW, Claireaux AE. Familial hemophagocytic reticulosis. Arch Dis Child 1952;27:519–25.
31. Gonzalez CL, Jaffe ES. The histiocytosis: clinical presentation and differential diagnosis. Oncology 1990;4:47–60.
32. Henter JI, Elinder G, Ost A. Diagnostic guidelines for hemophagocytic lymphohistiocytosis. The FHL Study Group of the Histiocyte Society. Semin Oncol 1991; 18:29–33.
33. Jaffe ES. Malignant histiocytosis and true histiocytic lymphomas. In: Jaffe ES, ed. Surgical pathology of lymph nodes and related organs. Philadelphia: WB Saunders, 1985:381–411.
34. Loy TS, Diaz-Arias AA, Perry MC. Familial erythrophagocytic lymphohistiocytosis. Semin Oncol 1991;18:34–8.
35. McClain K, Gehrz R, Grierson H, Purtilo D, Filipovich A. Virus-associated histiocytic proliferations in children. Frequent association with Epstein-Barr virus and congenital or acquired immunodeficiencies. Am J Pediatr Hematol Oncol 1988;10:196–205.
36. McKenna RW, Risdall RJ, Brunning RD. Virus associated hemophagocytic syndrome. Hum Pathol 1981;12:395–8.
37. Risdall RJ, Brunning RD, Sibley RK, Dehner LP, McKenna RW. Malignant histiocytosis. A light- and electron-microscopic and histochemical study. Am J Surg Pathol 1980;4:439–50.
38. _____, McKenna RW, Nesbit ME, et al. Virus-associated hemophagocytic syndrome: a benign histiocytic proliferation distinct from malignant histiocytosis. Cancer 1979;44:993–1002.
39. Rubin CM, Burke BA, McKenna RW, et al. The accelerated phase of Chediak-Higashi syndrome. An expression of the virus-associated hemophagocytic syndrome? Cancer 1985;56:524–30.
40. Simrell CR, Margolick JB, Crabtree GR, Cossman J, Fauci AS, Jaffe ES. Lymphokine-induced phagocytosis in angiocentric immunoproliferative lesions (AIL) and malignant lymphoma arising in AIL. Blood 1985; 65:1469–76.

Malignant Histiocytosis

41. Byrne GE Jr, Rappaport H. Malignant histiocytosis. In: Akazaki K, Rappaport H, Berard CW, Bennett JM, Ishikawa E, eds. Malignant diseases of the hematopoietic system. Tokyo: University of Tokyo Press, 1973:145–62. (Gann monograph on cancer research, No. 15)
42. Dehner LP. Morphologic findings in the histiocytic syndromes. Semin Oncol 1991;18:8–17.
43. Gonzalez CL, Jaffe ES. The histiocytosis: clinical presentation and differential diagnosis. Oncology 1990;4:47–60.
44. Jaffe ES. Malignant histiocytosis and true histiocytic lymphomas. In: Jaffe ES, ed. Surgical pathology of lymph nodes and related organs. Philadelphia: WB Saunders, 1985:381–411.
45. Kadin ME, Sako D, Berliner N, et al. Childhood Ki-1 lymphoma presenting with skin lesions and peripheral lymphadenopathy. Blood 1986;68:1042–9.
46. Kaneko Y, Frizzera G, Edamura S, et al. A novel translocation, t(2;5) (p23;q35), in childhood phagocytic large T-cell lymphoma mimicking malignant histiocytosis. Blood 1989;73:806–13.
47. Levine EG, Hanson CA, Jaszcz W, Peterson BA. True histiocytic lymphoma. Semin Oncol 1991;18:39–49.
48. Pileri S, Mazza P, Rivano MT, et al. Malignant histiocytosis (true histiocytic lymphoma clinicopathological study of 25 cases). Histopathology 1985;9:905–20.
49. Risdall RJ, Brunning RD, Sibley RK, Dehner LP, McKenna RW. Malignant histiocytosis. A light- and electron-microscopic and histochemical study. Am J Surg Pathol 1980;4:439–50.
50. _____, McKenna RW, Nesbit ME, et al. Virus-associated hemophagocytic syndrome: a benign histiocytic proliferation distinct from malignant histiocytosis. Cancer 1979;44:993–1002.
51 van der Valk P, Meijer CJ, Willemze R, van Oosterom AT, Spaander PJ, te Velde J. Histiocytic sarcoma (true histiocytic lymphoma): a clinicopathological study of 20 cases. Histopathology 1984;8:105–23.
52. van Heerde P, Feltkamp CA, Hart AA, Somers R, van Unnik JA, Vroom TM. Malignant histiocytosis and related tumors. A clinicopathologic study of 42 cases using cytological, histochemical and ultrastructural parameters. Hematol Oncol 1984;2:13–32.

METASTATIC TUMORS INVOLVING THE BONE MARROW

Definition. Neoplasms of nonhematopoietic tissues involving the bone marrow secondarily through spread from their site of origin.

Incidence and Clinical Findings. There is considerable variation in the incidence of bone marrow metastasis for different types of malignant neoplasms. Some of the more common tumors also have the highest frequency of bone marrow involvement. These include carcinomas of the breast, prostate, lung, and gastrointestinal tract in adults and neuroblastomas in children (1,15,27). There is variability in the reported incidence of bone marrow involvement for each of these. This may reflect differences in patient selection and in techniques for identifying marrow metastasis. In several reports only bone marrow aspirates were performed; the frequency of metastasis in these studies may be significantly underestimated.

In adult females, adenocarcinoma of the breast is the most common metastatic tumor in the bone marrow: up to 20 percent of patients with breast carcinoma manifest bone marrow metastasis (1,21). In adult male patients, carcinomas of the lung and prostate are most common (1,36). The incidence of bone marrow involvement in patients with lung cancer at the time of initial evaluation is 5 to 21 percent; the frequency varies with the histologic type (1). Small cell carcinoma has the highest incidence, approximately 20 percent (1,16,19,20). The incidence for squamous cell carcinoma and adenocarcinoma of the lung is 3 to 15 percent and 5 to 10 percent, respectively (1,16).

Carcinoma of the prostate may be found in bone marrow biopsies in 13 to 20 percent of patients prior to treatment and accounts for 18 to 39 percent of all marrow metastases in adult males (1,11, 25,36). Poorly differentiated prostatic carcinomas are more likely to involve the bone marrow than moderately or well-differentiated types (11).

Approximately 4 percent of patients with gastrointestinal cancer have bone marrow involvement at diagnosis (1). Adenocarcinomas of the stomach and colon are the most common (25). Several other tumors in adult patients have a relatively low incidence of bone marrow metastasis but occasionally spread to the marrow early in the clinical course. These include malignant melanoma, renal cell carcinoma, thyroid carcinoma, pancreatic carcinoma, ovarian and testicular carcinomas, transitional cell carcinomas, lymphoepitheliomas, rhabdomyosarcoma, Ewing sarcoma, and Kaposi sarcoma and other vascular tumors (1,25,37). Many other malignant tumors have been reported to occasionally metastasize to the bone marrow, usually in advanced or terminal stages of the disease.

In children neuroblastoma is the most common solid tissue tumor and has the highest frequency of bone marrow involvement: 50 to 60 percent of patients manifest bone marrow infiltration at the time of initial diagnosis and at least 70 percent have biopsy-demonstrable bone marrow metastasis at some time during their course (1,10,13,17,29). Bone marrow involvement is least common in patients under 1 year of age.

Several other childhood tumors have a relatively high incidence of bone marrow involvement. These include ganglioneuroblastoma, rhabdomyosarcoma, Ewing sarcoma, retinoblastoma, and medulloblastoma (1,10,13). Osteosarcoma, fibrosarcoma, and various carcinomas in children may involve the bone marrow late in the clinical course. Nephroblastomas, hepatoblastomas, and central nervous system tumors, except for medulloblastomas, rarely metastasize to the bone marrow (1,10,13).

Symptoms related to bone marrow metastasis are variable and nonspecific (26). Occasionally, thrombocytopenia-induced bleeding or symptoms related to anemia are presenting manifestations. In rare cases patients present with an infection due to neutropenia. Bone pain is a symptom of advanced malignancy and a strong indicator of bone marrow metastasis (6). Up to 75 percent of patients with documented bone marrow metastasis experience bone pain or tenderness (6). Bone marrow tumor necrosis is often associated with bone pain (24).

Physical findings referable to the primary neoplasm may include a palpable mass, an enlarged lymph node, or organomegaly. In advanced disease, physical signs of cachexia may be apparent.

Laboratory Findings. Hypercalcemia is associated with bone marrow metastasis in some cases. However, there are many causes for hypercalcemia in patients with cancer that are independent of bone marrow involvement. Serum calcium levels appear to have little value in predicting bone marrow metastasis (6).

Serum glutamic-oxaloacetic transaminase (SGOT), lactate dehydrogenase (LDH), and uric acid levels are higher in patients with bone marrow metastasis than in patients with advanced malignancy without marrow involvement (6). The elevation of serum LDH and SGOT is related to bone marrow necrosis in some cases. Serum uric acid elevations are caused by tumor necrosis and increased tumor cell proliferation (24).

Serum alkaline phosphatase and acid phosphatase values are often elevated in patients with a malignancy but abnormal levels have not been useful in predicting bone marrow involvement (6). Bone marrow alkaline and acid phosphatase determinations are of greater utility than serum levels, especially in patients with prostatic cancer (39). Tumor markers for specific types or groups of tumors, e.g., carcinoembryonic antigen (CEA), prostate-specific antigen (PSA), alpha-fetoprotein, estrogen receptors, and beta-human chorionic gonadotropin (β-hCG) are useful in designing therapy and, in some cases, in predicting tumor burden and recurrence; they are not especially helpful in identifying bone marrow involvement (18).

Various combinations of clinical, laboratory, and radiographic findings are useful indicators of bone marrow metastasis. A leukoerythroblastic reaction, a serum LDH level of greater than 500 IU/L, a platelet count less than 100×10^9/L, and bone pain are all strongly correlated with bone marrow metastasis in patients with malignant tumors. A positive bone scan, hematocrit of less than 30 percent, serum uric acid level of greater than 10 mg/dL, and blood urea nitrogen (BUN) of greater than 25 mg/dL are associated with bone marrow metastasis but are less reliable indicators (6).

Various radiographic techniques are useful in assessing the bone marrow for metastatic disease. Routine bone films identify osteolytic and osteoblastic lesions but small lesions and those in which bone changes are minimal or lacking are often not detected. Bone scans may show evidence of metastasis when random bone marrow biopsies are negative (3,6). Bone scans may fail to identify lesions in some patients with positive bone marrow biopsies, however, and should be used to complement, but not replace, the marrow biopsy (14). Computerized tomography (CT) scanning and magnetic resonance imaging (MRI) have added significantly to radiographic assessment of tumor metastasis in bone marrow (31).

Blood and Bone Marrow Findings. Anemia is present at diagnosis in most patients with bone marrow metastatic disease. Approximately 40 percent of patients have thrombocytopenia (6). Thrombocytosis is commonly associated with advanced malignancies and is present in some patients with bone marrow metastasis. Leukocytosis, leukopenia, eosinophilia, neutrophilia, lymphocytosis, and monocytosis may all be found (6). A leukoerythroblastic reaction with circulating erythroblasts and immature granulocytes is a relatively common finding (9). A leukoerythroblastic reaction may also be seen in several conditions associated with neoplastic disease including infection, hemorrhage, and megaloblastic and hemolytic anemias (38).

Microangiopathic hemolytic anemia may occur in patients with advanced malignancies, with or without bone marrow involvement. It is especially common in mucin-producing adenocarcinomas. Peripheral blood smears show red blood cell fragmentation, increased polychromatophilic red blood cells, usually thrombocytopenia, and frequently erythroblastemia. The finding of a leukoerythroblastic reaction and microangiopathic hemolytic anemia in a patient with a neoplastic disease is highly suggestive of bone marrow metastasis (fig. 504).

Occasionally, circulating metastatic tumor cells are found in blood smears. They are seen in small clusters or as scattered individual cells and may resemble lymphoma cells or myeloblasts (fig. 505). The patients generally have advanced disease with a heavily infiltrated bone marrow, blood cytopenias, and a leukoerythroblastic reaction. Metastatic tumor cells are most often observed in blood smears from children with neuroblastoma, but may be seen in adults with small cell carcinomas and, rarely, with other metastatic neoplasms.

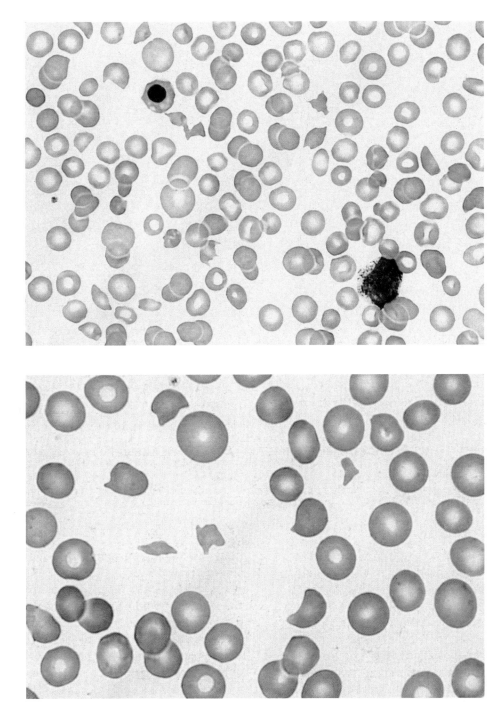

Figure 504
LEUKOERYTHROBLASTIC REACTION AND MICROANGIOPATHIC HEMOLYTIC ANEMIA
IN A PATIENT WITH BONE MARROW METASTASIS

A blood smear from a woman with carcinoma of the breast and disseminated intravascular coagulation (DIC). The bone marrow was heavily infiltrated with metastatic tumor. DIC and microangiopathic hemolytic anemia may be observed in many types of metastatic tumors but appear to be most common in cases of disseminated mucin-producing adenocarcinomas. (Wright-Giemsa stain)

Top: A nucleated red blood cell and neutrophil myelocyte are present in this field. The patient has marked thrombocytopenia and fragmented red blood cells.

Bottom: A higher magnification shows several red blood cell fragments typical of microangiopathic hemolytic anemia.

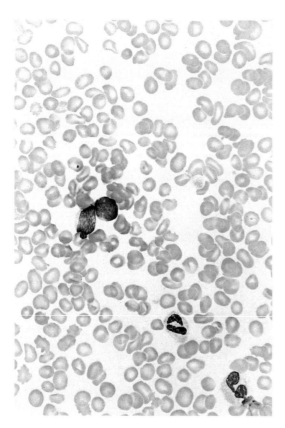 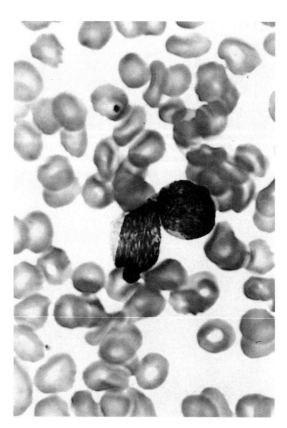

Figure 505

METASTATIC TUMOR CELLS ON A BLOOD SMEAR

A blood smear from a man with small cell carcinoma of the lung.

Left: Two tumor cells are clustered near the center of the field.

Right: The tumor cells have a high nuclear-cytoplasmic ratio and coarse nuclear chromatin. They are similar in size to hematopoietic cells and could be mistaken for lymphoma cells. (Wright-Giemsa stain)

Assessment for bone marrow metastasis is important in the initial staging of a malignant neoplasm, in monitoring response to therapy, and in identifying recurrent disease. A positive bone marrow biopsy at the time of diagnosis may advance the stage of disease and obviate the need for further diagnostic procedures. Occasionally, in patients undergoing evaluation for abnormal blood counts or a chest or abdominal mass, a bone marrow biopsy is the first material diagnostic of a malignant solid tissue tumor.

Trephine biopsies are more often positive for metastatic tumor than are bone marrow aspirates (8,16,25,28,33,35,36). This is primarily because many metastatic tumors induce fibrosis or osteosclerosis, which interferes with obtaining a satisfactory aspirate (25,36). Adenocarcinomas of the breast and prostate are particularly noto-

rious for causing desmoplastic reactions in the bone marrow (25). In pediatric patients, the most common metastatic neoplasms (neuroblastoma, rhabdomyosarcoma, Ewing sarcoma, and retinoblastoma) are usually present in both trephine sections and aspirate smears; occasionally, only the aspirates are diagnostic (19).

It is often possible to classify a metastatic tumor in trephine biopsy sections. This is particularly important in cases in which the primary neoplasm is unknown or inaccessible. The cytologic features of most metastatic tumors in bone marrow smears are not sufficiently distinctive to characterize the primary tumor (2,33).

Metastatic tumors are often focal in the marrow biopsies and may be localized to a specific anatomic region. It is important to obtain sufficient tissue, to diminish the likelihood of nondiagnostic biopsies

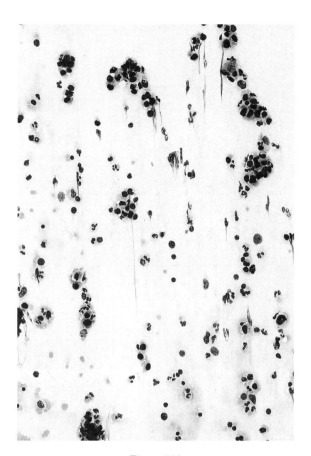

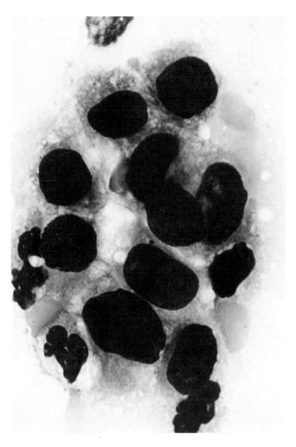

Figure 506
METASTATIC CARCINOMA
ON A BONE MARROW SMEAR

A low magnification of the thin edge of a bone marrow smear from a 58-year-old woman with metastatic carcinoma of the breast. Clumps and individual tumor cells are concentrated at the edge of the smear. This distribution is commonly found on marrow aspirate smears. (Wright-Giemsa stain)

Figure 507
METASTATIC CARCINOMA
ON A BONE MARROW SMEAR

A high magnification of a tumor clump from the smear illustrated in figure 506. The tumor cells are moderately heteromorphous. They have indistinct cell borders and condensed nuclear chromatin. The nuclei are larger than those of most hematopoietic cells. (Wright-Giemsa stain)

due to sampling inadequacy. Bilateral posterior iliac crest trephine biopsies provide a higher yield of tumor diagnosis than single biopsies and are recommended for the assessment of metastatic disease (5).

The bone marrow aspirate specimens from patients with metastatic tumor are often quantitatively small and diluted. Small clusters of metastatic tumor may be found in only one or two of several smears or predominate in all of the preparations. Metastatic tumor cells are usually concentrated in various sized clumps and clusters towards the thin edge and lateral aspects of the smear (figs. 506, 507). These areas should be carefully examined. Single intact metastatic cells, damaged cells, and swollen bare nuclei may be concentrated at the edge of the smear or scattered throughout. In some instances numerous damaged cells, proteinaceous material, and necrotic cell debris are abundant with a relative paucity of intact tumor cells. Clusters of osteoblasts are occasionally found and must be distinguished from neoplastic cells.

In cases of metastatic carcinoma, the neoplastic cells are usually larger than all hematopoietic cells except megakaryocytes. They are generally heteromorphous and vary in nuclear size and cytoplasmic volume. Nuclear eccentricity, prominent nucleoli, and cytoplasmic vacuolization are frequently observed. Individual cytoplasmic borders are not discernable in tumor clumps (fig. 507). Small cell carcinomas, neuroblastomas, retinoblastomas, embryonal rhabdomyosarcomas, and

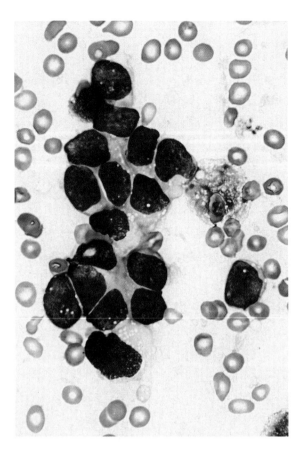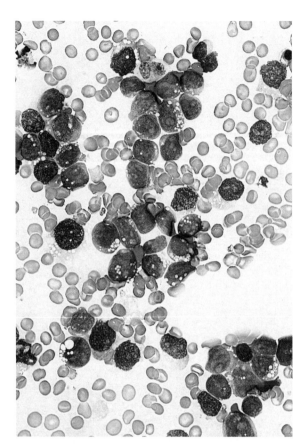

Figure 508
METASTATIC TUMOR ON BONE MARROW SMEARS

Left: A bone marrow aspirate smear from a 3-year-old child with neuroblastoma. A cohesive clump of tumor cells was found near the thin edge of the smear. The cells are approximately the size of lymphoblasts and have additional common cytologic features. Their clustered distribution on the smear is often a helpful feature in differentiating neuroblastoma from a hematopoietic tumor. (Fig. 31 (bottom) from McKenna RW. Disorders of bone marrow. In: Sternberg SS, ed. Diagnostic surgical pathology. New York: Raven Press, 1989:479–513.)

Right: A bone marrow smear from a child with medulloblastoma. The marrow is heavily infiltrated. The tumor cells are scattered as individual cells with distinct cell margins similar to a lymphoma or leukemia. In this case they resemble ALL-L3. (Wright-Giemsa stain) (Figures 508, right and 165 are from the same patient.)

Ewing sarcomas are often similar in size to large cell lymphomas, myeloblasts, or lymphoblasts (figs. 508, 509) (17). In patients with these small cell tumors, single, scattered neoplastic cells occasionally predominate in the marrow smears; in most cases at least a few tumor clumps are also observed.

In some instances the cytologic features of the metastatic tumor cells allow them to be characterized in bone marrow aspirate smears. One example is malignant melanoma cells which may contain blue-brown granular melanin pigment in their cytoplasm (fig. 510). In most cases, however,

metastatic tumor cells lack sufficient cytologic specificity in smear preparations to determine the primary neoplasm. Bone marrow smears are suitable, however, for cytochemical and immunocytochemical studies used to characterize metastases from an unknown primary tumor.

Histopathologic Findings. In trephine biopsy sections metastatic tumors manifest considerable morphologic variation. The pattern of infiltration in the biopsy section may be focal, diffuse, or a combination of both (figs. 511, 512). The extent of involvement varies from minute foci of tumor cells in one or two sections of the

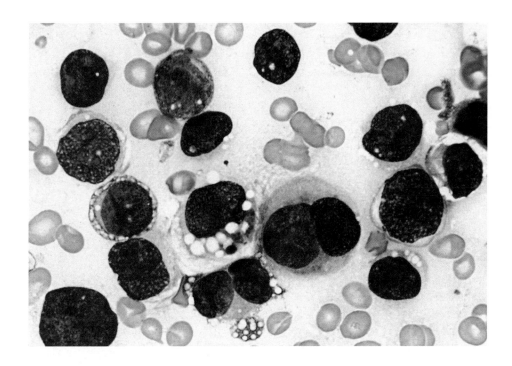

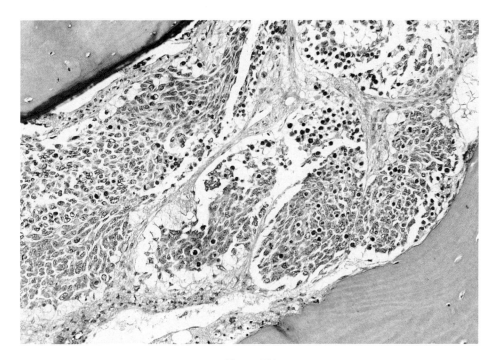

Figure 509
METASTATIC RHABDOMYOSARCOMA IN BONE MARROW

Top: A bone marrow aspirate smear from a 9-year-old boy with embryonal rhabdomyosarcoma. The tumor cells are heteromorphous and exhibit little cohesiveness. They have cytologic similarities to neoplastic hematopoietic cells. The vacuoles in the cytoplasm stained intensely with PAS. The cells also reacted weakly with antibodies to CD61 (antiglycoprotein IIIa), a characteristic usually specific for megakaryocytes and megakaryoblasts. (Wright-Giemsa stain)

Bottom. The bone marrow section in this case showed the histologic pattern of a small round cell metastatic tumor. (Hematoxylin and eosin stain)

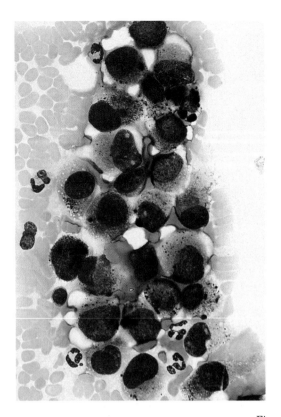
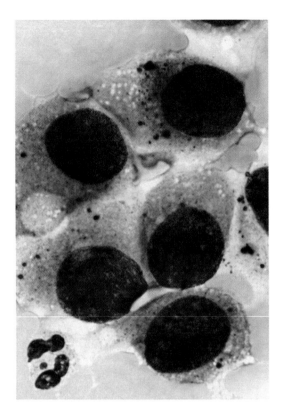

Figure 510
METASTATIC MELANOMA

A bone marrow aspirate smear from a 60-year-old man with melanoma.

Left: At the thin edge of the smear the tumor cells are clustered but have distinct cell borders. Dark granular melanin pigment is present in variable quantity in the cytoplasm.

Right: A higher magnification shows relative uniformity of cytologic features and granular pigment in all of the cells. The tumor cells are much larger than the neutrophil in the field. (Hematoxylin and eosin stain)

Figure 511
METASTATIC MELANOMA

A trephine biopsy section from the same case depicted in figure 510. Focal lesions of metastatic melanoma were scattered throughout the marrow biopsy section. They were encircled by normal hematopoietic tissue. (Hematoxylin and eosin stain)

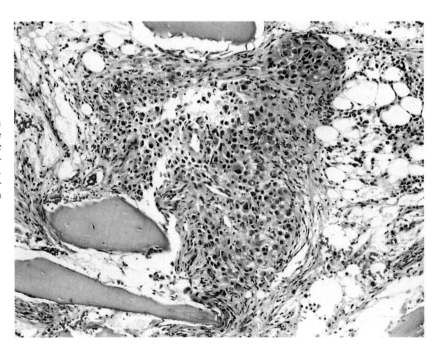

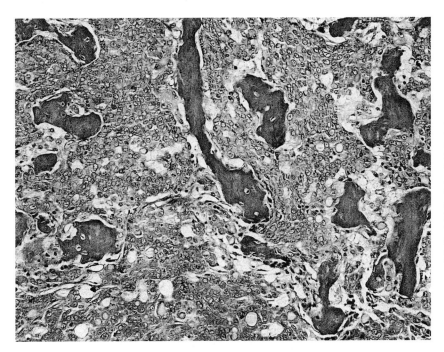

Figure 512
METASTATIC CARCINOMA
WITH DIFFUSE BONE
MARROW INVOLVEMENT
A trephine biopsy section from
a 51-year-old man with metastatic
carcinoma of the colon. There is
diffuse replacement of the bone
marrow with metastatic tumor.
The bone trabeculae are irregular
and show striking osteoclastic activity. (Hematoxylin and eosin
stain) (Fig. 5 (right) from Gale PF,
McKenna RW. Monitoring metastasis in bone marrow. In: Stoll GA,
ed. Screening and monitoring of
cancer. Chichester, England: John
Wiley and Sons, 1985:265–83.)

Figure 513
FOCAL BONE MARROW
INVOLVEMENT WITH
METASTATIC
NEUROBLASTOMA
A trephine biopsy section from
a 3-year-old male shows a small
focus of metastatic neuroblastoma.
The surrounding bone marrow is
normocellular. (Hematoxylin and
eosin stain) (Fig. 1 from Gale PF,
McKenna RW. Monitoring metas-
tasis in bone marrow. In: Stoll GA,
ed. Screening and monitoring of
cancer. Chichester, England: John
Wiley and Sons, 1985:265–83.)

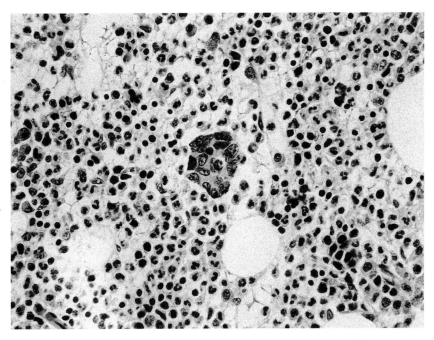

trephine biopsy to total replacement of the hematopoietic marrow (figs. 512, 513). Small foci of
metastatic tumor are usually sharply defined
from normal hematopoietic cells and are readily
recognized as clusters of cells foreign to the bone
marrow, with neoplastic cytologic features (fig.
513). Bone marrow adjacent to metastatic tumor

may be entirely normal or manifest nonspecific
changes such as generalized hyperplasia or increased eosinophils, lymphocytes, granulocytes,
or plasma cells (22). When infiltration is diffuse
and extensive, metastatic tumor may comprise
virtually all of the cellular elements of the bone
marrow biopsy (fig. 512).

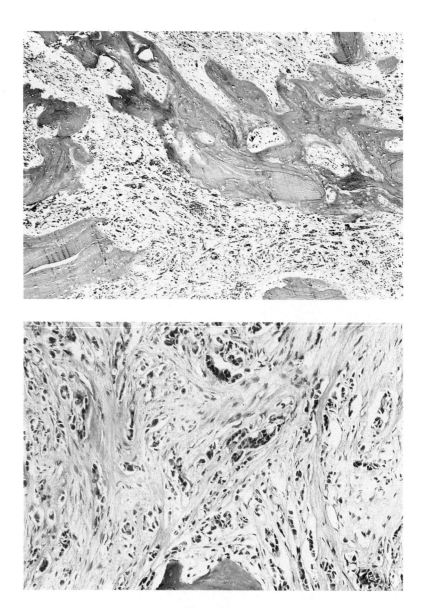

Figure 514
OSTEOBLASTIC LESION IN METASTATIC CARCINOMA

Top: A bone marrow section from a woman with carcinoma of the breast shows a profoundly osteoblastic and fibrotic metastatic lesion.

Bottom: Nests of tumor cells are encircled by dense fibrous connective tissue. (Hematoxylin and eosin stain)

Myelofibrosis is a feature common to many metastatic lesions in the bone marrow. The degree of fibrosis varies from a mild increase in reticulin fibers encircling clusters of neoplastic cells to extensive collagen fibrosis (figs. 514–516). When myelofibrosis is extensive it can mask the underlying malignancy and may be confused with primary myelofibrosis. A careful search for metastatic tumor cells in several sections of the trephine biopsy or a repeat biopsy may be necessary for diagnosis if the patient does not have a known primary neoplasm. The myelofibrosis associated with metastasis often reverses completely with a good response to therapy (23).

Bone structure abnormalities are found in many metastatic lesions. The bone changes include erosion of trabeculae, osteopenia with increased osteoclastic activity, and markedly

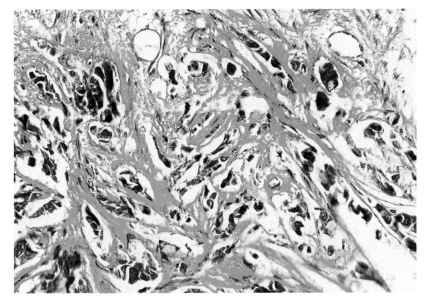

Figure 515
REACTIVE FIBROSIS IN
METASTATIC CARCINOMA
A collagen stain on the same biopsy as depicted in figure 514 shows
collagen fibrosis encircling nests of
tumor cells. (Collagen stain)

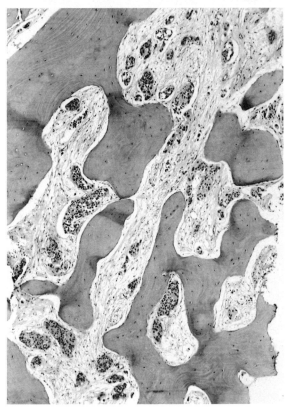

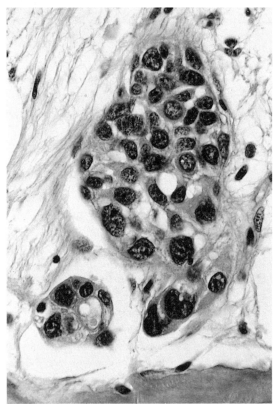

Figure 516
OSTEOBLASTIC LESION IN METASTATIC CARCINOMA

A trephine biopsy section from a woman with metastatic carcinoma of the breast. The bone marrow was extensively replaced by tumor metastasis.

Left: The bone trabeculae are markedly thickened. The carcinoma is scattered as small clusters in dense fibrous connective tissue.

Right: A higher magnification shows a nest of metastatic tumor adjacent to a bone trabeculum. Osteoblastic lesions are typical of several metastatic carcinomas, particularly carcinomas of the breast and prostate. (Hematoxylin and eosin stain) (Fig. 48 from McKenna RW. Disorders of bone marrow. In: Sternberg SS, ed. Diagnostic surgical pathology. 2nd ed. New York: Raven Press, 1994:623–72)

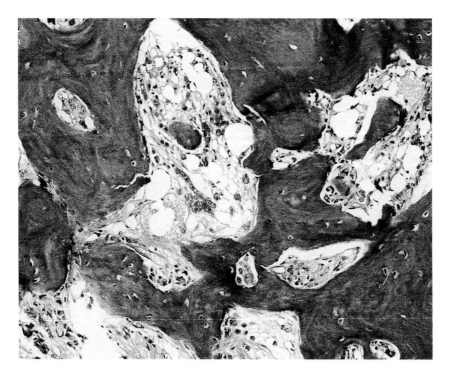

Figure 517
OSTEOBLASTIC LESION IN METASTATIC CARCINOMA
Bone marrow trephine biopsy from a man with carcinoma of the pancreas. The trabeculae are markedly thickened and irregular. Tumor cells are scattered in loose fibrous connective tissue. (Hematoxylin and eosin stain) (Fig. 5 (center) from Gale PF, McKenna RW. Monitoring metastasis in bone marrow. In: Stoll GA, ed. Screening and monitoring of cancer. Chichester, England: John Wiley and Sons, 1985:265–83.)

thickened, irregularly shaped bone trabeculae with profound osteoblastic reactions (figs. 512, 514, 516, 517). Osteoblastic bone lesions are typical of several neoplasms, most commonly, adenocarcinomas of the prostate and breast (32).

Metastatic lesions frequently contain necrotic tissue (24). The necrosis may be patchy with scattered necrotic foci throughout the involved bone marrow or the entire biopsy specimen may consist of necrotic tumor tissue (4). Additional biopsies at adjacent sites may be necessary when necrosis is extensive in patients without a primary diagnosis. Whenever unexplained necrosis is encountered in a bone marrow biopsy, metastatic tumor should be a major consideration (7).

Cytochemical and Immunohistochemical Findings. Cytochemical and immunohistochemical stains may be of value in characterizing a metastatic lesion when the site of origin is unknown (figs. 518–520) (29,30). Table 38 lists several of the more commonly employed antibodies used for characterizing metastatic tumors in trephine biopsy sections. Most of the antigens associated with a particular type of neoplasm are not restricted to that tumor. It is always necessary to apply an appropriate panel of antibodies directed at various antigens to characterize metastatic or undifferentiated tumors in bone marrow.

Differential Diagnosis. In most cases a metastatic lesion in the bone marrow is recognized by its histologic features, even when a primary tumor is not apparent. Occasionally, metastases simulate hematopoietic malignancies. In adults the lesions that are most problematic in the differential diagnosis are malignant lymphomas and primary myelofibrosis. In children lymphoblastic leukemia or lymphoma must be distinguished from metastatic tumors.

Malignant lymphomas, like solid tissue tumors, generally involve the bone marrow secondarily. The clinical presentation may be identical to that of a patient with metastatic tumor. Usually the

Table 38

SELECTED ANTIBODIES FOR CHARACTERIZATION OF METASTATIC TUMORS IN BONE MARROW BY IMMUNOHISTOCHEMICAL TECHNIQUES*

Antigen	Tumor Type
Actin	Rhabdomyosarcoma
Alpha-1-antichymotrypsin	Histiocytic tumors, mast cells
Alpha-fetoprotein	Germ cell tumors
Alpha-lactalbumin	Breast carcinoma
Carcinoembryonic antigen (CEA)	Adenocarcinomas of the gastrointestinal tract and lungs
Chromogranin	Neuroendocrine tumors
Cytokeratins	Epithelial tumors
Desmin	Rhabdomyosarcoma
Epithelial membrane antigen (EMA)	Epithelial tumors (some hematopoietic tumors are reactive, e.g., large cell anaplastic lymphoma)
HBA-71	Ewing sarcoma, peripheral primitive neuroectodermal tumors**
Immunoglobulins	Myeloma, immunoblastic lymphomas
Leu-M1 (CD15)	Reed-Sternberg cells (some carcinomas are reactive)
Leukocyte common antigen (LCA) (CD45)	Lymphomas
Lymphocyte subset antigens (B- and T-cell markers, e.g., UCHL-1, L26 [CD20])	Lymphomas
Lysozyme	Histiocytes
Myoglobin	Rhabdomyosarcoma
Neurofilaments	Tumors of neuronal origin (neuroblastoma, medulloblastoma, retinoblastoma)
Neuron-specific enolase (NSE)	Tumors of neuroectodermal and neuro-endocrine origin (neuroblastoma, small cell tumors)
Prostate-specific antigen (PSA)	Prostatic carcinoma
S-100 protein	Melanomas
Vimentin	Mesenchymal tumors

* From reference 34.
**From reference 12.

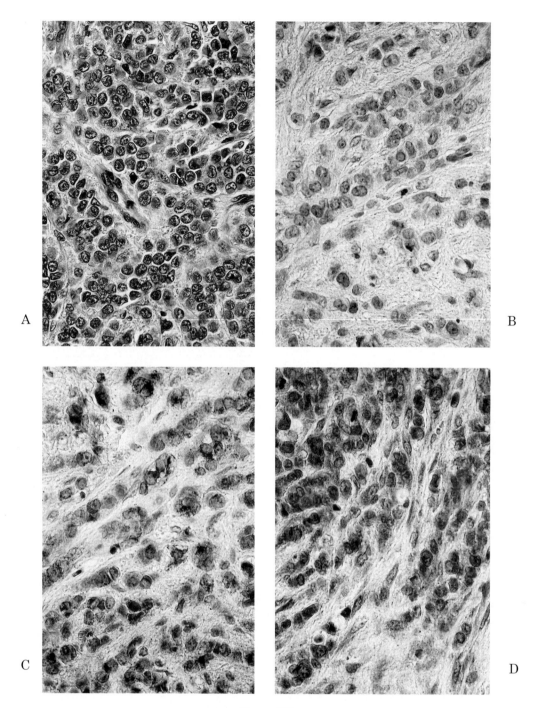

Figure 518
METASTATIC CARCINOMA INVOLVING BONE MARROW

A composite of four sections of bone marrow from a woman presenting with a metastatic tumor of unknown primary in the bone marrow.

A. The section shows relatively uniform tumor cells with eosinophilic cytoplasm and round to oval nuclei. (Hematoxylin and eosin stain)

B. A negative reaction with an antibody to leukocyte common antigen (LCA). (Immunoperoxidase stain)

C. A positive reaction with an antibody to epithelial membrane antigen (EMA). (Immunoperoxidase stain)

D. A positive reaction with an antibody to alpha-lactalbumin. (Immunoperoxidase stain)

A diagnosis of metastatic carcinoma of the breast was made. A small primary lesion was subsequently identified in the left breast by mammography.

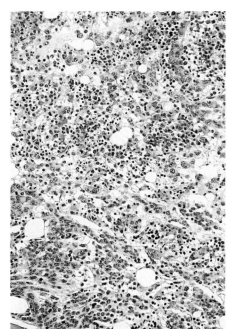

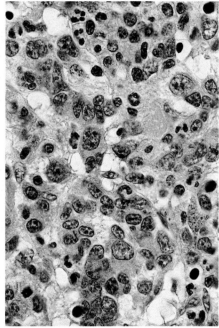

Figure 519
METASTATIC
NEUROBLASTOMA
INVOLVING
BONE MARROW

A bone marrow section from a boy with an abdominal mass.

Left: A low magnification of a routinely stained trephine biopsy section shows scattered clusters of metastatic tumor mixed with normal hematopoietic tissue.

Right: In a higher magnification the tumor cells blend with the hematopoietic tissue but are distinct by their large size and pleomorphic nuclei. (Hematoxylin and eosin stain)

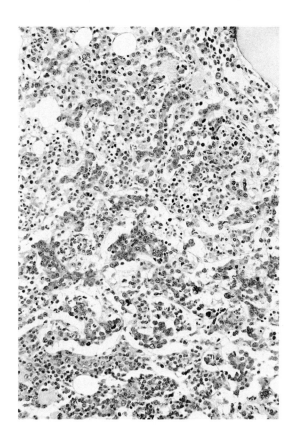

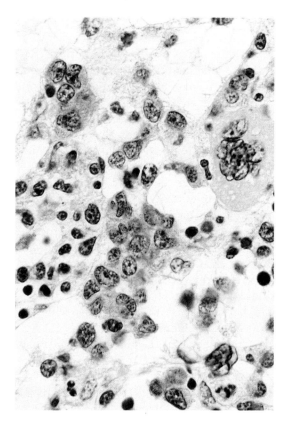

Figure 520
METASTATIC NEUROBLASTOMA INVOLVING BONE MARROW

Immunoperoxidase stains for neuron-specific enolase (NSE) on the same biopsy specimen as depicted in figure 519. The tumor cells react with the antibody. The stain clearly demarcates the tumor cells from adjacent normal hematopoietic cells. The patient had markedly elevated urinary catecholamines supporting the diagnosis of neuroblastoma. (Immunoperoxidase stain)

Table 39

USUAL IMMUNOHISTOCHEMICAL REACTIONS OF
METASTATIC ROUND CELL TUMORS IN CHILDREN*

	T- or B-cell Antigens	CD45 (LCA)	Neuro-filaments	Chromo-granin	Vimentin	Desmin	HBA-71
Lymphoblastic leukemia-lymphoma	+	+	−	−	−**	−	−
Neuroblastoma	−	−	+	+	−	−	−
Retinoblastoma	−	−	+	+	−	−	−
Rhabdomyosarcoma	−	−	−	−	+	+	−
Ewing sarcoma	−	−	−	−	+/−	−	+
Medulloblastoma	−	−	−**	+/−	+/−	−**	−

* Reactivity may be affected by method of fixation and decalcification.
**Rare cases are positive.

histopathology in the trephine biopsy and the cytology of the malignant cells in smear preparations readily distinguishes the two processes. In difficult cases immunophenotyping for lymphocyte antigens and enzyme immunohistochemistry using a panel of antibodies to various tumor types will generally provide the correct diagnosis (see chapter, Bone Marrow Lymphomas).

Myelofibrosis may be caused by several marrow invasive processes as well as primary myeloproliferative disorders, e.g., idiopathic myelofibrosis. The absence of definitive evidence of metastatic tumor cells in the trephine biopsy and the finding of changes in blood smears typical of a myeloproliferative disorder are most helpful in distinguishing primary myelofibrosis from a desmoplastic metastatic tumor (see chapter, Chronic Myeloproliferative Diseases).

In pediatric patients the differential diagnosis of a small cell undifferentiated neoplasm in the bone marrow may include lymphoblastic lymphoma and leukemia and several solid tissue tumors including neuroblastoma, retinoblastoma, rhabdomyosarcoma, medulloblastoma, and Ewing sarcoma. Careful evaluation of the clinical presentation and supplementary studies including electron microscopy, catecholamine levels, and immunohistochemistry are often necessary to distinguish these tumors. Table 39 summarizes the usual immunohistochemical reactions for several small round cell tumors in pediatric patients.

Treatment and Prognosis. Therapy is generally aimed at controlling the primary neoplasm. The most appropriate combination of chemotherapy, hormonal therapy, or radiotherapy for a particular neoplasm is used. Bone pain and tenderness from localized lesions may be improved by reducing the lesion size. The presence of bone marrow metastases is indicative of advanced disease and is generally a poor prognostic sign. Individual patients may experience a good treatment response.

REFERENCES

1. Anner RM, Drewinko B. Frequency and significance of bone marrow involvement by metastatic solid tumors. Cancer 1977;39:1337–44.

2. Bearden JD, Ratkin GA, Coltman CA. Comparison of the diagnostic value of bone marrow biopsy and bone marrow aspiration in neoplastic disease. J Clin Pathol 1974;27:738–40.

3. Broghamer WL Jr, Keeling MM. The bone marrow biopsy, osteoscan, and peripheral blood in non-hematopoietic cancer. Cancer 1977;40:836–40.

4. Brown CH III. Bone marrow necrosis. A study of seventy cases. Johns Hopkins Med J 1972;131:189–203.

5. Brunning RD, Bloomfield CD, McKenna RW, Peterson LA. Bilateral trephine bone marrow biopsies in lymphoma and other neoplastic diseases. Ann Intern Med 1975;82:365–6.

6. Chernow B, Wallner SF. Variables predictive of bone marrow metastasis. Cancer 1978;42:2373–8.

7. Colvin BT, Revell PA, Ibbotson RM, Turnbull Al. Necrosis of bone marrow and bone in malignant disease. Clin Oncol 1980;6:265–72.

8. Contreras E, Ellis LD, Lee RE. Value of the bone marrow biopsy in the diagnosis of metastatic carcinoma. Cancer 1972;29:778–83.

9. Delsol G, Guiu-Godfrin B, Guiu M, Pris J, Corberand J, Fabre J. Leukoerythroblastosis and cancer frequency, prognosis and physiopathologic significance. Cancer 1979;44:1009–13.

10. Delta BG, Pinkel D. Bone marrow aspiration in children with malignant tumors. J Pediatr 1964;64:542–6.

11. Duchek M, Lingardh G, Saterborg NE, Winblad B, Angstrom T. Bone marrow examination as a diagnostic tool in carcinoma of the prostate. Int Urol Nephrol 1975;7:59–64.

12. Fellinger EJ, Garin-Chesa P, Glasser DB, Huvos AG, Rettig WJ. Comparison of cell surface antigen HBA71 (p30/32MIC2), neuron-specific enolase, and vimentin in the immunohistochemical analysis of Ewing's sarcoma of bone. Am J Surg Pathol 1992;16:746–55.

13. Finkelstein JZ, Ekert H, Isaacs H Jr, Higgins G. Bone marrow metastases in children with solid tumors. Am J Dis Child 1970;119:49–52.

14. Fordham EW, Ali A. Radionucleotide imaging of bone marrow. Semin Hematol 1981;18:222–39.

15. Gale PF, McKenna RW. Monitoring metastasis in bone marrow. In: Stoll GA, ed. Screening and monitoring of cancer. Chichester, England: John Wiley and Sons, 1985:265–83.

16. Hansen HH, Muggia FM, Selawry OS. Bone-marrow examination in 100 consecutive patients with bronchogenic carcinoma. Lancet 1971;2:443–5.

17. Head DR, Kennedy PS, Goyette RE. Metastatic neuroblastoma in bone marrow aspirate smears. Am J Clin Pathol 1979;72:1008–11.

18. Hilf R. Biochemical markers in monitoring. In: Stoll BA, ed. Screening and monitoring of cancer. Chichester, England: John Wiley and Sons, 1985:47–56.

19. Hirsch FR, Hansen HH, Hainau B. Bilateral bone-marrow examinations in small-cell anaplastic carcinoma of the lung. Acta Pathol Microbiol Immunol Scand 1979;87:59–62.

20. Ihde DC, Simms EB, Matthews MJ, Cohen MH, Burn PA, Minna JD. Bone marrow metastases in small cell carcinoma of the lung: frequency, description, and influence on chemotherapeutic toxicity and prognosis. Blood 1979;43:677–86.

21. Ingle JN, Tormey DC, Tan HK. The bone marrow examination in breast cancer: diagnostic considerations and clinical usefulness. Cancer 1978;41:670–4.

22. Jakoubkova J, Hermansk Z, Bek V. Reaction of the bone marrow in malignant tumors of the kidney and testis. Neoplasma 1970;17:427–31.

23. Kiang DT, McKenna RW, Kennedy BJ. Reversal of myelofibrosis in advanced breast cancer. Am J Med 1978;64:173–6.

24. Kiraly JF III, Wheby MS. Bone marrow necrosis. Am J Med 1976;60:361–8.

25. Lake-Lewin D, Tang CK, Gray GF. Metastatic tumor in bone-marrow biopsy. NY State J Med 1975;75:1008–11.

26. Laszlo J, Huang AT. Anemia associated with marrow infiltration. In: Williams WJ, Beutler E, Erslev AJ, Lichtman MA, eds. Hematology. 4th ed. New York: McGraw-Hill, 1990:546–8.

27. Leland J, MacPherson B. Hematologic findings in cases of mammary cancer metastatic to bone marrow. Am J Clin Pathol 1979;71:31–5.

28. Mills AE. A study of the value of closed bone marrow biopsy. S Afr Med J 1976;50:1928–31.

29. Moss TJ, Reynolds CP, Sather HN, Romansky SG, Hammond GD, Seeger RC. Prognostic value of immunocytologic detection of bone marrow metastases in neuroblastoma. N Eng J Med 1991;324:219–26.

30. Osborne MP, Asina S, Wong GY, Old LJ, Cote RJ. Immunofluorescent monoclonal antibody detection of breast cancer in bone marrow: sensitivity in a model system. Cancer Res 1989;49:2510–3.

31. Parbhoo S. Serial monitoring in management of bone metastases. In: Stoll BA, ed. Screening and monitoring of cancer. Chichester, England: John Wiley and Sons, 1985:355–406.

32. Ridell B, Landys K. Incidence and histopathology of metastases of mammary carcinoma in biopsies from the posterior iliac crest. Cancer 1979;44:1782–8.

33. Roeckel IE. Diagnosis of metastatic carcinoma by bone marrow biopsy versus bone marrow aspiration. Ann Clin Lab Sci 1974;4:193–7.

34. Rosai J. Special techniques in surgical pathology. In: Rosai J, ed. Ackerman's surgical pathology, Vol. 1. 7th ed. St. Louis: CV Mosby, 1989:31–51.

35. Savage RA, Hoffman GC, Shaker K. Diagnostic problems involved in detection of metastatic neoplasms by bone-marrow aspirate compared with needle biopsy. Am J Clin Pathol 1978;70:623–7.

36. Singh G, Krause JR, Breitfeld V. Bone marrow examination for metastatic tumor: aspirate and biopsy. Cancer 1977;40:2317–21.

37. Suprun H, Rywlin AM. Metastatic carcinoma in histologic sections of aspirated bone marrow: a comparative autopsy study. South Med J 1976;69:438–9.

38. Weick JK, Hagedorn AB, Linman JW. Leukoerythroblastosis. Diagnostic and prognostic significance. Mayo Clin Proc 1974;49:110–3.

39. Yarrison G, Merterns BF, Mathies JC. New diagnostic use of bone marrow acid and alkaline phosphatase. Am J Clin Pathol 1976;66:667–71.

APPENDIX:
BONE MARROW SPECIMEN PROCESSING (5)

The study of neoplastic disorders involving the bone marrow optimally includes blood smears, bone marrow aspirate smears, particle crush preparations, and bone marrow trephine biopsies. The manner in which these bone marrow specimens are processed is of considerable importance to assuring optimal cytologic detail, a factor of critical importance to the diagnosis of leukemias and lymphomas. The procedures outlined in this chapter are intended to serve as general guidelines in the processing of the bone marrow specimen.

OBTAINING SPECIMENS

Several instruments are available for obtaining bone marrow biopsies; the most widely used are patterned on the needle introduced by Jamshidi and Swaim in 1971 (14). These instruments are available in a variety of adult and pediatric sizes, in both disposable and reusable types. They yield high quality specimens and have a wide margin of safety when properly used. Detailed instructions for the use of these needles are provided in the manufacturers' brochures.

The posterior superior iliac spine is the most commonly used site for trephine biopsies both in adults and children. The core biopsy should be obtained before aspirating the fluid portion of the specimen. Aspirating bone marrow with the trephine biopsy needle and then advancing the needle for the biopsy, a procedure advocated by some, may result in hemorrhage into the biopsy site, leading to difficulties in interpretation and, possibly, erroneous conclusions.

The optimal size of a trephine biopsy is 1 to 2 cm; specimens should be free of distortion and crush artifacts. Prior to placing the biopsy in fixative, several imprint preparations are made for routine Wright staining and other procedures such as terminal deoxynucleotidyltransferase (TdT), cytochemistry, and immunocytochemistry. Less damage to the biopsy specimen results if the imprint is made by gently touching a glass slide to the specimen rather than squeezing the specimen with a tweezers and touching it to a slide. The imprint preparations of the biopsy may occa-sionally serve as the single most important resource for the evaluation of cytologic, cytochemical, and immunocytochemical characteristics.

After the core biopsy, the aspiration is obtained through a separate puncture. Aspiration needles such as the Illinois needle or modifications of this instrument are ideal for aspiration of the fluid portion of the specimen and cause less discomfort to the patient than the larger trephine biopsy needles. The aspiration needle can be inserted through the same skin incision used for the trephine biopsy and placed on the periosteal surface at a distance of approximately 1 cm from the trephine biopsy site. Approximately 1 mL of fluid should be aspirated for morphologic studies. About 0.9 mL of this is placed in an appropriate anticoagulant; powdered disodium EDTA, 1 mg/1 mL of fluid marrow, is very satisfactory. The portion of the specimen remaining in the syringe is then used for making smears; this should be done as soon as possible before clotting occurs. These smears, which are free of anticoagulant artifact, frequently result in better preservation of nuclear and cytoplasmic detail than those made from the specimen placed in anticoagulant. They should be air dried as rapidly as possible immediately after they are made.

PROCESSING THE CORE BIOPSY

There are several choices of fixative for bone marrow biopsies. Because of the overriding importance of cytologic detail in the evaluation of hematopoietic tumors, the choice of fixative is one of the most crucial steps in the processing procedure. In laboratories that are dedicated to the processing of hematopoietic tissues, the mercury-based fixatives are generally preferred. In laboratories in which bone marrow biopsies are processed with other tissues, neutral buffered formalin is the preferred fixative. Because of restrictions on the disposal of the mercury-based fixatives such as Zenker and B5, routine buffered formalin is increasingly used. Fixatives using zinc instead of mercury are now available and the results with these reagents are very satisfactory.

Zenker fixative is prepared by adding 5 mL of glacial acetic acid to 95 mL of Zenker stock; the solution should be prepared each day. The biopsy is fixed in the Zenker for a minimum of 4 hours; overnight and over-weekend fixation has no adverse effect on the tissue. A core biopsy of 1 to 2 cm in length is placed in approximately 15 to 20 mL of fixative. Zenker fixative results in excellent preservations of cytology. A disadvantage is the nonreactivity of some monoclonal antibodies that react with paraffin-embedded specimens: L26 (CD20), which is a very good B-cell marker, does not react in Zenker-fixed tissue.

Specimens in neutral buffered formalin are fixed for at least 18 to 24 hours. There is no limit on the duration of fixation. Specimens in Bouin fixative should be fixed for 4 to 12 hours.

The optimal fixation period for bone marrow biopsies in B5 fixative is 2 to 4 hours, depending on the size of the biopsy. Specimens exposed to B5 for periods in excess of 5 hours may become hard and brittle; this may result in considerable difficulty in sectioning.

The following steps in the processing of bone marrow trephine biopsies are generally applicable to tissues fixed in Zenker, B5, neutral buffered formalin, and Bouin solutions. Following removal from the fixative:

1. Wash in deionized water for 30 to 60 minutes.
2. Decalcify for a period appropriate to the size of the biopsy. Decalcification in RDO (APB Engineering Products Corporation, Plainfield, IL), a commercially available dilute solution of hydrochloric acid (HCl) in coal tar base, for 30 to 60 minutes gives satisfactory results. Decalcification in Surgipath (Surgipath Medical Industries, Grayslake, IL) decalcifier for 90 minutes or in a HCl–formic acid solution for 2 1/2 hours is also satisfactory.
3. Wash 60 to 90 minutes with several changes of water. Avoid washing in running tap water as this may damage the specimen.

Steps 4 and 5 are eliminated if specimens are placed in an automated tissue processor.

4. Dehydration procedure:
   a. 30% alcohol for 30 to 60 minutes
   b. 50% alcohol for 30 to 60 minutes
   c. 70% alcohol for a minimum of 60 minutes. The specimen may be left in 70 percent alcohol for an extended period.
   d. 95% alcohol, two changes, 15 minutes each
   e. 100% alcohol, two changes, 15 minutes each
   f. 100% alcohol plus equal amounts of xylene for 15 minutes
   g. Xylene, two changes, 15 minutes each
5. Place in paraffin or Surgipath medium three times for 30 minutes each time (maximum total time of 90 minutes).
6. Embed in paraffin or Surgipath embedding medium.
7. Section the biopsies at 3 to 4 μm with a knife blade that is repeatedly checked for defects. If the biopsy is performed for determination of bone marrow involvement by lymphoma, metastatic tumor, or granulomatous inflammation, the biopsies should be completely sectioned and stepwise serial sections mounted.

The hematoxylin and eosin stain is the most widely used routine stain for bone marrow trephine biopsies. It is the one with which all pathologists are familiar and yields the most information. Several other stains are important in routine diagnostic work in hematopathology and although not used for all specimens, are applied with sufficient frequency to be detailed. These are the periodic acid–Schiff and Giemsa stains and the stains for reticulin and collagen. The periodic acid–Schiff is useful in the identification of maturing granulocytes and megakaryocytes and may also be used as an initial screening procedure for the detection of fungal organisms. The Giemsa stain may be used to accentuate granules in maturing neutrophils, eosinophils, and basophils; it will also highlight the mast cells in the lesions of mastocytosis. The reticulin and collagen stains are used to determine the degree of fibrosis in marrow sections. The reticulin stain is invaluable for demonstrating an increase in reticulin fibers. Frank collagen fibrosis is uncommon in hematopoietic disorders but occurs frequently in bone marrows involved by metastatic tumor.

BONE MARROW ASPIRATION SPECIMEN (5,6,19)

The major portion of the aspirated fluid specimen is immediately transferred from the syringe to a plastic or paraffin-coated glass vial containing powdered disodium EDTA, 1 mg/1 mL of fluid marrow; the vial is gently inverted several times to mix the fluid with the anticoagulant. The remaining portion of the specimen is used for making smears; approximately one drop of the marrow remaining in the syringe is placed at one end of a slide and smeared. The smear is immediately air dried. Proper drying of the smear is critical and is best accomplished by gentle waving or using a small portable electric fan. Approximately eight or nine slides are prepared from each specimen.

The anticoagulated specimen should be transferred as soon as possible after aspiration to the laboratory. The specimen is spread onto a clean glass Petri dish; the fluid from the specimen is then aspirated with a Pasteur pipette and transferred to a Wintrobe hematocrit tube. The particles remaining following this step are used for two purposes: particle crush preparations and particle sections. The particle crush preparations, approximately five to seven, are prepared by gently squashing a particle between two slides and sliding them over each other. The slides are immediately air dried in a manner similar to the smears.

The remaining particles, aided by the addition of two to three drops of 0.015 mol/L $CaCl_2$ to accelerate clotting, are aggregated into a clump and placed in fixative. With the exception of the decalcification step, these specimens are processed in a manner similar to the trephine biopsy.

The Wintrobe tube containing the fluid portion of the marrow aspirate is centrifuged at 850×g (2800 rpm) for 8 minutes in a tabletop centrifuge. Following centrifugation, the marrow specimen in the tube is layered into four major components, the relative amounts of which can be determined from the markings on the Wintrobe tube. The four layers from top to bottom are the fat and perivascular (F-PV), plasma (P), myeloid-erythroid (M-E) (nucleated cells), and erythrocyte (E) layers. The relative proportion of two of these components, the F-PV and M-E layers, in general, reflect the cellularity of the bone marrow. The F-PV from a normal marrow is usually 1 to 3 percent and the M-E layer is 5 to 8 percent. An increase in the M-E layer and a decrease in the F-PV layer is usually reflective of marrow hypercellularity; the reverse indicates a hypocellular marrow. An inadequate marrow aspirate is reflected by a decrease in both the F-PV and M-E layers.

After recording the amounts of each of the separate layers, the F-PV component is gently aspirated and placed on two or three slides and smeared. Because of the rich component of macrophages in the perivascular tissue, these preparations are ideal for staining with Prussian blue for the evaluation of iron stores.

Using a clean pipette, the plasma (P) layer is gently aspirated from the Wintrobe tube and set aside. Following this, using a clean pipette, the M-E (buffy coat) layer is removed from the Wintrobe tube and transferred to a clean watch glass. To this is added a portion of the plasma equal to twice the amount of the buffy coat layer. These two layers are then thoroughly, but gently, mixed. Using a Pasteur pipette, one drop of this mixture is then placed on slides and smears made; the slides are immediately air dried. Approximately 15 to 20 slides are prepared if sufficient specimen is available.

Three slides of the direct (D) smears (made at the bedside), particle crush preparations, and M-E smears are then stained with a routine Romanowsky stain. An adequate number of slides should be reserved for any cytochemical and immunocytochemical reactions appropriate to the disease process. Iron stains are routinely performed (8,28).

IRON STAIN (PRUSSIAN BLUE)

This is used for smear preparations of bone marrow, blood, or other body fluids.

1. Fix air-dried films of peripheral blood or bone marrow with absolute methanol for 15 to 20 minutes. Particle crush preparations are not satisfactory because fat is dissolved out by the methanol. Air dry slides only, do not wash.
2. Incubate the slides for 10 minutes in a 1% potassium ferrocyanide solution at 50° to 56°C. One percent potassium ferrocyanide solution: Mix equal volumes of 2% potassium ferrocyanide and 0.2N HCl acid. The 2% potassium ferrocyanide solution is good for 1 week and should be stored in the dark. It is pale to moderate yellow in color. The 1% potassium ferrocyanide in 0.1N HCl acid solution should be made up just before using and can be used only once. It is pale yellow. A smear with a previously determined increase in siderocytes or sideroblasts should be processed with each batch of slides as a

control. Excessive heat or prolonged incubation can alter the reaction.

3. Rinse with distilled or deionized water, wash in running tap water for 20 minutes, and rinse again in distilled or deionized water. Do not dry; drying before counterstaining may cause artifacts.
4. Weakly counterstain with 0.1% aqueous safranin or 0.1% aqueous eosin for 5 to 10 seconds. Safranin is preferred.
5. Rinse briefly with distilled or deionized water, air dry, and coverslip with permount or another solvent-soluble mounting media if desired.

Results

Diffuse and particulate iron is colored a vivid blue to blue-green.

IRON STAIN FOR PARTICLE CRUSH PREPARATIONS

1. Air dry specimen.
2. Fix with formalin by allowing specimen to stand in weak formalin vapors (10% formalin) for 10 minutes. A piece of filter paper is placed on the top of a Coplin jar and one drop of 10% formalin is placed on the filter paper. The cover is replaced and the slides are allowed to fix in the formalin vapor for 10 minutes. Do not wash. Excess formalin results in a black granular precipitate.
3. Immerse in Prussian blue reagent, made with 15 mL of 2% potassium ferrocyanide and 45 mL of 0.5% HCl acid, for 10 minutes. This solution is good for 1 hour and is a pale yellow color.
4. Wash thoroughly with deionized or distilled water, then running tap water for 2 minutes. Air dry.
5. Coverslip with permount or another solvent-soluble mounting media if desired.

Note: Do not put oil directly on these preparations. The material on the slide will be removed when xylol is used to remove the oil.

Results

Diffuse and particulate iron is colored a vivid blue or blue-green.

IRON STAIN FOR SECTIONS

1. Take tissue through xylol and decreasing strengths of alcohol to distilled or deionized water. Run Zenker-fixed tissue through iodine and sodium thiosulfate in the usual manner.
2. Stain for 30 minutes with the Prussian blue reagent.
3. Wash in distilled or deionized water, then running tap water for 2 minutes.
4. Counterstain with eosin for 8 to 10 seconds.
5. Dehydrate through 70%, 95%, and 100% ethanol to xylol.
6. Coverslip with permount or another solvent-soluble mounting media.

Note: The 2% potassium ferrocyanide (crystals) solution is good for 1 week and should be stored in the dark. The solution is a pale to moderate yellow color.

Results

Diffuse and particulate iron is colored a vivid blue or blue-green.

HEMATOXYLIN AND EOSIN STAINING PROCEDURE (20)

This procedure may be used for bone marrow biopsies fixed in Zenker, B5, neutral buffered formalin, or Bouin fixatives. If formalin is the fixative, omit steps 5 and 6.

Put mounted sections in 58° to 62°C oven for 40 minutes, cool, and then process with:

1. Xylol, two changes, 3 to 5 minutes each.
2. 100% alcohol, two changes, 3 to 5 minutes each.
3. 95% alcohol, two changes, 3 to 5 minutes each.
4. 70% alcohol for 3 to 5 minutes.
5. Alcoholic solution of iodine for 10 minutes (0.25% solution of iodine in 70% alcohol).
6. 5% aqueous solution of sodium thiosulfate for 10 minutes.
7. Running tap water wash for 5 to 10 minutes.
8. Bluing solution for 1 minute.
9. Deionized water, two changes for 10 dips each.
10. Hematoxylin, 5 minutes for particles and 30 to 40 minutes for trephine biopsies. Some trephine sections require a longer staining time. (With formalin and B5 fixatives, stain trephine 10 to 15 minutes in hematoxylin.)

11. Running water rinse for 5 minutes.
12. Differentiate in diluted acid alcohol, two dips.
13. Rinse twice in tap or deionized water.
14. Wash in running tap water for at least 20 minutes.
15. Bluing solution, 2 minutes and deionized water, two changes for 10 dips each.
16. 70% alcohol, 3 to 5 minutes. Check intensity of hematoxylin color. If hematoxylin is too light, place back into water for 2 minutes and hematoxylin for 10 to 20 minutes or longer. Then repeat steps 11 to 16. If stain is too dark, repeat steps 12 to 16.
17. Eosin-Y stain, 2 to 5 seconds depending on the age of the eosin, dilution of the solution, and intensity of counterstain desired. Dip several times before allowing sections to remain in solution. Usually, formalin and B5 fixatives need a longer time in eosin.
18. 70% alcohol, two to three changes, 4 dips each.
19. 95% alcohol, two changes, 15 dips each.
20. 100% alcohol, two changes, 3 to 5 minutes each.
21. 100% alcohol plus equal amounts of xylol, 3 to 5 minutes.
22. Xylol, three changes, 3 to 5 minutes each (or longer). Check eosin after first xylol. If too light, dip back through solutions of eosin and repeat steps 17 to 22. If the stain is too dark, dip back through solutions to first 95 percent alcohol (or 70% if very dark) and repeat steps 19 to 22.
23. Mount with permount or another solvent-soluble mounting media.

Solutions

Acid alcohol
1% hydrochloric acid in 70% alcohol
70% ethanol   950 mL
concentrated hydrochloric acid   9.5 mL

Dilute acid alcohol
Mix 1% HCl acid 1:1 with 70% alcohol.

Bluing reagent (0.2% sodium bicarbonate, 1.0% magnesium sulfate)
sodium bicarbonate   2 g
magnesium sulfate   10 g
Dilute to 1000 mL with deionized or distilled water.

GIEMSA STAIN FOR SECTIONS (20)

1. Process biopsy as for hematoxylin and eosin stain through step 7.
2. Place slides into Giemsa stain immediately after making solution. Leave sections 2 to 4 hours (or overnight) in the staining solution.
3. Place sections individually into deionized or distilled water, 8 to 10 dips.
4. Differentiate each slide individually in 95% ethyl alcohol, two quick dips. Section should turn a purplish-pink color.

Note: 95% ethyl alcohol is preferred to the originally described solution of 95% ethyl alcohol plus a few drops of 10% rosin solution in absolute alcohol.

5. Dehydrate sections in absolute alcohol, three to four quick dips.
6. Clear in xylol and mount in solvent-soluble mounting media.

Note: If sections are not differentiated enough, dip quickly back through alcohols to water and then back through alcohols to xylol. If over differentiated (too light), slides must go back to water and then into fresh Giemsa solution for 2 to 4 hours.

Preparation of Giemsa Stain

Dissolve 0.5 g powdered Giemsa blood stain in 33 mL glycerin at 55° to 60°C for 1.5 to 2 hours. To this add 33 mL absolute methyl alcohol and filter.

Working solution (make fresh each time)
stock Giemsa stain   1.25 mL
methyl alcohol   1.5 mL
deionized water   50 mL

PERIODIC ACID–SCHIFF REACTION (PAS STAIN) (17): FOR SECTIONS AND SMEARS

Procedure for Sections

Fixation: Formalin, Zenker, B5, or Bouin fixatives
1. Remove paraffin from sections in the usual manner and take slides through alcohols to distilled or deionized water. Run Zenker-fixed tissue through iodine and sodium thiosulfate in the usual manner.
2. Place slides in 0.5% periodic acid for 5 minutes. The periodic acid can be reused the same day.

3. Wash 5 minutes in running water.
4. Stain 30 minutes in Schiff reagent. This may be used several times during the day but should be prepared fresh each day.
5. Wash in tap water in staining dish for 5 to 10 minutes.
6. Rinse in distilled or deionized water. For section counterstain see step 7 below; for smear counterstain, see step 4 under smear procedures.
7. Stain with hematoxylin for 8 minutes.
8. Wash in running water 4 minutes.
9. Put in acid alcohol (1% HCl acid in 70% ethanol), 4 to 5 seconds (agitate up and down).
10. Wash in running water 10 minutes.
11. Put in 95% alcohol, two changes for 2 minutes each.
12. Put in 100% alcohol, two changes for 2 minutes each.
13. Put in 100% alcohol plus equal amount of xylol, 2 minutes.
14. Put in xylol, three changes for 2 minutes each.
15. Mount with permount or another solvent-soluble mounting media.

Procedure for Smears

1. Fix smear in strong formalin fumes for 10 minutes. Allow slides to air dry. Wipe off excess formalin.
2. Place in methanol for 10 minutes.
3. Rinse in running water for 10 minutes and place into 0.5% periodic acid solution. Process in same manner as sections until counterstain (see step 2 under sections).
4. Counterstain with hematoxylin for 6 to 8 minutes.
5. Rinse in running water for 5 to 10 minutes.
6. Rinse in distilled or deionized water and air dry.
7. Coverslip with permount or another solvent-soluble mounting media.

Results

Glycogen - dark red purple
Amyloid - light red
Mucin - dark red purple
Fibrinoid - red
Some fungi - red
Basement membrane and reticulin - red
Loose collagen - light red
Nuclei - blue

Solutions

Schiff reagent

basic fuchsin (pararosaniline)	32.0 g
sodium metabisulfite	60.8 g
1N hydrochloric acid	480.0 mL
Distilled or deionized water	2720.0 mL

Mix on magnetic stirrer for 2 to 3 hours.
Add approximately 32 g fresh powdered decolorizing charcoal.
Mix on magnetic stirrer for about 1 hour.
Filter. Use extra fine filter paper, double thickness.
Refrigerate.
The filtered solution must be colorless or pale straw colored. The solution has a usable period of approximately 1 month.

0.5% periodic acid

periodic acid	10 g
distilled or deionized water	2000 mL

Good for approximately 2 weeks.

RETICULIN STAIN (WILDER) (20)

Fixation: Formalin, Zenker, B5, or Bouin fixatives

1. Process as for hematoxylin and eosin stain through step 7.
2. Wash well in distilled or deionized water.
3. Place in phosphomolybdic acid solution for 1 minute; this should be prepared fresh each time.
4. Rinse well in running water for at least 1 minute.
5. Dip in 1% aqueous uranyl nitrate for 1 minute or less.
6. Wash in distilled or deionized water for 10 to 20 seconds.
7. Place in ammoniacal silver solution for 1 minute.
8. Dip very quickly in 95% alcohol and go immediately to step 9.
9. Put in reducing solution for 1 minute.
10. Rinse well in distilled or deionized water; dip several times.
11. Tone in gold chloride solution for 30 seconds or until sections lose their yellow color and turn lavender. Too much toning will make sections red. Check individually under microscope.
12. Dip once or twice in distilled or deionized water and then check.

13. Place in 5% sodium thiosulfate solution for 5 minutes.
14. Wash well in tap water.
15. If desired, counterstain with nuclear fast red or 0.1% aqueous safranin, 3 to 5 seconds. Rinse well in distilled water.
16. Dehydrate with 70, 95, and 100% alcohols to xylol. Mount in permount or another solvent-soluble mounting media.

Results

Reticulin fibers - black
Collagen - rose color
Other tissue elements - varies with counterstain used.

Solutions

Phosphomolybdic acid solution
The unused solution is good for 2 months; use fresh each time.

phosphomolybdic acid	10 g
(do not use metal spatula)	
deionized or distilled water	100 mL

1% uranyl nitrate solution
This solution is good for approximately 3 months (dispose the same way as with radioactive waste).

uranyl nitrate	1 g
deionized or distilled water	100 mL

Ammoniacal silver solution
Use at once.
10.2% aqueous solution of silver nitrate (10.2 g AgNO$_3$/100 mL H$_2$O)
28% (concentrated) ammonia water
3.1% sodium hydroxide
To 5 mL of 10.2% aqueous solution of silver nitrate add 28% ammonia water, drop by drop, until the precipitate that forms is almost dissolved. Add 5 mL of 3.1% sodium hydroxide and dissolve the resulting precipitate with a few drops of ammonia water. Make the solution up to 50 mL with distilled or deionized water.

Reducing solution
Make fresh just before use.

1% uranyl nitrate, aqueous solution	1.5 mL
deionized or distilled water	50.0 mL

40% neutral formaldehyde	0.5 mL

Calcium carbonate in excess: 1 g/10 mL
40% formaldehyde
Dispose the same as radioactive waste.

Gold chloride working solution
Make fresh each time.

1% gold chloride solution	10 mL
deionized or distilled water	40 mL

Sodium thiosulfate (hypo) solution

sodium thiosulfate	5 g
deionized or distilled water	100 mL

Nuclear fast red (Kernechtrot)
optional counterstain
Dissolve 0.1 g nuclear fast red in 100 mL of 5% solution of aluminum sulfate with aid of heat. Cool, filter, and add grain of thymol as a preservative.

MASSON TRICHROME STAIN FOR COLLAGEN (20)

Fixation: Bouin, 10% formalin, Zenker, or B5. Mordant sections of formalin and Zenker-fixed tissue in Bouin fluid for 1 hour at 56°C, or overnight at room temperature; see staining procedure.

1. Dehydrate sections to distilled or deionized water. Carry Zenker-fixed tissue through sodium thiosulfate and iodine process in the usual manner.
2. Mordant in Bouin fixative for 1 hour at 56°C, or overnight at room temperature. Do not reuse solution.
3. Cool and wash in running water until yellow color disappears. With bone marrow sections the yellow disappears in 3 to 5 minutes; however, washing for at least 15 minutes is recommended.
4. Place in Weigert iron hematoxylin solution for 10 minutes. Wash in running water 10 minutes.
5. Rinse in distilled or deionized water.
6. Place in Biebrich scarlet-acid fuchsin solution for 15 seconds. If a more intense red stain is desired the slides can be left in the solution longer. Save solution.
7. Rinse in running water for 3 minutes and rinse with deionized or distilled water.
8. Place in aqueous phosphotungstic acid 5% for 5 minutes. Do not wash. Discard solution.
9. Put in light green solution for 25 minutes. Save solution.

10. Dip once quickly in distilled or deionized water.
11. Dip twice quickly in acetic water, 1%. Discard solution.
12. Dip two to three times in 95% alcohol.
13. Dip four to five times in absolute alcohol.
14. Two changes in xylene.
15. Mount in permount or another organic solvent mounting media.

Results

Nuclei - black
Cytoplasm, keratin, muscle fibers, intracellular fibers - red.
Collagen, mucous - blue or green.

Solutions

Light green solution

light green	5 g
distilled or deionized water	250 mL
glacial acetic acid	2 mL

Heat water, dissolve light green, filter, and add acid. The stain is stable.

1% acetic water solution

glacial acetic acid	1 mL
distilled or deionized water	100 mL

Weigert iron hematoxylin

Solution A:

hematoxylin	1 g
alcohol, 95%	100 mL

Solution B:

29% ferric chloride, aqueous	4 mL

This heats up and fumes when water is added.

distilled or deionized water	95 mL
hydrochloric acid, concentrated	1 mL

Working solution

Equal parts of solution A and solution B. Solutions A and B are stable and can be made up in larger quantities. The working solution is good for 3 weeks.

Biebrich scarlet-acid fuchsin solution

1% aqueous Biebrich scarlet	90 mL
1% aqueous acid fuchsin	10 mL
glacial acetic acid	1 mL

The Biebrich scarlet is difficult to dissolve. This stain is extremely stable.

IMMUNOCYTOCHEMISTRY

Immunocytochemistry, as in other disciplines of pathology, is increasingly utilized in the evaluation of bone marrow biopsies (7,12,15,24). Immunocytochemical methodology can be applied to all types of bone marrow specimens including paraffin- and plastic-embedded biopsies, cryostat sections, and air-dried smears and cytospin preparations. The introduction of antibodies reactive with paraffin-embedded specimens, however, has greatly facilitated the application of immunocytochemistry to bone marrow biopsy sections (9–13,18,22–27,29). Although these antibodies have proven to be very useful in bone marrow diagnosis, considerable judgment must be exercised both in the selection of antibodies to be used and in the interpretation of the results. The type of fixative and the decalcification procedure may be limiting factors in the application of some antibodies to bone marrow biopsies.

The application of immunohistochemical methods using both monoclonal and nonmonoclonal antibodies on routinely processed paraffin-embedded biopsies has been greatly facilitated by the availability of kits using either the avidin-biotin complex (ABC) or peroxidase-antiperoxidase (PAP) techniques (16). These kits contain detailed instructions and it is important to carefully follow the manufacturers' directions. The immunoalkaline phosphatase technique, using either the avidin-biotin complex or alkaline phosphatase–antialkaline phosphatase (APAAP) methodologies, also gives very good results but is less widely used for sections (11). It is very important that each laboratory determine the reactivity pattern of the various antibodies in the specimens processed in that laboratory. Differences in fixatives and decalcification procedures may lead to very different results from those published in the literature or specified by the manufacturer. The most common problem is the loss of antigen reactivity due to the type of fixative or decalcification solution. Whenever a new antibody is introduced into a laboratory, the reactivity must be authenticated. This is accomplished by using tissue of known antigenicity.

One of the most useful roles of immunocytochemistry for bone marrow sections is the application of antibodies to kappa and lambda light chain immunoglobulins to determine relative proportions of kappa- and lambda-reacting cells in multiple myeloma or other immunoproliferative disorders (23). Although the antibodies to both kappa and lambda polypeptide chains react very well in Zenker- and B5-fixed, decalcified sections, the reactivity is restricted to cells that contain intracytoplasmic immunoglobulin; the technique is not sufficiently sensitive to determine clonality in the lymphoproliferative disorders characterized by the presence of only surface immunoglobulin. Uncommonly, the lymphocytes in a B-cell lymphoma will contain sufficient cytoplasmic immunoglobulin to be detected.

Several monoclonal antibodies to lymphocytes, both B and T, and granulocytes, which react in paraffin-embedded sections, have been developed (10,22,25–27,29). These various antibodies have two applications: determining the immunophenotype of the proliferative process and evaluating the extent of bone marrow involvement. Because these antibodies are not a determinant of clonality, they cannot be used to distinguish a malignant from a reactive process. In addition, because many of the B-cell and T-cell monoclonal antibodies react with varying types of lymphoproliferative disorders, reactivity must not be used as a determinant for classification. The pattern of the process in routinely stained sections must be used in conjunction with antibody studies to distinguish benign from malignant and well-differentiated from poorly differentiated processes. It is important that the immunophenotypic evaluation of a lymphoproliferative disorder include a panel of antibodies to all possible cell lines and not to just the suspected immunophenotype.

The adverse effects of fixatives and decalcification, as noted previously, must be considered in the evaluation of antibody reactions to B or T lymphocytes in bone marrow biopsies. L26 (CD20), a widely used monoclonal antibody for B lymphocytes does not react with Zenker-fixed, decalcified marrow biopsies. The antibody does work, however, in B5-fixed, decalcified marrow specimens.

Antibodies reactive with myeloid cells must be used with the same degree of caution as those for lymphocytes. Combinations of antibodies are necessary. Particularly useful are antibodies to lysozyme and myeloperoxidase (21,24). The antibody to lysozyme reacts with both neutrophils and monocytes. Antimyeloperoxidase antibody reacts principally with neutrophils and precursors in-cluding myeloblasts, but may show weak reactivity with monocytic cells (24). Commercially available polyclonal antibodies to myeloperoxidase generally give excellent results with most fixatives and are particularly useful in recognizing cells of neutrophil lineage. A limitation of these antibodies is failure to react with myeloblasts in some cases of acute myeloid leukemia without maturation (M1). Antibody to CD15 (Leu-M1) reacts with more mature neutrophils but is generally nonreactive with myeloblasts. Antibodies to hemoglobin A and antiglycophorin A can be used to identify erythroblasts; antihemoglobin A may not react with very primitive erythroblasts in which no or only minimal amounts of hemoglobin are present. Antibody to *Ulex e uropaeus* reacts with megakaryocytes but is not specific for this cell lineage and may also react with erythroid precursors and granulocytes. Anti–factor VIII antibody reacts with mature megakaryocytes.

In addition to the antibodies to hematopoietic cells reactive with paraffin-embedded bone marrow biopsies, there are several antibodies available that react with tumors that commonly metastasize to the bone marrow (4).

PLASTIC EMBEDDING

Paraffin embedding is the most widely used routine methodology for the processing of bone marrow. In certain instances, when it is desirable to perform cytochemical reactions that are ablated in the decalcification process used for paraffin-embedded specimens, it may be preferable to use a plastic embedding procedure that bypasses decalcification, or a decalcification process utilizing a nonrapid acid decalcifier such as EDTA (1,3). Virtually any enzymatic reaction can be performed on plastic-embedded tissue if it is properly processed. The processing includes the avoidance of the mercury-based fixatives which interfere with most enzymatic reactions and the performance of the major steps at 4°C. Neutral buffered formalin is the preferred fixative for this methodology. With the introduction of newer resins for plastic embedding, the processing, although more time consuming than paraffin embedding, has been improved and some laboratories prefer plastic embedding to paraffin for routine biopsies (12).

PLASTIC SECTIONS: ROUTINE STAINS AND CYTOCHEMISTRY (1,3)

1. Place specimen in cold 10% buffered formalin fixative overnight. Omit steps 2 and 3 for specimens not needing decalcification.
2. Rinse with EDTA decalcification solution a few seconds.
3. Put in fresh EDTA decalcification solution for 4 hours.
4. Wash with cold 0.1 mol/L phosphate buffer (pH 7.3) for 1 hour (change after 30 minutes).
5. Put in acetone and buffer (1:1) for 10 minutes.
6. Put in acetone and buffer (3:1) for 10 minutes.
7. Put in acetone for 10 minutes.
8. Put in acetone and JB-4 component A + catalyst (1:1) for 10 minutes.
9. Put in JB-4 component A + catalyst for 10 minutes and then in fresh JB-4 component A + catalyst overnight and one more day and night or over weekend.
   Use a hood for the rest of the procedure.
10. Prepare fresh JB-4 component A + catalyst.
11. To 25 mL JB-4 component A + catalyst, add 1 mL JB-4 component B. Mix well with applicator stick. Keep beaker on cold plate while preparing.
12. Pipette 1.5 mL of JB-4 component A + catalyst and JB-4 component B mixture into plastic block mold, drop section in and position. Keep plastic mold on cold plate. Solution does not thicken for 15 minutes or more; specimen may be manipulated during this time.
13. Place metal block holder on top.
14. Place embedded section into open slide box and set in refrigerator overnight. When ready to remove, gently loosen embedded tissue from plastic mold. There may be fluid around specimen; this can be ignored if the face of the block is hard. Cut within 48 hours as tissue becomes dry and hard.
15. After cutting, float sections on weak ammonia water: approximately four to five drops concentrated ammonia for 200 mL water. Do not use hot plate or oven for special stains. Dry; this may take 30 to 60 minutes. For hematoxylin and eosin and Giemsa stains, place in oven for 30 to 60 minutes; cool before staining.

Solutions

EDTA (versonate solution) saturated
Good for several months.

EDTA (versonate)	10 g
phosphate buffer (pH 6.4)	100 mL

Shake well (EDTA will not completely dissolve); refrigerate.

Phosphate buffer (pH 6.4)

potassium monobasic phosphate	6.63 g
sodium dibasic phosphate	2.56 g

Dilute to 1000 mL with distilled or deionized water.

Phosphate buffer (pH 7.3)

potassium monobasic phosphate	0.272 g
sodium dibasic phosphate	1.135 g

Dilute to 100 mL with distilled or deionized water; keep in refrigerator.

JB-4 component A + catalyst (use hood)

JB-4 component A (keep in refrigerator)	50 mL
catalyst	1/2 scoop (approx. 0.45 g)

Cover with parafilm and mix on automatic mixer with magnet for 15 minutes or until dissolved.
Refrigerate for 15 minutes before using.

HEMATOXYLIN AND EOSIN STAIN FOR PLASTIC SECTIONS

Fix mounted sections in oven at 58° to 62°C for 1/2 hour. Then process with:

1. Hematoxylin for 1 hour.
2. Water, two changes, 10 dips each.
3. Bluing solution for 2 minutes.
4. Water, two changes, 10 dips each.
5. 70 percent ethanol, 10 dips.
6. Eosin Y alcoholic for 6 to 7 minutes.
7. Absolute ethyl alcohol, two times, 10 dips.
8. Xylene, three changes, 3 to 5 minutes each.
9. Coverslip (solvent-soluble mounting media).

Solution

Bluing reagent (0.2% sodium bicarbonate, 1.0% magnesium sulfate)

sodium bicarbonate	2 g
magnesium sulfate	10 g

Dilute to 1000 mL with deionized water.

PLASTIC-EMBEDDED SECTIONS FOR IMMUNOHISTOCHEMISTRY

Plastic-embedding procedures have also been developed for immunohistochemistry (7). This methodology is used when bone marrow aspirates cannot be procured for flow cytometry studies or for immunohistochemistry on smears.

The following methodology for plastic embedding published by Casey et al. (7) can be used for both routine hematoxylin and eosin stained sections and cytochemical and immunohistochemical procedures.

Embedding Procedure

1. Collect bone marrow trephine biopsies or other specimens (2 to 3 mm sections) in 4°C acetone. Keep vial with acetone on ice while transporting specimens.
2. Place acetone and specimens in freezer (20°C) immediately upon receipt in the laboratory for overnight fixation.
3. Infiltrate the fixed samples the following day in 5 to 10 mL JB-4 component A with 5% methyl benzoate for 3 to 8 hours at 4°C.
4. Following infiltration, embed specimen in catalyzed JB-4 component A with JB-4 component B which is prepared as follows:

   Add 2.5 mL catalyzed JB-4 component A to 0.063 mL JB-4 component B.

   Pipette 1.5 mL of the solution into plastic molding cups, add specimen, and cover with appropriate plastic block holder.

   Polymerize overnight at 4°C in a desiccator.

   Following polymerization, store the block at -20°C until needed.

Sectioning Procedure

1. Allow blocks to come to room temperature in a desiccator.
2. Cut in 2 μm sections using a glass knife and a histology microtome.
3. Collect sections on an appropriate water bath. Sections to be used for immunohistochemistry are collected on a water bath prepared as follows:

   Add 25 mL acetone to 600 mL distilled or deionized water (total volume, 625 mL).

   Add 5 to 10 drops concentrated ammonium hydroxide.

   Allow sections to float on mixture for 15 minutes before transferring to coverslips.

   Discard mixture at end of day.
4. Transfer sections to labeled coverslips and allow to air dry overnight at room temperature. Sections should be collected 1 day prior to staining.

Immunohistochemistry Procedure

1. Using a fine tweezers, place the labeled coverslips containing tissue sections into staining rack; align sections to face in the same direction.
2. Place staining rack into beaker containing 0.05 mol/L Tris buffered saline (TBS) (pH 7.6) for 10 to 30 minutes at room temperature.
3. Blot coverslips vertically on absorbent paper and place section side down onto a parafilmed slide tray containing 100 μL of 2% normal swine serum for 30 minutes in a moist 37°C chamber.
4. Blot coverslips and place section side down on 100 μL of appropriate dilutions of mouse monoclonal antibody on parafilmed slide tray. Incubate for 2 hours at 37°C.

   Discard solutions at end of day.
5. Blot coverslips and perform two 5 minute washes by gently dipping staining rack into beaker containing TBS.
6. Blot coverslips and place section side down onto a parafilmed slide tray containing 100 μL of 0.1% sodium azide and 3% hydrogen peroxide for 10 minutes at room temperature.
7. Blot coverslips and perform two 5 minute washes in TBS.
8. Blot coverslips and place section side down on parafilmed slide tray containing 100 μL of 1:40 dilution of horseradish peroxidase conjugated rabbit antimouse antibody with 2.5% human antibody (AB) serum for 1 hour at 37°C. Discard remaining solution.
9. Blot coverslips and perform two 5 minute washes in TBS.
10. Blot coverslips and place section side down on parafilmed slide tray containing 100 μL of 1:40 dilution of horseradish peroxidase conjugated swine antirabbit antibody with 2.5% human AB serum for 1 hour at 37°C.

Discard remaining solution.

11. Blot coverslips and perform two 5 minute washes in TBS.

12. Wash coverslips in 0.1 mol/L acetate buffer, pH 5.2, for 5 minutes.

13. Incubate coverslips in small Coplin jars filled with aminoethylcarbizole in formamide for 15 minutes at 37°C.

14. Wash coverslips with distilled or deionized water two to three times; collect excess aminoethylcarbizole and all washings for proper disposal.

15. Counterstain with hematoxylin for 10 to 15 minutes at room temperature.

16. Wash coverslips in running tap water for 5 minutes.

17. Air dry coverslips and mount with glycergel or other water-based mounting media onto an appropriately labeled glass slide.

Embedding Materials

Embedding molds	Sorvall plastic block holder and molding for use on Sorvall microtome
Coverslips	Scientific Prod. cat. #M6050-2
JB-4 Embedding kit #0026:	Polysciences, Inc. Warrington, PA 18976
Individual components:	
JB-4 Component A	cat. #0226A
JB-4 Component B	cat. #0226B
JB-4 Catalyst	cat. #02618
Acetone	A.C.S. certified
Ammonium hydroxide	A.C.S. certified
Methyl benzoate	A.C.S. certified

Immunohistochemistry Reagents and Solutions

2% normal swine serum
normal swine serum	0.06 mL
TBS	2.94 mL

total volume - 3 mL
This amount is adequate for 25 coverslips. Discard solution at the end of the day.
Dilutions of mouse monoclonal antibody

TBS	95 mL
2% sodium azide	5 mL
bovine serum albumin	100 mg

This should be stored at 4°C.

1% sodium azide and 3% hydrogen peroxide
2% sodium azide	0.25 mL
30% hydrogen peroxide	0.05 mL
distilled or deionized water	4.70 mL

total volume - 5 mL

2.5% human AB serum in TBS
human AB serum	0.175 mL
TBS	6.825 mL

total volume - 7 mL
This volume is sufficient for 25 coverslips.

1:4 dilution of horseradish peroxidase conjugated rabbit antimouse antibody with 2.5% human AB serum
peroxidase conjugated rabbit antimouse antibody	0.075 mL
2.5% human AB serum in TBS	2.925 mL

total volume - 3 mL
This is sufficient for 25 coverslips.

1:40 dilution of horseradish peroxidase conjugated swine antirabbit antibody with 2.5% human antibody (AB) serum
peroxidase conjugated swine antirabbit antibody	0.075 mL
2.5% human AB serum in TBS	2.925 mL

total volume - 3 mL
This is sufficient for 25 coverslips.

Aminoethylcarbizole in formamide
aminoethylcarbizole (AEC)	2.034 mL
3% hydrogen peroxide	0.030 mL
0.1 mol/L acetate buffer	28.5 mL

Prepare this immediately prior to use.

JB-4 component A with 5% methyl benzoate
methyl benzoate	5 mL
JB-4 component A	95 mL

total volume - 100 mL
Store at 4°C. Expires in 3 to 4 weeks.

Catalyzed JB-4 component A
JB-4 catalyst	0.15 g
JB-4 component A	40 mL

Add magnet and place solution on magnetic mixer for 15 minutes or until catalyst is dissolved. Store at 4°C. Expires in 3 to 4 weeks.

CRYOSTAT SECTIONS

Cryostat sections have limited use in diagnostic bone marrow pathology; in most instances in which the marrow is infiltrated by proliferative cells, sufficient specimen can be aspirated for flow cytometry analysis, or touch imprint preparations of the core biopsy can be used for immunohistochemical studies. For those uncommon occasions when immunophenotyping is considered absolutely necessary and no specimens can be obtained by these methods, cryostat sections of a trephine core biopsy can be prepared (15,30). Alternatively, a core biopsy can be embedded in plastic and processed for immunohistochemistry as described previously.

Cryostat sections have a distinct advantage over paraffin-embedded sections for immunohistochemical procedures since there is complete preservation of surface antigens and membrane and cytoplasmic immunoglobulins. The disadvantages of cryostat sections, in addition to suboptimal cytology, relates to the difficulties encountered in cutting tissue with dense bone structure and the architectural distortion that may occur from compression or tearing of the specimen. Sections of one cell layer thickness are difficult to achieve. This may lead to considerable difficulties in interpretation and caution must be exercised in the evaluation of these specimens.

The trephine for cryostat sections is obtained in the same manner as for conventional processing. Immediately after it is obtained, the biopsy is placed on a saline soaked gauze and transported to the laboratory. Before freezing the biopsy specimen, it should be examined with a magnifying glass to determine if there is substantial cortical bone present. If cortical bone is present, it should be carefully dissected away without damaging the specimen and processed in a routine manner. The presence of cortical bone in a biopsy causes greater difficulty in sectioning and may lead to increased tissue distortion. The specimen to be frozen is then placed in a plastic specimen holder which is filled with OCT embedding compound (Tissue Tek II, Lab Tek Products Division, Miles Laboratories, Inc., Naperville, IL). The specimen holder is grasped with a long pair of tongs and gradually immersed in liquid nitrogen or isopentane. After immersion for a few minutes, the specimen is withdrawn, wrapped in aluminum foil, and stored at -70°C until sectioning is performed.

Prior to sectioning, the specimen is placed in the cryostat for approximately 15 to 20 minutes before the actual cutting. The chuck on which the specimen is mounted should be placed so that the long axis of the specimen is oriented vertically or at a diagonal to the cutting edge of the knife. The knife blade should be moved frequently as dulling of the blade occurs after only a few cuts. Because of damage to the knife blade, disposable knife blades should be used. The specimen is picked up on albumin coated slides that are placed in the cryostat 30 minutes prior to use. The sections are air dried for approximately 18 to 24 hours. Following drying, the sections are fixed in acetone at room temperature for approximately 10 minutes. The slides may then be immunostained by standard immunoperoxidase or immunoalkaline phosphatase methods. If the sections are to be immunostained at a later time, they should be wrapped in aluminum foil and stored at -20°C until used.

PREPARATION OF BONE MARROW SPECIMENS FOR ELECTRON MICROSCOPY

If electron microscopic studies are anticipated, an additional 1.0 to 2.0 mL of bone marrow should be aspirated. An anticoagulated specimen of bone marrow, using either powdered EDTA or heparin, is spun in a Wintrobe tube in the same manner as the anticoagulated routine marrow aspirate (see below). After the tube has been spun and the separated layers are identified, the F-PV and plasma layers are drawn off with a Pasteur pipette. Cold 2.5 percent glutaraldehyde fixative is layered over the M-E layer without disrupting this layer. Following 10 minutes of fixation, the Wintrobe tube is scored at the level of the interface of the M-E and erythrocyte layer. The tube is cracked and the portion of the tube with the M-E layer is placed in a vial of fresh cold glutaraldehyde so that the exposed portion of the M-E layer is in contact with the fixative. Following an additional 10 minutes of fixation, the M-E layer is gently ejected from the Wintrobe tube into a vial of fresh cold glutaraldehyde using a Pasteur pipette. After another 10 minutes of fixation, the M-E pellet is diced into 1 mm portions with a sharp blade. These portions are then placed into fresh cold glutaraldehyde and allowed to fix for at least 30 minutes. The particles are then processed for electron microscopy by standard techniques. The specimen may remain in fixative for up to 2 weeks at 4°C before processing.

As an alternative to using an M-E layer for electron microscopy, particles from the aspirated anticoagulated specimen can be separated from the fluid portion of the specimen and placed directly into cold glutaraldehyde for 1 hour. If the particles are large or clumped, they should be cut into 1 mm cubes.

If no aspirate can be obtained because of fibrosis, portions of the trephine biopsy specimen can be used. The biopsy specimen should be placed on saline soaked gauze and transferred to the laboratory immediately after the biopsy procedure. Small portions of the biopsy should be cut away with a sharp scalpel blade. These should be placed in cold glutaraldehyde for approximately 10 minutes. The specimens should then be cut into small cubes of 1 mm size and placed in fresh cold glutaraldehyde.

ULTRASTRUCTURAL PLATELET PEROXIDASE (2)

The diagnosis of acute megakaryoblastic leukemia (M7) is based on the demonstration of reactivity of cells with antibodies to platelet glycoproteins or ultrastructural demonstration of platelet peroxidase .

The blood or bone marrow specimen is prepared in the same manner as for routine transmission electron microscopy. However, if the primary purpose of the study is the demonstration of platelet peroxidase, tannic acid fixative is substituted for glutaraldehyde. The tannic acid is gently added over the M-E layer of the spun specimen; a fixation time of 10 minutes is optimal. The Wintrobe tube is then scored at the lower margin of the M-E layer and broken. The tube is then placed into a fresh vial of tannic acid with the exposed M-E layer down for 10 minutes. The slightly solidified M-E layer is then gently ejected into the fixative and allowed to fix for an additional 5 minutes. The specimen is then diced into 1 mm

cubes which are placed in a vial of fresh tannic acid for 5 minutes.

Following the 5 minute fixation, the specimen is washed three times in 0.05 mol/L of Tris-HCl buffer.

The specimen is then incubated in platelet peroxidase reaction mixture for 1 to 1.5 hours at room temperature; the specimen is gently agitated during the incubation.

Following this incubation the specimen is washed three times in 0.05 mol/L Tris-HCl buffer. The specimen is post-fixed in 1 percent buffered osmium tetroxide (OsO_4) for 1 hour at room temperature. It is then processed as for routine electron microscopy.

If the processing cannot be completed during one period, it may be interrupted at two points. The fixed cells can be held overnight in Tris wash buffer at 4°C and incubated with the platelet peroxidase reaction mixture the following day or following incubation can be held overnight in the Tris-HCl buffer at 4°C.

Reagents

Tannic acid fixative

Stock: 2% formaldehyde, 0.5% glutaraldehyde in 0.1 mol/L phosphate buffer.

16% formaldehyde	25 mL
25% glutaraldehyde	4 mL

Dilute up to 100 mL with 0.1 mol/L phosphate buffer (pH 7.4). Store in refrigerator.

On day of use:

Add: 0.25 g tannic acid to 25 mL of stock.

Adjust pH to 7.3 with 1N NaOH.

Filter and use same day.

Platelet peroxidase media (PPO)

Dissolve 20 mg DAB (diaminobenzidine tetrahydrochloride) in 10 mL 0.05 mol/L Tris-HCl acid buffer (pH 7.5).

Add 0.033 mL 3% H_2O_2 (fresh).

Adjust pH to 7.6 with 1N NaOH.

Control: Make up above media without the 3 percent H_2O_2

Note: Make up 3% H_2O_2 fresh from 30% H_2O_2. Use the PPO media the same day it is prepared.

REFERENCES

1. Beckstead JH, Bainton DF. Enzyme histochemistry on bone marrow biopsies: reactions useful in the differential diagnosis of leukemia and lymphoma applied to 2-micron plastic sections. Blood 1980;55:386–94.

2. Breton-Gorius J, Reyes F, Duhemal G, et al. Megakaryoblastic acute leukemia: identification by the ultrastructural demonstration of platelet peroxidase. Blood 1978;51:45–60.

3. Brinn NT, Pickett JP. Glycol methacrylate for routine, special stains, histochemistry, enzyme histochemistry and immunochemistry. A simplified cold method for surgical biopsy tissue. J Histotechnol 1979;2:125–30.

4. Brunning RD. Bone marrow. In: Rosai J, ed. Ackerman's surgical pathology, Vol. 2. 2nd ed. St. Louis: CV Mosby, 1989;1379–454.

5. _____. Bone marrow specimen processing. In: Knowles DM, ed. Neoplastic hematopathology. Baltimore: Williams and Wilkins, 1992:1081–95.

6. Brynes RK, McKenna RW, Sundberg RD. Bone marrow aspiration and trephine biopsy. An approach to a thorough study. Am J Clin Pathol 1978;70:753–9.

7. Casey TT, Olson SJ, Cousar JB, Collins RD. Plastic section immunohistochemistry in the diagnosis of hematopoietic and lymphoid neoplasma. Clin Lab Med 1990;10:199–213.

8. Dacie JV, Lewis SM. Practical haematology. London: J&A Churchill, 1968:85.

9. Davey FR, Olson S, Kurec AS, Eastman-Abaya J, Gottlieb AJ, Mason DY. The immunophenotyping of extramedullary myeloid cell tumors in paraffin-embedded tissue sections. Am J Surg Pathol 1988;12:699–707.

10. Epstein AL, Marder RJ, Winter JN, Fox RI. Two new monoclonal antibodies (LN-1, LN-2) reactive in B5 formalin-fixed, paraffin-embedded tissues with follicular center and mantle zone human B lymphocytes and derived tumors. J Immunol 1984;133:1028–36.

11. Falini B, Martelli MF, Tarallo F, et al. Immunohistological analysis of human bone marrow trephine biopsies using monoclonal antibodies. Br J Haematol 1984;365–86.

12. Frisch B, Bartl R. Atlas of bone marrow pathology. Boston: Kluwer Academic Publishers, 1990. (Greshman GA, ed. Current histopathology; Vol. 15).

13. Hall PA, d'Ardenne AJ, Stansfeld AG. Paraffin section immunocytochemistry. I. Non-Hodgkin's lymphoma. Histopathology 1988;13:149–60.

14. Jamshidi K, Swaim WR. Bone marrow biopsy with unaltered architecture: a new biopsy device. J Lab Clin Med 1971;77:335–42.

15. Kronland R, Grogan T, Spier C, et al. Immunotopographic assessment of lymphoid and plasma cell malignancies of the bone marrow. Hum Pathol 1985;16:1247–54.

16. Kubic VL, Brunning RD. Immunohistochemical evaluation of neoplasms in bone marrow biopsies using monoclonal antibodies reactive in paraffin-embedded tissue. Mod Pathol 1989;2:618–29.

17. Lillie RD. Histopathologic technic and practical histochemistry. 3rd ed. New York: McGraw Hill, 1965:194.

18. Linder J, Ye Y, Armitage JO, Weisenburger DD. Monoclonal antibodies marking B-cell non-Hodgkin's lymphoma in paraffin-embedded tissue. Mod Pathol 1988;1:29–34.

19. Lofsness KG, Spanjers EM. Preparation and evaluation of bone marrow. In: Lotspeich-Steininger CA, Stiene-Martin EA, Koepke JA, eds. Clinical hematology: principles, procedures, correlations. Philadelphia: JB Lippincott, 1992:366–78.

20. Luna LG, ed. Manual of histologic staining methods of the Armed Forces Institute of Pathology. 3rd ed. New York: McGraw-Hill, 1968.

21. Muller S, Sangster G, Crocker J, et al. An immunohistochemical and clinicopathological study of granulocytic sarcoma ("chloroma"). Hematol Oncol 1986;4:101–12.

22. Okon E, Felder B, Epstein A, Lukes RJ, Taylor CR. Monoclonal antibodies reactive with B-lymphocytes and histiocytes in paraffin sections. Cancer 1985;56:95–104.

23. Peterson LC, Brown BA, Crosson JT, Mladenovic J. Application of the immunoperoxidase technic to bone marrow trephine biopsies in the classification of patients with monoclonal gammopathies. Am J Clin Pathol 1986;85:688–93.

24. Pinkus GS, Pinkus JL. Myeloperoxidase: a specific marker for myeloid cells in paraffin sections. Mod Pathol 1991;4:733–41.

25. Poppema S, Hollema H, Visser L, Vos H. Monoclonal antibodies (MT1, MT2, MB1, MB2, MB3) reactive with leukocyte subsets in paraffin-embedded tissue sections. Am J Pathol 1987;127:418–29.

26. Said JW, Stoll PN, Shintaku P, Bindl JM, Butmarc JR, Pinkus GS. Leu 22: a preferential marker for T-lymphocytes in paraffin sections. Staining profile in T- and B-cell lymphomas, Hodkin's disease, other lymphoproliferative disorders, myeloproliferative diseases, and other various neoplastic processes. Am J Clin Pathol 1989;91:542–9.

27. Strickler JG, Weiss LM, Copenhaver CM, et al. Monoclonal antibodies reactive in routinely processed tissue sections of malignant lymphoma, with emphasis on T-cell lymphomas. Hum Pathol 1987;18:808–14.

28. Sundberg RD, Broman H. The application of the Prussian blue stain to previously stained films of blood and bone marrow. Blood 1955;10:160–6.

29. West KP, Warford A, Fray L, Allen M, Campbell AC, Lauder I. The demonstration of B-cell, T-cell and myeloid antigens in paraffin sections. J Pathol 1986;150:89–101.

30. Wood GS, Warnke RA. The immunologic phenotyping of bone marrow biopsies and aspirates: frozen section techniques. Blood 1982;59:913–22.

Index*

*Page numbers in boldface represent table and figure pages.

✧✧✧